PROGRESS IN BRAIN RESEARCH

VOLUME 103

NEURAL REGENERATION

Other Volumes in PROGRESS IN BRAIN RESEARCH

PROGRESS IN BRAIN RESEARCH

VOLUME 103

NEURAL REGENERATION

EDITED BY

FREDRICK J. SEIL

Office of Regeneration Research Programs, V.A. Medical Center, Portland, OR, USA

ELSEVIER
AMSTERDAM – LAUSANNE – NEW YORK – OXFORD – SHANNON – TOKYO
1994

ISBN 0-444-81727-1 (volume)
ISBN 0-444-80104-9 (series)

Published by:
Elsevier Science BV.
P.O. Box 211
1000 AE Amsterdam
The Netherlands

Printed in The Netherlands on acid-free paper

List of Contributors

A. Akaike, Department of Neuropharmacology, Faculty of Pharmacy and Pharmaceutical Sciences, Fukuyama University, Fukuyama 729-02, Japan
C. Andersson, Department of Cell Biology & Anatomy, Oregon Health Sciences University, Portland, OR 97201, USA
P.A. Anton, Department of Medicine, UCLA School of Medicine, Los Angeles, CA 90024, USA
J.S. Beckman, Department of Anesthesiology, University of Alabama at Birmingham, Birmingham, AL 25233, USA
A.M. Bedard, Department of Physiology and Neuroscience Research Institute, University of Ottawa, Ottawa, Ontario, Canada
A.P. Bentley, Department of Biology and Neuroscience Program, Williams College, Williamstown, MA 01267, USA
J. Bockaert, Center CNRS, INSERM, Departments of Pharmacology and Endocrinology, Montpellier, France 34094
P.C. Bridgman, Department of Anatomy and Neurobiology, Washington University School of Medicine, St. Louis, MO 63110, USA
K.K. Briggs, Department of Zoology and Genetics, Iowa State University, Ames, IA 50011, USA
S.L. Cassar, Department of Anatomy, Unversity of Calgary, Calgary, Alberta, Canada
A.C. Charles, Department of Neurology, UCLA School of Medicine, Los Angeles, CA 90024, USA
J. Chen, Department of Anesthesiology, University of Alabama at Birmingham, Birmingham, AL 25233, USA
J.P. Crow, Department of Anesthesiology, University of Alabama at Birmingham, Birmingham, AL 25233, USA
R. Curtis, Regeneron Pharmaceuticals Inc., Tarrytown, NY 10591, USA
T.M. Dawson, Departments of Neuroscience and Neurology, Johns Hopkins University School of Medicine, Baltimore, MD 21205, USA
V.L. Dawson, Departments of Neurology and Physiology, Johns Hopkins University School of Medicine, Baltimore, MD 21205, USA
P.S. DiStefano, Regeneron Pharmaceuticals Inc., Tarrytown, NY 10591, USA
M.T. Duffy, Department of Biological Science, University of Illinois at Chicago, Chicago, IL 60607, USA
F.P. Eckenstein, Departments of Cell Biology & Anatomy and Neurology, Oregon Health Sciences University, Portland, OR 97201, USA
P.B. Ehrhard, Department of Physiology, University of Basel, Basel, Switzerland
S. Eitan, Department of Neurobiology, The Weizmann Institute of Science, Rehovot, Israel
A. Elman-Faber, Department of Neurobiology, The Weizmann Institute of Science, Rehovot, Israel
P. Ernfors, Whitehead Institute for Biomedical Research and Department of Biology, MIT, Cambridge, MA 02142, USA

S. Erulkar, Department of Pharmacology, Biocenter, Basel, Switzerland
D.W. Ethell, Department of Zoology, University of British Columbia, Vancouver, British Columbia, Canada V6T 1Z4
L.L. Evans, Department of Anatomy and Neurobiology, Washington University School of Medicine, St. Louis, MO 63110, USA
L. Fagni, Center CNRS, INSERM, Departments of Pharmacology and Endocrinology, Montpellier, France 34094
D.G. Feiner, Department of Biology and Neuroscience Program, Williams College, Williamstown, MA 01267, USA
R.D. Fields, Laboratory of Developmental Neurobiology, National Institute of Child Health and Human Development, National Institutes of Health, Bethesda, MD 02892, USA
R.A. Gadient, Department of Physiology, University of Basel, Basel, Switzerland
G.T. Ghooray, Department of Cell Biology, Neurobiology and Anatomy, The Ohio State University, Columbus, OH 43210, USA
K.M.G. Giehl, Department of Physiology and Neuroscience Research Institute, University of Ottawa, Ottawa, Ontario, Canada
D.J. Goldberg, Department of Pharmacology & Center for Neurobiology and Behavior, Columbia University, New York, NY 10032, USA
T.M. Gomez, Department of Cell Biology and Neuroanatomy, University of Minnesota, Minneapolis, MN 55455, USA
A. Grabowska, Center for Neurologic Diseases, Department of Medicine, Division of Neurology, Brigham and Women's Hospital, and Department of Neurology, Harvard Medical School, Boston, MA 02115, USA
S.J. Hasan, Department of Zoology, University of British Columbia, Vancouver, British Columbia, Canada V6T 1Z4
T. Herdegen, II. Institute of Physiology, University of Heidelberg, Heidelberg, Germany 69120
J.R. Hering, Department of Biology and Neuroscience Program, Williams College, Williamstown, MA 01267, USA
D.L. Hirschberg, Department of Neurobiology, The Weizmann Institute of Science, Rehovot, Israel
L.J. Ignarro, Department of Pharmacology, UCLA School of Medicine, Los Angeles, CA 90024, USA
R. Jaenisch, Whitehead Institute for Biomedical Research and Department of Biology, MIT, Cambridge, MA 02142, USA
J. Jellies, Neurobiology Research Center, Department of Physiology and Biophysics, University of Alabama, Birmingham, AL 35294, USA
J. Johansen, Department of Zoology and Genetics, Iowa State University, Ames, IA 50011, USA
K.M. Johansen, Department of Zoology and Genetics, Iowa State University, Ames, IA 50011, USA
H.S. Keirstead, Department of Zoology, University of British Columbia, Vancouver, British Columbia, Canada V6T 1Z4
N.R. Kobayashi, Department of Physiology and Neuroscience Research Institute, Unversity of Ottawa, Ottawa, Ontario, Canada
J.D. Kocsis, Department of Neurology, Yale Unversity School of Medicine and Neuroscience Regeneration Research Center, VA Medical Center, West Haven, CT 06516, USA
D.M. Kopp, Neurobiology Research Center, Department of Physiology and Biophysics, University of Alabama, Birmingham, AL 35294, USA
K. Kuzis, Department of Cell Biology & Anatomy, Oregon Health Sciences University, Portland, OR 97201, USA

M.B. Lachyankar, The Worcester Foundation for Experimental Biology, Shrewsbury, MA 01545, USA
M. Lafon-Cazal, Center CNRS, INSERM, Departments of Pharmacology and Endocrinology, Montpellier, France 34094
L.A. Lampson, Center for Neurologic Diseases, Department of Medicine, Division of Neurology, Brigham and Women's Hospital, and Department of Neurology, Harvard Medical School, Boston, MA 02115, USA
L. Landmesser, Department of Neurosciences, Case Western Reserve University, Cleveland, OH 44106, USA
K. Lankford, Department of Neurology, Yale University School of Medicine and Neuroscience Regeneration Research Center, VA Medical Center, West Haven, CT 06516, USA
K.-F. Lee, Whitehead Institute for Biomedical Research and Department of Biology, MIT, Cambridge, MA 02142, USA
V.A. Lennon, Departments of Immunology, Neurology and Laboratory Medicine and Pathology, Mayo Clinic, Rochester, MN 55905, USA
M. Lerner-Natoli, Center CNRS, INSERM, Laboratory of Experimental Medicine, Montpellier, France 34000
P.C. Letourneau, Department of Cell Biology and Neuroanatomy, University of Minnesota, Minneapolis, MN 55455, USA
A.K. Lewis, Department of Anatomy and Neurobiology, Washington University School of Medicine, St. Louis, MO 63110, USA
R.M. Lindsay, Regeneron Pharmaceuticals Inc., Tarrytown, NY 10591, USA
S.A. Lipton, Department of Neurology, Harvard Medical School, Boston, MA 02115, USA
M. Lotan, Department of Neurobiology, The Weizmann Institute of Science, Rehovot, Israel
R. Loy, University of Rochester School of Medicine and Veterans Medical Center, Batavia, NY 14020, USA
O. Manzoni, Center CNRS, INSERM, Departments of Pharmacology and Endocrinology, Montpellier, France 34094
F.C. Martin, Department of Neurology, UCLA School of Medicine, Los Angeles, CA 90024, USA
G.F. Martin, Department of Cell Biology, Neurobiology and Anatomy, The Ohio State University, Columbus, OH 43210, USA
C.B. McBride, Department of Zoology, University of British Columbia, Vancouver, British Columbia, Canada V6T 1Z4
A.D. McClellan, Division of Biological Science, University of Missouri, Columbia, MO 65211, USA
J.E. Merrill, Department of Neurology, UCLA School of Medicine, Los Angeles, CA 90024, USA
D.J. Miller, Department of Immunology, Mayo Clinic, Rochester, MN 55905, USA
F.D. Miller, Center for Neuronal Survival, Department of Neurology and Neurosurgery, Montreal Neurological Institute, McGill Unversity, Montreal, Quebec, Canada H3A 2B4
B. Mitrovic, Department of Neurology, UCLA School of Medicine, Los Angeles, CA 90024, USA
G.D. Muir, Department of Zoology, University of British Columbia, Vancouver, British Columbia, Canada V6T 1Z4
N. Nakata, Department of Neuropharmacology, Faculty of Pharmacy and Pharmaceutical Sciences, Fukuyama University, Fukuyama 729-02, Japan
J.G. Nicholls, Department of Pharmacology, Biocenter, Basel, Switzerland
U. Otten, Department of Physiology, University of Basel, Basel, Switzerland

D.M. Pataky, Department of Zoology, University of British Columbia, Vancouver, British Columbia, Canada V6T 1Z4
B. Petrausch, Department of Zoology, University of British Columbia, Vancouver, British Columbia, Canada V6T 1Z4
D.K. Poluha, The Worcester Foundation for Experimental Biology, Shrewsbury, MA 01545, USA
B.J. Prendergast, Department of Biology and Neuroscience Program, Williams College, Williamstown, MA 01267, USA
M.N. Rand, Department of Neurology, Yale University School of Medicine and Neuroscience Regeneration Research Center, VA Medical Center, West Haven, CT 06516, USA
H.I. Rieff, Department of Biology and Neuroscience Program, Williams College, Williamstown, MA 01267, USA
M.W. Rochlin, Department of Anatomy and Neurobiology, Washington University School of Medicine, St. Louis, MO 63110, USA
M. Rodriguez, Departments of Neurology and Immunology, Mayo Clinic, Rochester, MN 55905, USA
G. Rondouin, Center CNRS, INSERM, Laboratory of Experimental Medicine, Montpellier, France 34000
A.H. Ross, The Worcester Foundation for Experimental Biology, Shrewsbury, MA 01545, USA
N.R. Saunders, Department of Physiology, University of Tasmania, Hobart, Tasmania 7001, Australia
M. Schwartz, Department of Neurobiology, The Weizmann Institute of Science, Rehovot, Israel
J.L. Scully, Department of Physiology, University of Basel, Basel, Switzerland
F. Shanahan, Department of Medicine, UCLA School of Medicine, Los Angeles, CA 90024, USA
S.B. Simpson, Jr., Department of Biological Science, University of Illinois at Chicago, Chicago, IL 60607, USA
D.J. Singel, Department of Chemistry, Harvard University, Boston, MA 02115, USA
T. Sivron, Department of Neurobiology, The Weizmann Institute of Science, Rehovot, Israel
D.M. Snow, Department of Cell Biology and Neuroanatomy, University of Minnesota, Minneapolis, MN 55455, USA
S.H. Snyder, Departments of Neuroscience, Pharmacology and Molecular Sciences, Psychiatry and Behavioral Sciences, Johns Hopkins University School of Medicine, Baltimore, MD 21205, USA
N.C. Spitzer, Department of Biology and Center for Molecular Genetics, University of California at San Diego, La Jolla, CA 92093 USA
J.S. Stamler, Departments of Respiratory and Cardiovascular Medicine, Harvard Medical School, Boston, MA 02115, USA
J.D. Steeves, Departments of Zoology and Anatomy, University of British Columbia, Vancouver, British Columbia, Canada V6T 1Z4
Y. Tamura, Department of Neuropharmacology, Faculty of Pharmacy and Pharmaceutical Sciences, Fukuyama University, Fukuyama 729-02, Japan
K. Terada, Department of Neuropharmacology, Faculty of Pharmacy and Pharmaceutical Sciences, Fukuyama University, Fukuyama 729-02, Japan
W. Tetzlaff, Department of Physiology and Neuroscience Research Institute, University of Ottawa, Ottawa, Ontario, and Department of Anatomy, University of Calgary, Calgary, Alberta, Canada
B.J. Tsui, Department of Anatomy, University of Calgary, Calgary, Alberta, Canada
Z. Varga, Department of Pharmacology, Biocenter, Basel, Switzerland
H. Vischer, Department of Pharmacology, Biocenter, Basel, Switzerland

X.M. Wang, Department of Cell Biology, Neurobiology and Anatomy, The Ohio State University, Columbus, OH 43210, USA

S.G. Waxman, Department of Neurology, Yale University School of Medicine and Neuroscience Regeneration Research Center, VA Medical Center, West Haven, CT 06516, USA

J.P. Whelan, Center for Neurologic Diseases, Department of Medicine, Division of Neurology, Brigham and Women's Hospital, and Department of Neurology, Harvard Medical School, Boston, MA 02115, USA

W.R. Woodward, Departments of Neurology and Biochemistry & Molecular Biology, Oregon Health Sciences University, Portland, OR 97201, USA

D.-Y. Wu, Department of Pharmacology and Center for Neurobiology and Behavior, Columbia University, New York, NY 10032, USA

X.M. Xu, The Miami Project to Cure Paralysis, University of Miami, Miami, FL 33136, USA

Y.Z. Ye, Department of Anesthesiology, University of Alabama at Birmingham, Birmingham, AL 25233, USA

J. Zhang, Department of Neuroscience, Johns Hopkins University School of Medicine, Baltimore, MD 21205, USA

M. Zimmermann, II. Institute of Physiology, University of Heidelberg, Heidelberg, Germany 69120

S.J. Zottoli, Department of Biology and Neuroscience Program, Williams College, Williamstown, MA 01267, USA

X.C. Zou, Department of Cell Biology, Neurobiology and Anatomy, The Ohio State University, Columbus, OH 43210, USA

T.J. Zwimpfer, Departments of Zoology and Surgery, University of British Columbia, Vancouver, British Columbia, Canada V6T 1Z4

Preface

Much has happened since publication of the previous volume (71) on neural regeneration in this series in 1987. Some of the progress in research in this field is reflected in the present volume, which incorporates the proceedings of the Fifth Internationl Symposium on Neural Regeneration held at the Asilomar Conference Center, Pacific Grove, California from December 8–12, 1993. The symposium was cosponsored by the US Department of Veterans Affairs (Medical Research Service), the Paralyzed Veterans of America (Spinal Cord Research Foundation), the National Institutes of Health (National Institute of Neurological Disorders and Stroke), the American Paralysis Association and the Eastern Paralyzed Veterans Association. The Program Planning Committee for the symposium included Drs. Harry Goshgarian (Wayne State University), Jeffrey D. Kocsis (VA Medical Center, West Haven and Yale University), Anthony L. Mescher (Indiana University), Monica M. Oblinger (The Chicago Medical School), Inder Perkash (VA Medical Center, Palo Alto and Stanford University), Fredrick J. Seil (VA Office of Regeneration Research Programs, VA Medical Center, Portland and Oregon Health Sciences University), Frank R. Sharp (VA Medical Center and University of California, San Francisco), Marion E. Smith (VA Medical Center, Palo Alto and Stanford University) and Roy A. Tassava (The Ohio State University). Guest participants during the planning process were Dr. Margaret Gianinni and Mr. David D. Collins of the Paralyzed Veterans of America.

The volume is organized into six topic sections, including Neurotrophins and Receptors, Axonal Outgrowth and Pathfinding, Calcium and Gene Expression, Models of Spinal Cord Regeneration, Cross Talk Between Nervous and Immune Systems in Response to Injury, and Nitric Oxide in the Central Nervous System. The first chapter in each section, whose title reflects that of the section heading, is an introduction to and an overview of the topic. The senior authors of these chapters chaired the corresponding sessions at the symposium. The subsequent section chapters were contributed by the invited session speakers and their co-workers. Although not included in this volume, the symposium was enriched by an inspired keynote address by Dr. Hans Thoenen (Max Planck Institute for Psychiatry, Planegg-Martinsried), by featured talks by Drs. Donald S. Faber (Medical College of Pennsylvania) and Constantino Sotelo (INSERM, Paris) and by the many poster presenters who displayed their work throughout the symposium.

No single symposium can cover the entire field of neural regeneration research. For this reason the topics chosen for presentation at successive international neural regeneration symposia are varied, so that eventually the spectrum of neural regeneration research is covered. Topics are also selected on the basis of what is current, and sometimes even on an expectation of what will be relevant to regeneration, such as the subject of nitric oxide in the present volume. The highlights presented here reflect some of the more important recent advances, such as characterization of the increasingly complex family of the neurotrophins and their receptors, definition of the molecular mechanisms that encourage and guide axon growth, including immediate early gene activation and calcium signals, and elucidation of the many ways in which the nervous and immune systems are interactive. The section on models of spinal cord regeneration is phylogenetically organized to provide comparisons between lower animals that can and higher animals that cannot regenerate their spinal cords. In this context, the role of inhibitory factors in discouraging regeneration is becoming increasingly clear. There are no illusions that all aspects of neural regeneration are addressed in this volume, but the rich sample presented here should give the reader a strong sense of the excitement and the hope that have come to pervade this field.

Fredrick J. Seil, M.D.
Director, VA Office of
Regeneration Research Programs
Portland, OR

Contents

Section III: Calcium and Gene Expression

Section IV: Models of Spinal Cord Regeneration

Section VI: Nitric Oxide in the Central Nervous System

SECTION I

Neurotrophins and Receptors

F.J. Seil (Ed.)
Progress in Brain Research, Vol 103

CHAPTER 1

Neurotrophins and receptors

Ronald M. Lindsay

Regeneron Pharmaceuticals Inc., Tarrytown, NY 10591, USA

Introduction

Our extensive knowledge on the biological properties and structure of the prototypical neurotrophic factor, nerve growth (NGF), is largely based on the relative ease in purifying substantial amounts of this protein from natural sources. NGF purified from the salivary gland of the male mouse has provided adequate material for: (a) extensive characterization of the neuronal specificity of this neurotrophic factor using both in vitro and in vivo approaches; and (b) determination of the primary, secondary and tertiary structure of this protein. Such information permitted cloning of the murine NGF gene and subsequently the human NGF gene. As determined from tissue culture studies, studies of chicken development in ovo, and most recently from NGF transgenic and gene knockout studies in the mouse, NGF is essential for the development and maintenance of sympathetic neurons, subpopulations of neural crest-derived sensory neurons and cholinergic neurons of the basal forebrain. The restricted specificity of NGF for these neuronal classes prompted the search for other neurotrophic factors. Although a number of such 'neurotrophic activities' have been identified in the last 20 years, it is only recently that full molecular characterization of several of these factors has been achieved. Some of these factors such as CNTF (ciliary neurotrophic factor; a member of the LIF, OSM, IL-6 cytokine family), FGFV (a member of the fibroblast growth factor family) and GDNF (glia-derived neurotrophic factor; a member of the transforming growth factor superfamily) are quite distinct from NGF in structure and function, but interestingly it has now been established that NGF is but one member of a gene family, the *neurotrophins*. Currently four members of this family have been identified, including NGF, brain-derived neurotrophic factor (BDNF), neurotrophin-3 (NT-3) and neurotrophin-4/5 (NT-4/5). This article describes some of the similarities and differences in the biological properties of the neurotrophins, especially in relation to their specificity for a recently described family of neurotrophin receptors, the trk family of receptor tyrosine kinases.

The neurotrophin family

As noted, the neurotrophin family currently compromises four members. At the level of the amino acid sequence of the mature proteins, there is 50–60% identity between any two members of this family (Fig. 1). The neurotrophins are highly basic proteins (p*I* 9–10.5) of around 120 amino acids in length and each is processed from a larger precursor. The three disulphide bridges which were originally identified in the structure of NGF appear to be retained in each of the neurotrophins and each of the six contributing cystine residues is flanked by regions of high homology. Functionally the neurotrophins act as

```
NGF       SSSHPIFHRGEFSVCDSVSVWVG--DKTTATDIKGKEVMVLGEVN
BDNF        HSDPARRGELSVCDSISEWVTAADKKTAVDMSGGTVTVLEKVS
NT-3       YAEHKSHRGEYSVCDSESLWVT--DKSSAIDIRGHQVTVLGEIG
NT-4    GVSETAPASRRGELAVCDAVSGWVT--DRRTAVDLRGREVEVLGEVP

NGF     NIN-SVFKQYFFETKCRDPNPVDS-------GCRGIDSKHWNSYCTT
BDNF    PVK-GQLKQYFYETKCNPMGYTKE-------GCRGIDKRHWNSQCRT
NT-3    KTN-SPVKQYFYETRCKEARPVKN-------GCRGIDDRHWNSQCKT
NT-4    AAGGSPLRQYFFETRCKADNAEEGGPGAGGGGCRGVDRRHWVSECKA

NGF     THTFVKAMLTDG-KQAAWRFIRIDTACVCVLSRKAVRRA
BDNF    TQSYVRAMLTDSKKRIGWRFIRIDTSCVCILTIKRGR
NT-3    SQTYVRASLTENNKLVGWRWIRIDTSCVCALSRKIGRT
NT-4    KQSYVRALTADAQGRVGWRWIRIDTACVCTLLSRTGRA
```

Fig. 1. Primary amino acid sequence of the four members of the neurotrophin family. The aligned sequences are of the human proteins.

homodimers, and may also be found naturally as heterodimers.

Nerve growth factor

The biology of NGF has been extensively reviewed elsewhere (Levi-Montalcini and Angeletti, 1968; Thoenen and Barde, 1980), but as the prototypical neurotrophic factor, detailed study of the biological properties of this protein has served as the model with which to test various hypotheses on the role of neurotrophic factors in development and maintenance of peripheral (PNS) and central nervous system (CNS) neurons. Perhaps as a consequence of the history of its discovery, NGF is usually considered as the major proof of the target-derived neurotrophic factor hypothesis, whereby strictly limited amounts of neuronal survival factors in target tissues are thought to regulate the type and density of neuronal innervation of that tissue. From in vitro and in vivo studies, it is clear that the neuronal specificity of NGF is restricted to sympathetic neurons, certain subpopulations of neural crest-derived sensory neurons and, within the CNS, cholinergic neurons of the basal forebrain and striatum. Much of the compelling evidence for a critical role of NGF in vivo was originally derived from studies in which endogenous NGF was neutralized by heterologous or maternal anti-NGF antibody approaches. More recently, null mutation or 'gene-knockout' of the NGF gene in mice has elegantly confirmed the earlier immunodepletion studies, such that homozygote NGF knockout mice have virtually no sympathetic neurons and > 70% depletion of dorsal root ganglion neurons (Crowley et al., 1994). Interestingly, initial reports indicate that these animals have a relatively normal complement of basal forebrain cholinergic neurons. This contrasts with established findings that NGF rescues adult rat septal cholinergic neurons from axotomy-induced cell death and the fact that during late development NGF promotes the survival of these neurons in vitro (for review see Hefti et al., 1993).

Brain-derived neurotrophic factor

Although first purified from porcine brain in 1982 (Barde et al., 1982), it was only upon the subsequent molecular cloning of BDNF (Liebrock et al., 1989) that it emerged that this protein was related to NGF, as the mature human NGF and BDNF proteins were found to share more than 55% sequence identity (for a recent review of the biology of BDNF see Lindsay, 1993). In contrast to an abundant source of NGF in the mouse salivary gland, initial studies of the neuronal biology of BDNF were greatly hampered by the very small amounts of this protein that could be purified from natural sources. Despite this, even prior to the availability of recombinantly produced BDNF it was established that BDNF and NGF had both distinct as well as overlapping neuronal specificities. For example, unlike NGF, BDNF was found to promote the survival in vitro of sensory neurons of placode-derived cranial ganglia, such as the nodose ganglion of the vagus nerve, and in contrast to NGF, BDNF appears to have no affect on sympathetic neurons (reviewed in Lindsay, 1993). NGF and BDNF do appear, however, to have overlapping actions on dorsal root ganglion sensory neurons and basal forebrain cholinergic neurons, although the exact degree and the temporal aspect of this overlap remains to be determined. A summary of the known specificity of the neurotrophin family toward PNS and motor neurons is shown in Table I.

TABLE I

Neurotrophin specificity: PNS and motor neurons

	NGF	BDNF	NT-3
Sensory			
Neural Crest			
DRG Small Neurons	***	—	—
DRG Medium Neurons	—	**	—
DRG Large Neurons	—	—	**
Neural Placode			
Nodose	—	**	**
Sympathetic	***	—	*
Parasympathetic	—	—	—
Motor Neurons	—	***	***

The production of recombinant BDNF has been critical to recent rapid advances in defining the neuronal specificity of BDNF in comparison to NGF and other members of the neurotrophin family. It is now quite clear, however, that in contrast to the very restricted specificty of NGF, BDNF has actions on many classes of CNS neurons in vitro and in vivo, including basal forebrain cholinergic neurons (Alderson et al., 1990; Knüsel et al., 1991), nigral dopaminergic (Hyman et al., 1991) and GABAergic neurons (Hyman et al., 1994), spinal motor neurons (Henderson et al., 1993; Wong et al., 1993), various classes of hippocampal neurons (Ip et al., 1993a), retinal photoreceptors (LaVail et al., 1992), striatal GABAergic and calbindin containing neurons (Ventimiglia et al., 1993), raphe serotonergic neurons (Siuciak et al., 1994), cerebellar Purkinje and granule neurons (Segal et al., 1992; Lärkfors et al., 1994), and cortical NPY containing neurons (Nawa et al., 1993).

Effects of BDNF on basal forebrain cholinergic neurons

Only in the case of basal forebrain cholinergic neurons is there an observed overlap in the neuronal specificity of BDNF and NGF toward CNS neurons. In culture, both BDNF and NGF promote the survival of late embryonic rat septal cholinergic neurons (Alderson et al., 1990). In terms of survival, their effects are not additive, suggesting effects on the same population of neurons. However, when combined, there is a synergistic effect on the upregulation of choline acetyltransferase (ChAT) levels in septal cultures. As mentioned above, it is interesting to note that basal forebrain cholinergic neurons are not evidently depleted in the NGF knockout mice (Crowley et al., 1994). Perhaps BDNF can substitute for NGF during the ontogeny of these neurons or perhaps, of the two factors, BDNF (or NT-4/5; see below) is the more critical survival factor and NGF is more involved in regulation of the mature phenotype of cholinergic neurons.

Although still at an early stage, in vivo studies with BDNF have begun to confirm the neuronal actions of BDNF defined using tissue culture approaches. For example, infusion of BDNF from an implanted osmotic pump into the brains of adult rats has now been shown to rescue basal forebrain cholinergic neurons from axotomy-induced atrophy and cell death which results from fimbria-fornix lesion (Morse et al., 1993). When delivered into the parenchyma at the level of the septum, the effects of BDNF are comparable to those previously reported for NGF delivered by an intracerebroventricular route. However, in contrast to NGF, which diffuses well from the CSF space into the brain parenchyma, BDNF exhibits only very limited penetration through the ependymal cells and glial end feet which comprise the ventricular lining. This is thought to be due to a high level of expression of a truncated form of the BDNF high-affinity receptor, trkB, on astrocytes and ependymal cells (Frisén et al., 1993; Morse et al., 1993; Valenzuela et al., 1993; Lindsay et al., 1994; Rudge et al., 1994).

Given that loss of basal forebrain cholinergic neurons has been implicated as a major cause of cognitive decline in Alzheimer's disease, the finding that NGF promotes the survival of developing cholinergic neurons in vitro, and is able to rescue mature cholinergic neurons from axotomy-induced cell death in vivo, has created a lot of interest in exploring the clinical potential of NGF in Alzheimer's disease (Hefti and Weiner, 1986). On the one hand, the restricted specificty of NGF may be an attractive feature in terms of there being little expectation of side effects of infusing NGF into the human brain, but on the other hand, the fact that many neuronal systems which are not responsive to NGF are affected in Alzheimer's disease is likely to limit the efficacy of NGF. In this context, the much broader spectrum of action of BDNF toward CNS neurons may make this neurotrophin a more interesting candidate for assessment in Alzheimer's disease. However, much more basic research needs to be done to support this idea, studies which will undoubtedly be problematic in the absence of any suitable animal model of Alzheimer's disease.

In the absence of any relevant animal models of Alzheimer's disease, one approach to assessing agents that might have therapeutic benefit is to apply them locally to multiple brain regions and assess their effects on morphology, neurochemistry and behavior. In this context, infusion of BDNF within the hippocampus, cortex or striatum of adult rats has been found to induce marked changes in the levels of several important neuroactive peptides, including substance P, dynorphin and cholecystokinin, and the mRNA encoding the precursors of these peptides (Croll et al., 1993). Interestingly, the increases or decreases in peptide levels produced by BDNF were largely in a direction that was opposite to changes in these peptides that have been observed in Alzheimer's disease. Studies are also in progress to assess the effects of BDNF in cognitively impaired aged rats, or animals impaired by chemical lesions.

Effects of BDNF on spinal motor neurons

Although it was first suggested that developing motor neurons did not respond to BDNF (Arakawa et al., 1990), it is now clear that the survival and differentiation of motor neurons is affected by a number of neurotrophic factors, including BDNF, NT-3, NT-4/5 and CNTF. Although CNTF was the first neurotrophic factor shown to promote the survival of developing motor neurons in culture (Arakawa et al., 1990) and in vivo (rescue of axotomized facial nerve motor neurons; Sendtner et al., 1990), it was first evident from retrograde axonal transport studies (DiStefano et al., 1992) that motor neurons were likely to be responsive to BDNF and NT-3. Wong et al. (1993) have shown that not only do BDNF, NT-3 and NT-4/5 act independently to increase ChAT levels in cultured rat embryo motor neurons, but also that combinations of neurotrophins with each other (e.g., BDNF and NT-3) or with CNTF exhibit synergistic effects on the levels of ChAT activity in motor neurons.

A number of recent studies have shown that not only can BDNF reduce naturally occurring cell death of developing motor neurons (Oppenheim et al., 1992) but as with CNTF, BDNF can attenuate the loss of facial nerve nucleus or spinal motor neurons in the early postnatal rat following axotomy of either the facial nerve or the sciatic nerve, respectively (Sendtner et al., 1992a; Yan et al., 1992). The effects of BDNF on motor neurons are not confined to development, as either local or systemic application of BDNF in adult rats can attenuate the loss of ChAT levels observed in spinal cord motor neurons following sciatic nerve transection (Friedman et al., 1994). CNTF has been shown to attenuate neuromuscular deficits in three quite distinct strains of mutant mice: Mnd, pmn and Wobbler (Helgren et al., 1992; Sendtner et al., 1992b; Mitsumoto et al., 1994). None of these mutants could be described as a model of human motor neuron disease, but taken together the effects of CNTF in altering the course of disease progression in affected animals has provided a strong rationale for initiating clinical trials of CNTF in amyotrophic lateral sclerosis (ALS). In the Wobbler mouse, a recessive disorder where affected mice show deficits primarily of the forelimbs as a result of cervical cord motor neuron loss and atrophy of forelimb musculature, BDNF treatment has now been found to have effects similar to CNTF (Ikeda et al., 1993). Over a 4-week treatment period, the effects of subcutaneous injections of BDNF include attenuation of grip strength loss and attenuation of progressive paw position abnormalities.

Most interestingly, a very recent study has found that, as suggested from in vitro experiments, the effects of combined CNTF and BDNF treatment of affected Wobbler mouse has a much more pronounced effect in slowing disease progression than either factor alone (Mitsumoto et al., 1993). Potential efficacy of BDNF in ALS is currently at the stage of a Phase I clinical trial, whereas a trial of CNTF in the same disease is already at the Phase III stage. If either neurotrophic factor shows efficacy alone, a combination trial should be initiated.

Effects of BDNF on dopaminergic and GABAergic neurons of the substantia nigra

Although little is known about the etiology of the disease, loss of dopaminergic neurons in the substantia nigra is the primary cause of the symptoms and progressive nature of Parkinson's disease. This fact has prompted the search for trophic factors that might influence the survival or maintenance of dopaminergic neurons. Although several 'trophic activities' which enhance the survival or differentiation of developing mesencephalic dopamine neurons have been described (reviewed in Lindsay et al., 1993), BDNF was the first fully characterized neurotrophic factor found to promote the survival of embryonic rat nigral dopaminergic neurons (Hyman et al., 1991). Furthermore, BDNF has been shown to protect these neurons in vitro from the toxicity of either 6-hydroxydopamine (6-OHDA) or methylphenyl-tetrahydropyridinium (MPTP). The latter findings are of particular interest as these two neurotoxins are widely used in rodent and primate models to create Parkinsonian-like symptoms. The mechanism of action of both toxins is thought to be a result of inhibition of mitochondrial function and the creation of free radicals that ultimately lead to oxidative damage. Although direct evidence is still lacking, there is a lot of current interest in the hypothesis that oxidative stress may be a component of various neurodegenerative disorders, including Parkinson's disease. Thus the finding that BDNF protects dopaminergic neurons from 6-OHDA toxicity by a mechanism which decreases oxidative stress may have important implications (Spina et al., 1992). In addition to effects on cultured nigral dopaminergic neurons, it has recently been shown that BDNF also promotes the survival of nigral GABAergic neurons (Hyman et al., 1994).

Based on the survival promoting and neuroprotective effects of BDNF toward nigral dopaminergic neurons discussed above, studies are in progress to determine whether BDNF displays similar effects in vivo. In the first attempt to demonstrate protective effects in vivo, infusion of BDNF into the brain was not found to protect dopamine neurons from a relatively standard unilateral 6-OHDA medial forebrain bundle lesion (S.J. Wiegand, unpublished observations). The extent and acute nature of this lesion may, however, make it unrealistic to expect any protection. More promisingly, however, when infused directly above the nigra of intact adult rats there was both biochemical and behavioral evidence to suggest that BDNF can produce hypertrophy of undamaged nigral dopamine neurons (Altar et al., 1992). For a more detailed account of studies of the effects of BDNF and other neurotrophins on nigral neurons in vitro or in vivo, the reader is referred to a recent review (Lindsay et al., 1993).

Effects of BDNF on striatal neurons

The loss of medium spiny GABAergic neurons of the human striatum is a hallmark of the pathology of Huntington's disease, and although the disease has recently been linked to a specific gene defect, 'huntingtin', and appears to be one of several diseases now associated with aberrant nucleotide triplet repeats, the function of the normal gene is unknown, and thus the disease process remains to be elucidated. Until recently there was little clear evidence of effects of any known neurotrophic factors on cultured striatal neurons, although the relatively small population of striatal cholinergic neurons have been shown to be responsive to NGF. Interestingly, in the adult rodent brain, levels of BDNF and other neurotrophins are conspicuously low in the striatum.

Ventimiglia et al. (1993) have recently found that BDNF not only promotes the survival of cultured striatal GABAergic neurons but has a pronounced effect on morphological differentiation of these neurons. A careful morphometric analysis indicates that BDNF increases cell soma size, total neuritic length and area of neuritic arbor by 2-fold or more in each case.

In rodents quinolinic acid treatment is routinely used to produce excitoxic lesions to the striatum. We are currently exploring the protective or attenuating potential of BDNF infusion in such lesions.

Expression of BDNF within BDNF responsive neurons—autocrine function?

Localization of the expression of BDNF mRNA by in situ hybridization methods (Ernfors et al., 1990; Gall et al., 1992) has not only confirmed earlier Northern analyses which indicated widespread expression of BDNF in many brain regions (Maisonpierre et al., 1990a), but has revealed that several classes of neurons that respond to BDNF also appear to synthesize BDNF. This has important implications for how we think about the role of neurotrophic factors both in development and maintenance of the PNS and CNS.

Based almost entirely on the biology of NGF, the classical view of the primary function of neurotrophic factors is their role as target-derived factors. The widespread distribution of BDNF mRNA within many classes of CNS neurons may be consistent with a target-derived role, in which BDNF produced by one type of neuron acts as the target-derived factor for afferent inputs to that neuron. However, in light of the demonstration of BDNF synthesis within BDNF responsive neurons, it seems likely that neurotrophic factors may also have important paracrine and/or autocrine functions. The presence of BDNF mRNA in a subpopulation of sensory neurons of the dorsal root ganglion (DRG) is a particular case in which the site of synthesis of a neurotrophin seems incompatible with a purely target-derived role, especially as DRG neurons have no afferent inputs. Consistent with the possibility that BDNF expression in adult sensory neurons may serve an autocrine function, we have recently shown that specific disruption of BDNF synthesis in isolated, purified adult rat DRG neurons using antisense oligonucleotides leads to selective neuronal cell death (Acheson et al., 1994). Sense oligonucleotides were without effect, but most importantly the neuronal death produced by antisense disruption of endogenous BDNF could be rescued by applying exogenous BDNF to the cultured DRG neurons.

We postulate that in the adult CNS and PNS, autocrine neurotrophic factor loops may be a common mechanism to ensure neuronal survival once the appropriate complement of CNS and PNS neurons has been selected during development, i.e. once the period of so-called naturally occurring neuronal cell death is complete. If this idea is valid, it is interesting to speculate that any decrease in autocrine neurotrophic factor levels, as a result of ageing, disease or trauma, in the adult brain may precipitate neuronal loss and possibly be a component of the etiology of one or more neurodegenerative diseases. In this context it should be noted that a significant loss of BDNF mRNA levels has been revealed in the hippocampal formation of postmortem tissue from Alzheimer's patients (Phillips et al., 1991).

Neurotrophin-3 and neurotrophin-4 / 5

The cloning of BDNF revealed the homology of BDNF to NGF and therefore the existence of a NGF-related gene family. This rapidly lead several groups to identify a third family member, NT-3, using homology cloning strategies (Hohn et al., 1990; Maisonpierre et al., 1990b). A fourth family member, NT-4/5, was initially cloned from *Xenopus* (Hallböök et al., 1991), with the subsequent cloning of the human gene, which has been referred to either as NT-4 (Ip et al., 1992) or NT-5 (Berkemeier et al., 1991). The two nomenclatures do refer to the same mammalian gene and currently, therefore, the terminology NT-4/5 has been adopted.

In tissue culture studies with many classes of CNS neurons, there is very marked overlap between the effects of BDNF and NT-3. This probably reflects not only the colocalization of the preferential BDNF and NT-3 high-affinity receptors (trkB and trkC, respectively) on many CNS neurons but also the fact that NT-3 can act at the BDNF receptor, albeit requiring much higher concentrations of NT-3 than BDNF. The latter is perhaps evident when examining, for example, the effect of NT-3 on basal forebrain cholinergic neurons; in vitro NT-3 is much less potent than BDNF in promoting the survival and differentiation of these neurons and in vivo NT-3 is less robustly transported than BDNF to septal cholinergic neurons by retrograde axonal transport following intrahippocampal injection of either ligand (Alderson et al., 1990; DiStefano et al., 1992).

Within the PNS, retrograde axonal transport studies have indicated that following injection into the sciatic nerve, radiolabeled NT-3 is preferentially transported to motor neurons and to large diameter sensory neurons (DiStefano et al., 1992). The finding that NT-3 supports the survival and differentiation of developing motor neurons (Henderson et al., 1993; Wong et al., 1993) with equivalent potency to BDNF would suggest colocalization of trkB and trkC. This indeed is the case in vitro, and also explains the observation that combinations of BDNF and NT-3 upregulate ChAT levels in cultured motor neurons to a greater degree that saturating levels of either factor alone (Wong et al., 1993).

When the neurite outgrowth promoting effects of NGF, BDNF and NT-3 were first compared side by side on cultured explants of chick embryo DRG, all three neurotrophins produced fiber outgrowth. However, there was a clear difference in the extent of fiber outgrowth and the thickness of fibers produced by each factor, suggesting specificity for subpopulations of sensory neurons, rather than a broadly overlapping spectrum of action (Maisonpierre et al., 1990b). This has now been confirmed by several studies, such that it is now clear that NGF is primarily specific for small sensory neurons (unmyelinated nociceptive sensory neurons; numerically the largest subpopulation of DRG neurons), BDNF shows effects on small to medium sized DRG neurons, and NT-3 is specific for the largest (proprioceptive) sensory neurons, the latter being more abundant in lumbar and cervical level DRG than in thoracic or sacral DRG (Hory-Lee et al., 1993). A number of laboratories are at the early stage of analysis of mice in which either NGF, BDNF, NT-3 or NT-4/5 or their cognate receptors (trk A, B and C) have been knocked out, and preliminary unpublished results from these animals are entirely consistent with the above findings.

The specificity of NT-3 for proprioceptive sensory neurons has been exploited in an animal model directed at assessing the potential efficacy of neurotrophic factors in large fiber peripheral neuropathy arising from chemotherapy drugs such as cisplatin. In this model, systemic NT-3 treatment has been found to attenuate deficits in locomotion that result from specific large fiber sensory neuron atrophy produced by multiple daily dosing with pyridoxine (Helgren, M., unpublished results). Other interesting effects of NT-3 in vivo are beginning to emerge, including the recent report by Schwab and colleagues that NT-3 treatment enhances sprouting of severed corticospinal tract neurons in the adult rat (Schnell et al., 1994).

As a consequence of being a ligand for trkB, with potency on trkB fibroblasts at least equivalent to BDNF (Ip et al., 1993b), NT-4/5 has been shown both in vitro and in vivo to have effects that are in many ways similar to BDNF (e.g., Henderson et al., 1993; Wong et al., 1993). However, there are now several observations on cultured CNS neurons that clearly distinguish the actions of BDNF and NT-4/5. For example, in cultures of embryonic rat ventral mesencephalon, NT-4/5 promotes survival of dopaminergic neurons to an even greater degree than BDNF, and the potency of NT-4/5 is approximately an order of magnitude greater than that of BDNF. In the same cultures, BDNF increases both dopamine content and dopamine uptake in the cultures; NT-4/5 increases dopamine content but has no effect on dopamine uptake (Hyman et al., 1994).

Neurotrophin receptors

The low-affinity neurotrophin receptor, p75

Early binding studies with radiolabeled NGF revealed the presence of both low- and high-affinity NGF binding sites, with dissociation constants on the order of 10^{-9} and 10^{-11}, respectively (Herrup and Shooter, 1975). Subsequent studies led to the identification and cloning of a protein with the properties of a low-affinity NGF receptor (Chao et al., 1986; Radeke et al., 1987), referred to alternately as LNGFR or p75LNGFR or simply p75. Although capable of binding NGF, and indeed all of the neurotrophins with nM affinity, the role of p75 is still unclear. p75 is expressed on several classes of neurons and non-neuronal cells but does not appear by itself to transduce signaling upon ligand binding (for review see Meakin and Shooter, 1992). Suggested roles for p75 include sequestration or localization of secreted NGF, presentation of NGF to high-affinity receptors, functioning as an essential component of a high-affinity NGF receptor complex, and serving as a modulator of the specificity of action of the neurotrophins on different classes of neurotrophins (see reviews by Chao, 1992; Meakin and Shooter, 1992).

The trk family of high-affinity neurotrophin receptors

Quite independent of the discovery of the neurotrophin family, the last few years have seen the discovery of a family of receptor tyrosine kinases, the trks, which are high-affinity neurotrophin receptors (for review see Chao, 1992; Meakin and Shooter, 1992; Glass and Yancopoulos, 1993). The specificity of each of the neurotrophins for the receptors encoded by the three known mammalian trk genes, trkA, trkB and trkC, is summarized in Fig. 2. In addition to proteins which

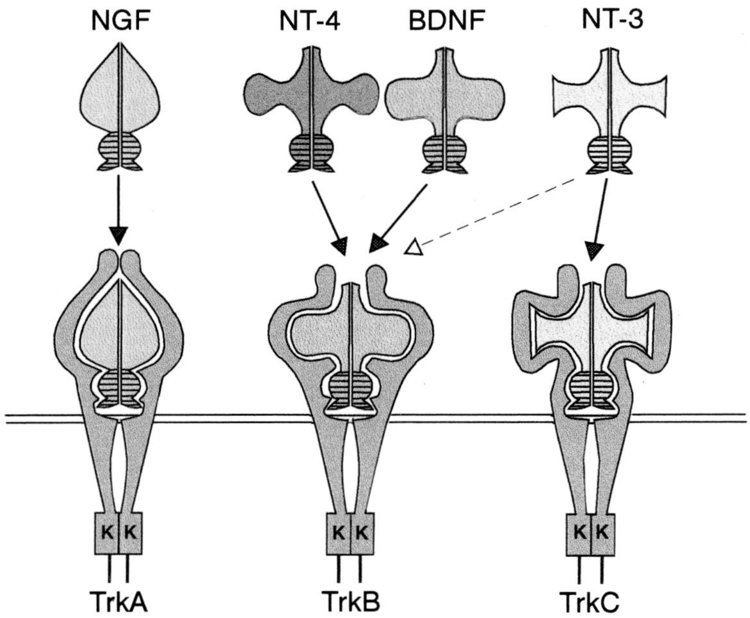

Fig. 2. Schematic diagram showing the preferred specificity of each of the neurotrophins for members of the trk family of neurotrophin high-affinity receptors. NGF is a unique ligand at trkA, whereas NT-3 is a unique ligand for trkC. BDNF and NT-4/5 show similar affinity for trkB (although not always identical biological effects upon cultured neurons which express trkB; see text), whereas NT-3 is a weaker ligand for trkB. K = kinase.

display variants in their kinase domains, trkB and trkC receptors also exist as truncated proteins which lack intracellular kinase domains. The neurotrophins exist naturally as homodimers (and possibly heterodimers) and, as with ligands for other tyrosine kinase receptors, activate signal transduction by inducing dimerization and autophosphorylation of the appropriate trk (Jing et al., 1992).

Consistent with the restricted neuronal specificity of NGF, high-affinity NGF binding sites and trkA mRNA are localized to only a very few neuronal types in the CNS and PNS. In marked contrast to trkA, transcripts for trkB and trkC are widely distributed throughout the brain (Klein et al., 1989, 1990, 1991; Middlemas et al., 1991; Merlio et al., 1992; Valenzuela et al., 1993). In situ hybridization studies indicate that full length, kinase containing forms of trkB or trkC are expressed, possibly often coexpressed, on the majority of CNS neurons but not on non-neuronal elements such as astrocytes, oligodendrocytes, ependyma or cells of the choroid plexus. trkA is not found in any truncated form and does not appear to be expressed in neuroglia. In contrast, truncated forms of trkB and trkC that lack intracellular kinase domains are expressed at very high levels in the CNS, with truncated trkB localized predominantly to non-neuronal cells (Frisén et al., 1993). Taken together, the very widespread distribution of trkB and trkC throughout the CNS and a similar widespread distribution of their ligands (Maisonpierre et al., 1990a) has predicted that the actions of BDNF and NT-3 in the CNS will be much more diverse than those of NGF. This appears to be borne out by many recent in vitro studies, as discussed earlier. In addition, the high levels of expression of truncated forms of trkB and trkC (but not trkA) indicate that there may be mechanisms to restrict the distribution (Morse et al., 1993) or otherwise modulate the action of BDNF or NT-3 following release from sites of synthesis (Klein et al., 1990; Middlemas et al., 1991; Frisén et al., 1993). In the case of BDNF, the presence of truncated trkB receptors on astrocytes may serve to produce high local concentrations through sequestration on the cell surface or, through internalization and degradation, to inactivate this neurotrophin, and thereby prevent its spread to inappropriate sites of action, analogous to the function of neurotransmitter high-affinity reuptake systems (see Lindsay et al., 1994).

Conclusions

For many years our understanding of the biology of neurotrophic factors was restricted to concepts that arose from the study of NGF. It is perhaps fitting that NGF should turn out to be but one member of a gene family whose members are proving to have more diverse biological actions than NGF itself. The cloning and production of recombinant BDNF, NT-3 and NT-4/5 is bringing rapid advances to this field, not least of which is the ability to carry out in vivo studies that would have been inconceivable a few years ago.

Although there is only limited evidence to implicate a neurotrophic factor deficit as a component of any neurological disorder, there is a growing body of animal data to support the idea that pharmacological doses of several neurotrophic factors, may prove useful in the treatment of a number of neurodegenerative diseases. Currently, BDNF, CNTF and insulin-like growth factor 1 (IGF-1) are being evaluated as therapeutic agents in ALS, while NGF is being assessed for the treatment of toxic neuropathies.

Acknowledgements

The material summarized in this article is largely the work of many of my colleagues at Regeneron, whom I thank for many fruitful discussions, critical comments and enthusiasm. I also thank Rhonda Littlefair for help in preparing the manuscript.

References

Acheson, A., Fandl, J.P., Yancopoulos, G.D. and Lindsay, R.M. (1994) An autocrine loop mediates BDNF-dependent survival of adult sensory neurons. Submitted to *Nature*, under revision.

Alderson, R.F., Alterman, A.L., Barde, Y.-A. and Lindsay, R.M. (1990) Brain-derived neurotrophic factor increases survival and differentiated functions of rat septal cholinergic neurons in culture. *Neuron,* 5: 297–306.

Altar, C.A., Boylan, C.B., Jackson, C., Hershenson, S., Miller, J., Wiegand, S.J., Lindsay, R.M. and Hyman, C. (1992) Brain-derived neurotrophic factor augments rotational behavior and nigrostriatal dopamine turnover in vivo. *Proc. Natl. Acad. Sci. USA*, 89: 11347–11351.

Arakawa, Y., Sendtner, M. and Thoenen, H. (1990) Survival effect of ciliary neurotrophic factor (CNTF) on chick embryonic motoneurons in culture: comparison with other neurotrophic factors and cytokines. *J. Neurosci.,* 10: 3507–3515.

Barde, Y.-A., Edgar, D. and Thoenen, H. (1982) Purification of a new neurotrophic factor from mammalian brain. *EMBO J.*, 1: 549–553.

Berkemeier, L.R., Winslow, J.W., Goeddel, D.V. and Rosenthal, A. (1991) Neurotrophin-5: a novel neurotrophic factor that activates trk and trkB. *Neuron,* 7: 857–866.

Chao, M.V. (1992) Neurotrophin receptors: a window into neuronal differentiation. *Neuron,* 9: 583–593.

Chao, M.V., Bothwell, M.A., Ross, A.H., Koprowski, H., Lanahan, A.A., Buck, C.R. and Sehgal, A. (1986) Gene transfer and molecular cloning of the human NGF receptor. *Science,* 232: 518–521.

Croll, S.D., Wiegand, S.J., Anderson, K.D., Lindsay, R.M. and Nawa, H. (1993) Neuropeptide regulation by BDNF and NGF in adult rat forebrain. *Soc. Neurosci. Abstr.,* 19: 662.

Crowley, C., Spencer, S.D., Nishimura, M.C., Chen, K.S., Pitts-Meek, S., Armanini, M.P., Ling, L.H., McMahon, S.B., Shelton, D.L., Levinson, A.D. and Phillips, H.S. (1994) Mice lacking nerve growth factor display perinatal loss of sensory and sympathetic neurons yet develop basal forebrain cholinergic neurons. *Cell,* 76: 1001–1012.

DiStefano, P.S., Friedman, B., Radziejewski, C., Alexander, C., Boland, P., Schick, C.M., Lindsay, R.M. and Wiegand, S.J. (1992) The neurotrophins BDNF, NT-3, and NGF display distinct patterns of retrograde axonal transport in peripheral and central neurons. *Neuron,* 8: 983–993.

Ernfors, P., Wetmore, C., Olson, L. and Persson, H. (1990) Identification of cells in rat brain and peripheral tissues expressing mRNA for members of the nerve growth factor family. *Neuron,* 5: 511–526.

Friedman, B., Kleinfeld, D., Ip, N.Y., Verge, V.M.K., Moulton, R., Boland, P., Zlotchenko, E., Lindsay, R.M. and Liu, L. (1994) BDNF and NT-4/5 exert neurotrophic influences on injured adult spinal motor neurons. *J. Neurosci.,* in press.

Frisén, J., Verge, V.M.K., Fried, K., Risling, M., Persson, H., Trotter, J., Hkfelt, T. and Lindholm, D. (1993) Characterization of glial trkB receptors: differential response to injury in the central and peripheral nervous systems. *Proc. Natl. Acad. Sci. USA*, 90: 4971–4975.

Gall, C.M., Gold, S.J., Isackson, P.J. and Seroogy, K.B. (1992) Brain-derived neurotrophic factor and neurotrophin-3 mRNAs are expressed in ventral midbrain regions containing dopaminergic neurons. *Mol. Cell. Neurosci.*, 3: 56–63.

Glass, D.J. and Yancopoulos, G.D. (1993) The neurotrophins and their receptors. *Trends Cell Biol.*, 3: 262–268.

Hallböök, F., Ibáñez, C.F. and Persson, H. (1991) Evolutionary studies of the nerve growth factor family reveal a novel member abundantly expressed in *Xenopus* ovary. *Neuron,* 6: 845–858.

Hefti, F. and Weiner, W.J. (1986) Nerve growth factor and Alzheimer's disease. *Ann. Neurol.*, 20: 275–281.

Hefti, F., Denton, T.L., Knüsel, B. and Lapchak, P.A. (1993) Neurotrophic factors: what are they and what are they doing? In: S.E. Loughlin and J.H. Fallon (Eds.), *Neurotrophic Factors*, Academic Press, New York, pp. 25–49.

Helgren, M.E., Friedman, B., Kennedy, M., Mullholland, K., Messer, A., Wong, V. and Lindsay, R.M. (1992) Ciliary neurotrophic factor (CNTF) delays motor impairments in the Mnd mouse, a genetic model of motor neuron disease. *Soc. Neurosci. Abstr.*, 18: 618.

Henderson, C.E., Camu, W., Mettling, C., Gouin, A., Poulsen, K., Karihaloo, M., Rullamas, J., Evans, T., McMahon, S.B., Armanini, M.P., Berkemeier, L., Phillips, H.S. and Rosenthal, A. (1993) Neurotrophins promote motor neuron survival and are present in embryonic limb bud. *Nature (Lond.),* 363: 266–270.

Herrup, K. and Shooter, E.M. (1975) Properties of the beta-nerve growth factor receptor in development. *J. Cell Biol.*, 67: 118–125.

Hohn, A., Leibrock, J., Bailey, K. and Barde, Y.-A. (1990) Identification and characterization of a novel member of the nerve growth factor/brain-derived neurotrophic factor family. *Nature (Lond.)*, 344: 339–341.

Hory-Lee, R., Russell, M., Lindsay, R.M. and Frank, E. (1993) Neurotrophin 3 supports the survival of developing muscle sensory neurons in culture. *Proc. Natl. Acad. Sci. USA*, 90: 2613–2617.

Hyman, C., Hofer, M., Barde, Y.-A., Juhasz, M., Yancopoulos, G.D., Squinto, S.P. and Lindsay, R.M. (1991) BDNF is a neurotrophic factor for dopaminergic neurons of the substantia nigra. *Nature (Lond.)*, 350: 230–232.

Hyman, C., Juhasz, M., Jackson, C., Wright, P., Ip, N.Y. and Lindsay, R.M. (1994) Overlapping and distinct actions of the neurotrophins, BDNF, NT-3 and NT-4/5, on cultured dopaminergic and GABAergic neurons of the ventral mesencephalon. *J. Neurosci.*, 14: 335–347.

Ikeda, K., Mitsumoto, H., Wong, V., Cedarbaum, J.M. and Lindsay, R.M. (1993) Brain-derived neurotrophic factor (BDNF) slows the progression of Wobbler mouse motor neuron disease. *Soc. Neurosci. Abstr.*, 19:199.

Ip, N.Y., Ibáñez, C.F., Nye, S.H., McClain, J., Jones, P.F., Gies, D.R., Beluscio, L., Le Beau, M.M., Espinosa, R., III, Squinto, S.P., Persson, H. and Yancopoulos, G.D. (1992)

Mammalian neurotrophin-4: structure, chromosomal localization, tissue distribution and receptor specificity. *Proc. Natl. Acad. Sci. USA*, 89: 3060–3064.

Ip, N.Y., Li, Y., Yancopoulos, G.D. and Lindsay, R.M. (1993a) Cultured hippocampal neurons show responses to BDNF, NT-3, and NT-4, but not NGF. *J. Neurosci.,* 13: 3394-3405.

Ip, N.Y., Stitt, T.N., Tapley, P., Klein, R., Glass, D.J., Fandl, J., Greene, L.A., Barbacid, M. and Yancopoulos, G.D. (1993b) Similarities and differences in the way neurotrophins interact with the trk receptors in neuronal and nonneuronal cells. *Neuron,* 10: 137–149.

Jing, S., Tapley, P. and Barbacid, M. (1992) Nerve growth factor mediates signal transduction through trk homodimer receptors. *Neuron,* 9: 1067–1079.

Klein, R., Parada, L.F., Boulier, F. and Barbacid, M. (1989) trkB, a novel tyrosine protein kinase receptor expressed during mouse neural development. *EMBO J.*, 8: 3701–3709.

Klein, R., Conway, D., Parada, L.F. and Barbacid, M. (1990) The trk B tyrosine protein kinase gene codes for a second neurogenic receptor that lacks the catalytic kinase domain. *Cell,* 61: 647–656.

Klein, R., Nanduri, V., Jing, S., Lamballe, F., Tapley, P., Bryant, S., Cordon-Cardo, C., Jones, K.R., Reichardt, L.F. and Barbacid, M. (1991) The trkB tyrosine protein kinase is a receptor for brain-derived neurotrophic factor and neurotrophin-3. *Cell,* 66: 395–403.

Knüsel, B., Winslow, J.W., Rosenthal, A., Burton, L.E., Seid, D.P., Nikolics, K. and Hefti, F. (1991) Promotion of central cholinergic and dopaminergic neuron differentiation by brain-derived neurotrophic factor but not neurotrophin-3. *Proc. Natl. Acad. Sci. USA*, 88: 961–965.

Lärkfors, L., Lindsay, R.M. and Alderson, R.A. (1994) Ciliary neurotrophic factor enhances the survival of Purkinje cells in vivo. *Eur. J. Neurosci.,* in press.

LaVail, M.M., Unoki, K., Yasumura, D., Matthes, M.T., Yancopoulos, G.D. and Steinberg, R.H. (1992) Multiple growth factors, cytokines, and neurotrophins rescue photoreceptors from the damaging effects of constant light. *Proc. Natl. Acad. Sci. USA,* 89: 11249–11253.

Levi-Montalcini, R. and Angeletti, P.U. (1968) Nerve growth factor. *Physiol. Rev.*, 48: 534-569.

Liebrock, J., Lottspeich, F., Hohn, A., Hofer, M., Hengerer, B., Masiakowski, P., Thoenen, H .and Barde, Y.-A. (1989) Molecular cloning and expression of brain-derived neurotrophic factor. *Nature (Lond.)*, 341: 149–152.

Lindsay, R.M. (1993) Brain derived neurotrophic factor: an NGF-related neurotrophin. In: S.E. Loughlin and J.H. Fallon (Eds.), *Neurotrophic Factors*, Academic Press, New York, pp. 257–284.

Lindsay, R.M., Altar, C.A., Cedarbaum, J.M., Hyman, C. and Wiegand, S.J. (1993) The therapeutic potential of neurotrophic factors in the treatment of Parkinson's disease. *Exp. Neurol.*, 124: 103–118.

Lindsay, R.M., Wiegand, S.J., Altar, C.A.and DiStefano, P.S. (1994) Neurotrophic factors: from molecule to man. *Trends Neurosci.*, 17: 182–190.

Maisonpierre, P.C., Belluscio, L., Friedman, B., Alderson, R.F., Wiegand, S.J., Furth, M.E., Lindsay, R.M. and Yancopoulos, G.D. (1990a) NT-3, BDNF, and NGF in the developing rat nervous system: parallel as well as reciprocal patterns of expression. *Neuron*, 5: 501–509.

Maisonpierre, P.C., Belluscio, L., Squinto, S., Ip, N.Y., Furth, M.E., Lindsay. R.M.. and Yancopoulos, G.D. (1990b) Neurotrophin-3: a neurotrophic factor related to NGF and BDNF. *Science,* 247: 1446–1451.

Meakin, S.O. and Shooter, E.M. (1992) The nerve growth factor family of receptors. *Trends Neurosci.*, 15: 323–331.

Merlio, J.P., Ernfors, P., Jaber, M. and Persson, H. (1992) Molecular cloning of rat trkC and distribution of cells expressing messenger RNAs for members of the trk family in the rat central nervous system. *Neuroscience,* 51: 513–532.

Middlemas, D.S., Lindberg, R.A.and Hunter, T. (1991) trkB, a neural receptor protein-tyrosine kinase: evidence for a full-length and two truncated receptors. *Mol. Cell. Biol.*, 11: 143–153.

Mitsumoto, H., Ikeda, K., Wong, V., Cedarbaum, J.M. and Lindsay, R.M. (1993) Ciliary neurotrophic factor (CNTF) and brain-derived neurotrophic factor (BDNF) co-administration arrests loss of motor function in wobbler mice. *Soc. Neurosci. Abstr.*, 19: 199.

Mitsumoto, H., Ikeda, K., Holmlund, T., Greene, T., Cedarbaum, J.M., Wong, V. and Lindsay, R.M. (1994) The effects of ciliary neurotrophic factor (CNTF) on motor dysfunction in wobbler mouse motor neuron disease. *Ann. Neurol.*, in press.

Morse, J.K., Wiegand, S.J., Anderson, K.A., You, Y., Cai, N., DiStefano, P.S., Altar, C.A., Lindsay, R.M. and Alderson, R.F. (1993) Brain-derived neurotrophic factor (BDNF) increases the survival of basal forebrain cholinergic neurons following a fimbria-fornix transection. *J. Neurosci.*, 13: 4146–4156.

Nawa, H., Bessho, Y., Carnahan, J., Nakanishi, S.and Mizuno, K. (1993) Regulation of neuropeptide expression in cultured cerebral cortical neurons by brain-derived neurotrophic factor. *J. Neurochem.*, 60: 772–775.

Oppenheim, R.W., Qin-Wei, Y., Prevette, D. and Yan, Q. (1992) Brain-derived neurotrophic factor rescues developing avian motoneurons from cell death. *Nature (Lond.),* 360: 755–757.

Phillips, H.S., Hains, J.M., Armanini, M., Laramee, G.R., Johnson, S.A. and Winslow, J.W. (1991) BDNF mRNA is decreased in the hippocampus of individuals with Alzheimer's disease. *Neuron,* 7: 695–702.

Radeke, M.J., Misko, T.P., Hsu, C., Herzenberg, L.A. and Shooter, E.M. (1987) Gene transfer and molecular cloning of the rat nerve growth factor receptor. *Nature (Lond.),* 325: 593–897.

Rudge, J.S., Li, Y., Pasnikowski, E.M., Mattson, K., Pan, L., Yancopoulos, G.D., Wiegand, S.J., Lindsay, R.M. and Ip, N.Y. (1994) Neurotrophic factor receptors and their signal transduction capabilities in rat astrocytes. *Eur. J. Neurosci.*, 6: 693–705.

Schnell, L., Schneider, R., Kolbeck, R., Barde, Y.-A. and Schwab, M.E. (1994) Neurotrophin-3 enhances sprouting of corticospinal tract during development and after adult spinal cord lesion. *Nature (Lond.),* 367: 170–173.

Segal, R.A., Takahashi, H. and McKay, R.D.G. (1992) Changes in neurotrophin responsiveness during the development of cerebellar granule neurons. *Neuron,* 9: 1041–1052.

Sendtner, M., Kreutzberg, G.W.and Thoenen, H. (1990) Ciliary neurotrophic factor prevents the degeneration of motor neurons after axotomy. *Nature (Lond.)*, 345: 440–441.

Sendtner, M., Holtmann, B., Kolbeck, R., Thoenen, H. and Barde Y.-A. (1992a) Brain-derived neurotrophic factor prevents the death of motoneurons in newborn rats after nerve section. *Nature (Lond.),* 360: 757–758.

Sendtner, M., Schmalbruch, H., Stöckli, K.A., Carroll, P., Kreutzberg, G.W. and Thoenen, H. (1992b) Ciliary neurotrophic factor prevents degeneration of motor neurons in mouse mutant progressive motor neuronopathy. *Nature (Lond.),* 358: 502–504.

Siuciak, J.A., Altar, C.A., Wiegand, S.J. and Lindsay, R.M. (1994) Antinociceptive effect of brain-derived neurotrophic factor and neurotrophin-3. *Brain Res.*, 633: 326–330.

Spina, M.B., Squinto, S.P., Miller, J., Lindsay, R.M. and Hyman, C. (1992) Brain-derived neurotrophic factor protects dopamine neurons against 6-hydroxydopamine and *n*-methly-4-phenylpyridinium ion toxicity: involvement the glutathione system. *J. Neurochem.*, 59: 99106.

Thoenen, H. and Barde, Y.-A. (1980) Physiology of nerve growth factor. *Physiol. Rev.*, 60: 1284–1335.

Valenzuela, D.M., Maisonpierre, P.C., Glass, D.J., Rojas, E., Nuñez, L., Kong, Y., Gies, D.R., Stitt, T.N., Ip, N.Y. and Yancopoulos, G.D. (1993) Alternative forms of rat trkC with different functional capabilities. *Neuron,* 10: 1–20.

Ventimiglia, R., Mather, P. and Lindsay, R.M. (1993) Brain derived neurotrophic factor promotes survival and biochemical and morphological differentiation of striatal GABA neurons in vitro. *Soc. Neurosci. Abstr.*, 19: 666.

Wong, V., Arriaga, R., Ip, N.Y. and Lindsay, R.M. (1993) The neurotrophins BDNF, NT-3 and NT-4/5, but not NGF, up-regulate the cholinergic phenotype of developing motor neurons. *Eur. J. Neurosci.*, 5: 466–474.

Yan, Q., Elliott, J. and Snider, W.D. (1992) Brain-derived neurotrophic factor rescues spinal motor neurons from axotomy-induced cell death. *Nature (Lond.),* 360: 753–755.

F.J. Seil (Ed.)
Progress in Brain Research, Vol 103

CHAPTER 2

Axonal transport of the trkA high-affinity NGF receptor

Alonzo H. Ross[1], Mahesh B. Lachyankar[1], Dorota K. Poluha[1] and Rebekah Loy[2]

[1]*The Worcester Foundation for Experimental Biology, Shrewsbury, MA 01545 and* [2]*University of Rochester School of Medicine and Veterans Administration Medical Center, Batavia, NY, U.S.A.*

Introduction

Neurotrophic factors (NTFs) are required for growth, differentiation and survival of neurons and are particularly important during embryonic development of the nervous system (Purves and Lichtman, 1985). NTFs are produced in limited amounts by target tissues and are taken up by responsive neurons at the synapses. As a normal part of development, the neurons which do not make proper connections do not receive sufficient NTFs and die. In this way, nature selects for only those neurons which form functional synapses with correct targets. In adults, NTFs maintain normal neurophysiological function and survival of mature neurons. Following injury, expression of NTFs and NTF receptors is upregulated (Taniuchi et al., 1986; Sobue et al., 1988; Ernfors et al., 1989; Frisén et al., 1992; Merlio et al., 1993).

Nerve growth factor (NGF) is the best characterized NTF. NGF is a 26,000-Da polypeptide which modulates differentiation of rat pheochromocytoma PC12 cells to sympathetic neuron-like cells (Greene and Tischler, 1976) and can act as a chemoattractant (Gunderson and Barrett, 1980). NGF is a survival factor for sympathetic and sensory neurons (Johnson et al., 1986). NGF also is thought to be a trophic factor for CNS neurons of the basal forebrain (Gnahn et al., 1983; Hartikka and Hefti, 1986) and the striatum (Mobley et al., 1985; Hartikka and Hefti, 1986). In addition to its role as a trophic factor, NGF may regulate the electrophysiological properties of septal neurons (Palmer et al., 1993).

NGF receptors

All of the actions of NGF are thought to be mediated by two cell surface receptors (Chao, 1992; Barbacid, 1993). The low-affinity NGF receptor (NGFR) is a 75,000-Da protein with a cysteine-rich extracellular domain, a single transmembrane domain and a 155-amino acid cytoplasmic domain. The second NGF receptor is trkA, a 140,000-Da transmembrane protein with an intracellular tyrosine-specific kinase domain. Binding of NGF activates the trkA kinase and initiates the signal transduction cascade (Kaplan et al., 1991; Klein et al., 1991)

The functional relation between these two receptors is complex and controversial (Chao, 1992; Barbacid, 1993). TrkA can mediate many responses in the absence of the low-affinity NGFR (Birren et al., 1992; Barbacid, 1993), but the low-affinity NGFR also must play an important role, since transgenic mice lacking low-affinity NGFR have neuronal deficits, particularly in the sensory nervous system (Lee et al., 1992). Current data suggest that the low-affinity NGFR may play a dual role in signal transduction. First, the low-affinity NGFR may form a complex with trkA and, thereby, increase the affinity of NGF binding (Hempstead et al., 1991). Second, the low-affinity NGFR also may initiate signal transduction (Yan et al., 1991). The low-affinity NGFR can induce apoptosis of neural cell lines (Rabizadeh et al., 1993) and can modulate the activity of adenyl cyclase (Knipper et al., 1993a,b). The mechanism of signal transduction is not clear, but the low-affinity NGFR does have a mastoparan-like domain which might interact with G proteins (Feinstein and Larhammer, 1990). In addition, a protein kinase N (PKN)-like kinase and extracellular signal regulated kinases are associated with the low-affinity NGFR (Volonte et al., 1993a,b). Activation of the associated kinases seems to require trkA, suggesting a cross talk between trkA and the low-affinity NGFR.

NGF and retrograde transport

While some effects of NGF are elicited directly at nerve terminals, the longer-term responses to NGF require retrograde transport of a signaling molecule to the cell body (Thoenen and Barde, 1980; Hendry, 1993). Because of the extreme length of the axon, special mechanisms have developed for the delivery of materials from the cell body to the synapse (anterograde transport) and from the synapse to the cell body (retrograde transport). For transport in both directions, proteins are packaged into vesicles which are transported by molecular motors along the microtubules (Jahn and Sudhof, 1993). Blockage of retrograde transport by ligation of the axon or with drugs which disrupt microtubules results in death of the neuron, but such isolated neurons can be rescued by addition of NGF directly to the cell bodies (Purves, 1976).

What is the neurotrophic signal which is retrogradely transported to the cell body and allows survival of the neuron? NGF is retrogradely transported to the cell body but does not appear to be the signal. NGF microinjected into the cytoplasm or nucleus does not induce a biological response, and microinjection of anti-NGF antibodies into the nucleus does not block the response to exogenous NGF (Heumann et al., 1981; Seeley et al., 1983). The low-affinity NGFR also is transported to the cell body (Johnson et al., 1987) but does not appear to allow neuronal survival in the absence of trkA. Hence, we have to consider other candidates for the neurotrophic signal, such as trkA.

Preparation and characterization of anti-trkA antibodies

Anti-trkA antibodies were prepared using synthetic peptides. Sequences for immunization were chosen based on the antigenicity index (Jameson and Wolf, 1988) as calculated with the PEPTIDESTRUCTURE program in the Genetics Computer Group package. As additional criteria, sequences were chosen which lack glycosylation sites and which are distinct from the trkB and trkC sequences (Fig. 1). Peptides were coupled to bovine serum albumin (BSA) and used to immunize and boost rabbits. The resulting sera reacted in ELISA with peptides coupled to ovalbumin, displaying titers of 1:500 to 1:1000. The sera were absorbed on a BSA-Sepharose column and passed over a peptide-ovalbumin-Sepharose column. Specific antibody was eluted with 4.5 M $MgCl_2$ and then immediately diluted and dialyzed. As judged by ELISA, this is a gentle procedure with no loss of antibody activity during purification and elution. The anti-peptide 679 antibody and the anti-peptide 683 antibody are referred to as IA679 and IA683. Both of these antibodies reacted with trkA but not with trkB (summarized in Table I).

IA679 and IA683 were used to stain sections of adult rat brain. Immunostaining with IA683 was more intense than that with IA679. A number of brain regions known by in situ hybridization to express trkA were immunostained with IA683 (Fig. 2). Cell bodies in the diagonal band and the

```
peptide 679: human TrkA amino acids 160-176
rat TrkA       Q R W E Q E D L C G V Y T Q K L Q
human TrkA     Q R W E E E G L G G V P E Q K L Q
mouse TrkB     K T L Q E - T K S S P D T Q D L Y
porcine TrkC   Q L W Q E Q G E A K L N S Q S L Y

peptide 683: human TrkA amino acids 379-394
rat TrkA       M D N P - - - F E F N P E D P - - - - - - - - - - - - - I P V S
human TrkA     M D N P - - - F E F N P E D P - - - - - - - - - - - - - I P D T
mouse TrkB     M E R P G V D Y E T N P N Y P E V L Y E D W T T P T D L G D T
porcine TrkC   L K E P - - - - - - - - - - F P E S T - D N F V S F Y E V S P T
```

Fig. 1. Peptide 679 consists of amino acids 160–176, and peptide 683 consists of amino acids 379–394, both from human trkA. These regions are quite homologous for rat and human trkA, but only slightly resemble the corresponding trkB and trkC sequences. The 679 peptide matches the trkB sequence at only three of 17 amino acids and matches the trkC sequence at five amino acids. The 683 peptide matches the trkB sequence at nine of 16 amino acids and matches the trkC sequence at three amino acids. TrkB and trkC also include additional sequence not present in trkA. Gaps to keep the sequences in frame are shown as dashes.

caudate/putamen were positive for trkA. In addition, cerebellar Purkinje cells were immunostained with both IA683 (Fig. 2) and the weaker antibody IA679 (not shown). Other studies have suggested that Purkinje cells are responsive to NGF. NGF is present in several Purkinje cell target regions (Nishio et al., 1992), and Purkinje cells retrogradely transport ^{125}I-NGF (Aloe and Vigneti, 1992). Anti-NGF antibodies alter Purkinje cell morphogenesis (Legrand and Clos, 1991), and for cultured Purkinje cells, NGF enhances neurite outgrowth, cell survival and morphological differentiation (Cohen-Cory et al., 1991; Aloe and Vigneti, 1992). The receptors mediating these responses to NGF are not clearly identified. Adult Purkinje cells express the low-affinity NGF receptor (Koh et al., 1989; Pioro and Cuello, 1990). Although Purkinje cells show high-affinity binding of ^{125}I-NGF (Altar et al., 1991), the mRNA for trkA has not been detected by in situ hybridization. Given the biological and immunohistochemical data, it seems likely that the sensitivity of in situ hybridization is not sufficient to detect the trkA message in Purkinje cells.

TABLE I

Properties of anti-trkA antibodies. The reactivities with trkA and trkB were determined by Western blotting. IA679 was used at a dilution of 1:100 and IA683 was used at a dilution of 1:20. For immunocytochemistry, the antibodies were used at 1:50 or 1:200 dilution.

Antibody	Reactivity with trkA	Reactivity with trkB	Efficacy for immunocytochemistry
IA679	+ +	−	+
IA683	+ +	−	+ +

Axonal transport of trkA

The anti-trkA antibodies were used to test for axonal transport of trkA. The fimbria-fornix was bilaterally transected at the level at which it joins the rostral pole of the hippocampus. At 8–12 h following transection, the animals were sacrificed and used for immunostaining for trkA. Cut fibers on both the distal and proximal sides of the transection stained with IA679, IA683 and 1088, a pan trk antibody (Fig. 3). On the distal side (retrograde transport), fibers were relatively short and varicose, while on the proximal side (anterograde transport) the fibers were more numerous, less varicose and stained for longer distances. In no case was trkA immunoreactivity detected in cellular elements adjacent to the transection site. Hence, there seems no possibility that the trkA immunoreactivity results from glial cells. The

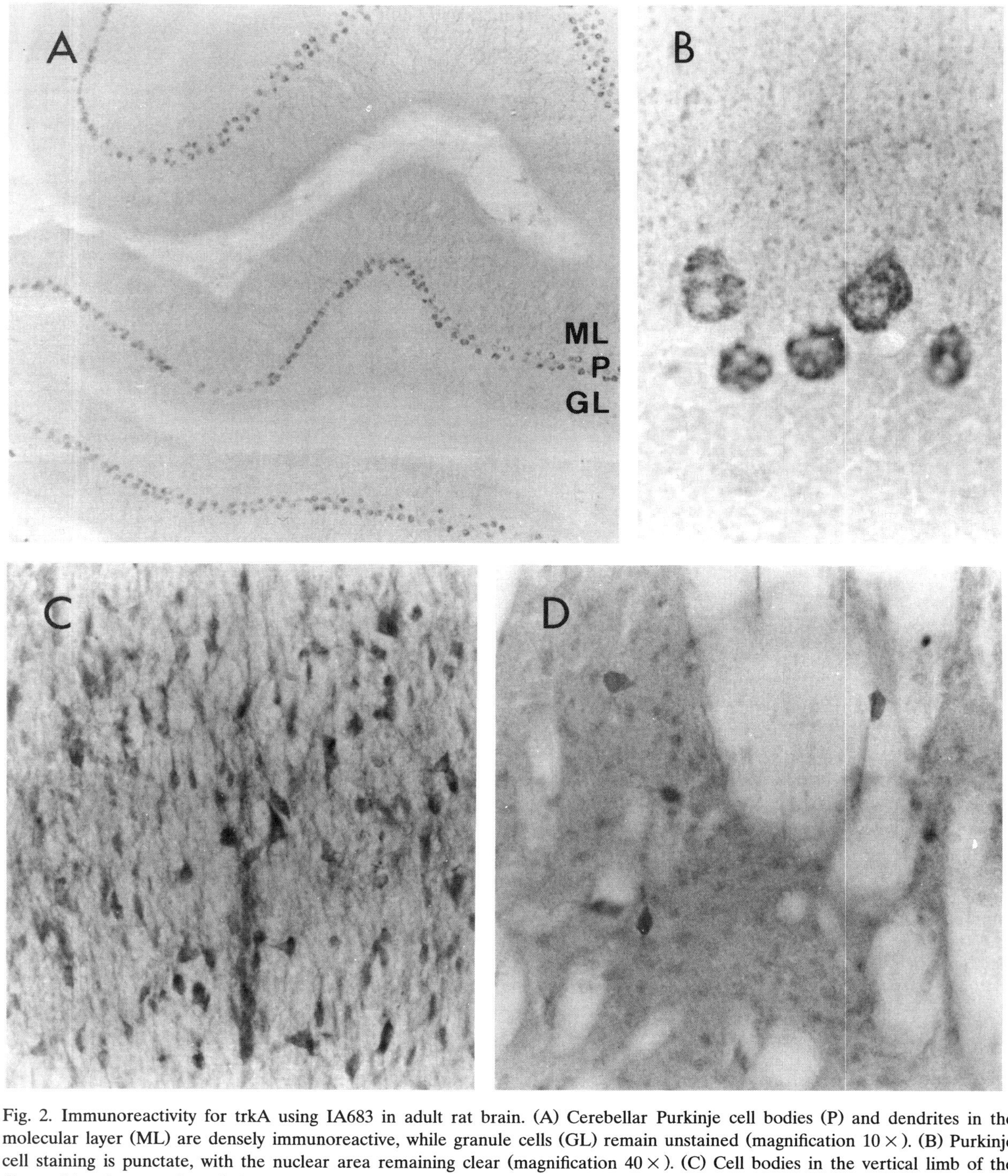

Fig. 2. Immunoreactivity for trkA using IA683 in adult rat brain. (A) Cerebellar Purkinje cell bodies (P) and dendrites in the molecular layer (ML) are densely immunoreactive, while granule cells (GL) remain unstained (magnification 10 ×). (B) Purkinje cell staining is punctate, with the nuclear area remaining clear (magnification 40 ×). (C) Cell bodies in the vertical limb of the diagonal band are moderately immunoreactive for trkA. The staining is most dense in clusters or as punctate grains around nuclei (magnification 20 ×). (D) Large cell bodies within the caudate/putamen are moderately immunoreactive for trkA (magnification 20 ×).

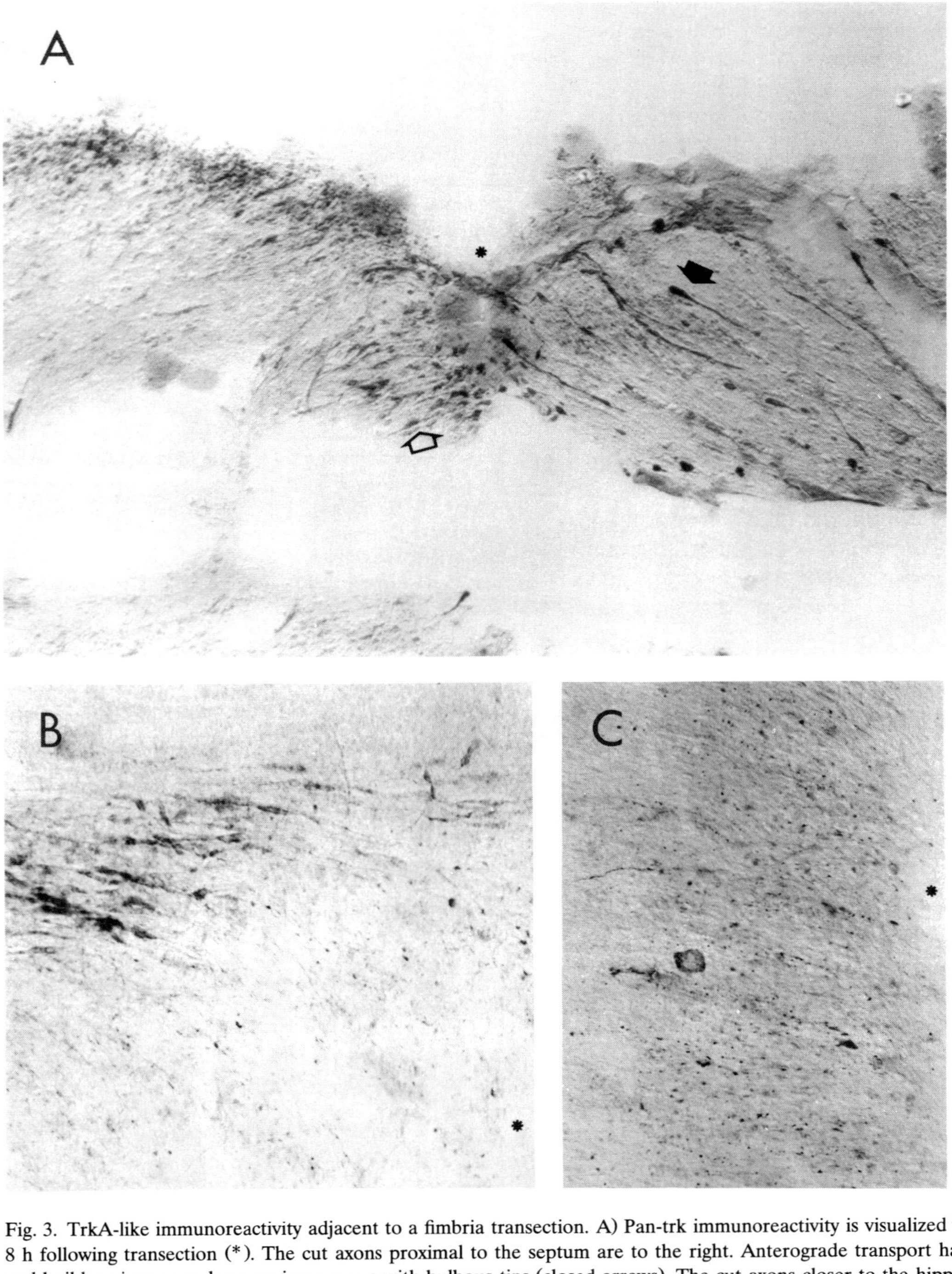

Fig. 3. TrkA-like immunoreactivity adjacent to a fimbria transection. A) Pan-trk immunoreactivity is visualized with antibody 1088, 8 h following transection (*). The cut axons proximal to the septum are to the right. Anterograde transport has been interrupted and build-up is seen as long, varicose axons with bulbous tips (closed arrows). The cut axons closer to the hippocampus are to the left; these have immunoreactive varicosities suggestive of build-up of retrogradely transported trkA-like material (open arrows)(magnification 20 ×). (B) and (C) Immunoreactivity for trkA using IA683. Both micrographs show immunoreactive fibers on the distal side of transections (*), with varicosities characteristic of retrograde transport (magnification 20 ×).

build-up of trkA immunoreactivity indicates that trkA is transported in both the retrograde and anterograde directions.

Implications of these studies

In these recent studies, we discovered that trkA is retrogradely transported along axons in the fimbria/fornix region of the brain. We hypothesize that an NGF-trkA complex (or NGF-trkA-low-affinity NGFR complex) is transported to the cell body and that the activated trkA kinase is the signal for survival of the neuron.

In proposing that the trkA kinase remains activated during retrograde transport, one must consider the mechanisms by which trkA might be inactivated. For several receptors, activation of the tyrosine kinase results in activation of other kinases which phosphorylate the receptor and, thereby, inactivate the receptor kinase domain (Friedman et al., 1984). However, trkA does not appear to undergo this type of feedback regulation (Heasley and Johnson, 1992; Qiu and Green, 1992). Another mechanism of inactivation is simple dissociation of ligand from the receptor. However, in the proposed model, NGF is trapped in the vesicle and cannot diffuse away from the receptor. Finally, some internal vesicles are acidic, triggering the dissociation of ligand from internalized receptors. Although the pH of vesicles undergoing retrograde transport has not been measured, it is likely that they resemble early endosomes (Jahn and Sudhof, 1993) which are only mildly acidic and would not dissociate NGF from its receptor (Vale and Shooter, 1985). Hence, none of the obvious mechanisms for inactivation appear to be applicable to trkA, and this model will be tested in further experiments.

References

Aloe, L. and Vigneti, E. (1992) In vivo and in vitro NGF studies on developing cerebellar cells. *NeuroReport,* 3: 279–282.

Altar, C.A., Burton, L.E., Bennett, G.L. and Dugich-Djordjevic, M. (1991) Recombinant human nerve growth factor is biologically active and labels novel high-affinity binding sites in rat brain. *Proc. Natl. Acad. Sci. USA*, 88: 281–285.

Barbacid, M. (1993) Nerve growth factor: a tale of two receptors. *Oncogene,* 8: 2033–2042.

Birren, S.J., Verdi, J.M. and Anderson, D.J. (1992) Membrane depolarization induces $p140^{trk}$ and NGF responsiveness, but not $p75^{LNGFR}$ in MAH cells. *Science,* 257: 395–397.

Chao, M.V. (1992) Neurotrophin receptors: a window into neuronal differentiation. *Cell,* 9: 583-593.

Cohen-Cory, S., Dreyfus, C. F. and Black, I. B. (1991) NGF and excitatory neurotransmitters regulate survival and morphogenesis of cultured cerebellar Purkinje cells. *J. Neurosci.,* 11: 462–471.

Ernfors, P., Henschen, A., Olson, L. and Persson, H. (1989) Expression of nerve growth factor receptor mRNA is developmentally regulated and increased after axotomy in rat spinal cord motoneurons. *Neuron,* 2: 1605–1613.

Feinstein, D.L. and Larhammer, D. (1990) Identification of a conserved protein motif in a group of growth factor receptors. *FEBS Lett.*, 272: 7-11.

Friedman, B., Frackelton, A.R., Ross, A.H., Connors, J.M., Fujiki, H., Sugimura, T. and Rosner, M.R. (1984) Tumor promoters block tyrosine-specific phophorylation of the epidermal growth factor receptor. *Proc. Natl. Acad. Sci. USA,* 81: 3034–3038.

Frisén, J., Verge, V. M. K., Cullheim, S., Persson, H., Fried, K., Middlemas, D.S., Hunter, T., Hökfelt, T. and Risling, M. (1992) Increased levels of trkB mRNA and trkB protein-like immunoreactivity in the injured rat and cat spinal cord. *Proc. Natl. Acad. Sci. USA,* 89: 11282–11286.

Gnahn, H., Hefti, F., Heumann, R., Schwab, M. and Thoenen, H. (1983) NGF-mediated increase of choline acetyltransferase (ChAT) in the neonatal forebrain: evidence for a physiological role of NGF in the brain? *Dev. Brain Res.,* 9: 45–52.

Greene, L.A. and Tischler, A.S. (1976) Establishment of a noradrenergic clonal line of rat adrenal pheochromocytoma cells which respond to nerve growth factor. *Proc. Natl. Acad. Sci. USA,* 73: 2424–2428.

Gunderson, R.W. and Barrett, J.N. (1980) Characterization of the turning response of dorsal root neurites toward nerve growth factor. *J. Cell Biol.,* 87: 546–554.

Hartikka, J. and Hefti, F. (1986) Comparison of nerve growth factor's effects on development of septum, striatum, and nucleus basalis cholinergic neurons in vitro. *J. Neurosci. Res.*, 21: 352–364.

Heasley, L.E. and Johnson, G.L. (1992) The beta-PDGF receptor induces neuronal differentiation of PC12 cells. *Mol. Biol. Cell,* 3: 545-553.

Hempstead, B.L., Martin-Zanca, D., Kaplan, D.R., Parada, L.F. and Chao, M.V. (1991) High-affinity NGF binding requires coexpression of the *trk* proto-oncogene and the low-affinity NGF receptor. *Nature (Lond.),* 350: 678–683.

Hendry, I. A. (1993) Retrograde factors in peripheral nerves. *Pharmacol. Ther.*, 56: 265–285.

Heumann, R., Schwab, M. and Thoenen, H. (1981) A second

messenger required for nerve growth factor biological activity? *Nature (Lond.),* 292: 838–840.

Jahn, R. and Sudhof, T.C. (1993) Synaptic vesicle traffic: rush hour in the nerve terminal. *J. Neurochem.*, 61: 12–21.

Jameson, B.A. and Wolf, H. (1988) The antigenic index: a novel algorithm for predicting antigenic determinants. *CABIOS,* 4: 181–186.

Johnson, E.M., Rich, K.M. and Yip, H.K. (1986) The role of NGF in sensory neurons in vivo. *Trends Neurosci.*, 9: 33–37.

Johnson, E.M., Taniuchi, M., Clark, H.B., Springer, J.E., Koh, S., Tayrien, M.W. and Loy, R. (1987) Demonstration of the retrograde transport of nerve growth factor receptor in the peripheral and central nervous system. *J. Neurosci.,* 7: 923–929.

Kaplan, D.R., Hempstead, B.L., Martin-Zanca, D., Chao, M. V. and Parada, L.F. (1991) The *trk* proto-oncogene product: a signal transducing receptor for nerve growth factor. *Science,* 252: 554-558.

Klein, R., Jing, S., Nanduri, V., O'Rourke, E. and Barbacid, M. (1991) The *trk* proto-oncogene encodes a receptor for nerve growth factor. *Cell,* 65: 189–197.

Knipper, M., Beck, A., Rylett, J. and Breer, H. (1993a) Neurotrophin induced cAMP and IP3 responses in PC12 cells. *FEBS Lett.*, 324: 147–152.

Knipper, M., Beck, A., Rylett, J. and Breer, H. (1993b) Neurotrophin induced second messenger responses in rat brain synaptosomes. *NeuroReport,* 4: 483486.

Koh, S., Oyler, G.A. and Higgins, G.A. (1989) Localization of nerve growth factor receptor messenger RNA and protein in the adult rat brain. *Exp. Neurol.,* 106: 209–221.

Lee, K.-F., Li, E., Huber, J., Landis, S.C., Sharpe, A.H., Chao, M.V. and Jaenisch, R. (1992) Targeted mutation of the gene encoding the low affinity NGF receptor p75 leads to deficits in the peripheral sensory nervous system. *Cell,* 69: 737–749.

Legrand, C. and Clos, J. (1991) Biochemical, immunocytochemical and morphological evidence for an interaction between thyroid hormone and nerve growth factor in the developing cerebellum of normal and hypothyroid rats. *Dev. Neurosci.*, 13: 382–396.

Merlio, J.-P., Ernfors, P., Kokaia, Z., Middlemas, D. S., Bengzon, J., Kokaia, M., Smith, M.-L., Siesjo, B.K., Hunter, T., Lindvall, O. and Persson, H. (1993) Increased production of the trkB protein tyrosine kinase receptor after brain insults. *Neuron,* 10: 151–164.

Mobley, W.C., Rutkowski, J.L., Tennekoon, G.I., Buchanan, K. and Johnston, M. V. (1985) Choline acetyltransferase activity in striatum of neonatal rats increased by nerve growth factor. *Science,* 229: 284–287.

Nishio, T., Akiguch, I. and Furukawa, S. (1992) Detailed distribution of nerve growth factor in rat brain determined by a highly sensitive enzyme immunoassay. *Exp. Neurol.*, 116: 76–84.

Palmer, M.R., Eriksdotter-Nilsson, M., Henschen, A., Ebendal, T. and Olson, L. (1993) Nerve growth factor-induced excitation of selected neurons in the brain which is blocked by a low- affinity receptor antibody. *Exp. Brain Res.,* 93: 226–230.

Pioro, E.P. and Cuello, A.C. (1990) Distribution of nerve growth factor receptor-like immunoreactivity in the adult rat central nervous system. *Neuroscience,* 34: 89–110.

Purves, D. (1976) Functional and structural changes in mammalian sympathetic neurons following colchicine applications to post-ganglionic nerves. *J. Physiol.*, 259: 159–175.

Purves, D. and Lichtman, J.W. (1985) *Principles of Neural Development*, Sinauer Associates, Sunderland, MA.

Qiu, M.-S. and Green, S.H. (1992) PC12 cell neuronal differentiation is associated with prolonged $p21^{ras}$ activity and consequent prolonged ERK activity. *Neuron,* 9: 705–717.

Rabizadeh, S., Oh, J., Zhong, L., Yang, J., Bitler, C. M., Butcher, L. L. and Bredesen, D. E. (1993) Induction of apoptosis by the low-affinity NGF receptor. *Science,* 261: 345–348.

Seeley, P.J., Keith, C.H., Shelanski, M.L. and Greene, L.A. (1983) Pressure microinjection of nerve growth factor and anti-nerve growth factor into the nucleus and cytoplasm: lack of effects on neurite outgrowth from pheochromocytoma cells. *J. Neurosci.,* 3: 1488–1494.

Sobue, G., Yasuda, T., Mitsuma, T., Ross, A. H. and Pleasure, D. (1988) Expression of nerve growth factor receptor in human peripheral neuropathies. *Ann. Neurol.*, 24: 64–72.

Taniuchi, M., Clark, H. B. and Johnson, E. M. (1986) Induction of nerve growth factor receptor in Schwann cells after axotomy. *Proc. Natl. Acad. Sci. USA,* 83: 4094–4098.

Thoenen, H. and Barde, Y.-A. (1980) Physiology of nerve growth factor. *Physiol. Rev.*, 60: 1284–1335.

Vale, R.D. and Shooter, E.M. (1985) Assaying binding of nerve growth factor to cell surface receptors. *Methods Enzymol.,* 109: 21–39.

Volonte, C., Angelastro, J.M. and Greene, L.A. (1993a) Association of protein kinases ERK1 and ERK2 with p75 nerve growth factor receptors. *J. Biol. Chem.*, 268: 21410–21415.

Volonte, C., Ross, A.H. and Greene, L.A. (1993b) Association of a purine-analog-sensitive protein kinase activity with p75 NGF receptors. *Mol. Biol. Cell,* 4: 71–78.

Yan, H., Schlessinger, J. and Chao, M.V. (1991) Chimeric NGF-EGF receptors define domains responsible for neuronal differentiation. *Science,* 252: 561–563.

F.J. Seil (Ed.)
Progress in Brain Research, Vol 103

CHAPTER 3

Nerve growth factor and neuronal gene expression

Freda D. Miller

Center for Neuronal Survival, Department of Neurology and Neurosurgery, Montreal Neurological Institute, McGill University, Montreal, PQ, Canada H3A 2B4

Introduction

Interactions between a developing peripheral neuron and its target organ are believed to partially determine the phenotype of that neuron and to play an important role in neuronal competition and cell death. Nerve growth factor (NGF) is a neurotrophic factor involved in the survival and differentiation of developing sympathetic and neural crest-derived sensory neurons. NGF given systemically promotes growth of nerve terminals and dendritic arborization of developing sympathetic neurons (Levi-Montalcini and Booker, 1960a; Snider, 1988) and affects neurotransmitter phenotype in both developing sensory and sympathetic neurons (Thoenen et al., 1971; Kessler and Black, 1980). Conversely, antibodies to NGF lead to the death of embryonic sensory neurons (Johnson et al., 1980; Carroll et al., 1992) and neonatal sympathetic neurons (Levi-Montalcini and Booker, 1960b; Angeletti et al., 1971), and inhibit the sprouting of both sensory (Diamond et al., 1987, 1992) and sympathetic (Gloster and Diamond, 1992) neurons, although cross-reactivity with other members of the neurotrophin family could have contributed to the observed effects (Acheson et al., 1991). Locally increased NGF also leads to spatially regulated growth of developing sympathetic neurons both in vivo (Edwards et al., 1989) and in culture (Campenot, 1982).

Neuronal responses to NGF are believed to be mediated by a high-affinity membrane-bound NGF receptor (Green et al., 1986). The molecular components of this high-affinity receptor are controversial, but they include trkA, a tyrosine kinase protooncogene that activates cellular signalling events upon NGF binding (Cordon-Cardo et al., 1991; Kaplan et al., 1991a, b; Klein et al., 1991; Jing et al., 1992) and may or may not include the p75 NGF receptor (Johnson et al., 1986; Radeke et al., 1987; Berg et al., 1991; Hempstead et al., 1991; Ibanez et al., 1992; Battleman et al., 1993). This latter receptor, which, in addition to NGF, binds the other members of the neurotrophin family (Rodriguez-Tebar et al., 1990, 1992), is a transmembrane glycoprotein that also exists in an extracellular, truncated form generated by post-translational cleavage (DiStefano and Johnson, 1988; Barker et al., 1991). Although the functional role of the p75 NGF receptor remains undefined, recent studies disrupting this gene in transgenic mice indicate that it plays an important physiological role (Lee et al., 1992).

This review summarizes our studies examining the mechanisms whereby NGF regulates gene expression in developing and mature sympathetic neurons. These studies demonstrate that NGF specifically up-regulates the expression of a subset of genes important to the growth and differentiation of neonatal sympathetic neurons, including those encoding the p75 NGF receptor, Tα1 α-tubulin, and tyrosine hydroxylase. These increases are independent of neuronal survival, and occur in a graded fashion at concentrations of NGF that preclude simple models based upon activation of the trkA NGF receptor alone. Furthermore, the magnitude of the increases in gene expression are a function of the spatial location of the increased NGF, with NGF exposure on distal axons eliciting less of an increase than NGF exposure on cell bodies. Our studies also indicate that such NGF-induced changes in gene expression are not limited to developing neurons; increased NGF derived from the terminals of mature sympathetic neurons in vivo distally increases synthesis of the p75 NGF receptor relative to the trkA receptor, leading to an increased density of p75 NGF receptors on terminal neurites.

Together, our data support a model wherein the availability of target-derived NGF distally regulates the expression of a subset of genes important to neuronal growth and differentiation in both the developing and mature animal, providing a cellular mechanism for coupling neuronal synthesis of axonal proteins to alterations in size of the innervated target territory. Furthermore, we postulate that the p75 NGF receptor modulates the function of the trkA receptor in sympathetic neurons and that the NGF-induced upregulation of p75 NGF receptor synthesis that we have described provides a potential molecular substrate for a modulatory feedback loop. More specifically, an increased ratio of membrane-bound p75 to trkA NGF receptors may serve to attenuate the function of the trkA tyrosine kinase receptor by sequestering NGF from a productive high-affinity complex, thereby increasing the range of effective NGF concentrations to which a neuron could respond. Such a modulatory feedback loop might play a role not only during the period of neuronal competition and cell death, but may also effectively modify neuronal responsiveness to NGF itself as a function of the amount of available target tissue and/or trophic support.

Concentration-dependent regulation of neuronal gene expression by NGF

Administration of NGF to neonates has dramatic effects on sympathetic neurons, causing increased terminal sprouting (Levi-Montalcini and Bockel, 1960a), increased dendritic arborization (Snider, 1988), and increased activity of enzymes involved in catecholamine biosynthesis (Thoenen et al., 1971). To determine whether NGF similarly regulated the expression of proteins that play a role in neuronal differentiation, we injected neonatal animals with NGF from postnatal days 2 to 11, isolated RNA from the superior cervical ganglia (SCG) at postnatal day 12, and examined the expression of p75 NGF receptor (Fig. 1) and Tα1 α-tubulin (Fig. 2) mRNAs, the latter of which is

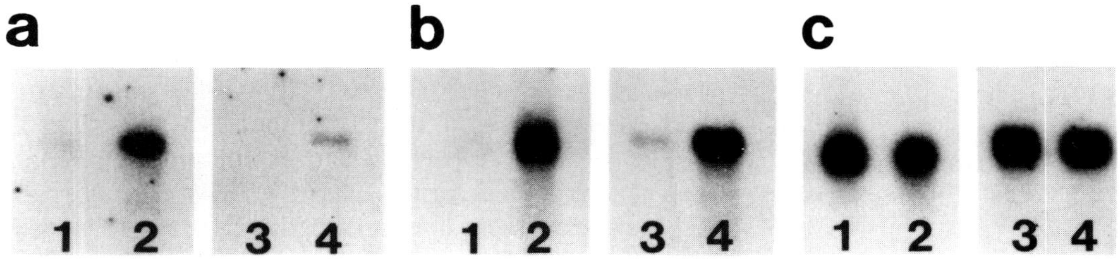

Fig. 1. Expression of the p75 NGF receptor, tyrosine hydroxylase, and neuropeptide Y mRNAs in the postnatal day 1 SCG with and without NGF treatment. Northern blot analysis of (a) p75 NGF receptor, (b) tyrosine hydroxylase, and (c) neuropeptide Y mRNAs in equal amounts of total RNA from the SCG of an animal treated with 10 mg/kg NGF (lane 2) and its control littermate (lane 1), and equal amounts of total RNA from an animal treated with 5 mg/kg NGF (lane 4) and its control littermate (lane 3). Note that lanes 1 and 2 are not directly comparable with lanes 3 and 4 in the amount of RNA analysed, the specific activity of the probe, or in the exposure time (from Miller et al., 1991).

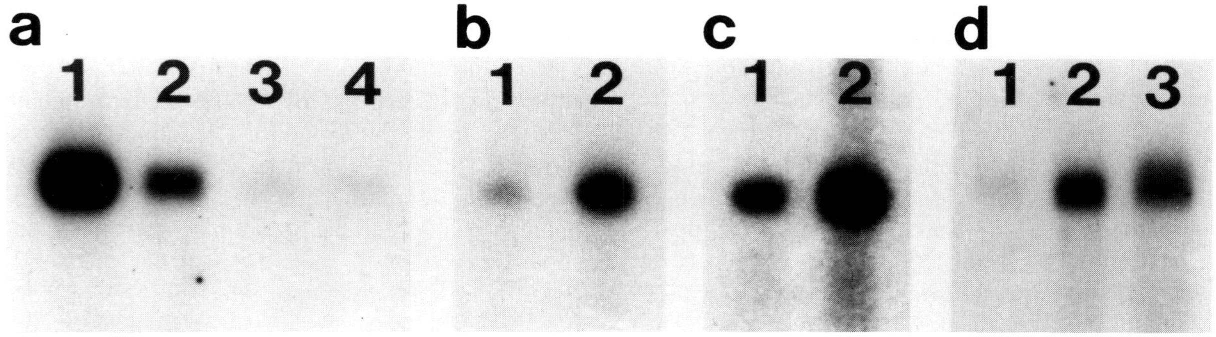

Fig. 2. Northern blot analysis of Tα1 α-tubulin mRNA in the superior cervical ganglion (a) during postnatal development, and (b–d) following systemic NGF treatment for 10 days. (a) Total cytoplasmic RNA from the SCG of developing rats at (1) postnatal day 5, (2) postnatal day 10, (3) postnatal day 30, and (4) postnatal day 45. (b and c) Total cytoplasmic RNA from the SCG of two different postnatal day 12 rats that were treated with NGF from postnatal days 2-11 (lane 2 in each of b and c) versus their age-matched control litter-mates (lane 1 in each of b and c). (d) Equal amounts of total cytoplasmic RNA from the SCG of (1) a control postnatal day 12 animal, (2) a NGF-treated postnatal day 12 animal, and (3) a control postnatal day 5 animal (from Mathew and Miller, 1990).

regulated as a function of neuronal growth (Fig. 2a; Miller et al., 1987, 1989). Northern blot analysis revealed that levels of p75 NGF receptor mRNA increased 5–10-fold relative to total RNA synthesis in NGF-treated versus control SCG (Fig. 1a; Miller et al., 1991), while levels of Tα1 α-tubulin mRNA increased at least 10-fold (Fig. 2b, c; Mathew and Miller, 1990). To determine whether these NGF-induced increases were specific to a subset of neuronal genes, we also examined the expression of tyrosine hydroxylase and neuropeptide Y mRNAs, both of which are associated with the transmitter phenotype of sympathetic neurons. Northern blot analysis demonstrated that tyrosine hydroxylase (Fig. 1b) mRNA increased at least 10-fold in the SCG, while neuropeptide Y mRNA levels remained constant (Fig. 1c). Further analysis indicated that, in the case of both p75 NGF receptor and tyrosine hydroxylase mRNAs, NGF treatment dramatically increased levels over normal neonatal levels (Miller et al., 1991), whereas NGF prevented a developmentally programmed decrease in Tα1 α-tubulin mRNA (Fig. 2d). Thus, systemic NGF directly or indirectly regulated the developmental expression of a number of genes associated with neuronal differentiation. Support for the hypothesis that these increases are at least partially transcriptional derives from data demonstrating that transcription of all three of these genes is increased by NGF in PC12 cells (Gizang-Ginsberg and Ziff, 1990; Miller et al., 1991; J. Toma and F. Miller, unpublished data).

On the basis of these data, we hypothesized that initial exposure of a developing sympathetic neuron to target-derived NGF would lead to increased p75 NGF receptor and tyrosine hydroxylase mRNAs, and maintain elevated levels of Tα1 α-tubulin mRNA. The increased mRNA levels could provide protein essential for expansion of the terminal arbor, and/or for neuronal maturation. Such a graded induction of neuronal gene expression by target-derived NGF could provide a mechanism for coupling neuronal synthesis of axonal proteins to increases in size of innervated target territory. Furthermore, increased levels of either membrane-bound p75 NGF receptor or truncated p75 NGF receptor secreted into the terminal microenvironment in response to initial target contact could provide a 'sink' for NGF, which might allow early arriving neurons to compete more effectively than later arriving neurons for limiting concentrations of target-derived NGF.

This hypothesis predicts that NGF regulates

gene expression in sympathetic neurons in a concentration-dependent fashion, independent of its effects upon neuronal survival. To test this prediction, we examined the effects of different NGF concentrations on gene expression in pure cultures of neonatal sympathetic neurons (Ma et al., 1992). These studies demonstrated that when sympathetic neurons were cultured in the presence of 10–200 ng/ml NGF for 5 days, levels of p75 NGF receptor, tyrosine hydroxylase, and Tα1 α-tubulin mRNAs all increased in a graded fashion over the entire concentration range, with the steepest increase occurring between 10 and 50 ng/ml. To ensure that the observed effects were due to effects on gene expression, and not on neuronal survival, neurons were maintained for 5 days in 10 ng/ml NGF and, in some dishes, the NGF concentration was subsequently raised to 200 ng/ml. Northern blot analysis (Fig. 3; Ma et al., 1992) revealed that levels of both p75 NGF receptor (Fig. 3a) and tyrosine hydroxylase (Fig. 3c) mRNAs were increased approximately 4-fold, while Tα1 α-tubulin mRNA (Fig. 3b) levels increased only 2-fold in response to increased NGF. Thus, independent of survival effects, different concentrations of NGF differentially regulated the development of sympathetic neurons in culture. Although the molecular mechanisms underlying these graded changes remain undefined, it is unlikely that activation of the trkA tyrosine kinase receptor alone is sufficient to explain these observations, since in PC12 cells tyrosine phosphorylation of trkA by NGF is maximal at 1–10 ng/ml (Kaplan et al., 1991b), whereas the concentration-dependent effects described here occurred from 10 to 200 ng/ml.

NGF derived from neuronal terminals selectively upregulates the ratio of p75 to trkA NGF receptors

These studies indicated that alterations in NGF concentration regulated synthesis of the p75 NGF receptor in developing sympathetic neurons both in vivo and in culture. Furthermore, as described above, neonatal sympathetic neurons respond to NGF over a broader concentration range than predicted by the affinity of the trkA receptor alone (Chun and Patterson, 1977a, b; Ma et al., 1992). On the basis of these observations, we hypothesized that the p75 NGF receptor might function in an NGF-induced feedback loop to modulate the function of the trkA tyrosine kinase receptor by regulating the amount of NGF available to trkA, thereby broadening the NGF response range of sympathetic neurons. This hypothesis predicts that target-derived NGF differentially regulates the synthesis of its two characterized receptors, leading to an increased ratio of p75 to trkA receptors on terminal neurites. To directly test this prediction, we developed a model system that allowed us to deliver exogenous NGF to the terminals of intact, mature sympathetic neurons in vivo, and to subsequently examine both cell body gene expression and local sprouting (Miller et al., 1994). To perform these studies, we turned to the SCG, which has two major postganglionic nerve branches that innervate specific target organs, one of which is the iris (Lichtman et al., 1979). This system allowed us to differentially label two target-specific populations of neurons in the same ganglion and to administer exogenous NGF to the terminals of one of these populations. Sympathetic neurons that project via the internal carotid nerve to the eye were retrogradely labeled with Fast Blue (eye neurons), while those neurons of the same ganglion that project via the external carotid nerve to the pinna of the ear were retrogradely labeled with Fluoro-Gold (ear neurons) (see Mathew and Miller, 1993). Five to seven days later, NGF was injected daily into the anterior chamber of one eye, thereby exposing the terminals of the eye neurons (which project unilaterally) to an increased local concentration of trophic factor. As a control for any systemic effects of the locally administered NGF, and for any injury due to the daily injection protocol, phosphate buffered saline (PBS) or cytochrome C was injected daily into the other eye of the same animal. The effectiveness of this experimental paradigm was evidenced by the fact that neuronal hypertrophy was only observed in the NGF-treated eye neurons, and was not

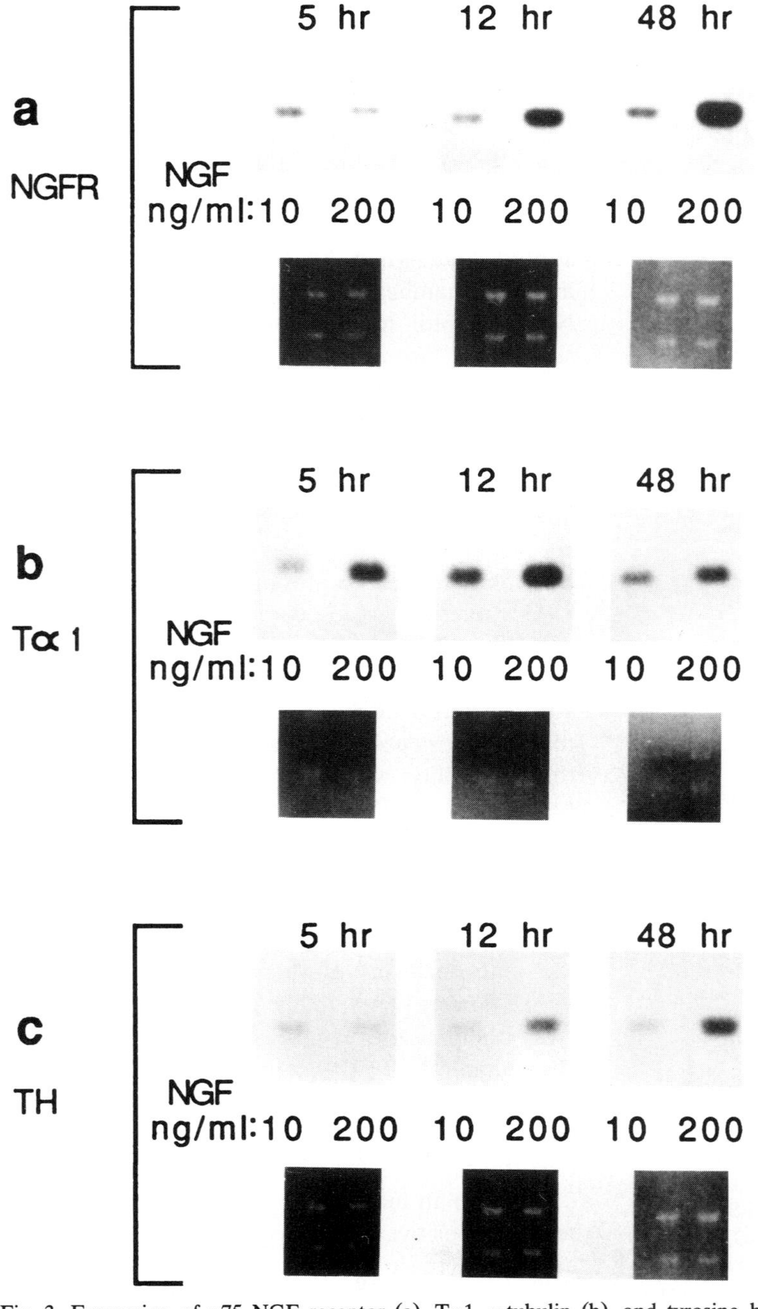

Fig. 3. Expression of p75 NGF receptor (a), Tα1 α-tubulin (b), and tyrosine hydroxylase (c) mRNAs in neonatal sympathetic neurons cultured in the presence of 10 ng/ml NGF for 5 days, followed by the addition of 200 ng/ml NGF for 5, 12, or 48 h. The upper panels are photographs of autoradiographs produced by hybridizing Northern blots with radiolabeled probes specific for each mRNA. The lower panels are photographs of the original agarose gels with the samples electrophoressed in the presence of ethidium bromide to demonstrate that equivalent amounts of total RNA were loaded in each lane (from Ma et al., 1992).

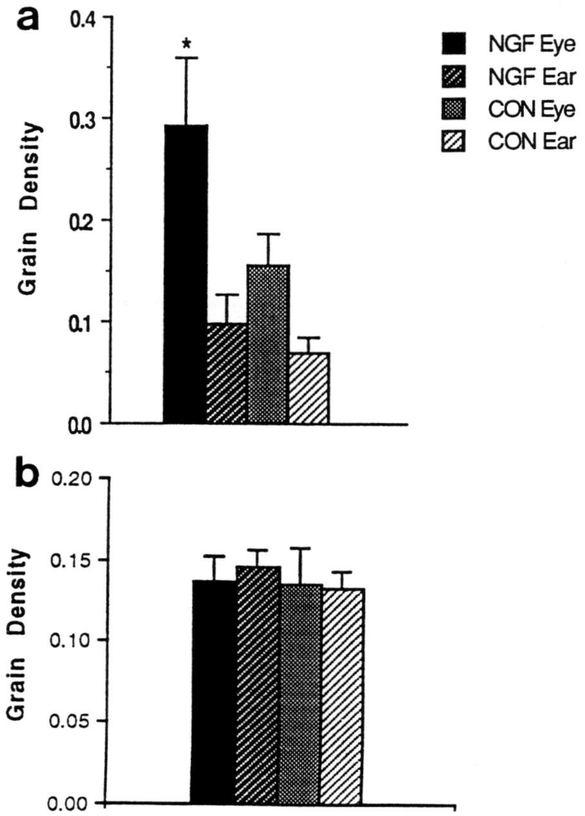

Fig. 4. Expression of p75 NGF receptor (a) and trkA (b) mRNAs in eye neurons exposed to exogenous, terminally derived NGF. In both panels, the error bars represent the standard error of the mean and the asterisks denote values that are significantly different from controls, as indicated by Student's *t*-test. (a) Mean p75 NGF receptor mRNA grain densities for a representative animal. Neurons that project to the eye were retrogradely labeled with Fast Blue, and those that project to the ear were retrogradely labeled with Fluoro-Gold. Exogenous NGF was injected into the anterior chamber of one eye, and the levels of p75 NGF receptor mRNA in NGF-treated eye neurons (NGF Eye) and control ear neurons of the same ganglion (NGF Ear) were analysed by in situ hybridization. From the same animal, contralateral eye neurons (CON Eye) that had been exposed to PBS at their terminals, and contralateral ear neurons (CON Ear) were also analysed. For each neuron analysed, grain counts were divided by cross-sectional area to obtain grain densities, thereby compensating for the neuronal hypertrophy caused by terminally derived NGF. Levels of p75 NGF receptor mRNA were significantly higher in the NGF-treated eye neurons. (b) Mean trkA mRNA grain densities for NGF-treated eye neurons (NGF Eye), control ear neurons of the same ganglion (NGF Ear), contralateral eye neurons that were exposed to cytochrome C injected into the anterior chamber (CON Eye), and contralateral ear neurons (CON Ear) from one representative animal. All four neuronal populations expressed statisticaly similar levels of trkA mRNA (modified from Miller et al., 1994).

observed in any of the control populations (Miller et al., 1994).

To determine whether exogenous, terminally derived NGF could distally regulate synthesis of the p75 and trkA NGF receptors, levels of these two mRNAs in retrogradely labeled eye and ear neurons were determined using in situ hybridization and image analysis. This analysis demonstrated that, when NGF was injected into the anterior chamber of the eye, grain counts for p75 NGF receptor mRNA in eye neurons increased significantly from 2- to 6-fold relative to control neurons (Fig. 4a). Grain densities, which account for neuronal hypertrophy, were also increased significantly in the NGF-treated neurons. In contrast, levels of trkA mRNA were not altered (Fig. 4b). Thus, increased terminally derived NGF specifically up-regulated expression of one of its two characterized receptors.

The gene expression data suggested that neuronal synthesis of the p75 NGF receptor was selectively increased to levels high enough to result in a net increase in the density of p75 NGF receptors on the neuronal surface. To directly address this possibility, we performed immunocytochemistry for the p75 NGF receptor on the NGF-treated irides with the monoclonal antibody IgG 192 (Chandler et al., 1985) (Fig. 5). In the normal iris, NGF receptor-positive fibers were detected throughout its width, from the pupillary margin to the outer margins of the dilater (Miller et al., 1994). These fibers likely derive both from the sympathetic neurons of the ipsilateral SCG (Lichtman et al., 1979), and from NGF responsive sensory neurons of the trigeminal ganglion (Cuello et al., 1978; Miller et al., 1981). Injection of NGF into the anterior chamber of the eye for 3 or 5 days led to an increase in the density of p75 NGF receptor-positive fibers (Fig. 5), as well as a generalized increase in the intensity of IgG 192 staining on virtually all positive fibers, relative to cytochrome C-injected irides from the same animals. Thus, local administration of NGF resulted in both an increase in the number of p75 NGF receptor-positive fibers and in an increase in the density of receptor per fiber, suggesting that terminally derived NGF distally regulates the ratio of p75 to trkA receptors on the surface of mature sympathetic neurons, while locally regulating terminal sprouting.

Interestingly, the magnitude of the changes in gene expression observed in this study were significantly lower than those observed with systemic NGF injection in neonatal animals (Fig. 1). These differences in gene expression could be due to developmental differences or, alternatively, could reflect a difference in neuronal responses to systemic versus local NGF administration. We have recently obtained evidence supporting the latter alternative: NGF application to axons versus cell bodies of cultured sympathetic neurons differentially regulates neuronal gene expression (Toma et al., 1993). In these experiments, sympathetic neurons were established in a compartmented culture system (Campenot, 1982) that allows manipulation of the environment of distal axons independently of the environment of cell bodies and proximal axons. Neonatal sympathetic neurons were maintained in these compartmented cultures in 10 ng/ml NGF for 7 days, and then 200 ng/ml NGF was added (a) to the entirety of the neuronal surface, (b) to distal axons only, or (c) to cell bodies and proximal axons only. These studies demonstrated that increased NGF applied to distal axons was sufficient to elicit an increase in the expression of p75 NGF receptor and tyrosine hydroxylase mRNAs, but that the magnitude of these increases was much smaller than when NGF was applied to cell bodies and proximal axons alone. Furthermore, when neurons were responding maximally to distally applied NGF, further increases in expression of p75 NGF receptor and tyrosine hydroxylase mRNAs could be elicited by NGF application to cell bodies and proximal axons. Thus, the nuclear response to NGF, at least as monitored by these two genes,

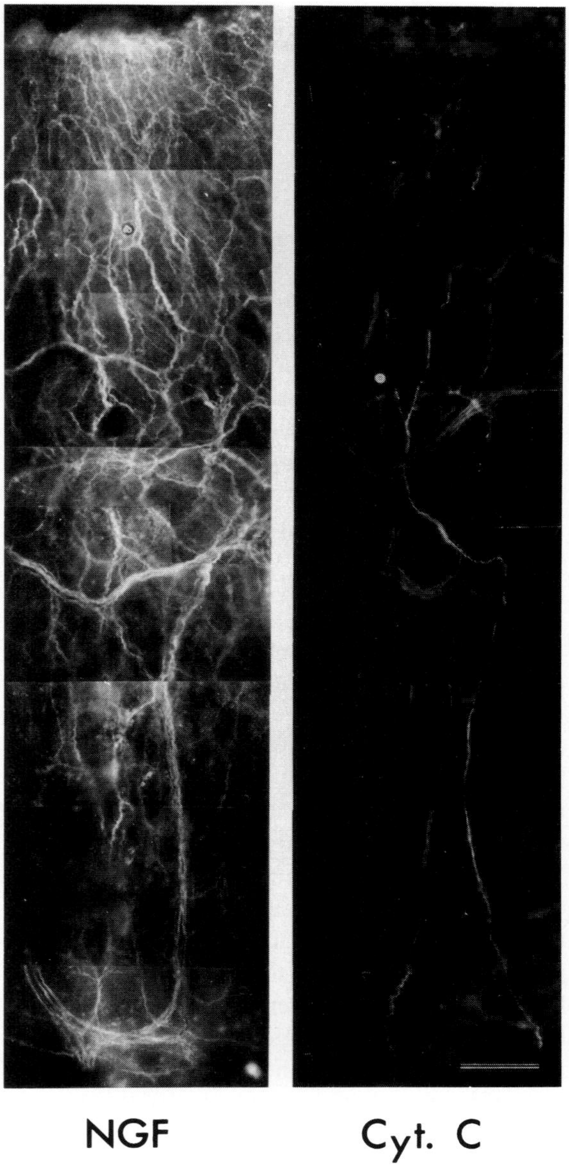

Fig. 5. Immunocytochemical detection of p75 NGF receptor in an iris exposed to daily injections of 2.5S NGF (NGF) versus one exposed to cytochrome C (Cyt. C). The immunocytochemistry was performed for both irides at the same time. Furthermore, the irides were photographed at the same exposure times, the printing was optimized for the NGF-treated iris, and the cytochrome C pictures were printed identically. Note the presence of significantly more fibers in the NGF-treated iris than in the cytochrome C-treated iris. Moreover, there is an increase in the intensity of IgG-192 immunostaining in the NGF-treated iris. The pupillary margin is at the top of the figure. Bar is 150 μm (from Miller et al., 1994).

was a function of the spatial location of the activated ligand:receptor complex.

Discussion

The studies reviewed here support a number of major conclusions. First, developing sympathetic neurons respond, both in vivo and in culture, to a broad range of NGF concentrations with graded alterations in the expression of genes important to neuronal differentiation, including those encoding the p75 NGF receptor, tyrosine hydroxylase, and Tα1 α-tubulin. Second, these NGF-induced alterations in gene expression are not limited to developing sympathetic neurons, but can be elicited in mature neurons in vivo. Third, NGF exposure on distal axons and neuronal terminals is sufficient to elicit increases in both p75 NGF receptor and tyrosine hydroxylase mRNAs, but the magnitude of these increases is less than when NGF is applied to cell bodies and proximal axons, indicating that neuronal responses to NGF are spatially regulated. Finally, NGF derived at neuronal terminals differentially regulates the synthesis of its two characterized receptors, leading to a net increase in the ratio of p75 to trkA on terminal neurites.

These results raise a number of questions about the receptor mechanisms that underly this relatively complex pattern of NGF-induced gene expression in sympathetic neurons. First, NGF elicits graded increases in gene expression at concentrations significantly higher than those required for maximal trkA autophosphorylation in a PC12 cell environment (Kaplan et al., 1991b), suggesting either the presence of a second, lower-affinity signal transducing receptor and/or cellular mechanisms that modulate and extend the trkA response range. Second, activation of NGF:receptor complexes on the distal axon elicit less of a nuclear response than does activation of NGF:receptor complexes on the cell body and proximal axons. Thus, either the receptor complexes on the distal axon differ from those on the cell body, or the distal signalling mechanism itself is responsible for these spatial differences.

To at least partially explain these observations, we propose that the p75 NGF receptor modulates the function of the trkA receptor, and that the ratio of p75 to trkA on the neuronal surface plays a critical role in determining neuronal responsiveness to NGF. More specifically, we propose, for postnatal sympathetic neurons, which express a relatively large amount of p75, that p75 NGF receptor either on the neuronal surface, or secreted into the microenvironment as a truncated receptor (DiStefano and Johnson, 1988) could serve to attenuate the effects of NGF by sequestering NGF from a productive, high-affinity receptor and/or complex. Thus, the NGF- induced increase in the ratio of p75 to trkA could serve to ensure that occupancy of the productive signalling complex would occur over a much broader concentration range than predicted by the number of high-affinity binding sites alone. Such a mechanism could explain the graded increases in gene expression that we observe at relatively high NGF concentrations, if activation of the trkA complex results in multiple signalling pathways that then converge onto these genes at the transcriptional and/or posttranscriptional levels.

Such a mechanism would have implications for the mechanisms whereby target-derived NGF regulates neuronal competition and cell death. Initial exposure of a developing sympathetic neuron to target-derived NGF would selectively up-regulate the levels of the p75 NGF receptor on the terminal arbor, and potentially increase the amount of truncated p75 secreted into the local microenvironment. The increase in membrane-bound and/or truncated p75 NGF receptor may serve to allow an early arriving neuron to sequester limiting concentrations of target-derived NGF, thereby creating an unfavorable microenvironment for later arriving neurons, and conferring a competitive advantage on the early arriving neurons.

This NGF-induced modulatory feedback loop also makes biological sense for postnatal sympathetic neurons following the period of neuronal cell death. During normal development and growth of the animal, target tissues that are innervated by the sympathetic nervous system, such as the vasculature, grow many fold. Since the number of sympathetic neurons in, for example, the superior cervical ganglion, remain constant after postnatal day 20 (Wright et al., 1983), any individual neuron is faced with innervating an increasingly large target area, and must therefore have in place receptor mechanisms that allow it to respond, in a graded fashion, to large variations in NGF concentration. Similar mechanisms would come into play in the mature nervous system during collateral sprouting of sympathetic neurons, which is known to be dependent upon NGF (Gloster and Diamond, 1992).

This proposed cellular mechanism, whereby the p75 NGF receptor modulates the activity of the trkA tyrosine kinase, thereby regulating the responsiveness of the neuron itself, has a number of additional implications. First, since the p75 NGF receptor is in actuality a 'pan-neurotrophin' receptor, such a mechanism suggests that neurotrophins other than NGF may modulate neuronal responsiveness to NGF in the absence of their cognate trk receptor. For example, brain-derived neurotrophic factor (BDNF), by displacing NGF from the p75 NGF receptor, might regulate neuronal responses to NGF by effectively altering the ratio of available p75 to trkA receptors. Second, the fact that the p75 NGF receptor is expressed developmentally late relative to the trkA receptor (Wyatt et al., 1990) suggests that NGF responsive neurons may respond differently to NGF at different developmental stages, as a consequence of the receptor repertoire that they express (e.g., embryonic versus postnatal sympathetic neurons). Finally, since the p75 NGF receptor is expressed on neurons that are not NGF targets, it is possible that it may modulate the response of other trk receptors to their cognate neurotrophin ligands.

In summary, our data suggest that target-derived NGF regulates the expression of genes that are important to the growth and differentiation of sympathetic neurons in a graded, concentration dependent fashion. Furthermore, increased terminally derived NGF specifically upregulates the ratio of p75 to trkA NGF receptors, a phenomenon which we postulate provides a molecular mechanism for a modulatory feedback loop that regulates neuronal responses to NGF itself.

Acknowledgements

We wish to thank Grace Dotto, Dwight Draker, and Audrey Speelman for excellent technical assistance over the course of these experiments; T.C. Mathew, Y. Ma, D. Rogers, J. Fabian, E. Chang, C. Pozniak, and J. Toma for their participation in these experiments; and Bob Campenot for his collaboration in many of these studies. F.M. is supported by grants from the Medical Research Council of Canada and the NCE for Neural Regeneration and Functional Recovery.

References

Acheson, A., Barker, P.A., Alderson, R.F., Miller, F.D. and Murphy, R.A. (1991) Detection of brain-derived neurotrophic factor-like activity in fibroblasts and Schwann cells: inhibition by antibodies to nerve growth factor. *Neuron*, 7: 265–275.

Angeletti, P.U., Levi-Montalcini, R. and Caramia, F. (1971) Analysis of the effects of the antiserum to the nerve growth factor in adult mice. *Brain Res.*, 92: 343–355.

Barker, P., Miller, F.D., Large, T.H. and Murphy, R.A. (1991) Generation of the truncated form of the NGF receptor by rat Schwann cells: evidence for post-translational processing. *J. Biol. Chem.*, 266: 19113–19119.

Battleman, D.S., Geller, A.I. and Chao, M.V. (1993) HSV-1 vector-mediated gene transfer of the human nerve growth factor receptor p75hNGFR defines high-affinity NGF binding. *J. Neurosci.*, 13: 941–951.

Berg, M.M., Sternberg, D.W., Hempstead, B.L. and Chao, M.V. (1991) The low-affinity p75 nerve growth factor (NGF) receptor mediates NGF-induced tyrosine phosphorylation. *Proc. Natl. Acad. Sci. USA*, 88: 7106–7110.

Campenot, R.B. (1982) Development of sympathetic neurons in compartmentalized cultures. I. Local control of neurite growth by nerve growth factor. *Dev. Biol.*, 93: 1-12.

Carroll, S.L., Silos-Santiago, I., Frese, S.E., Ruit, K.G., Milbrandt, J. and Snider, W.D. (1992) Dorsal root ganglion neurons expressing trk are selectively sensitive to NGF deprivation in utero. *Neuron*, 9: 779–788.

Chandler, C.E., Parsons, L.M., Hosang, M. and Shooter, E.M. (1985) A monoclonal antibody modulates the interaction of nerve growth factor with PC12 cells. *J. Biol. Chem.*, 259: 6882–6889.

Chun, L.L.Y. and Patterson, P.H. (1977a) Role of nerve growth factor in the development of rat sympathetic neurons in vitro. I. Survival, growth, and differentiation of catecholamine production. *J. Cell Biol.*, 75: 694–704.

Chun, L.L.Y. and Patterson, P.H. (1977b) Role of nerve growth factor in the development of rat sympathetic neurons in vitro. II. Developmental studies. *J. Cell Biol.*, 75: 705–711.

Cordon-Cardo, C., Tapley, P., Jing, S.Q., Nanduri, V., O'Rourke, E., Lamballe, F., Kovary, K., Klein, R., Jones, K.R., Reichard, L.F. and Barbacid, M. (1991) The trk tyrosine protein kinase mediates the mitogenic properties of nerve growth factor and neurotrophin-3. *Cell*, 66: 173–183.

Cuello, A.C., Delfiacco, M. and Paxinos, G. (1978) The central and peripheral ends of the substance P-containing sensory neurones in the rat trigeminal system. *Brain Res.*, 152: 499–509.

Diamond, J., Coughlin, M., MacIntyre, L., Holmes, M. and Visheau, B. (1987) Evidence that endogenous β nerve growth factor is responsible for the collateral sprouting, but not the regeneration, of nociceptive axons in the adult rats. *Proc. Natl. Acad. Sci. USA*, 84: 6596–6600.

Diamond, J., Holmes, M. and Coughlin, M. (1992) Endogenous NGF and nerve impulses regulate the collateral sprouting of sensory axons in the skin of the adult rat. *J. Neurosci.*, 12: 1454–1466.

DiStefano, P. and Johnson, E.M,. Jr. (1988) Identification of a truncated form of the nerve growth factor receptor. *Proc. Natl. Acad. Sci. USA*, 85: 270–274.

Edwards, R.M., Rutter, W.J. and Hanahan, D. (1989) Directed expression of NGF to pancreatic β cells in transgenic mice leads to selective hyperinnervation of the islets. *Cell*, 58: 161–170.

Gizang-Ginsberg, E. and Ziff, E.B. (1990) Nerve growth factor regulates tyrosine hydroxylase gene transcription through a nucleoprotein complex that contains c-Fos. *Genes Dev.*, 4: 477–491.

Gloster, A. and Diamond, J. (1992) Sympathetic nerves in adult rats regenerate normally and restore pilomotor function during an anti-NGF treatment that prevents their collateral sprouting. *J. Comp. Neurol.*, 326: 363–374.

Green, S.M., Rydel, R.M., Connolly, J.L. and Greene, L.A. (1986) PC12 mutants that possess low- but not high-affinity nerve growth factor receptors neither respond to nor internalize nerve growth factor. *J. Cell Biol.*, 102: 830–843.

Hempstead, B.L., Martin-Zanca, D., Kaplan, D.R., Parada, L.F. and Chao, M.V. (1991) High-affinity NGF binding requires coexpression of the trk proto-oncogene and the low-affinity NGF receptor. *Nature, (Lond.)*, 350: 678–682.

Ibanez, C.F., Ebendal, T., Barbany, G., Murray-Rust, J., Blundell, T.L. and Persson, H. (1992) Disruption of the low affinity receptor-binding site in NGF allows neuronal survival and differentiation by binding to the trk gene product. *Cell*, 69: 329–341.

Jing, S., Tapley, P. and Barbacid, M. (1992) Nerve growth factor mediates signal transduction through trk homodimer receptors. *Neuron*, 9: 1067–1079.

Johnson, D., Lanahan, A., Buck, C.R., Sehgal, A., Morgan, C., Mercer, E., Bothwell, M. and Chao, M. (1986) Expression and structure of the human NGF receptor. *Cell*, 47: 545–554.

Johnson, E.M., Gorin, P.D., Brandeis, L.D. and Pearson, J. (1980) Dorsal rat ganglion neurons are destroyed by exposure in utero to maternal antibody to nerve growth factor. *Science*, 210: 916–913.

Kaplan, D.R., Hempstead, B.L., Martin-Zanca, D., Chao, M.V. and Parada, L.F. (1991a) The trk proto-oncogene product: a signal transducing receptor for nerve growth factor. *Science*, 252: 554–558.

Kaplan, D.R., Martin-Zanca, D. and Parada, L.F. (1991b) Tyrosine phosphorylation and tyrosine kinase activity of the trk proto-oncogene product induced by NGF. *Nature*, (Lond.), 350: 158–160.

Kessler, J.A. and Black, I.B. (1980) Nerve growth factor stimulates the development of substance P in sensory ganglia. *Proc. Natl. Acad. Sci. USA*, 77: 649–652.

Klein, R., Jing, S., Nanduri, V., O'Rourke, E. and Barbacid, M. (1991) The trk protooncogene encodes a receptor for nerve growth factor. *Cell*, 65: 189–197.

Lee, K., Li, E., Huber, L.J., Landis, S.C., Sharpe, A.H., Chao, M.V. and Jaenisch, R. (1992) Targeted mutation of the gene encoding the low affinity NGF receptor p75 leads to deficits in the peripheral sensory nervous system. *Cell*, 69: 737–749.

Levi-Montalcini, R. and Booker, B. (1960a) Excessive growth of the sympathetic ganglia evoked by a protein isolated from mouse salivary glands. *Proc. Natl. Acad. Sci. USA*, 42: 373–384.

Levi-Montalcini, R. and Booker, B. (1960b) Destruction of the sympathetic ganglia in mammals by an antiserum to the nerve-growth promoting factor. *Proc. Natl. Acad. Sci. USA*, 42: 384–391.

Lichtman, J.W., Purves, D. and Yip, J.W. (1979) On the purpose of selective innervation of guinea pig superior ganglion cells. *J. Physiol. (London)*, 292: 69–84.

Ma, Y., Campenot, R.B. and Miller, F.D. (1992) Concentration-dependent regulation of neuronal gene expression by nerve growth factor. *J. Cell Biol.*, 117: 135–141.

Mathew, T.C. and Miller F.D. (1990) Increased expression of Tα1 α-tubulin mRNA during collateral and NGF-induced sprouting of sympathetic neurons. *Dev. Biol.*, 141: 84–92.

Mathew, T.C. and Miller F.D. (1993) Induction of Tα1 α-tubulin mRNA during neuronal regeneration is a function of the amount of axon lost. *Dev. Biol.*, 158: 467–474.

Miller, A., Costa, M., Furness, J.B. and Chubb, J.W. (1981) Substance P immunoreactive sensory nerves supply the rat iris and cornea. *Neurosci. Lett.*, 23: 243–249.

Miller, F.D., Naus, C.C.G., Durand, M., Bloom, F.E. and Milner, R.J. (1987) Isotypes of α-tubulin are differentially regulated during neuronal maturation. *J. Cell Biol.*, 105: 3065–3073.

Miller, F.D., Tetzlaff, W., Bisby, M.A., Fawcett, J.W. and Milner, R.J. (1989) Rapid induction of the major embryonic α-tubulin mRNA, Tα1, during nerve regeneration in adult rats. *J. Neurosci.*, 9: 1452–1463.

Miller, F.D., Mathew, T.C. and Toma, J.G. (1991) Regulation of nerve growth factor receptor gene expression by NGF in the developing peripheral nervous system. *J. Cell Biol.*, 112: 303–312.

Miller, F.D., Speelman, A., Mathew, T.C., Fabian, J., Chang, E., Pozniak, C. and Toma, J.G. (1994) Nerve growth factor derived from terminal selectively increases the ratio of p75 to trkA NGF receptors on mature sympathetic neurons. *Dev. Biol.*, 161: 206–217.

Radeke, M.J., Misko, T.P., Hsu, C., Herzenberg, L.A. and Shooter, E.M. (1987) Gene transfer and molecular cloning of the rat nerve growth factor receptor. *Nature, (Lond.)*, 325: 593–597.

Rodriguez-Tebar. A., Dechant, G. and Barde, Y.-A. (1990) Binding of brain-derived neurotrophic factor to the nerve growth factor receptor. *Neuron*, 4: 487–492.

Rodriguez-Tebar, A., Dechant, G., Gotz, R. and Barde, Y.-A. (1992) Binding of neurotrophin-3 to its neuronal receptors and interactions with nerve growth factor and brain-derived neurotrophic factor. *EMBO J.*, 11: 917–922.

Snider, W.D. (1988) Nerve growth factor enhances dendritic arborization of sympathetic ganglion cells in developing mammals. *J. Neurosci.*, 8: 2628–2634.

Toma, J.G., Rogers, D., Campenot, R.B. and Miller, F.D. (1993) Neuronal responses to NGF are spatially regulated: NGF exposure at terminals versus cell bodies differentially alters neuronal gene expression. *Soc. Neurosci. Abstr.*, 19: 1305.

Thoenen, H., Angeletti, P.V., Levi-Montalcini, R. and Kettler, R. (1971) Selective induction by nerve growth factor of tyrosine hydroxylase and dopamine-β-hydroylase in the rat superior cervical ganglia. *Proc. Natl. Acad. Sci. USA*, 68: 1598–1602.

Wright, L., Cunningham, T.J. and Smolen, A.J. (1983) Developmental neuron death in the rat superior cervical sympathetic ganglion: cell counts and ultrastructure. *J. Neurocytol.*, 12: 727–738.

Wyatt, S., Shooter, E.M. and Davies, A.M. (1990) Expression of the NGF receptor gene in sensory neurons and their cutaneous targets prior to and during innervation, *Neuron*, 2: 421–427.

F.J. Seil (Ed.)
Progress in Brain Research, Vol 103

CHAPTER 4

Receptor mediated retrograde axonal transport of neurotrophic factors is increased after peripheral nerve injury

Peter S. DiStefano and Rory Curtis

Regeneron Pharmaceuticals, Inc., 777 Old Saw Mill River Road Tarrytown, NY 10591-6707, U.S.A.

Introduction

Target-derived neurotrophic factors are produced in limiting quantities and thus regulate the survival of developing neurons. In the mature nervous system certain neuronal populations may depend upon a continued supply of these factors for survival and maintenance of phenotype. In general, neurotrophic factors are thought to exert their effects on neurons by binding to high affinity receptors on axons, followed by receptor-mediated uptake and retrograde transport back to the cell body. Beyond this, little is known of how they further transduce their signals to mediate trophism.

Receptor-mediated retrograde axonal transport to sensory neurons of the dorsal root ganglia (DRG) has been demonstrated for the neurotrophins, nerve growth factor (NGF), brain-derived neurotrophic factor (BDNF), neurotrophin-3 (NT-3) and neurotrophin-4 (NT-4), as well as the neuroactive cytokines, ciliary neurotrophic factor (CNTF) and leukemia inhibitory factor (LIF) (DiStefano et al., 1992; Curtis et al., 1993a, b, 1994). The receptor-mediated nature of these transport events has been demonstrated by a pharmacological approach. For example, retrograde transport of ^{125}I-labeled BDNF to sensory neurons is blocked by an excess of unlabeled BDNF, NT-3 and NT-4, all known to interact with the high affinity receptor for BDNF, namely trkB. Conversely, NGF is unable to compete for this transport, consistent with the lack of NGF binding to trkB. Accordingly, retrograde transport of ^{125}I-NGF is not blocked by an excess of BDNF, which does not bind to the high affinity NGF receptor, trkA (Squinto et al., 1991; DiStefano et al., 1992; Ip et al., 1992).

With respect to the cytokines, recent studies have shown that a functional CNTF receptor is composed of the CNTF binding protein, CNTFRα, and two 'β' components designated LIFRβ and gp130 (Davis and Yancopoulos, 1993). Interestingly, LIFRβ and gp130 comprise a functional LIF receptor (Gearing et al., 1992), predicting overlapping but distinct patterns of competition for retrograde transport of these factors. Indeed, excess unlabeled CNTF and LIF compete equally for the transport of ^{125}I-labeled CNTF to sensory neurons, but ^{125}I-labeled LIF transport is not blocked by CNTF (Curtis et al., 1993a, 1994). Furthermore, related cytokines that bind to gp130 are incapable of blocking the transport of either CNTF or LIF. Thus, as for the retrograde transport of the neurotrophins, transport of CNTF and LIF also occurs via specific receptor-mediated mechanisms.

Trophic factor expression after nerve injury

Loss of target-derived trophic support as a result of axotomy can result in altered phenotype or cell death. The successful regeneration of peripheral neurons may be related to the production of neurotrophic factors in compartments other than the target. Recent evidence has shown that Schwann cells distal to the site of peripheral nerve injury increase their expression of the neurotrophins NGF, BDNF and NT-4 (Fig. 1), factors that are normally found in neuronal target tissues (Heumann et al., 1987; Meyer et al., 1992; Funakoshi et al., 1993). LIF, which is also expressed in distal nerve Schwann cells after axotomy, does not appear to be synthesized in target tissues and may represent a lesion factor expressed exclusively by glia in response to injury (Curtis et al., 1994). In contrast to the aforementioned factors, expression of CNTF and NT-3 is decreased in distal nerve Schwann cells after axotomy (Fig. 1; Friedman et al., 1992; Sendtner et al., 1992; Funakoshi et al., 1993). CNTF is unique in that it is expressed at extraordinarily high levels in normal nerve, where it is stored in the cytoplasm of myelinating Schwann cells. Although down-regulation of CNTF mRNA occurs distal to nerve injury, considerable levels of CNTF protein remain within the nerve (Friedman et al., 1992; Sendtner et al., 1992). Due to the lack of a consensus signal sequence, the mechanism by which CNTF is released from Schwann cells is unknown; however, immunocytochemical evidence suggests that injury results in deposition of CNTF into the extracellular space. Thus, CNTF sequestered in Schwann cells may act as another

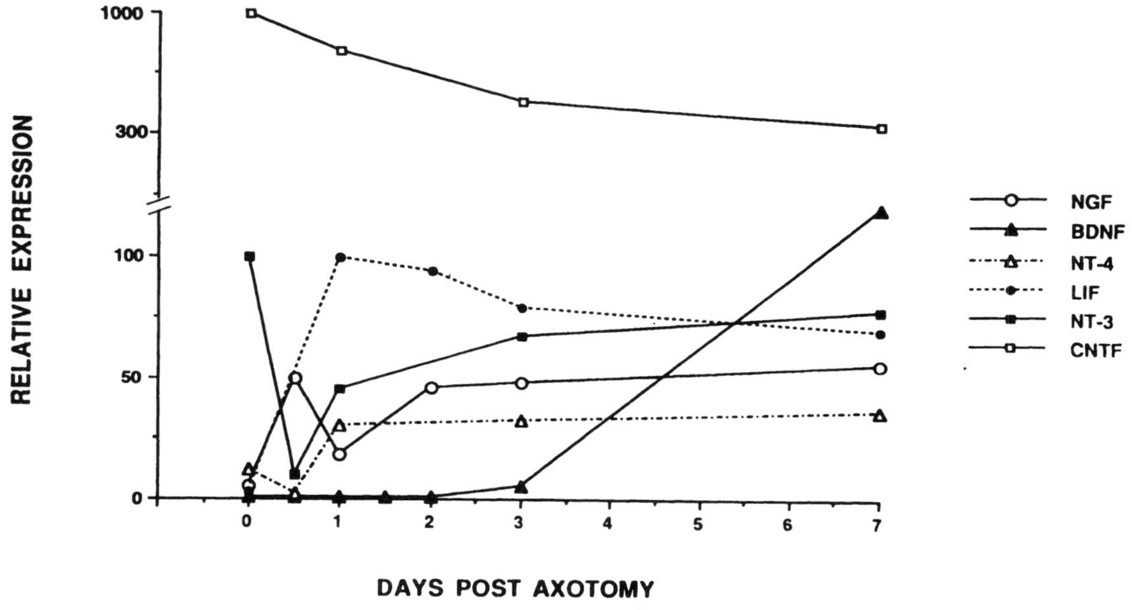

Fig. 1. Expression of known neurotrophic molecules in distal regions of peripheral nerve with time after injury. Relative levels are approximated from Northern blot analyses or from protein levels. Note that whereas levels of NGF (Heumann et al., 1987), BDNF (Meyer et al., 1992; Funakoshi et al., 1993), LIF (Curtis et al., 1994) and NT-4 (Funakoshi et al., 1993) are increased with time after axotomy, levels of CNTF (Friedman et al., 1992; Sendtner et al., 1992) and NT-3 (Funakoshi et al., 1993) are diminished. Also note that, although CNTF levels are decreased after injury, they are still probably higher than levels of other factors, even at 7 days.

lesion factor, becoming accessible to CNTF responsive neurons shortly after nerve injury.

The multitude of factors with altered expression in distal Schwann cells after axotomy strongly suggests that they play a critical role in peripheral nerve regeneration. As shown in Fig. 1, these factors appear to be regulated in a temporally coordinated fashion, suggesting that each factor plays a distinct role at critical times during regeneration. The expression of each factor may be intrinsically programmed as part of the Schwann cell response to injury or may depend on synthesis of a previously expressed factor, suggestive of an autocrine cascade.

The model

Previous work from this laboratory has shown that retrograde transport of ^{125}I-labeled CNTF by normal, uninjured sensory neurons of the DRG is modest and that transport by normal motor neurons is not detectable. However, 24 h after a crush lesion of the sciatic nerve, CNTF is robustly transported by both sensory and motor neurons (Curtis et al., 1993a). Similar lesion-induced increases in retrograde transport were observed with the CNTF-related molecule, LIF (Curtis et al., 1994). This prompted us to determine whether peripheral nerve injury resulted in the increased retrograde transport of the neurotrophins or whether this phenomenon was specific for the neuroactive cytokines, CNTF and LIF. The methodology employed in the present studies involved a crush of the sciatic nerve at the level of the tendon of the obturator internus muscle (see Curtis et al., 1993a, 1994). After a period of 1, 3 or 7 days, ^{125}I-labeled neurotrophins were injected into the crush site in the presence or absence of excess unlabeled neurotrophins (Fig. 2). This particular injection paradigm was chosen since it most closely approximates the site where axons encounter trophic support after a lesion, namely the distal nerve segments. At survival times of 6, 14 and 20 h after the injections, rats were sacrificed and the lumbar 4th and 5th (L4, L5) DRG and L4, L5 spinal cord segments were

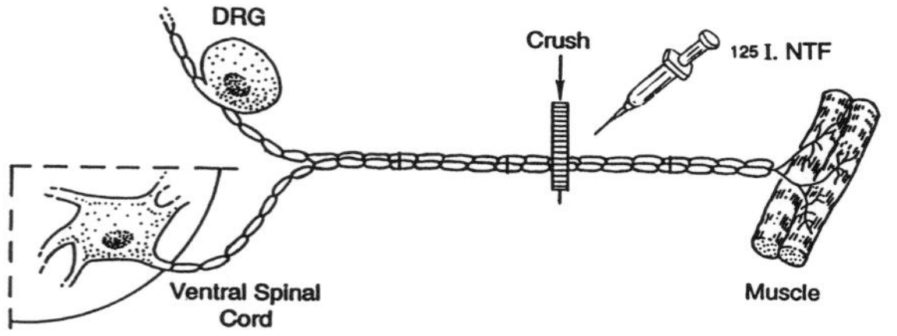

Fig. 2. Schematic depicting the methodology employed in retrograde transport studies. Crush (shaded region) is made at the site where the sciatic nerve overlies the tendon of the obturator internus muscle. Solutions containing ^{125}I-labeled neurotrophins (e.g., BDNF) with or without unlabeled factors are injected directly into the nerve. After various survival times the L4 and L5 DRG and corresponding spinal cord region (left) are dissected, counted and processed for emulsion autoradiography. Intraneural injection best approximates the site of neurotrophic factor acquisition after injury.

collected in 4% paraformaldehyde and counted in a gamma counter to quantify retrograde transport. Also, fixed tissues were sectioned at 10 μm on a cryostat and ^{125}I-labeled neurotrophins were localized in cell bodies by emulsion autoradiography.

Lesion-induced increases in retrograde transport

BDNF

The time course of BDNF transport to DRG in normal rats indicates detectable accumulation by 6 h and a peak between 14 and 20 h after an intraneural injection. In rats whose sciatic nerves were crushed 24 h prior to injection of ^{125}I-labeled BDNF, transport at all survival times was elevated 3–4-fold. Three days after a crush lesion, retrograde transport to sensory neurons subsided but remained elevated compared with non-lesioned animals. By 7 days, transport was not different from normal and at 14 days a significant decrease in sensory neuron transport of BDNF was evident. BDNF is also robustly transported by spinal cord motor neurons (DiStefano et al., 1992). As observed in the DRG, dramatically increased levels of ^{125}I-labeled BDNF accumulation were observed in motor neurons with time after a crush lesion; however, unlike sensory neurons, the peak transport of BDNF to motor neurons did not occur until 3 days after the crush injury. Nonetheless, these observations suggest that similar mechanisms of lesion-induced transport were operable in both sensory and motor neurons.

The increases in transport to both DRG and spinal cord were visualized by emulsion autoradiography and revealed an intense cellular labeling pattern in lesioned DRG and motor neurons compared with their normal counterparts. Both increased numbers of labeled cells and greater intensity of labeling per cell were observed with the emulsion autoradiography.

We have previously shown that the retrograde transport of BDNF in normal sensory and motor neurons occurs via a distinct receptor-mediated mechanism, consistent with the known pharmacology of the trkB receptor (DiStefano et al., 1992). Thus, BDNF transport is completely blocked by BDNF and to a lesser extent by NT-3, whereas NGF has little effect on BDNF transport. To show that the lesion-induced increase in transport to both sensory and motor neurons was receptor-mediated and not due to non-specific events caused by the lesion, we performed similar pharmacological (cross-competition) experiments. Consistent with our previous results in normal animals, BDNF transport, assessed 24 h after a crush lesion, was blocked by the trkB-interactive ligands but not NGF, with the rank order of potency: BDNF $\geq$ NT-4 $>$ NT-3 $\gg$ NGF.

One potential mechanism for the lesion-induced increase in retrograde transport is an increased expression of high affinity receptors for this molecule. To test this, Northern blot analysis was performed on DRG and ventral spinal cord tissues as a function of time after a sciatic nerve crush lesion using a cDNA directed towards the kinase domain of trkB. The results showed that trkB mRNA in both tissues was not increased after the lesion. In fact, trkB mRNA levels actually decreased slightly 7–14 days after the lesion. We conclude that de novo synthesis of receptors need not be invoked as the mechanism for increased transport after lesion, suggesting that alterations in the existing transport machinery predominate.

NGF

We compared the transport properties of ^{125}I-labeled NGF with those of ^{125}I-labeled BDNF after peripheral nerve injury. Although lesion-induced increases in NGF transport to DRG neurons were strikingly evident, the time course characteristics varied somewhat from those of BDNF. As with BDNF, transport of NGF was most robustly increased 24 h after the lesion; however, the peak of transport was evident at an earlier survival time (6 h). This increased transport was accompanied by extraordinarily heavy labeling of DRG neurons, as assessed by emulsion autoradiography. Another feature distinct from BDNF was that the increased transport of NGF to the DRG was more short-lived compared with BDNF. Whether this shift in the time course of NGF transport represents an increased rate of transport, an increased coupling of NGF receptor complexes to the axonal transport machinery, an altered presentation of NGF to regenerating axons by neurotrophin receptors on glial cells (Johnson et al., 1988; Frisén et al., 1993), or a more rapid turnover of ligand at the cell body, remains to be elucidated.

Since the levels of accumulation of ^{125}I-labeled NGF were so high 24 h after the lesion, we determined, as for BDNF, that this transport of NGF was mediated by specific NGF receptors (e.g., trkA) and was not a result of non-specific uptake and transport. Consistent with a receptor-mediated mechanism we demonstrated that NGF transport was blocked by an excess (30-fold) of unlabeled NGF but was unaltered by coinjection of the trkB ligand, BDNF. These observations were corroborated by emulsion autoradiography of DRG sections from animals injected with ^{125}I-labeled NGF and the corresponding unlabeled neurotrophins.

A common theme observed thus far for lesion-induced increases in the retrograde transport of BDNF, as well as the neuroactive cytokines CNTF and LIF, is that steady state expression of receptor mRNAs in cells responding to the factors is unaltered (Curtis et al., 1993a), obviating de novo synthesis of receptor molecules as a mechanism to account for increased transport. NGF receptor expression was no different in this regard in that mRNA for trkA in DRG was unaltered with time after sciatic nerve crush.

In contrast to BDNF and NT-3, whose receptors (trkB and trkC) are expressed by normal adult motor neurons (Merlio et al., 1992), studies have shown that NGF is not retrogradely transported by normal adult motor neurons. Indeed, it is generally perceived that NGF does not exert positive trophic influences on adult motor neurons. However, early postnatal motor neurons have the capacity to retrogradely accumulate NGF after injection into the foot pad (Yan et al., 1988). To determine if this developmental characteristic is recapitulated in the adult after nerve injury, we monitored the retrograde transport of NGF by motor neurons with time after a sciatic nerve crush. Surprisingly, transport of NGF to spinal cord motor neurons was evident by 24 h, and peaked approximately 3 days after lesion. This transport of NGF was assessed by measuring counts in lumbar cord segments and by visualization using emulsion autoradiography. The transport of ^{125}I-labeled NGF to motor neurons was completely blocked by unlabeled NGF but only partially so by the other neurotrophins, indicating a potentially complex receptor mechanism that may involve the low affinity neurotrophin receptor, which is known to be up-regulated in motor neurons within 1 day after sciatic nerve lesion (Ernfors et al., 1989; Rende et al., 1992). Involvement of trkA in this response is difficult to postulate since expression of this receptor is extremely low, if detectable at all, in ventral spinal cord motor neurons. These results with NGF are reminiscent of those observed for the transport of CNTF to motor neurons, which is detectable only after nerve injury (Curtis et al., 1993a). In summary, several neurotrophic molecules, expressed in nerve and retrogradely transported by motor and sensory neurons, may play roles during repair of damaged neurons, as well as in the maintenance of the mature nervous system.

WGA

The retrograde axonal transport of lectins, such as wheat germ agglutinin (WGA), is well established and is thought to occur through the interaction with complex carbohydrates located on a multitude of cell surface proteins. We utilized ^{125}I-labeled WGA as a tool to discern whether increased axonal transport after axotomy was specific for neurotrophic factors. Two major observations arose from the ^{125}I-labeled WGA transport studies. First, transport of this lectin was increased with time after lesion, like many neurotrophic factors studied. Second, although retrograde transport was robustly increased after trauma, the time course of transport following intraneural injection of ^{125}I-labeled WGA was drastically different from that of any neurotrophic factor described thus far. It is difficult to ascertain whether WGA transport is truly a receptor-mediated process, since there is no defined, specific receptor for this molecule. However, ^{125}I-labeled WGA transport was blocked by excess unlabeled WGA and was, therefore, saturable. Thus, WGA may represent a 'non-specific' indicator of the increased retrograde transport machinery that is engaged shortly after the onset of motor and sensory neuron trauma. Nonetheless, the results with neurotrophic factors and WGA point to the inescapable fact that the increase in retrograde transport of each factor after lesion occurs with a distinct time course and a different peak accumulation time, indicating a level of specificity for transport of different factors (Fig. 3).

Derivation of trophic support: different compartments

The site from which a neuron derives its trophic support can be significantly altered, depending on the developmental or pathological state of the neuron (Johnson et al., 1988; DiStefano, 1993; Lindsay et al., 1994). For instance, the production

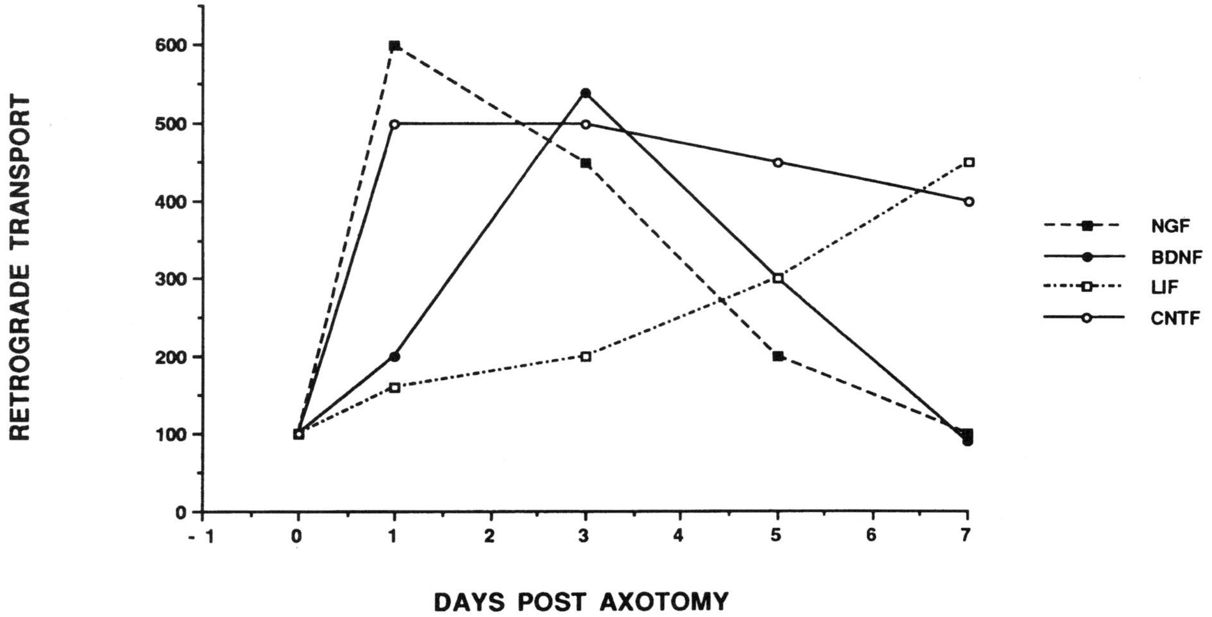

Fig. 3. Relative time courses of retrograde transport of ^{125}I-labeled NGF, BDNF, CNTF and LIF by DRG neurons after sciatic nerve crush. The graph shows that profound differences in the times of peak transport occur between classes of neurotrophic molecules (neurotrophins versus neuroactive cytokines) and among members of a given class (NGF versus BDNF; CNTF versus LIF).

of many different neurotrophic molecules by Schwann cells is increased in distal nerve, as discussed above. The present results demonstrate that several trophic factors, including the neurotrophins, show dramatically increased uptake and retrograde axonal transport by different classes of neurons after injury. We propose that, following peripheral nerve damage, the glial cell becomes an alternate 'target' for regenerating neurons and that the mechanisms driving the machinery for increased transport are enhanced. This increase comes at a time when neurons are probably in most need of trophic support, namely, immediately following axotomy. That the increased transport of the neurotrophins in DRG neurons is short-lived compared with that for CNTF (Curtis et al., 1993a) or LIF (Curtis et al., 1994) may indicate that neurons derive the neurotrophins from yet additional compartments, such as the cell soma. In support of this, BDNF and NT-3 are expressed by both sensory and motor neurons, raising the possibility of autocrine/paracrine actions of these factors (Acheson et al., 1993; Lindsay et al., 1994).

Receptor-mediated retrograde transport

While the mechanisms of lesion-induced increases in transport remain unknown, pharmacological experiments have shown that the increases in transport of CNTF (Curtis et al., 1993a) and LIF (Curtis et al., 1994), as well as BDNF and NGF (present work) are receptor-mediated. The time course of retrograde accumulation at the cell body is also consistent with an active, receptor-mediated process. Accumulation by diffusion, based on theoretical calculations, would occur over the course of days instead of hours. Bulk flow of materials at damaged nerve terminals is also not a mechanism by which a lesion could cause increased transport. With bulk flow there would be no competition in the pharmacologically distinct manner observed here and transport would not be a saturable process. We have indeed shown that the retrograde transport of neurotrophins by DRG neurons is a saturable process (DiStefano et al., 1991).

From Northern blot analyses of receptor expression in DRG and spinal cord, it is highly unlikely that increased receptor expression is responsible for the lesion-induced increase in retrograde transport of the neurotrophins or of CNTF and LIF (Curtis et al., 1993a). Previous investigations have revealed that the retrograde axonal transport of proteins, in general, is increased upon injury to peripheral nerve (Bulger and Bisby, 1978; Bisby, 1984). Thus, neurons may possess the intrinsic capacity to increase the transport of several molecules in response to damage.

The increased level of transport of the neurotrophins, CNTF, LIF and even WGA, after sciatic nerve crush indicates that a general increase in the uptake/transport machinery is operable within the first 24 h after a lesion. However, the time courses of transport for these factors are quite distinct (see Fig. 3), suggesting that there exists an element of specificity for the transport of different factors. It is tempting to speculate that different factors may actually be transported at different rates. After injury, the different time courses of retrograde transport suggest that neurons respond in an orchestrated manner to temporally distinct patterns of neurotrophic factor expression by Schwann cells (compare Figs. 1 and 3).

Implications of increased retrograde transport after neuronal injury

We have previously discussed that increased transport of CNTF after peripheral nerve lesion may be an intrinsically programmed cellular mechanism for increasing the accumulation of much needed neurotrophic factors after neuronal damage (Curtis et al., 1993a). Further, injured or otherwise compromised neurons (by genetic lesion or toxic insult) may show a selective responsiveness to neurotrophic factors by virtue of their increased retrograde transport. This is of significance when considering therapeutic intervention with pharmacological doses of neurotrophic factors for peripheral neuropathies (DiStefano, 1993). It now becomes necessary to determine how the increased retrograde flow of neurotrophic signals is processed and what molecular mechanisms are operable in the transduction of these retrograde signals. Experiments are in progress to determine if receptor molecules, as well as the ligands themselves, are retrogradely transported and what auxiliary molecules are potentially transported with this complex.

Acknowledgements

The authors thank K. Adryan, J. Stark and Y. Zhu for excellent technical assistance and Dr R.M. Lindsay for criticism, advice and support for these studies.

References

Acheson, A., Ip, N.Y., Squinto, S.P. and Lindsay, R.M. (1993) BDNF antisense oligonucleotides elicit selective neuronal death in cultures of adult rat sensory neurons: evidence that a neurotrophin autocrine loop sustains neuronal survival. *Soc. Neurosci. Abstr.*, 19: 442.

Bisby, M.A. (1984) Retrograde axonal transport and nerve regeneration. In: J.S. Elam and P. Cancalon (Eds.), *Axonal Transport In Growth and Regeneration*, Plenum Press, New York, pp. 45–67.

Bulger, V.T. and Bisby, M.A. (1978) Reversal of axonal transport in regenerating nerves. *J. Neurochem.*, 31: 1411–1418.

Curtis, R., Adryan, K.M., Zhu, Y., Harkness, P.J., Lindsay, R.M. and DiStefano, P.S. (1993a) Retrograde axonal transport of ciliary neurotrophic factor is increased by peripheral nerve injury. *Nature, (Lond.)*, 365: 253–255.

Curtis, R., Lee, K.-F., Jaenisch, R., Huber, J., Chao, M.V., Lindsay, R.M. and DiStefano, P.S. (1993b) Potential involvement of p75LNGFR in retrograde transport of neurotrophin-4 (NT-4). *Soc. Neurosci. Abstr.*, 19: 1476.

Curtis, R., Scherer, S.S., Somogyi, R., Adryan, K.M., Ip, N.Y., Zhu, Y., Lindsay, R.M. and DiStefano, P.S. (1994) Retrograde axonal transport of LIF is increased by peripheral nerve injury: correlation with increased LIF expression in distal nerve. *Neuron*, 12: 191–204.

Davis, S. and Yancopoulos, G.D. (1993) The molecular biology of the CNTF receptor. *Curr. Opin. Neurobiol.*, 3: 20–24.

DiStefano, P.S. (1993) Neurotrophic factors in the treatment of motor neuron disease and trauma. *Exp. Neurol.*, 124: 56–59.

DiStefano, P.S., Friedman, B., Wiegand, S.J. and Lindsay, R.M. (1991) Retrograde axonal transport of ^{125}I-labeled neurotrophins in peripheral neurons. *Soc. Neurosci. Abstr.*, 17: 1121.

DiStefano, P.S., Friedman, B., Radziejewski, C., Alexander, C., Boland, P., Schick, C.M., Lindsay, R.M. and Wiegand, S.J. (1992) The neurotrophins BDNF, NT-3, and NGF display distinct patterns of retrograde axonal transport in peripheral and central neurons. *Neuron*, 8: 983–993.

Ernfors, P., Henschen, A., Olson, L. and Persson, H. (1989) Expression of nerve growth factor receptor mRNA is developmentally regulated and increased after axotomy in rat spinal cord motoneurons. *Neuron*, 2: 1605–1613.

Friedman, B., Scherer, S.S., Rudge, J.S., Helgren, M., Morrisey, D., McClain, J., Wang, D.-y., Wiegand, S.J., Furth, M.E., Lindsay, R.M. and Ip, N.Y. (1992) Regulation of ciliary neurotrophic factor expression in myelin-related Schwann cells in vivo. *Neuron*, 9: 295–305.

Frisén, J., Verge, V.M.K., Fried, K., Risling, M., Persson, H., Trotter, J., Hökfelt, T. and Lindholm, D. (1993) Characterization of glial trkB receptors: differential response to injury in the central and peripheral nervous systems. *Proc. Natl. Acad. Sci. USA*, 90: 4971–4975.

Funakoshi, H., Frisén, J., Barbany, G., Timmusk, T., Zachrisson, O., Verge, V.M.K. and Persson, H. (1993) Differential expression of mRNAs for neurotrophins and their receptors after axotomy of the sciatic nerve. *J. Cell Biol.*, 123: 455–465.

Gearing, D.P., Comeau, M.R., Friend, D.J., Gimpel, S.D., Thut, C.J., McGourty, J., Brasher, K.K., King, J.A., Gillis, S., Mosley, B., Ziegler, S.F. and Cosman, D. (1992) The IL-6 signal transducer, gp130 - an oncostatin M receptor and affinity converter for the LIF receptor. *Science*, 255: 1434–1437.

Heumann, R., Lindholm, D., Bandtlow, C., Meyer, M., Radeke, M.J., Misko, T.P., Shooter, E. and Thoenen, H. (1987) Differential regulation of mRNA encoding nerve growth factor and its receptor in rat sciatic nerve during development, degeneration, and regeneration: role of macrophages. *Proc. Natl. Acad. Sci. USA*, 84: 8735–8739.

Ip, N.Y., Ibanez, C.F., Nye, S.H., McClain, J., Jones, P.F., Gies, D.R., Belluscio, L., Lebeau, M.M., Espinosa, R., Squinto, S.P., Persson, H. and Yancopoulos, G.D. (1992) Mammalian neurotrophin-4: structure, chromosomal localization, tissue distribution, and receptor specificity. *Proc. Natl. Acad. Sci. USA*, 89: 3060–3064.

Johnson, E.M., Jr., Taniuchi, M. and DiStefano, P.S. (1988) Expression and possible function of nerve growth factor receptors on Schwann cells. *Trends Neurosci.*, 11: 299–304.

Lindsay, R.M., Wiegand, S.J., Altar, C.A. and DiStefano, P.S. (1994) Neurotrophic factors: from molecule to man. *Trends Neurosci.*, 17: 182–190.

Merlio, J.P., Ernfors, P., Jaber, M. and Persson, H. (1992) Molecular cloning of rat trkC and distribution of cells expressing messenger RNAs for members of the trk family in the rat central nervous system. *Neuroscience*, 51: 513–532.

Meyer, M., Matsuoka, I., Wetmore, C., Olson, L. and Thoenen, H. (1992) Enhanced synthesis of brain-derived neurotrophic factor in the lesioned peripheral nerve; different mechanisms are responsible for the regulation of BDNF and NGF mRNA. *J. Cell Biol.*, 119: 45–54.

Rende, M., Hagg, T., Manthorpe, M. and Varon, S. (1992) Nerve growth factor receptor immunoreactivity in neurons of the normal adult rat spinal cord and its modulation after peripheral nerve lesions. *J. Comp. Neurol.*, 319: 285–298.

Sendtner, M., Stöckli, K.A. and Thoenen, H. (1992) Synthesis and localization of ciliary neurotrophic factor in the sciatic nerve of the adult rat after lesion and during regeneration. *J. Cell Biol.*, 118: 139–148.

Squinto, S.P., Stitt, T.N., Aldrich, T.H., Davis, S., Bianco, S.M., Radziejewski, C., Glass, D.J., Masiakowski, P., Furth, M.E., Valenzuela, D.M., DiStefano, P.S. and Yancopoulos, G.D. (1991) trkB encodes a functional receptor for brain-derived neurotrophic factor and neurotrophin-3 but not nerve growth factor. *Cell*, 65: 885–893.

Yan, Q., Snider, W.D., Pinzone, J.J. and Johnson, E.M. (1988) Retrograde transport of nerve growth factor (NGF) in motoneurons of developing rats: assessment of potential neurotrophic effects. *Neuron*, 1: 335–343.

F.J. Seil (Ed.)
Progress in Brain Research, Vol 103

CHAPTER 5

Target derived and putative local actions of neurotrophins in the peripheral nervous system

Patrik Ernfors, Kuo-Fen Lee and Rudolf Jaenisch

Whitehead Institute for Biomedical Research and Department of Biology, MIT, Nine Cambridge Center, Cambridge, MA 02142, U.S.A.

Introduction

In the developing vertebrate nervous system, neurons are produced in vast excess and within a restricted time period a majority undergo naturally occurring cell death (Oppenheim, 1985; Barde, 1989), which begins shortly after innervation of the target fields (Davies and Lumsden, 1984). A given target field supports the survival of only a fraction of neurons, due to limited amounts of neurotrophic factors synthesized by the target (Levi-Montalcini, 1987; Barde, 1989). This process is thought to ensure that target cells are innervated by the correct number and type of nerve fibers.

Nerve growth factor (NGF) is the prototype of a family of growth factors including four structurally related proteins known as the neurotrophins. Other members of this family are brain-derived neurotrophic factor (BDNF) (Barde et al., 1982; Leibrock et al., 1989), neurotrophin-3 (NT-3) (Ernfors et al., 1990a; Hohn et al., 1990; Jones and Reichardt, 1990; Kaisho et al., 1990; Maisonpierre et al., 1990; Rosenthal et al., 1990) and neurotrophin-4/5 (NT-4/5 or NT-4) (Berkemeier et al., 1991; Hallbook et al., 1991; Ip et al., 1992).

In the peripheral nervous system the neurotrophins influence a partially overlapping population of neurons. In in vitro neurite outgrowth or cell survival assays, NGF stimulates embryonic sensory and sympathetic neurons of neural crest origin. BDNF and NT-3 influence certain populations of both neural crest and placode derived sensory neurons. NT-3, but not BDNF, elicits a weak response from sympathetic neurons (Davies and Lindsay, 1985; Davies et al., 1986; Leibrock et al., 1989; Ernfors et al., 1990a; Hohn et al., 1990; Jones and Reichardt, 1990; Maisonpierre et al., 1990; Rosenthal et al., 1990; Berkemeier et al., 1991; Hallbook et al., 1991; Ip et al., 1992). It is clear that NGF and BDNF are also important in vivo, because administration of anti-NGF antibodies shortly after the period of cell death substantially increases the loss of spinal sensory neurons (Gorin and Johnson, 1979; Johnson et al., 1980; Aloe et al., 1982), whereas exogenous administration of NGF or BDNF at the time of naturally occurring cell death markedly reduces the loss of dorsal root or nodose ganglion neurons (Hamburger et al., 1981; Kalcheim et al., 1987; Hofer and Barde, 1988). In addition, developing or lesioned motor neurons can be rescued by administration of BDNF (Oppenheim et al., 1992; Sendtner et al., 1992; Yan et al., 1992; Koliatsos et al., 1993).

Although little is known about the mechanisms of action of BDNF, NT-3 and NT-4 in vivo, there is considerable support for the concept that neurotrophins act in a target derived, retrograde fashion, since enlargement of the target field reduces the loss of neurons during naturally occurring cell death (Hollyday and Hamburger, 1976; Narayan and Narayan, 1978; Boydston and Sohal, 1979). Conversely, extirpation of the target field results in excessive loss of innervating neurons (Hamburger, 1958; Prestige, 1967; Carr and Simpson, 1978; Chu-Wang and Oppenheim, 1978). In addition, NGF, BDNF and NT-3 are retrogradely transported from the target of innervation to the cell bodies of neuronal populations that respond to the neurotrophins (Hendry et al., 1974a, b; Stöckel and Thoenen, 1975; Johnson et al., 1978; Schwab et al., 1979; Richardson and Riopelle, 1984; Seiler and Schwab, 1984; DiStefano et al., 1992). Furthermore, the tissue-specific expression of both NGF mRNA and protein correlates with the innervation of responsive neurons (Heumann et al., 1984; Shelton and Reichardt, 1984; Davies et al., 1987; Ayer-LeLievre et al., 1988; Ernfors et al., 1989a; Phillips et al., 1990).

In addition to promoting the survival of neurons during development, neurotrophins have been implicated in neuronal proliferation (Cattaneo and McKay, 1990), differentiation (Cattaneo and McKay, 1990; Sieber-Blum, 1991; Wright et al., 1992) and in guiding and stimulating growth of axons (Johnson et al., 1988). NGF also appears to influence collateral sprouting in the peripheral (Diamond et al., 1987) and central nervous system (Ernfors et al., 1989a; Hagg et al., 1990).

Neurotrophins exert their physiological effects by binding to receptors with different affinities (Banerjee et al., 1973; Herrup and Shooter, 1973; Sutter et al., 1979; Richardson et al., 1986). All neurotrophins bind a 75,000-Da receptor, p75, with similar low affinities (Ernfors et al., 1990a; Rodrigues-Tebar et al., 1990, 1992; Hallbook et al., 1991; Squinto et al., 1991). p75 is expressed in the populations of neurons known to respond to the neurotrophins (Hefti et al., 1986; Ernfors et al., 1988, 1989b, 1990b, 1991; Koh et al., 1989; Hallbook et al., 1990; Pioro and Cuello, 1990). The biological role of the p75 has not been resolved yet since signal transduction is mediated only by binding of the ligands to the high affinity receptors. However, the phenotype of mice carrying a mutation of the p75 gene suggests that the low affinity receptor is also important for neurotrophin interactions in vivo (Lee et al., 1992). Furthermore, recent reports have shown that it affects the survival of peripheral neurons in culture (Davies et al., 1993) (see below). The high affinity receptors are restricted to a subpopulation of neurons expressing p75 (Banerjee et al., 1973; Herrup and Shooter, 1973; Sutter et al., 1979; Richardson et al., 1986) and are members of the trk protooncogene family of tyrosine kinase receptors (Meakin and Shooter, 1991). In fibroblast cell lines, NGF binds and activates the high affinity receptor, trkA (Cordon-Cardo et al., 1991; Kaplan et al., 1991; Klein et al., 1991a). BDNF and NT-4 share the signal transducing receptor, trkB (Berkemeier et al., 1991; Glass et al., 1991; Klein et al., 1991b; Soppet et al., 1991; Squinto et al., 1991) and NT-3 binds and activates trkC (Lamballe et al., 1991). There are conflicting results whether NT-3 also interacts with the trkA and trkB receptors (Cordon-Cardo et al., 1991; Glass et al., 1991; Klein et al., 1991b; Soppet et al., 1991; Squinto et al., 1991). However, in a more neuronal-like context of PC12 cells, NT-3 insufficiently activates the trkA and trkB receptors (Ip et al., 1993). In addition, NGF deprivation in utero leads to a selective loss of neurons expressing trkA (Carroll et al., 1992), arguing that trkA is not used by NT-3 for stimulating survival.

Target derived actions of neurotrophins

Neurotrophin mRNA expression and survival activity in the trigeminal system

The primary sensory part of the trigeminal system consists mainly of cell bodies located in the trigeminal ganglion, with a small number of cells located in the mesencephalic trigeminal nucleus. Neurons in the trigeminal ganglion are derived from both neural crest and placode epithelium (Narayanan and Narayanan, 1980; D'Amico-Martel and Noden, 1983), and neurons of the mesencephalic trigeminal nucleus are likely of neural crest origin (Narayanan and Narayanan, 1978). The trigeminal ganglion becomes discernible at embryonic day 9 (E9) in the mouse, and at E9.5 the first nerve processes grow out of the ganglion (Davies and Lumsden, 1984; Stainier and Gilbert, 1991). The majority of the trigeminal ganglion neurons are born between E10 and E12 in the mouse (E13–14 in the rat), as shown by [^{3}H]thymidine birth-dating, neuronal cell counts and immunohistochemical studies (Altman and Bayer, 1982; Davies and Lumsden, 1984; Stainier and Gilbert, 1991). Axons of the trigeminal ganglion neurons reach their targets, the facial skin and mucous membranes of the mouth and nose, through three nerve branches, the maxillary, mandibular and ophthalmic nerves. The initial target encounter occurs at E10.5 and peaks at E12, but new fibers are recruited until E15 (Davies and Lumsden, 1984). More than 50% of the neurons degenerate during the period of naturally occurring cell death, which peaks between E13 and E15, but cell loss continues until birth (Davies and Lumsden, 1984).

Several lines of evidence support a target-derived mode of action of NGF during development of trigeminal ganglion neurons. NGF mRNA and protein are expressed in the target fields of the maxillary branch, the epithelium, mesenchyme and whisker follicles, the onset of expression correlating with the arrival of the first nerve fibers (Davies and Lumsden, 1984; Bandtlow et al., 1987; Davies et al., 1987). However, the finding that NGF is a member of a family of neurotrophic factors with overlapping biological activities in culture suggests that a more complex set of target derived neurotrophic effects may be required during development of the trigeminal system. In agreement with this, both NGF and BDNF have been shown to stimulate fiber outgrowth and the survival of trigeminal ganglion neurons in culture (Lindsay et al., 1985; Davies et al., 1986).

Using in situ hybridization, the temporal and spatial expression of mRNAs for all four neurotrophins (Bandtlow et al., 1987; Davies et al., 1987; Ernfors et al., 1992; Ibanez et al., 1993) and their receptors, trk, trkB and trkC (Klein et al., 1989, 1990; Martin-Zanca et al., 1990; Ernfors et al., 1992) have been characterized. Most, if not all, of the neurons in the trigeminal ganglion express trk mRNA at E13 in the rat, and the expression persists at least until birth. In contrast, only a subpopulation of the cells express trkB and trkC mRNAs at E13. A similar number of cells containing trkB mRNA at E13 is present at E16 and E18. However, the number of cells expressing trkC mRNA decreases between E13 and E16 (Ernfors et al., 1992).

At E13, NGF, NT-3 and NT-4 mRNAs are expressed in the surface epithelium and proximal mesenchyme of the maxillary and mandibular processes in the rat. At later stages of embryonic development, the levels are markedly decreased in these structures (Ernfors et al., 1992; Ibanez et al., 1993). However, at later stages (E16 and E18), high levels of both NT-3 and NT-4 mRNAs are expressed in whisker follicles (Ernfors et al., 1992). NT-4 mRNA is expressed in both the external and internal root sheath (ERS and IRS, respectively), while NT-3 mRNA is detected only in the ERS. BDNF mRNA is expressed throughout the deep mesenchyme in the maxillary process at E13, after which it decreases several-fold (schematically depicted in Fig. 1).

Expression of high affinity receptors for neurotrophins by trigeminal ganglion neurons and presence of the four ligands in the target suggest a role for all the neurotrophins in development of the trigeminal system. Accordingly, all four neurotrophins rescue trigeminal ganglion neurons in culture. However, responsiveness to a particular neurotrophin depends on developmental stages. NGF, BDNF, NT-3 and NT-4 substantially promote survival of mouse trigeminal ganglion neurons at E11. At E12 and E13, BDNF, NT-3 and NT-4 support the survival of relatively fewer neurons in culture, and at E14 virtually all trigeminal ganglion neurons depend on NGF only (Fig. 2) (Buchman et al., 1993; Ernfors, Lee and Jaenisch, unpublished data). At the time of onset of naturally occurring cell death (E12), NGF, BDNF, NT-3 and NT-4 rescue approximately 80%, 15%,

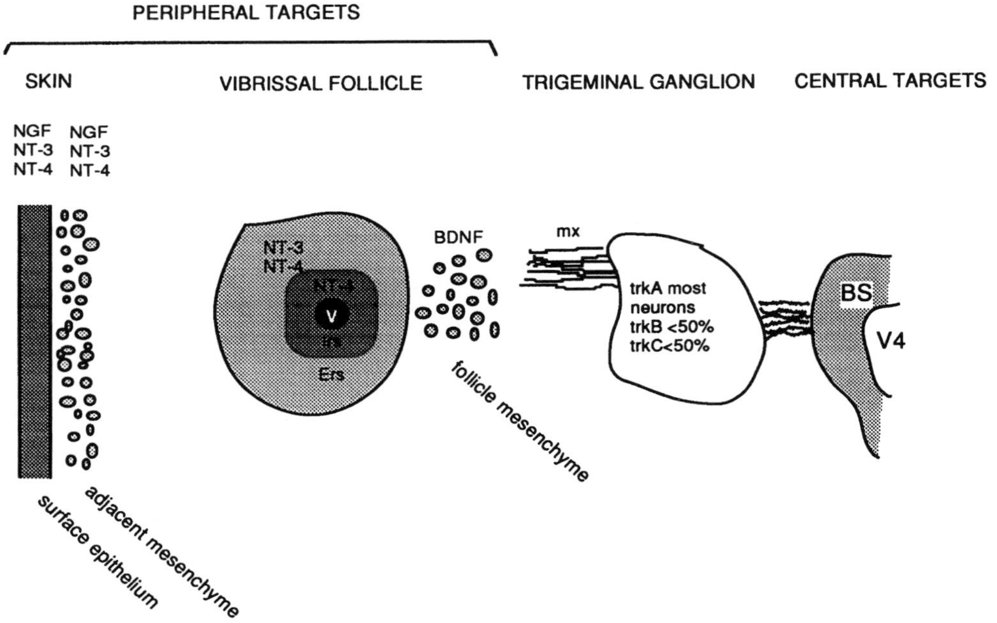

Fig. 1. Expression of neurotrophins and their receptor mRNAs in the targets of the trigeminal ganglion of E16 rat as revealed by in situ hybridization. BS, brainstem; Ers, external root sheath; Irs, internal root sheath; mx, maxillary nerve; V, hair shaft; V4, fourth ventricle.

35% and 60%, respectively, of mouse trigeminal ganglion neurons (Fig. 3). All neurotrophins show a partial additative effect when combined, except for NGF or BDNF, with NT-4 (Fig. 3). Thus, neurotrophins are likely to sustain innervation in a cooperative way in vivo, although specific subpopulations appear, at least in culture, to respond to one or a selective set of neurotrophins. BDNF

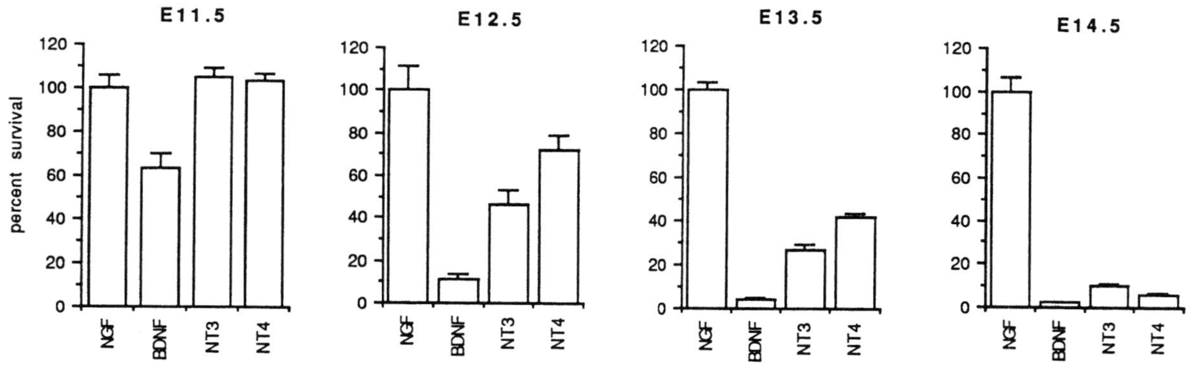

Fig. 2. Survival effects of NGF, BDNF, NT-3 and NT-4 (30 ng/ml) on dissociated mouse trigeminal ganglion neurons in culture at various embryonic stages. NGF survival was arbitrarily set as 100%. Note gradual decline of the number of neurons supported by BDNF, NT-3 and NT-4 at later developmental stages, and almost complete loss of survial effects by E14.5.

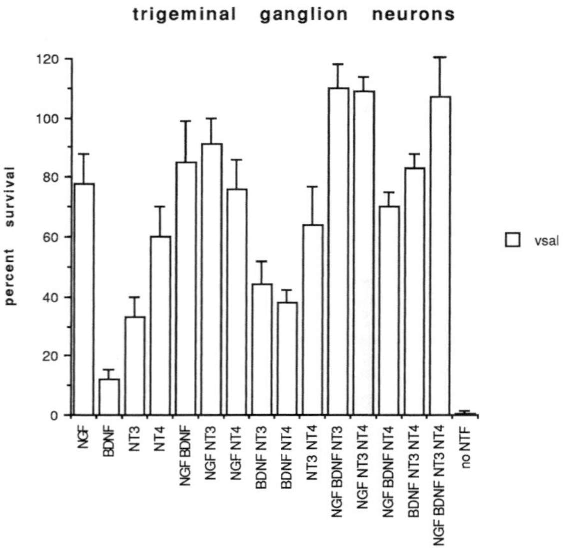

Fig. 3. Survival of dissociated mouse E12 trigeminal ganglion neurons in culture with a single or combinations of neurotrophins added to the medium (30 ng/ml). Note additative effects of all neurotrophins except NT-4 combined with NGF or BDNF.

has also been shown to be necessary for the survival of trigeminal ganglion neurons in vivo. Mice carrying a deletion in the BDNF locus by gene targeting have sensory deficits, including the loss of approximately 50% of the trigeminal ganglion neurons (Ernfors et al., 1994).

Neurotrophin mRNA expression and survival activity in the auditory and vestibular systems

The cell bodies of the primary sensory neurons in the auditory system are located in either the vestibular or the spiral (cochlear) ganglia and most, if not all, neurons originate from the otic placode (D'Amico-Martel and Noden, 1983). Shortly after the otic vesicle is formed, two waves of cells are detached from the external part of the vesicle. The first wave coincides with the formation of the vestibular ganglion and the second wave with the formation of the spiral ganglion (Altman and Bayer, 1982). The eighth cranial nerve innervates the sensory epithelia involved in hearing and equilibrium and coordination of movements. The cochlear sensory epithelium is innervated by both the spiral ganglion neurons and, to a lesser degree, vestibular ganglion neurons. The vestibular ganglion neurons mainly innervate the vestibule sensory epithelia, including the macula of the sacculus and utriculus, and the ampullary cristae of the semicircular ducts. Innervation of the cochlea occurs between E17 and E21 in the rat (Pirvola et al., 1991).

The peripheral targets of the cochleovestibular ganglion contain trophic activity which supports the survival of these neurons in culture (Hauger et al., 1989; Hemond and Morest, 1992). Although NGF has been suggested to play a role as a trophic factor during the development of the inner ear, at least the vestibular component of the vestibuloacoustic ganglion is unresponsive to NGF in culture (Davies and Lindsay, 1985). In agreement with this, vestibular and spiral ganglion neurons have subsequently been shown to express trkB and trkC mRNAs, but not trk mRNA (Ernfors et al., 1992), and the sensory epithelia of the inner ear contain mRNAs for BDNF and NT-3 but not NGF or NT-4 (Ernfors et al., 1992; Pirvola et al., 1992). As with the target fields of the trigeminal ganglion neurons, BDNF and NT-3 mRNAs are localized in a partially overlapping pattern. Sensory epithelia of the cochlea and vestibule express both BDNF and NT-3 mRNAs (Ernfors et al., 1992; Pirvola et al., 1992), although not in a completely overlapping pattern. NT-3 mRNA is localized to both the differentiating hair cells and surrounding supporting cells of the cochlea and vestibule sensory epithelia, whereas BDNF mRNA is localized exclusively to the differentiating hair cells (Pirvola et al., 1992). In addition, BDNF, but not NT-3 mRNA, is expressed in the crista of the semicircular ducts (Ernfors et al., 1992; Pirvola et al., 1992; schematically depicted in Fig. 4). Expression first appears at E11 and persists to at least postnatal day 7. As in the trigeminal ganglion, neurotrophins act sequentially in the vestibular system to promote neuronal survival. Both spiral and vestibular ganglion neurons respond to BDNF and NT-3 at the

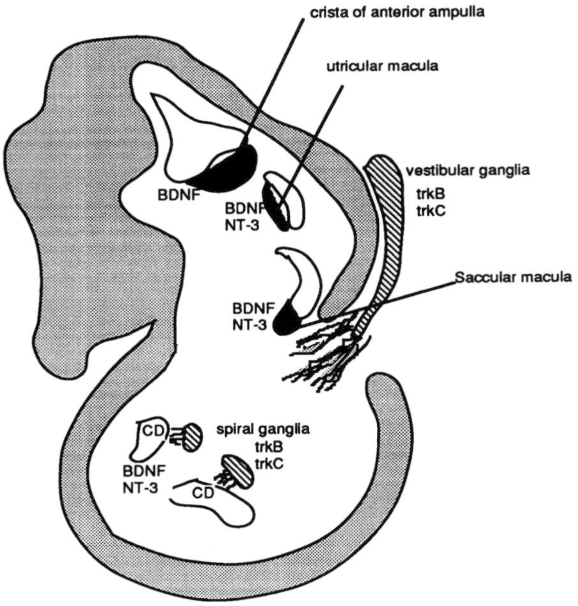

Fig. 4. Expression of neurotrophins and their receptor mRNAs in the inner ear of the E16 rat as revealed by in situ hybridization. BDNF and NT-3 mRNAs are expressed in the sensory epithelia of all compartments of the inner ear except the crista of the semicircular ducts, where only BDNF mRNA is expressed. CD, cochlear duct.

time of target encounter and innervation. However, at later stages, the neuronal survival is virtually only promoted by BDNF (Avila et al., 1993).

A role for BDNF in vivo for the survival of vestibular ganglion neurons and innervation of the inner ear has now been firmly established. Mice with an inactivated BDNF locus by gene targeting display severe deficits in coordination of movements and in balance. Lack of BDNF mRNA expression does not affect the developmental course of formation of cranial ganglia, extension of nerve processes or target encounter, but leads to the loss of more than 80% of the vestibular ganglion neurons at later developmental stages. The remaining axons fail to reach the vestibular hair cells, and terminate in the adjacent connective tissue (Ernfors et al., 1994).

In conclusion, in both the trigeminal and vestibular system, neurotrophins are expressed in a cell-specific, partially overlapping pattern in peripheral targets of innervation. The expression is temporally regulated, and the neurotrophins act in a developmental sequence to sustain survival of cultured neurons. At critical stages, such as the time of target encounter, innervation and cell death, several neurotrophins promote survival in a partially additive way. Thus, it is possible that additative and non-additive actions of neurotrophins in a developmental sequence is a general mechanism for regulating programmed cell death and establishment of the appropriate number and pattern of innervation in a given target field.

Putative role of p75 in neurotrophin interactions assessed by gene targeting

To elucidate the role of p75 in neural development, mice carrying a null mutation by gene targeting in the p75 locus have been generated (Lee et al., 1992). Dorsal root and trigeminal senory ganglia of mutant mice are reduced in size and the mice exhibit decreased cutaneous sensory innervation and pain sensitivity (Lee et al., 1992). In addition, sympathetic innervation of a number of target tissues was altered: pineal glands lacked innervation, and sweat gland innervation was reduced or absent in a subset of footpads (Lee et al., 1994a). These results indicate that p75 is required during development for sensory and sympathetic innervation of specific targets.

The absence of sensory and sympathetic innervation in adults reflects the failure during development of axons to reach these targets. The failure of innervation is unlikely, due to a lack of trophic support from targets, as demonstrated by the finding that pineal glands explanted from p75 deficient mice elicited neurite outgrowth from sympathetic ganglia in vitro. In cultures, the responses of p75 deficient dorsal root ganglion (DRG), trigeminal ganglion (TG) and superior cervical ganglion (SCG) neurons to different neurotrophins were altered. p75 deficient DRG, TG and SCG neurons displayed a 2–3-fold decreased sensitivity to NGF at E15 (DRG and TG neurons) and postnatal day 3 (SCG neurons), ages which coincide with the peak of programmed cell death (Davies et al., 1993; Lee et al., 1994b). Because the concentration of NGF in the target field is limiting, decreased sensitivity likely leads to excess loss of neurons. Furthermore, while p75 deficient E15 DRG and TG neurons had no change in their response specificity to BDNF, NT-3 and NT-4, postnatal day 3 SCG neurons became more responsive to NT-3 at higher concentrations.

In conclusion, studies of the p75 deficient mice have shown that p75 is necessary for particular axons to reach their targets. This is in agreement with a role for the reported non-neuronal expression of p75 in peripheral nerves (Ernfors et al., 1988; Yan and Johnson, 1988) and targets of innervation (Hallbook et al., 1990; Wyatt et al., 1990; Von Bartheld et al., 1991) in concentrating NGF, and thereby facilitating embryonic outgrowth of nerves and regeneration of injured nerves (Johnson et al., 1988). p75 has also been suggested to have an axon guidance function as a part of axon guidance by promoting Schwann cell migration (Anton and Matthew, 1992). In addition, studies of the p75 deficient mice have shown that neuronal expression of p75 increases the responsiveness of neurons to certain neurotrophins. Because p75 mRNA expression is upregulated in neurons at the time of target encounter during development, it may increase responsiveness of a neuron to a particular neuorotrophin at this developmental stage. Thus, p75 may restrict the ability of a neuron at a certain developmental stage to respond to a particular neurotrophin, and thereby may be involved within the target in guiding the innervation of a target cell.

Putative local action of neurotrophins

In addition to the target derived mode of action, the role for a local action of neurotrophins in the peripheral (Ernfors et al., 1990a, 1992; Ernfors and Persson, 1991; Schecterson and Bothwell, 1992) and central (Ceccatelli et al., 1991; Kokaia et al., 1993; Miranda et al., 1993) nervous system has been suggested. This hypothesis emerges from neurotrophin and receptor mRNA localization. Using oligonucleotide probes for in situ hybridization, BDNF mRNA was found expressed in the dorsal root ganglion of the adult rat (Ernfors et al., 1990c). More recently, neurotrophins have also been reported to be expressed in neurons during development. Embryonic and adult rat and mouse dorsal root ganglion neurons express both BDNF and NT-3 mRNAs (Ernfors et al., 1990c, 1992; Ernfors and Persson, 1991; Schecterson and Bothwell, 1992). In addition, nodose, superior and jugular ganglia neurons express BDNF mRNA, and geniculate and petrose ganglia neurons express NT-3 mRNA in the rat embryo (Ernfors et al., 1992; schematically depicted in Fig. 5). Using riboprobes for in situ hybridization, BDNF and NT-3 mRNAs have also been reported in sympathetic neurons and BDNF mRNA in trigeminal and petrose ganglia neurons of mice (Schecterson and Bothwell, 1992).

In several peripheral ganglia, the ligand and its corresponding receptor are coexpressed, including the trigeminal, geniculate, nodose and dorsal root ganglia (Ernfors et al., 1992; Schecterson and Bothwell, 1992; see Fig. 5). In agreement with a local role for neurotrophins, the maturation of cultured embryonic dorsal root ganglion neurons has been shown to be retarded by antisense BDNF oligonucleotides (Wright et al., 1992). In addition to an auto- or paracrine mode of action of neurotrophins for neuronal maturation, it is possible to envision a local mode of action for proliferation of neuronal precursor cells, since at least NGF has been shown to affect proliferation of central neuronal precursor cells in culture (Cattaneo and McKay, 1990). Consistent with a local action of neurotrophins, cells detached from the external part of the otic vesicle, which have been suggested to contribute to the spiral ganglion, express BDNF mRNA during migration (Ernfors et al., 1992).

If neurotrophins are released within the ganglia, a local auto- or paracrine neurotrophic action occurs in most cranial and spinal sensory and sympathetic ganglia. However, other mechanisms

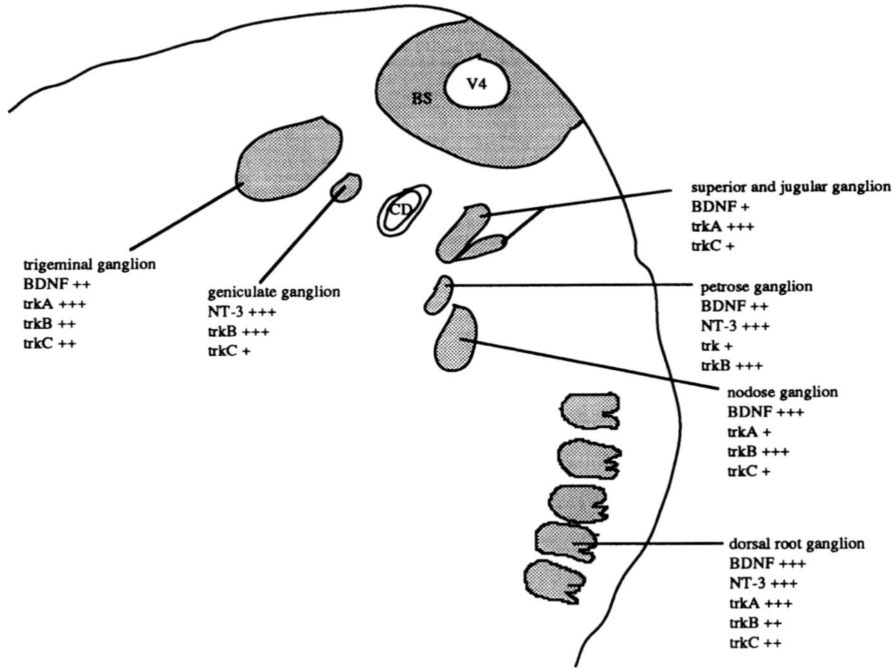

Fig. 5. Expression of neurotrophin and receptor mRNAs in cranial ganglia and dorsal root ganglion of the E14 rat as revealed by in situ hybridization. + + +, most or all neurons labeled; + + less than 50% of the neurons labeled; +, less than 10% of the neurons labeled. BS, brain stem; CD, cochlear duct; V4, 4th ventricle.

of actions are also possible, where neurotrophins may act in an orthograde fashion for neuron to target signaling, or may be involved in regulation of Schwann cell activity (Schecterson and Bothwell, 1992).

References

Aloe, L., Calissano, P. and Levi-Montalcini, R. (1982) Effect of oral administration of nerve growth factor and its antiserum on sympathetic ganglia of neonatal mice. *Nature (London)*, 291: 413–415.

Altman, J. and Bayer, S. (1982) Development of the cranial nerve ganglia and related nuclei in the rat. *Adv. Anat. Embryol. Cell Biol.*, 74: 1–90.

Anton, E.S. and Matthew, W.D. (1992) A novel function for NGF and NGF receptors expressed on Schwann cells: a role in Schwann cell migration. *Soc. Neurosci. Abstr.*, 18: 615.

Avila, M.A., Varela-Nieto, I., Romero, G., Mato, J.M., Giraldez, F., Van De Water, T.R. and Represa, J. (1993) Brain-derived neurotrophic factor and neurotrophin-3 support survival and neuritogenesis response of developing cochleovestibular ganglion neurons. *Dev. Biol.*, 159: 266–275.

Ayer-LeLievre, C., Olson, L., Ebendal, T., Seiger, Å. and Persson, H. (1988) Expression of the β-nerve growth factor gene in hippocampal neurons. *Science*, 240: 1339–1341.

Bandtlow, C.E., Heumann, R., Schwab, M.E. and Thoenen, H. (1987) Cellular localization of nerve growth factor synthesis by in situ hybridization. *EMBO J.*, 6: 891–899.

Banerjee, S.P., Snyder, S.H., Cuatrecasas, P. and Greene, L.A. (1973) Binding of nerve growth factor receptor in sympathetic ganglia. *Proc. Natl. Acad. Sci. USA*, 70: 2519–2523.

Barde, Y.-A. (1989) Trophic factors and neuronal survival. *Neuron*, 2: 1525–1534.

Barde, Y.-A., Edgar, D. and Thoenen, H. (1982) Purification of a new neurotrophic factor from mammalian brain. *EMBO J.*, 1: 549–553.

Berkemeier, L., Winslow, J., Kaplan, D., Nicolics, K., Goeddel, D. and Rosenthal, A. (1991) Neurotrophin-5: a novel neurotrophic factor that activates trk and trkB. *Neuron*, 7: 857–866.

Boydston, W. and Sohal, G. (1979) Grafting of additional periphery reduces embryonic loss of neurons. *Brain Res.*, 178: 403–410.

Buchman, V.L. and Davies, A.M. (1993) Different neurotrophins are expressed and act in a developmental sequence to promote the survival of embryonic sensory neurons. *Development*, 118: 989–1001.

Carr, V. and Simpson, S. (1978) Proliferative and degenerative events in the early development of chick dorsal root ganglia. II. Response to altered peripheral fields. *J. Comp. Neurol.*, 182: 741–756.

Carroll, S., Silos-Santiago, I., Frese, S., Ruit, K., Milbrandt, J. and Snider, W. (1992) Dorsal root ganglion neurons expressing trk are selectively sensitive to NGF deprivation in utero. *Neuron*, 9: 779–788.

Cattaneo, E. and McKay, R. (1990) Proliferation and differentiation of neuronal stem cells regulated by nerve growth factor. *Nature (London)*, 347: 762–765.

Ceccatelli, S., Ernfors, P., Villar, M.J., Persson, H. and Hökfelt, T. (1991) Expanded distribution of MRNA for nerve growth factor, brain-derived neurotrophic factor, and neurotrophin-3 in the rat brain after colchicine-treatment. *Proc. Natl. Acad. Sci. USA* 88: 10352–10356.

Chu-Wang, V. and Oppenheim, R. (1978) Cell death of motoneurones in the chick embryo spinal cord. I. A light and electron microscopy study of naturally occurring and induced cell loss during development. *J. Comp. Neurol.*, 177: 33–58.

Cordon-Cardo, C., Tapley, P., Jing, S., Nanduri, V., O'Rourke, E., Lamballe, F., Kovary, K., Klein, R., Jones, K., Reichardt, L. and Barbacid, M. (1991) The trk tyrosine kinase mediates the mitogenic properties of nerve growth factor and neurotrophin-3. *Cell*, 66: 173–183.

D'Amico-Martel, A. and Noden, D.M. (1983) Contributions of placodal and neural crest cells to avian cranial peripheral ganglia. *Am. J. Anat.*, 166: 445–468.

Davies, A. and Lindsay, R. (1985) The cranial sensory ganglia in culture: differences in the response of placode-derived and neural crest-derived neurons to nerve growth factor. *Dev. Biol.*, 111: 62–72.

Davies, A. and Lumsden, A. (1984) Relation of target encounter and neuronal death to nerve growth factor responsiveness in the developing mouse trigeminal ganglion. *J. Comp. Neurol.*, 223: 124–137.

Davies, A.M., Thoenen, H. and Barde, Y.-A. (1986) The response of chick sensory neurons to brain-derived neurotrophic factor. *J. Neurosci.*, 6: 1897–1904.

Davies, A.M., Bandtlow, C., Heumann, R., Korsching, S., Rohrer, H. and Thoenen, H. (1987) Timing and site of nerve growth factor synthesis in developing skin in relation to innervation and expression of the receptor. *Nature (London)*, 326: 353–358.

Davies, A.M., Lee, K.F. and Jaenisch, R. (1993) p75-Deficient trigeminal sensory neurons have an altered response to NGF but not to other neurotrophins. *Neuron*, 11: 565–574.

Diamond, J., Coughlin, M., Macintyre, L., Holmes, M. and Visheau, B. (1987) Evidence that endogenous nerve growth factor is responsible for the collateral sprouting, but not the regeneration, of nociceptive axons in adult rats. *Proc. Natl. Acad. Sci. USA*, 84: 6596–6600.

DiStefano, P., Friedman, B., Radziejewski, C., Alexander, C., Boland, P., Schick, C., Lindsay, R. and Wiegand, S. (1992) The neurotrophins BDNF, NT3 and NGF display distinct patterns of retrograde axonal transport in peripheral and central neurons. *Neuron*, 8: 983–993.

Ernfors, P. and Persson, H. (1991) Developmentally regulated expression of HDNF/NT-3 mRNA in rat spinal cord motoneurons and detection of BDNF mRNA in embryonic dorsal root ganglion. *Eur. J. Neurosci.*, 3: 953–961.

Ernfors, P., Hallbook, F., Ebendal, T., Shooter, E., Radeke, M.J., Misko, T.P. and Persson, H. (1988) Developmental and regional expression of β-nerve growth factor receptor mRNA in the chick and rat. *Neuron*, 1: 983–996.

Ernfors, P., Ebendal, T., Olson, L., Mouton, P., Strömberg, I. and Persson, H. (1989a) A cell line producing recombinant nerve growth factor evokes growth responses in intrinsic and grafted central cholinergic neurons. *Proc. Natl. Acad. Sci. USA*, 86: 4756–4760.

Ernfors, P., Henschen, A., Olson, L. and Persson, H. (1989b) Expression of nerve growth factor receptor mRNA is developmentally regulated and increased after axotomy in rat spinal cord motoneurons. *Neuron*, 2: 1605–1613.

Ernfors, P., Ibanez, C.F., Ebendal, T., Olson, L. and Persson, H. (1990a) Molecular cloning and neurotrophic activities of a protein with structural similarities to nerve growth factor: developmental and topographical expression in the brain. *Proc. Natl. Acad. Sci. USA*, 87: 5454–5458.

Ernfors, P., Lindefors, N., Chan-Palay, V. and Persson, H. (1990b) Cholinergic neurons of nucleus basalis express elevated levels of nerve growth factor receptor mRNA in senile demential of the Alzheimer type. *Dementia*, 1: 138–145.

Ernfors, P., Wetmore, C., Olson, L. and Persson, H. (1990c) Identification of cells in rat brain and peripheral tissues expressing mRNA for members of the nerve growth factor family. *Neuron*, 5: 511–526.

Ernfors, P., Wetmore, C., Eriksdotter-Nilsson, M., Bygdeman, M., Strömberg, I., Olson, L. and Persson, H. (1991) The nerve growth factor receptor gene is expressed in both neuronal and non-neuronal tissues in the human fetus. *Int. J. Dev. Neurosci.*, 9: 57–66.

Ernfors, P., Merlio, J.-P. and Persson, H. (1992) Cells expressing mRNA for neurotrophins and their receptors during embryonic rat development. *Eur. J. Neurosci.*, 4: 1140–1158.

Ernfors, P., Lee, K.-F. and Jaenisch, R. (1994) Mice lacking brain derived neurotrophic factor develop with sensory deficits. *Nature (London)*, 368: 147–150.

Glass, D.J., Nye, S.H., Hantzopoulos, P., Macchi, M.J., Squinto, S.P., Goldfarb, M. and Yancopoulos, G.D. (1991) TrkB mediates BDNF/NT-3-dependent survival and proliferation in fibroblasts lacking the low affinity NGF receptor. *Cell*, 66: 405–413.

Gorin, P. and Johnson, E. (1979) Experimental autoimmune

model of nerve growth factor deprivation: effects on developing peripheral sympathetic and sensory neurons. *Proc. Natl. Acad. Sci. USA*, 76: 5382–5386.

Hagg, T., Vahlsing, H.L., Manthorpe, M. and Varon, S. (1990) Nerve growth factor infusion into the denervated adult rat hippocampus formation promotes its cholinergic reinnervation. *J. Neurosci.*, 10: 3087–3092.

Hallbook, F., Ayer-LeLievre, C., Ebendal, T. and Persson, H. (1990) Expression of nerve growth factor receptor mRNA during early development of the chicken embryo: emphasis on cranial ganglia. *Development*, 108: 693–704.

Hallbook, F., Ibanez, C.F. and Persson, H. (1991) Evolutionary studies of the nerve growth factor family reveal a novel member abundantly expressed in *Xenopus* ovary. *Neuron*, 6: 845–58.

Hamburger, V. (1958) Repression versus peripheral control of differentiation in motor hypoplasia. *Am. J. Anat.*, 102: 365–410.

Hamburger, V., Brunso-Bechtold, J.K. and Yip, J.W. (1981) Neuronal death in the spinal ganglia of the chick embryo and its reduction by nerve growth factor. *J. Neurosci.*, 1: 60–71.

Hauger, S., Book, K. and Morest, D. (1989) Trophic support of the developing cochleovestibular ganglion by its peripheral target in vitro does not depend on neuronal cell division. *Neuroscience*, 33: 241–251.

Hefti, F., Hartikka, J., Salvatierra, A., Weiner, W.J. and Mash, D.C. (1986) Localization of nerve growth factor receptors in cholinergic neurons of the human basal forebrain. *Neurosci. Lett.*, 69: 37–41.

Hemond, S.G. and Morest, D.K. (1992) Trophic effects of otic epithelium on cochleo-vestibular ganglion fiber growth in vitro. *Anat. Rec.*, 232: 273–284.

Hendry, I., Stach, R. and Herrup, K. (1974a) Characteristics of the retrograde axonal transport system for nerve growth factor in the sympathetic nervous system. *Brain Res.*, 82: 117–128.

Hendry, I.A., Stöckel, K., Thoenen, H. and Iversen, L.L. (1974b) The retrograde axonal transport of nerve growth factor. *Brain Res.*, 68: 103–121.

Herrup, K. and Shooter, E.M. (1973) Properties of the B-nerve growth factor receptor of avian dorsal root ganglia. *Proc. Natl. Acad. Sci. USA*, 70: 3884–3888.

Heumann, R., Korsching, S., Scott, J. and Thoenen, H. (1984) Relationship between levels of nerve growth factor and its messenger RNA in sympathetic ganglia and peripheral target tissues. *EMBO J.*, 3: 3183–3189.

Hofer, M.M. and Barde, Y.-A. (1988) Brain-derived neurotrophic factor prevents neuronal death in vivo. *Nature (London)*, 331: 261–262.

Hohn, A., Leibrock, J., Bailey, K. and Barde, Y.A. (1990) Identification and characterization of a novel member of the nerve growth factor/brain-derived neurotrophic factor family. *Nature (London)*, 344: 339–341.

Hollyday, M. and Hamburger, V. (1976) Reduction of naturally occurring motor neuron loss by enlargement of the periphery. *J. Comp. Neurol.*, 170: 311–320.

Ibanez, C.F., Ernfors, P., Timmusk, T., Ip, N.Y., Arenas, E., Yancopolous, G.D. and Persson, H. (1993) Neurotrophin-4 is a target-derived neurotrophic factor for neurons of the trigeminal ganglion. *Development*, in press,

Ip, N., Ibanez, C., Nye, S., McClain, J., Jones, P., Gies, D., Belluscio, L., Le Beu, M., Espinosa III, M., Squinto, R., Persson, H. and Yancopolous, G. (1992) Mammalian neurotrophin-4: structure, distribution and receptor specificity. *Proc. Natl. Acad. Sci. USA*, 89: 3060–3064.

Ip, N., Stitt, T.N., Tapley, P., Klein, R., Glass, D., Fandl, J., Greene, L., Barbacid, M. and Yancopolous, G. (1993) Similarities and differences in the way neurotrophins interact with the trk receptors in neuronal and nonneuronal cells. *Neuron*, 10: 137–149.

Johnson, E.J., Andres, R.Y. and Bradshaw, R.A. (1978) Characterization of the retrograde transport of nerve growth factor (NGF) using high specific activity (^{125}I) NGF. *Brain Res.*, 150: 319–331.

Johnson, E., Gorin, P., Brandeis, L. and Pearson, J. (1980) Dorsal root ganglion neurons are destroyed by exposure in utero to maternal antibodies to nerve growth factor. *Science*, 210: 916–918.

Johnson, E.M., Taniuchi, M. and DiStefano, P.S. (1988) Expression and possible function of nerve growth factor receptors on Schwann cells. *Trends Neurosci.*, 11: 299–304.

Jones, K. and Reichardt, L. (1990). Molecular cloning of a human gene that is a member of the nerve growth factor family. *Proc. Natl. Acad. Sci. USA*, 87: 8060–8064.

Kaisho, Y., Yoshimura, K. and Nakahama, K. (1990) Cloning and expression of a cDNA encoding a novel human neurotrophic factor. *FEBS Lett.*, 266: 187–191.

Kalcheim, C., Barde, Y.-A., Thoenen, H. and LeDouarin, N.M. (1987) In vivo effect of brain-derived neurotrophic factor on the survival of developing dorsal root ganglion cells. *EMBO J.*, 6: 2871–2873.

Kaplan., Martin-Zanca, D. and Parada, L. (1991) Tyrosine phosphorylation and tyrosine kinase activity of the trk proto-oncogene produced by NGF. *Nature (London)*, 350: 158–160.

Klein, R., Parada, L., Moulier, F. and Barbacid, M. (1989) TrkB, a novel tyrosine kinase receptor expressed during mouse neural development. *EMBO J.*, 8: 3701–3709.

Klein, R., Martin-Zanca, D., Barbacid, M. and Parada, L.F. (1990) Expression of the tyrosine kinase gene trkB is confined to the murine embryonic and adult nervous system. *Development* 109: 845–850.

Klein, R., Jing, S.Q., Nanduri, V., O'Rourke, E. and Barbacid, M. (1991a) The trk proto-oncogene encodes a receptor for nerve growth factor. *Cell*, 65: 189–971.

Klein, R., Nanduri, V., Jing, S., Lamballe, F., Tapley, P., Bryant, S., Cordon-Cardi, C., Jones, K., Reichardt, L. and

Barbacid, M. (1991b) The trkB tyrosine protein kinase is a receptor for brain-derived neurotrophic factor and neurotrophin-3. *Cell*, 66: 395–403.

Koh, S., Oyler, G.A., and Higgins, G.A. (1989) Localization of nerve growth factor receptor messenger RNA and protein in the adult rat brain. *Exp. Neurol.*, 106: 209–226.

Kokaia, Z., Bengzon, J., Metsis, M., Kokaia, M., Persson, H. and Lindvall, O. (1993) Coexpression of neurotrophins and their receptors in neurons of the central nervous system. *Proc. Natl. Acad. Sci. USA*, 90: 6711–6715.

Koliatsos, V.E., Clatterbuck, R.E., Winslow, J.W., Cayouette, M.H. and Price, D.L. (1993) Evidence that brain-derived neurotrophic factor is a trophic factor for motor neurons in vivo. *Neuron*, 10: 359–367.

Lamballe, F., Klein, R. and Barbacid, M. (1991) trkC, a new member of the trk family of tyrosine protein kinases, is a receptor for neurotrophin-3. *Cell*, 66: 967–979.

Lee, K.-F., Li, E., Huber, L., J., Landis, S.C., Sharpe, A.H. and Chao, M.C.J. (1992) Targeted mutation of the gene encoding the low affinity NGF receptor p75 leads to deficits in the peripheral sensory nervous system. *Cell*, 69: 737–749.

Lee, K.-F., Bachman, K., Landis, S. and Jaenisch, R. (1994a) Dependence on P75 for innervation of some sympathetic targets. *Science*, 263: 1447–1449.

Lee, K.-F., Davies, A.M. and Jaenisch, R. (1994b) P-75 deficient dorsal root sensory and neonatal sympathetic neurons display a decreased sensitivity to NGF. *Development*, 120: 1027–1033.

Leibrock, J., Lottspeich, F., Hohn, A., Hofer, M., Hengerer, B., Masiakowski, P., Thoenen, H. and Barde, Y.A. (1989) Molecular cloning and expression of brain-derived neurotrophic factor. *Nature (London)*, 341: 149–151.

Levi-Montalcini, R. (1987) The nerve growth factor 35 years later. *Science*, 237: 1154–1162.

Lindsay, R.M., Thoenen, H. and Barde, Y.-A. (1985) Placode and neural crest-derived sensory neurons are responsive at early developmental stages to brain-derived neurotrophic factor. *Dev. Biol.*, 112: 319–328.

Maisonpierre, P.C., Belluscio, L., Squinto, S., Ip, N.Y., Furth, M.E., Lindsay, R.M. and Yancopoulos, G.D. (1990) Neurotrophin-3: a neurotrophic factor related to NGF and BDNF. *Science*, 247: 1446–1451.

Martin-Zanca, D., Barbacid, M. and Parada, L.F. (1990) Expression of the trk proto-oncogene is restricted to the sensory cranial and spinal ganglia of neural crest origin in mouse development. *Genes Dev.*, 4: 683–942.

Meakin, S. and Shooter, E. (1991) Molecular investigation on the high-affinity nerve growth factor receptor growth. *Neuron*, 6: 153–156.

Miranda, R.C., Sohrabji, F. and Toran-Allerand, C.D. (1993) Neuronal colocalization of mRNAs for neurotrophins and their receptors in the developing central nervous system suggests a potential for autocrine interactions. *Proc. Natl. Acad. Sci. USA*, 90: 6439–6443.

Narayanan, C.H. and Narayanan, Y. (1978) Determination of the embryonic origin of the mesencephalic nucleus of the trigeminal nerve in birds. *J. Embryol. Exp. Morphol.*, 43: 85–105.

Narayanan, C.H. and Narayanan, Y. (1980) Neural crest and placodal contributions in the development of the glossopharyngeal-vagal complex in the chick. *Anat. Res.*, 196: 71–82.

Oppenheim, R.W. (1985) Naturally occurring cell death during neuronal development. *Trends Neurosci.*, 9:487–493.

Oppenheim, R.W., Qin-Wei, Y., Prevette, D. and Yan, Q. (1992) Brain-derived neurotrophic factor rescues developing avian motoneurons from cell death. *Nature (London)*, 360: 755–757.

Phillips, H.S., Hains, J.M., Laramee, G.R., Rosenthal, A. and Winslow, J.W. (1990) Widespread expression of BDNF but not NT-3 by target areas of basal forebrain cholinergic neurons. *Science*, 250: 290–294.

Pioro, E.P. and Cuello, A.C. (1990) Distribution of nerve growth factor receptor-like immunoreactivity in the adult rat central nervous system. Effect of colchicine and correlation with the cholinergic system — I. Forebrain. *Neuroscience*, 34: 57–87.

Pirvola, U., Lehtonen, E. and Ylikoski, J. (1991) Spatiotemporal development of cochlear innervation and hair cell differentiation in the rat. *Hear. Res.*, 52: 345–355.

Pirvola, U., Ylikoski, J., Palgi, J., Lethonen, E., Arumäe, U. and Saarma, M. (1992) Brain-derived neurotrophic factor and neurotrophin 3 mRNAs in the peripheral target fields of developing inner ear ganglia. *Proc. Natl. Acad. Sci. USA*, 89: 9915–9919.

Prestige, M. (1967) The control of cell numbers in the spinal ganglia of *Xenopus laevis* tadpoles. *J. Embryol. Exp. Morphol.*, 17: 453–471.

Richardson, P.M. and Riopelle, R.J. (1984) Uptake of nerve growth factor along peripheral and spinal axons of primary sensory neurons. *J. Neurosci.*, 4: 1683–1689.

Richardson, P.M., Verge, V.M.K. and Riopelle, R.J. (1986) Distribution of neuronal receptors for nerve growth factor in the rat. *J. Neurosci.*, 6: 2312–2321.

Rodrigues-Tebar, A., Dechant, G., and Barde, Y.-A. (1990) Binding of brain-derived neurotrophic factor to the nerve growth factor receptor. *Neuron*, 4: 487–492.

Rodrigues-Tebar, A., Dechant, G., Götz, R. and Barde, Y.-A. (1992) Binding of neurotrophin 3 to trk neuronal receptors and interactions with nerve growth factor and brain-derived neurotrophic factor. *EMBO J.*, 11: 917–922.

Rosenthal, A., Goeddel, D.V., Nguyen, T., Lewis, M., Shih, A., Laramee, G.R., Nikolics, K. and Winslow, J.W. (1990) Primary structure and biological activity of a novel human neurotrophic factor. *Neuron*, 4: 767–773.

Schecterson, L.C. and Bothwell, M. (1992) Novel roles for neurotrophins are suggested by BDNF and NT3 mRNA expression in developing neurons. *Neuron*, 9: 449–463.

Schwab, M.E., Otten, U., Agid, Y. and Thoenen, H. (1979) Nerve growth factor (NGF) in the rat CNS: absence of specific retrograde axonal transport and tyrosine hydroxylase induction in locus coeruleus and substantia nigra. *Brain Res.*, 168: 473–483.

Seiler, M. and Schwab, M.E. (1984) Specific retrograde transport of nerve growth factor (NGF) from neocortex to nucleus basalis in the rat. *Brain Res.*, 300: 33–39.

Sendtner, M., Holtmann, B., Kolbeck, R., Thoenen, H. and Barde, Y. (1992) Brain-derived neurotrophic factor prevents the death of motoneurons in newborn rats after nerve section. *Nature (London)*, 360: 757–759.

Shelton, D.J. and Reichardt, L.F. (1984) Expression of the nerve growth factor gene correlates with the density of sympathetic innervation in effector organs. *Proc. Natl. Acad. Sci. USA*, 81: 7951–7955.

Sieber-Blum, M. (1991) Role of neurotrophic factors BDNF and NGF in commitment of pluripotent neural creast cells. *Neuron*, 6: 949–955.

Soppet, D., Escandon, E., Maragos, J., Middlemas, D.S., Reid, S. W., Blair, J., Burton, L.E., Stanton, B.R., Kaplan, D.R., Hunter, T., Nikolics, K. and Parada, L.F. (1991) The neurotrophic factors brain-derived neurotrophic factor and neurotrophin-3 are ligands for the trkB tyrosine kinase receptor. *Cell*, 65: 895–903.

Squinto, S.P., Stitt, T.N., Aldrich, T.H., Davis, S., Bianco, S.M., Radziejewski, C., Glass, D.J., Masiakowski, P., Furth, M.E., Valenzuela, D.M., DiStefano, P.S. and Yancopoulos, G.D. (1991) trkB encodes a functional receptor for brain-derived neurotrophic factor and neurotrophin-3 but not nerve growth factor. *Cell*, 65: 885–893.

Stainier, D. and Gilbert, W. (1991) Neuronal differentiation and maturation in the mouse trigeminal sensory system, in vivo and in vitro. *J. Comp. Neurol.*, 311: 300–312.

Stöckel, K. and Thoenen, H. (1975) Retrograde axonal transport of nerve growth factor and biological importance. *Brain Res.*, 85: 337–341.

Sutter, A., Riopelle, R.J., Harris-Warrick, R.M. and Shooter, E.M. (1979) Nerve growth factor receptors: characterization of two distinct classes of binding sites on chick embryo sensory ganglia cells. *J. Biol. Chem.*, 254: 5972–5982.

Von Bartheld, C., Patterson, S., Heuer, J., Wheeler, E., Bothwell, M. and Rubel, E. (1991) Expression of nerve growth factor (NGF) receptors in the developing inner ear of chick and rat. *Development*, 113: 455–470.

Wright, E.M., Vogel, K.S. and Davies, A.M. (1992) Neurotrophic factors promote the maturation of developing neurons before they become dependent on these factors. *Neuron*, 9: 139–150.

Wyatt, S., Shooter, E. and Davies, A. (1990) Expression of the NGF receptor gene in sensory neurons and their cutaneous target prior to and during innervation. *Neuron*, 2: 421–427.

Yan, Q., and Johnson, E.M., Jr. (1988) An immunohistochemical study of the nerve growth factor receptor in developing rats. J. *Neurosci.*, 8: 3481–3498.

Yan, Q., Elliot, J. and Snider, W.D. (1992) Brain-derived neurotrophic factor rescues spinal motor neurons from axotomy-induced cell death. *Nature (London)*, 360: 753–755.

F.J. Seil (Ed.)
Progress in Brain Research, Vol 103

CHAPTER 6

Distribution of acidic and basic fibroblast growth factors in the mature, injured and developing rat nervous system

Felix P. Eckenstein[1,2], Candace Andersson[1], Karl Kuzis[1] and William R. Woodward[2,3]

[1]*Department of Cell Biology and Anatomy,* [2]*Department of Neurology, and* [3]*Department of Biochemistry and Molecular Biology, Oregon Health Sciences University, Portland, OR 97201, U.S.A.*

Introduction

Fibroblast growth factors (FGFs) comprise a family of polypeptides ranging from about 16 kDa to about 30 kDa in molecular weight. Currently, nine members of this family are known (Burgess and Maciag, 1989; Marics et al., 1989; Haub et al., 1990; Miyamoto et al., 1993), which are structurally related as indicated by the 30–50% homology of their amino acid sequence. Interest in the neurobiology of FGFs was greatly stimulated by observations that two prominent members of this family, acidic and basic FGF (aFGF and bFGF, respectively), are present in the adult central nervous system (CNS) and that these two FGF family members can support the fiber outgrowth and survival of a variety of peripheral and central neurons in vitro. For example, such trophic effects of FGFs have been observed on neurons from cerebral cortex (Morrison et al., 1986), hippocampus (Walicke et al., 1986), retina (Lipton et al., 1988), cerebellum (Hatten et al., 1988), the septal area (Grothe et al., 1989), the ciliary ganglion (Unsicker et al., 1987; Eckenstein et al., 1990), and sympathetic and sensory ganglia (Eckenstein et al., 1990). In addition, application of exogenous FGF is able to rescue lesioned neurons from retrograde degeneration in vivo (Anderson et al., 1988). Also, as their name implies, FGFs are potent mitogens for fibroblasts and a variety of other other non-neuronal cells including astrocytes (Pettmann et al., 1985), oligodendrocytes (Eccleston and Silberberg, 1985) and Schwann cells (Davis and Stroobant, 1990).

Biological actions of the FGFs

The neurotrophic and mitogenic actions of the FGFs are mediated by a family of high affinity receptors (FGFRs). Currently, at least four different genes coding for FGFRs are known (referred to as FGFR1 to FGFR4). All FGFRs show substantial sequence homology and appear similar in their general structure (Dionne et al., 1990; Keegan et al., 1991; Partanen et al., 1991). For example, all four genes code for transmembrane molecules with one membrane spanning domain, and two or three extracellular immunoglobulin (Ig)-like domains. The intracellular aspect of all FGFRs contain a split tyrosine kinase domain, which is stimulated upon binding of FGFs to the extracellular domain of the receptor. Such receptor activation also involves dimerization and auto-tyrosine phosphorylation of the receptor. Interestingly, differential splicing of mRNA coding for FGFRs can result in a large number of different FGFRs being expressed from a single gene. For example, the first Ig-like domain of FGFR1 or FGFR2 can be removed by RNA splicing, resulting in the aforementioned two or three Ig domain forms of a given FGFR gene (Reid et al., 1990). Other important splice variants occur in the third Ig domain, where different exons can be employed to code for the part of the domain (Johnson et al., 1991). In addition, secreted FGFR splice variants that lack the transmembrane and intracellular aspects of FGFRs are known, as are variants lacking the extracellular domain. FGFR1 to FGFR4 appear to have distinct but overlapping ligand affinities for the different members of the FGF family (Ornitz and Leder, 1992), although this has not yet been exhaustively determined for all nine members of the FGF family. However, different genes may show significant selectivity for a subgroup of FGFs, with binding affinities varying as much as 20-fold. Differential splicing of a given receptor also appears to affect ligand binding. For example, the three Ig domain form of the FGFRs may show significantly lower affinity binding of FGFs then the two-domain form (Shi et al., 1993), and splice variants in the third Ig domain significantly affect the selectivity of binding of different FGFs to the receptor (Bottaro et al., 1990).

FGFs are known to bind not only to FGFRs but also to the sulfated glycosaminoglycan, heparin, and are also referred to as heparin binding growth factors (HBGFs). Interestingly, the biological action of FGFs appears to depend on the presence of extracellular heparin/heparan sulfate, as demonstrated by the observations that enzymatic removal of heparin/heparan sulfate from the cell surface or inhibition of sulfation both result in abolishing the mitogenic action of FGFs (Klagsbrun and Baird, 1991; Rapraeger et al., 1991; Yayon et al., 1991). These findings led to the hypothesis that binding to a cell surface heparan sulfate may lead to a change in FGF structure, resulting in the active conformation of FGF, which is then presented by a cell surface heparan sulfate proteoglycan (HSPG) to the transmembrane FGFR. It is currently unknown which of the characterized cell surface HSPGs can function in this manner, but syndecan (Kiefer et al., 1990) has been proposed as a candidate. It is possible that different HSPGs may exhibit differential abilities to activate different FGFs, as indicated by observations that aFGF often requires the presence of exogenous heparin in order to act on cells that respond to bFGF even in the absence of exogenous heparin (Eckenstein et al., 1991).

Thus, while many of the molecular features of the FGF system have become known over the last few years, the normal physiological role of FGFs is still not well understood. The main problem posed appears to be the relatively non-selective wide spectrum of mitogenic and neurotrophic activities of different FGFs observed in in vitro assays. For example, aFGF and bFGF have been shown to be highly potent neurotrophic factors for developing sympathetic neurons in vitro (Eckenstein et al., 1990), but the survival of the same neurons in vivo clearly depends on the availability of endogenous nerve growth factor (NGF), as the blocking of NGF action during development results in significant losses of sympathetic neurons. We have thus hypothesized that the specificity of FGF actions in vivo is defined primarily by a combination of when, where and how FGFs become available, and, secondly, by the pattern of expression of FGFRs and HSPGs by potential FGF responsive cells. In order to test this hypothesis, the pattern of distribution of FGFs and their extracellular availability have to be characterized. It is of particular interest in this regard that aFGF and bFGF, the main members of the FGF family present in CNS, lack hydrophobic signal sequences, which are thought to be necessary for the sorting of proteins into the secretory pathway (Walter and Lingappa, 1986). Indeed, the very abundance of aFGF and bFGF suggests that the main bulk of the factors may not be present in the extracellular space, but may be stored in an intracellular compartment (see Vlodavsky et al., 1991 for an opposing view). The following is a summary of our efforts to define FGF expression patterns in the rat CNS (Eckenstein et al., 1991; Stock et al., 1992; Woodward et al., 1992). Similar work has also been undertaken by other groups, resulting in observations both similar (Ferrara et al., 1988; Emoto et al., 1989; Elde et al., 1991; Gomez-Pinilla et al., 1992), and dissimilar (Pettmann et al., 1986; Unsicker et al., 1987; Grothe et al., 1991; Wilcox and Unnerstall, 1991) to ours. The likely reason behind such conflicts is the differing specificities of FGF probes used, and the interested reader is referred to Stock et al. (1992) for a more detailed discussion of this topic.

Analysis of the distribution of aFGF and bFGF in adult rat nervous system

A bioassay was developed in order to quantify the levels of aFGF- and bFGF-like activity in extracts prepared from CNS tissue. The assay consists of determining the potency of extracts in stimulating mitogenesis in a mouse fibroblast cell line, as measured by standard methods quantifying tritiated thymidine incorporation into DNA (Shipley, 1986). The main advantages of this assay are that it is reasonably simple, rapid and quantitative. In addition, the assay can be used to differentiate between aFGF and bFGF, as bFGF requires no exogenous heparin in order to be active in the assay, while aFGF activity depends on heparin (Eckenstein et al., 1991). Using this approach, we determined that bFGF-like bioactivity was relatively evenly distributed throughout the CNS, but not detectable in the peripheral nervous system (PNS). In contrast, aFGF-like bioactivity was very high in the periphery, such as sciatic nerve, and unevenly distributed in the CNS, with the highest aFGF levels being observed in spinal cord (Fig. 1). One interesting finding is that FGF levels, when expressed in biological units per gram of tissue, appears to be about 500 times (for bFGF) to 5000 times (for aFGF) higher than those of NGF in relevant tissues (for NGF data see Shelton and Reichardt, 1984; Korsching et al., 1985).

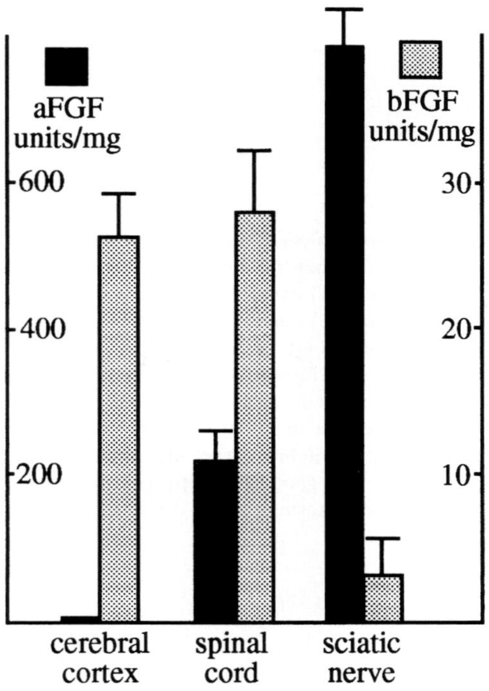

Fig. 1. The levels of aFGF- and bFGF-like biological activity in three areas of the adult rat nervous system are shown, as measured by bioassay (see text for details of assay). Note that similar levels of bFGF-like activity (shaded bars) are found in the two CNS areas shown (spinal cord and cerebral cortex), while the level of bFGF in the periphery (sciatic nerve) is very low. In contrast, aFGF-like activity (black bars) is very high in sciatic nerve, and the two CNS areas differ in their aFGF content, which is high in spinal cord and not detectable in cerebral cortex.

The primary weakness of the bioassay is that the cell line employed (AKR-2B) responds equally well to mitogens that are different from FGFs, such as epidermal growth factor (EGF) and platelet derived growth factor (PDGF). Therefore, additional experiments will always have to be performed in conjunction with this assay, in order to define the molecular identity of the mitogen. We performed Western blot experiments, using aFGF- and bFGF-specific antibodies, to determine the presence of these factors in extracts analysed by the bioassay. Figure 2

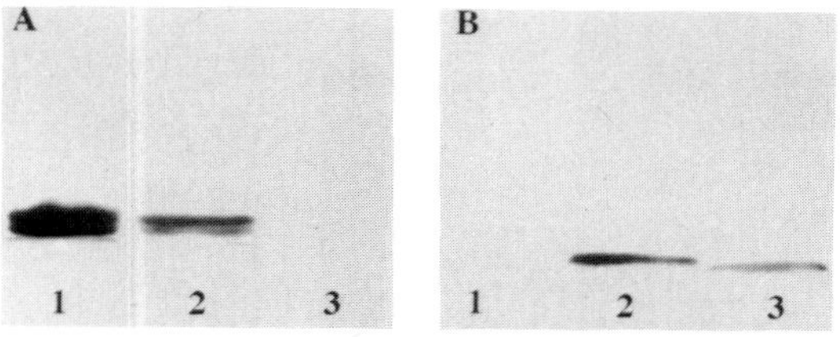

Fig. 2. A Western blot analysis of aFGF and bFGF presence in three areas of the adult rat nervous system is shown. Similar amounts of cerebral cortex (lane 1), spinal cord (lane 2) and sciatic nerve (lane 3) were extracted, and the presence of bFGF (panel A) and aFGF (panel B) in the extracts was characterized by heparin chromatography followed by Western blot analysis using aFGF- and bFGF-specific antibodies. Note that aFGF is present in spinal cord and sciatic nerve, while bFGF is present in cerebral cortex and spinal cord. This pattern of expression is in good agreement with the distribution of biological activity shown in Fig. 1. (From Eckenstein et al., 1991.)

shows that Western blot analysis indicates that the biological activity determined by bioassay indeed represented largely aFGF and bFGF. For example, bFGF immunoreactivity was found in all CNS areas analysed, whereas aFGF immunoreactivity was highest in spinal cord and sciatic nerve, and was not detectable in cerebral cortex. Additional conformation for the bioassay data was obtained by specific immunoprecipitation of aFGF and bFGF activity from extracts.

The effect of nerve transection on FGF levels

Both sciatic nerve and optic nerve transections were performed in adult rats in order to analyse whether the cellular changes induced by the lesions resulted in a regulation of FGF levels in the nerves. FGF levels were analysed by the bioassay method described above. Normal optic nerve appeared to contain mostly bFGF, in contrast to normal sciatic nerve, which contained bFGF exclusively. Interestingly, the lesion-affected FGF levels in the distal stump of the transected nerves in opposite directions: the high levels of aFGF were irreversibly and completely lost from sciatic nerve, while bFGF increased close to two-fold in optic nerve (Fig. 3). This differential regulation

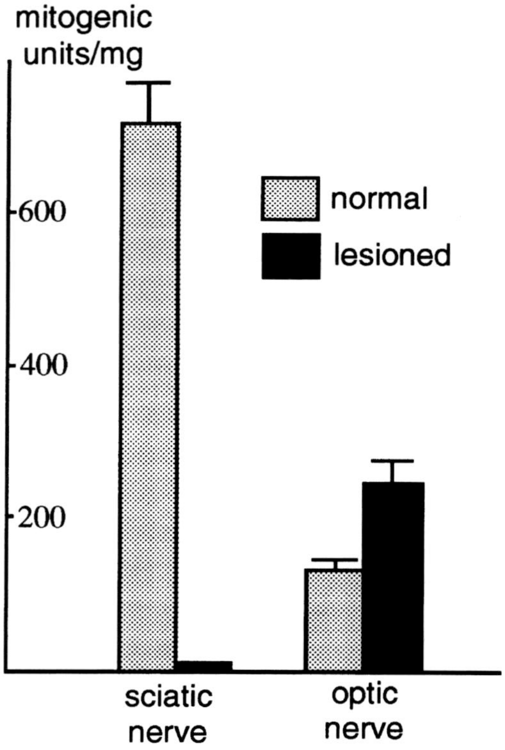

Fig. 3. The effect of transsection of a central (optic) nerve and a peripheral (sciatic) nerve on the overall levels of FGF-like activity in the distal stump seven days after the transection is shown. Levels of FGF-like bioactivity were quantified using a bioassay (see text for details of assay). Note that the lesion leads to the complete loss of FGF-like activity from the distal stump of sciatic nerve, while causing a significant increase in FGF-like activity in the optic nerve. The activity in optic nerve exhibits predominantly bFGF characteristics, while the activity in sciatic nerve has aFGF characteristics (not shown).

likely reflects the fact that aFGF appears to be expressed by specific neuronal populations, and bFGF by astrocytes, as detected by immunohistochemical methods (see below).

Immunohistochemical localization of aFGF in adult rat brain

Immunohistochemical localization of specific members of a polypeptide family that exhibits significant sequence homology is made difficult by the possibility that antibodies prepared against one family member may cross-react with other members. To rule out such a problem, we preadsorbed the antiserum used for aFGF immunohistochemistry with bFGF (the most closely related family member), and demonstrated that such preadsorption did not affect results observed (Stock et al., 1992). Immunoreactivity for aFGF was observed exclusively in specific populations of neurons, including their axons and dendrites. No staining of non-neuronal cells was observed. The strongest aFGF immunoreactivity was found in all motor neurons and the primary sensory neurons in the mesencephalon. Several other neuronal populations also contained significant aFGF immunoreactivity, including basal forebrain cholinergic neurons, the caudate nucleus and neurons the substantia nigra (Fig. 4; see Stock et al., 1992 for details). Only a low number of isolated aFGF-positive neurons were found in cerebral cortex and hippocampus. This distribution of aFGF-positive neurons is in good agreement with the levels of aFGF detected by bioassay and Western blot, as described above.

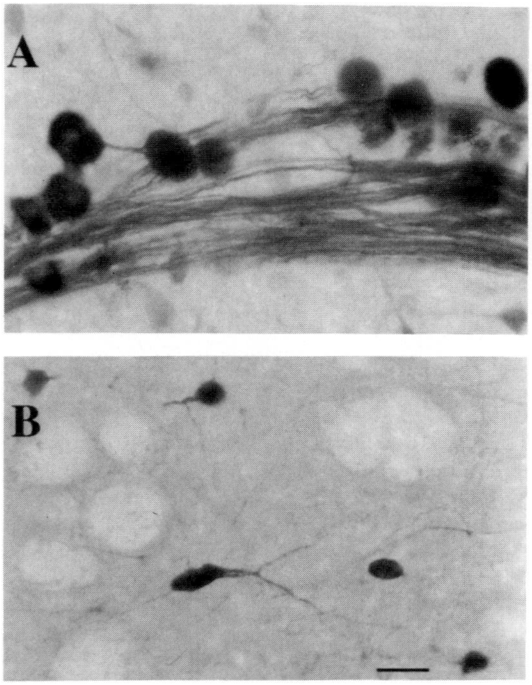

Fig. 4. Immunohistochemical localization of aFGF in coronal sections of rat brain is illustrated. An immunoperoxidase method was used for detection of aFGF. Panel A shows intensely labeled primary sensory neurons and their axons in the mesencephalic trigeminal nucleus. Panel B demonstrates the strong aFGF staining observed in a population of large neurons in the caudate nucleus. aFGF immunoreactivity is evenly distributed throughout the cytoplasm of the labeled cells, including dendrites and axons. Bar equals 20 μm.

Immunohistochemical detection of bFGF in the adult rat brain

bFGF immunoreactivity was localized using a monoclonal antibody that does not cross-react with aFGF (Eckenstein et al., 1991; a gift from Dr C. Hart). In all areas of the CNS, relatively small cells contained bFGF immunoreactivity. These cells were identified as astrocytes by double immunofluorescent localization of bFGF and the astrocyte marker, glial fibrillary acidic polypeptide (GFAP, Fig. 5). A specific neuronal population in the CA2 area of hippocampus was also bFGF-positive (Fig. 6), and additionally, more faintly stained neurons were observed in the cingulate cortex. Surprisingly, bFGF staining appeared stronger over the nucleus of labeled cells, but, although faint, was also detectable in their cytoplasm (Woodward et al., 1992). In addition, bFGF label in cultured astrocytes was also found to be mostly nuclear, with particularly heavy labeling of presumptive nucleoli in many cells (Fig. 7). Nuclear extracts prepared from adult rat brain also contained high levels of bFGF bioactivity and immunoreactivity, as detected by bioassay and Western blot (Fig. 8; see also Woodward et al., 1992). Three forms of bFGF (18, 21.5 and 22.5 kDa in molecular weight) were present in the cytoplasmic fraction, whereas only the two larger forms were found in the nuclear fraction. The three different forms of bFGF are known to be synthesized through use of alternate initiation of translation, with the two larger forms possessing nuclear translocation sequences (Florkiewicz and Sommer, 1989; Bugler et al., 1991).

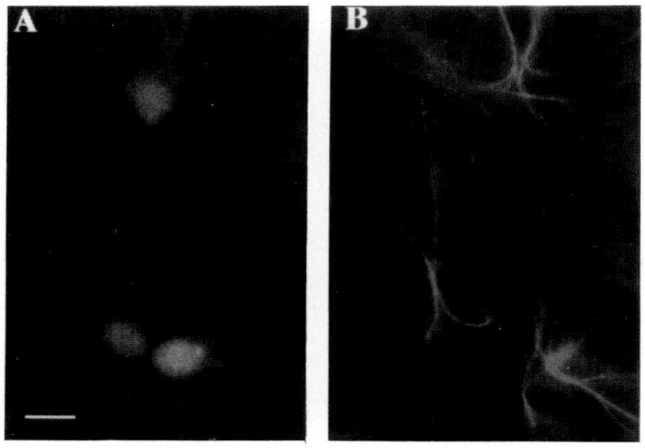

Fig. 5. Double immunofluorescence staining for bFGF (panel A, using a mouse monoclonal antibody to bFGF, followed by a fluorescein labeled anti-mouse antibody) and GFAP (panel B, using a rabbit antiserum to GFAP, followed by a rhodamine-labeled anti-rabbit antibody) is shown in a section through adult rat entorhinal cortex. All bFGF-positive cells are astrocytes, as they also contain GFAP immunoreactivity. bFGF immunoreactivity appears especially strong over the nuclei of GFAP-positive cells, but bFGF immunoreactivity is also observed in the processes of the cells. Bar equals 8 μm. (Modified from Woodward et al., 1992.)

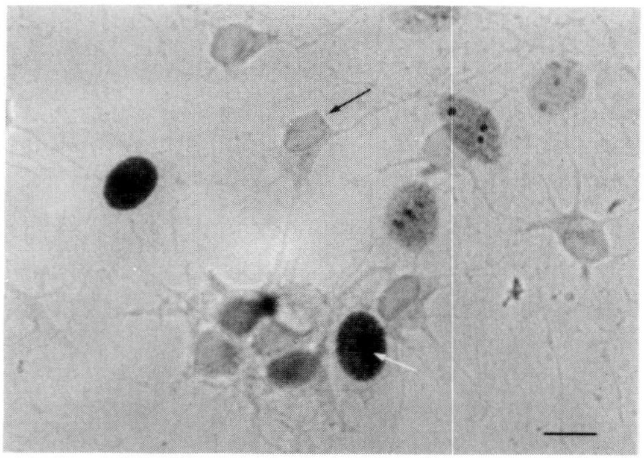

Fig. 7. Immunohistochemical localization of bFGF in cultured astrocytes is shown, using an immunoperoxidase method for bFGF detection. This photomicrograph was taken using phase contrast optics in order to visualize both bFGF-positive (white arrow) and bFGF-negative cells (solid black arrow). bFGF immunoreactivity appears to be most intense in large flat cells with the morphology of type 1 astrocytes. In these cells, staining appears confined to the area of the nucleus, with particularly intense immunoreactivity in the putative nucleolus. The unstained cells appear to have long processes indicative of type 2 astrocytes. Cells of either morphology were found to be GFAP-positive in parallel experiments (not shown).

The developmental distribution of aFGF and bFGF

The bioassay, Western blot and immunohistochemical tools described above were used in conjunction for analysing the distribution of the two FGFs during development. No detectable aFGF or bFGF bioactivity was found in the CNS at embryonic days 16 and 18 (E16 and E18), with very low levels being detectable at the day of birth. From then on, FGF levels were found to show a continuous increase until adult levels are reached at postnatal day 28 (P28). Similar data were obtained by Western blot. In general, the distribution of aFGF during all the analysed times (E16, E18, P0, P17, P14, P21, P28) reflected that seen in adult animals, with spinal cord showing the highest levels, followed by midbrain, while levels in cerebellum and forebrain were low. A more detailed picture emerged from immunohistochemical analysis. The onset of detectable aFGF immunoreactivity being present in specific neuronal populations was very distinct. The first neurons to become aFGF-positive were mesencephalic sensory neurons (by E18), followed by

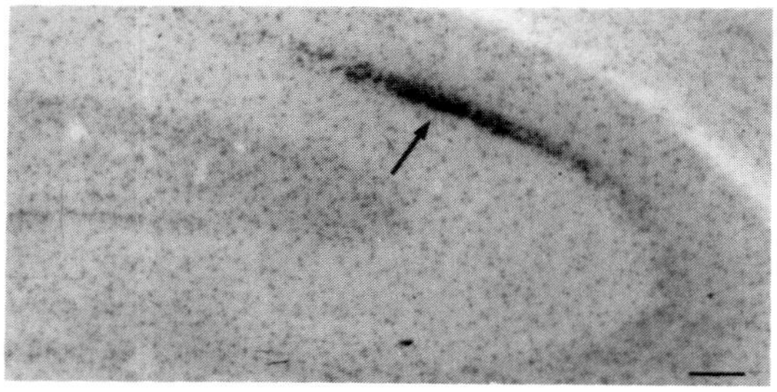

Fig. 6. Immunohistochemical localization of bFGF is shown in coronal section through adult rat hippocampus, using an immunoperoxidase method for bFGF detection. Numerous small, round profiles are stained in all areas of hippocampus. These profiles represent the nuclei of astrocytes, as shown in Fig. 5. Intense bFGF immunoreactivity is also found in neurons in area CA2 (indicated by a solid arrow). Bar equals 250 μm.

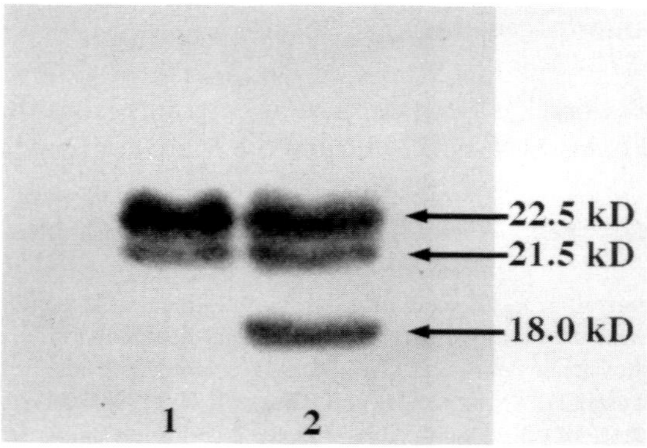

Fig. 8. Analysis by Western blot of the presence of bFGF in nuclear (lane 1) and cytoplasmic (lane 2) fractions prepared from adult rat brain. Three specific forms of bFGF are detected (22.5 kDa, 21.5 kDa and 18 kDa in molecular weight). The 18-kDa form, which lacks a nuclear translocation signal, is present exclusively in the cytoplasmic fraction. (From Woodward et al., 1992.)

motor neurons and septal cholinergic neurons (by P0), and most other neuronal populations, including the one in the substantia nigra (by P7). Adult levels of aFGF immunoreactivity were observed by P7 in the sensory neurons, by P14 in motor neurons and between P21 and P28 in all other labeled groups. No cellular populations were observed that showed transient expression of aFGF immunoreactivity during development, as only neuronal populations labeled in the adult were found to be aFGF-positive at the developmental time points analysed.

bFGF bioactivity was also not detectable before the day of birth, and showed a constant increase from then on in all four CNS areas, reaching adult levels between P21 and P28, a time course that is consistent with the maturation of astrocytes throughout the CNS. bFGF immunoreactivity was first detected in CA2 hippocampal neurons at P0, followed by the staining of hippocampal astrocytes at P7 and of all other astrocytes at P14. Adult levels of immunoreactivity appeared to be present in all labeled cells by P28.

The levels of mRNAs coding for FGFR1 and FGFR2 were analysed by Northern blot methods in spinal cord, midbrain/medulla, cerebellum and forebrain during the same time points. Both FGFR1 and FGFR2 were found to be expressed at detectable to significant levels in all areas at all times.

Discussion

In summary, the results presented above indicate that aFGF and bFGF are expressed in non-overlapping cellular populations in the CNS, with bFGF being present in most, if not all, astrocytes and a specific hippocampal neuronal population, and aFGF being present in a select set of neurons, including some that are at risk for neurodegenerative diseases such as Alzheimer's disease (magnocellular forebrain cholinergic neurons), Parkinson's disease (substantia nigra neurons) and amyotrophic lateral sclerosis (motor neurons). In addition, the levels of aFGF and bFGF in normal adult CNS are exceedingly high, so high indeed that if all the FGF were available in the extracellular space, it would be sufficient to activate all the FGFRs present in brain. This is unlikely, and common indicators of FGF action, such as astrocyte mitogenesis, are rare in adult CNS. Thus it seems likely that aFGF and bFGF are stored in intracellular compartments, such as the cytoplasm or the nucleus (for the larger forms of bFGF). The factors are likely to become available in the extracellular space after compromise of the cell membrane caused by a variety of events, such as mechanical injury, neurodegenerative disease and stroke. In support of this notion, we have, in a preliminary study, not been able to detect bFGF release from healthy astrocytes in vitro, although high levels of bFGF could be extracted from the cultures by detergent treatment. Clearly, more extensive studies will be required to fully determine the mode of release of bFGF and aFGF from astrocytes and neurons.

During development, both aFGF and bFGF appear to be expressed at high levels in the CNS only after the period of programmed cell death (PCD) has passed. It is possible that the onset of aFGF expression correlates with the termination of PCD. However, in motor neurons, PCD appears to have ceased well before reasonably high levels of aFGF are detected in the cells. It is interesting in this regard that postnatal motor neurons remain vulnerable to injury for a time span past PCD, as demonstrated by observations that motor neurons axotomized in a newborn rat will die, while they will regenerate in an adult animal (Sendtner et al., 1990). As motor neuron survival in vitro can be supported by FGFs (Arakawa et al., 1990; Hughes et al., 1993), it is possible that aFGF leaking from an injured motor neuron may be involved in initiating repair responses in the motor neuron in an autocrine manner. Simultaneously, this aFGF may also initiate additional responses in neighboring Schwann cells, possibly including the regulation of NGF and ciliary neurotrophic factor (CNTF). A similar hypothesis can be formulated for bFGF which may leak from injured mature astrocytes, resulting in the stimulation of mitogenesis in astrocytes and the survival of neurons adjacent to the injured astrocyte. Such a model hypothesis suggests that the main function of aFGF and bFGF may be the early signaling of injury affecting specific cell types, which initiates a widespread repair program. In this model, the source of FGF is likely to disappear significantly before the termination of a repair response, as the plasma membrane of the injured cell will either seal or the cell will die. Thus, FGFs may not function to guide any specific repair process to the end, a role which is more likely to be filled by other growth factors. This model is in good agreement with the observed widespread actions of FGFs and the likely intracellular localization of aFGF and bFGF.

In contrast to aFGF and bFGF, FGFRs are expressed in the developing nervous system during periods of neurogenesis and PCD (Heuer et al., 1990; Wanaka et al., 1991). It is possible that these FGFRs mediate the action of other members of the FGF family which may be expressed in relevant tissues during these earlier developmental time points.

Acknowledgements

This work has been supported by grants from the NIH (AG7424, NS17493) and the March of Dimes.

References

Anderson, K.J., Dam, D., Lee, S. and Cotman, C.W. (1988) Basic fibroblast growth factor prevents death of lesioned cholinergic neurons in vivo. *Nature (London)*, 332: 360–361.

Arakawa, Y., Sendtner, M. and Thoenen, H. (1990) Survival effect of ciliary neurotrophic factor (CNTF) on chick embryonic motoneurons in culture: comparison with other neurotrophic factors and cytokines. *J. Neurosci.*, 10: 3507–3515.

Bottaro, D.P., Rubin, J.S., Ron, D., Finch, P.W., Florio, C. and Aaronson, S.A. (1990) Characterization of the receptor for keratinocyte growth factor. Evidence for multiple fibroblast growth factor receptors. *J. Biol. Chem.*, 265: 12767–12770.

Bugler, B., Amalric, F. and Prats, H. (1991) Alternative initiation of translation determines cytoplasmic or nuclear localization of basic fibroblast growth factor. *Mol. Cell. Biol.*, 11: 573–577.

Burgess, W.H. and Maciag, T. (1989) The heparin-binding (fibroblast) growth factor family of proteins. *Annu. Rev. Biochem.*, 58: 575–606.

Davis, J.B. and Stroobant, P. (1990) Platelet-derived growth factors and fibroblast growth factors are mitogens for rat Schwann cells. *J. Cell Biol.*, 110: 1353–1360.

Dionne, C.A., Crumley, G., Bellot, F., Kaplow, J.M., Searfoss, G., Ruta, M., Burgess, W.H., Jaye, M. and Schlessinger, J. (1990) Cloning and expression of two distinct high-affinity receptors cross-reacting with acidic and basic fibroblast growth factors. *EMBO J.*, 9: 2685–2692.

Eccleston, P.A. and Silberberg, D.H. (1985) Fibroblast growth factor is a mitogen for oligodendrocytes in vitro. *Brain Res.*, 353: 315–318.

Eckenstein, F.P., Esch, F., Holbert, T., Blacher, R.W. and Nishi, R. (1990) Purification and characterization of a trophic factor for embryonic peripheral neurons: Comparison with fibroblast growth factors. *Neuron*, 4: 623–631.

Eckenstein, F.P., Shipley, G.D. and Nishi, R. (1991) Acidic and basic fibroblast growth factors in the nervous system: distribution and differential alteration of levels after injury of central versus peripheral nerve. *J. Neurosci.*, 11: 412–419.

Elde, R., Cao, Y., Cintra, A., Brelje, T.C., Pelto, H.M., Junttila, T., Fuxe, K., Pettersson, R.F. and Hökfelt, T. (1991) Prominent expression of acidic fibroblast growth factor in motor and sensory neurons. *Neuron*, 7: 349–364.

Emoto, N., Gonzalez, A.-M., Walicke, P.A., Wada, E., Simmons, D.M., Shimasaki, S. and Baird, A. (1989) Basic fibroblast growth factor (FGF) in the central nervous system: identification of specific loci of basic FGF expression in the rat brain. *Growth Factors*, 2: 21–29.

Ferrara, N., Ousley, F. and Gospodarowicz, D. (1988) Bovine brain astrocytes express basic fibroblast growth factor, a neurotropic and angiogenic mitogen. *Brain Res.*, 462: 223–232.

Florkiewicz, R.Z. and Sommer, A. (1989) Human basic fibroblast growth factor gene encodes four polypeptides: three initiate translation from non-AUG codons. *Proc. Natl. Acad. Sci. USA*, 86: 3978–3981.

Gomez-Pinilla, F., Lee, J.W. and Cotman, C.W. (1992) Basic FGF in adult rat brain: cellular distribution and response to entorhinal lesion and fimbria-fornix transsection. *J. Neurosci.*, 12: 345–355.

Grothe, C., Otto, D. and Unsicker, K. (1989) Basic fibroblast growth factor promotes in vitro survival and cholinergic development of rat septal neurons: comparison with the effects of nerve growth factor. *Neuroscience*, 31: 649–661.

Grothe, C., Zachmann, K. and Unsicker, K. (1991) Basic FGF-like immunoreactivity in the developing and adult rat brainstem. *J. Comp. Neurol.*, 305: 328–336.

Hatten, M.E., Lynch, M., Rydel, R.E., Sanchez, J., Joseph, S.J., Moscatelli, D. and Rifkin, D.B. (1988) In vitro neurite extension by granule neurons is dependent upon astroglial-derived fibroblast growth factor. *Dev. Biol.*, 125: 280–289.

Haub, O., Drucker, B. and Goldfarb, M. (1990) Expression of the murine fibroblast growth factor 5 gene in the adult central nervous system. *Proc. Natl. Acad. Sci. USA*, 87: 8022–8026.

Heuer, J.G., von Bartheld, C.S., Kinoshita, Y., Evers, P.C. and Bothwell, M. (1990) Alternating phases of FGF receptor and NGF receptor expression in the developing chicken nervous system. *Neuron*, 5: 283–296.

Hughes, R.A., Sendtner, M., Goldfarb, M., Lindholm, D. and Thoenen, H. (1993) Evidence that fibroblast growth factor 5 is a major muscle-derived survival factor for cultured spinal motoneurons. *Neuron*, 10: 369–377.

Johnson, D.E., Lu, J., Chen, H., Werner, S. and Williams, L.T. (1991) The human fibroblast growth factor receptor genes: a common structural arrangement underlies the mechanisms for generating receptor forms that differ in their third immunoglobulin domain. *Mol. Cell. Biol.*, 11: 4627–4634.

Keegan, K., Johnson, D.E., Williams, L.T. and Hayman, M.J. (1991) Isolation of an additional member of the fibroblast growth factor receptor family, FGFR-3. *Proc. Natl. Acad. Sci. USA*, 88: 1095–1099.

Kiefer, M.C., Stephans, J.C., Crawford, K., Okino, K. and Barr, P.J. (1990) Ligand-affinity cloning and structure of a cell surface heparan sulfate proteoglycan that binds basic fibroblast growth factor. *Proc. Natl. Acad. Sci. USA*, 87: 6985–6989.

Klagsbrun, M. and Baird, A. (1991) A dual receptor system is required for basic fibroblast growth factor activity. *Cell*, 67: 229–231.

Korsching, S., Auburger, G., Heumann, R., Scott, J. and Thoenen, H. (1985) Levels of nerve growth factor and its mRNA in the central nervous system of the rat correlate with cholinergic innervation. *EMBO J.*, 4: 1389–1393.

Lipton, S.A., Wagner, J.A., Madison, R.D. and D'Amore, P.A. (1988) Acidic fibroblast growth factor enhances regeneration of processes by postnatal mammalian retinal ganglion cells in culture. *Proc. Natl. Acad. Sci. USA*, 85: 2388–2392.

Marics, I., Adelaide, J., Raybaud, F., Mattei, M.-G., Coulier, F., Planche, J., De Lapeyriere, O. and Birnbaum, D. (1989) Characterization of the HST-related FGF 6 gene, a new member of the fibroblast growth factor gene family. *Oncogene*, 4: 335–340.

Miyamoto, M., Naruo, K., Seko, C., Matsumoto, S., Kondo, T. and Kurokawa, T. (1993) Molecular cloning of a novel cytokine cDNA encoding the ninth member of the fibroblast growth factor family, which has a unique secretion property. *Mol. Cell. Biol.*, 13: 4251–4259.

Morrison, R.S., Sharma, A., deVellis, J. and Bradshaw, R.A. (1986) Basic fibroblast growth factor supports the survival of cerebral cortical neurons in primary culture. *Proc. Natl. Acad. Sci. USA*, 83: 7537–7541.

Ornitz, D.M. and Leder, P. (1992) Ligand specificity and heparin dependence of fibroblast growth factors receptors 1 and 3. *J. Biol. Chem.*, 267: 16305–16311.

Partanen, J., Mèkelè, T.P., Eerola, E., Korhonen, J., Hirvonen, H., Claesson, W.L. and Alitalo, K. (1991) FGFR-4, a novel acidic fibroblast growth factor receptor with a distinct expression pattern. *EMBO J.*, 10: 1347–1354.

Pettmann, B., Weibel, M., Sensenbrenner, M. and Labourdette, G. (1985) Purification of two astroglial growth factors from bovine brain. *FEBS Lett.*, 189(1): 102–108.

Pettmann, B., Labourdette, G., Weibel, M. and Sensenbrenner, M. (1986) The brain fibroblast growth factor (FGF) is localized in neurons. *Neurosci. Lett.*, 68: 175–180.

Rapraeger, A.C., Krufka, A. and Olwin, B.B. (1991) Requirement of heparan sulfate for bFGF-mediated fibroblast growth and myoblast differentiation. *Science*, 252: 1705–1708.

Reid, H.H., Wilks, A.F. and Bernard, O. (1990) Two forms of the basic fibroblast growth factor receptor-like mRNA are expressed in the developing mouse brain. *Proc. Natl. Acad. Sci. USA*, 87: 1596–1600.

Sendtner, M., Kreutzberg, G.W. and Thoenen, H. (1990) Ciliary neurotrophic factor prevents the degeneration of motor neurons after axotomy. *Nature (London)*, 345: 440–441.

Shelton, D.L. and Reichardt, L.F. (1984) Expression of the beta-nerve growth factor gene correlates with the density of sympathetic innervation in effector organs. *Proc. Natl. Acad. Sci. USA*, 81: 7951–7955.

Shi, E., Kan, M., Xu, J., Wang, F., Hou, J. and McKeehan, W.L. (1993) Control of fibroblast growth factor receptor kinase signal transduction by heterodimerization of combinatorial splice variants. *Mol. Cell. Biol.*, 13: 3907–3918.

Shipley, G.D. (1986) A serum-free [3H] thymidine incorporation assay for the detection of transforming growth factors. *J. Tiss. Cult. Methods*, 10: 117–123.

Stock, A., Kuzis, K., Woodward, W.R., Nishi, R. and Eckenstein, F. (1992) Localization of acidic fibroblast growth factor in specific subcortical neuronal populations. *J. Neurosci.*, 12: 4688–4700.

Unsicker, K., Reichert-Preibsh, H., Schmidt, R., Pettmann, B., Labourdette, G. and Sensenbrenner, M. (1987) Astroglial and fibroblast growth factors have neurotrophic functions for cultured peripheral and central nervous system neurons. *Proc. Natl. Acad. Sci. USA*, 84: 5459–5463.

Vlodavsky, I., Fuks, Z., Ishai, M.R., Bashkin, P., Levi, E., Korner, G., Bar, S.R. and Klagsbrun, M. (1991) Extracellular matrix-resident basic fibroblast growth factor: implication for the control of angiogenesis. *J. Cell. Biochem.*, 45: 167–176.

Walicke, P., Cowan, W.M., Ueno, N., Baird, A. and Guillemin, R. (1986) Fibroblast growth factor promotes survival of dissociated hippocampal neurons and enhances neurite extension. *Proc. Natl. Acad. Sci. USA*, 83: 3012–3016.

Walter, P. and Lingappa, V.R. (1986) Mechanisms of protein translocation across the endoplasmic reticulum membrane. *Annu. Rev. Cell. Biol.*, 2: 499–516.

Wanaka, A., Milbrandt, J. and Johnson, E.J. (1991) Expression of FGF receptor gene in rat development. *Development*, 111: 455–468.

Wilcox, B.J. and Unnerstall, J.R. (1991) Expression of acidic fibroblast growth factor mRNA in the developing and adult rat brain. *Neuron*, 6: 397–409.

Woodward, W.R., Nishi, R., Meshul, C.K., Williams, T.E., Coulombe, M. and Eckenstein, F.P. (1992) Nuclear and cytoplasmic localization of basic fibroblast growth factor in astrocytes and CA2 hippocampal neurons. *J. Neurosci.*, 12: 142–152.

Yayon, A., Klagsbrun, M., Esko, J.D., Leder, P. and Ornitz, D.M. (1991) Cell surface, heparin-like molecules are required for binding of basic fibroblast growth factor to its high affinity receptor. *Cell*, 64: 841–848.

SECTION II

Axonal Outgrowth and Pathfinding

F.J. Seil (Ed.)
Progress in Brain Research, Vol 103

CHAPTER 7

Axonal outgrowth and pathfinding

Lynn Landmesser

Department of Neurosciences, Case Western Reserve University, School of Medicine, Cleveland, OH 44106-4975, U.S.A.

Introduction

During development many neurons must extend axons over relatively long distances to reach their proper target regions, where they then branch and form synapses with appropriate postsynaptic cells. During these initial stages of axonogenesis, the nerve cells are in a growth mode producing large amounts of cytoskeletal components such as tubulin and other growth associated proteins. In addition they must have on their cell surfaces the receptors and other cell adhesion/signaling molecules that allow their growth cones both to extend and to navigate by reading a variety of extrinsic guidance cues (for reviews see Bixby and Harris, 1991; Goodman and Shatz, 1993). Upon making synaptic contacts, many of the genes for these growth associated proteins are downregulated. Thus for a mature axon to regenerate, it must be switched into a growth mode for a period of time that is correlated with the length of the axon to be regenerated. We know today that some mature mammalian central nervous system (CNS) neurons can be induced to grow long distances (So and Aguayo, 1985; Carter et al., 1994), and as more is learned about the signals regulating the relevant genes, this growth process should be able to be enhanced. However, it is legitimate to question the extent to which initial axon outgrowth, studied either in the embryo or in culture, can serve as a useful model for regeneration.

Clearly there are a number of differences. First, the distances over which the axons must grow and detect signals differ. Many major fiber tracts, both in the periphery and in the CNS, are laid down over millimeters rather than centimeters. Some extrinsic guidance mechanisms that are known to operate during embryogenesis, such as chemotaxis (Lumsden, 1992; Tessier-Lavigne, 1992), operate effectively only over millimeters. Secondly, many neural cell adhesion molecules are developmentally regulated in both space and time (Bixby and Harris, 1991). For example, TAG-1 (Dodd et al., 1988), SC-1/DM-GRASP (Burns et al., 1991; Tanaka et al., 1991), and polysialic acid on NCAM (Landmesser et al., 1990; Tang et al., 1992) are downregulated on some classes of neurons shortly after they form their initial projections. We do not yet know if these and other as yet uncharacterized molecules are always reexpressed following axotomy. Furthermore, even if axotomy were to reinduce expression of all the relevant molecules, the environment encountered by the regenerating axons is very different. In the periphery, embryonic axons often navigate through a loose array of relatively undifferentiated mesenchyme cells, with many naked axons growing in close apposition to other axons while presumptive glial cells are sparse (Tosney and Landmesser, 1985). In contrast, following axotomy, growth cones must navigate down old Schwann cell tubes. In the CNS there are obvious changes in the glial environment, with mature oligodendrocytes and central myelin being inhibitory to growth cones (Bandtlow et al., 1990, 1993). A clear change in the ability of chick spinal cord neurons to regenerate and restore locomotor ability is at least correlated with the onset of myelination (Steeves et al., 1994).

Despite these differences, there is little doubt that a better understanding of the cellular mechanisms used by embryonic growth cones to establish their initial projections will enable us better to enhance appropriate regeneration. In the last 5 years, major strides have been made in determining the molecules involved in cell adhesion and recognition and how these transduce specific signals to allow both axon outgrowth and pathfinding. The following four chapters provide good examples of the advances that have been made. They also illustrate the complexity of the growth cone, which is capable of transducing and integrating multiple signals, both positive and negative. This chapter will present a brief overview of our current understanding of this fascinating structure first described and christened by Ramón y Cajal (1890) some 100 years ago.

Growth cone motility and the cytoskeleton

Three classes of cytoskeletal elements are believed to be important for growth cone advance: actin, myosin, and microtubules. Bundles of actin filaments extend to the tips of filopodia and the more sheet-like lamellipodia and are the basis for their protrusive motility, since cytochalasin, a drug which results in actin depolymerization, causes alteration of the growth cone structure and cessation of this type of motility (Letourneau et al., 1987). However, to sustain axon elongation, microtubules must continue to advance into the base of the growth cone, either by translocation or by new polymerization onto the distally directed, plus ends of the microtubules (Joshi and Bass, 1993). Much more remains to be known about how these two cytoskeletal components interact with each other, with molecules in the plasma membrane, and with myosin (Bridgman and Daily, 1989; Bridgman et al., Ch. 10, this volume) to provide the forces that actually allow the growth cone to advance over a substratum.

Even more challenging is to understand how growth cones alter their direction in response to extrinsic guidance cues. Although the growth cone must make some form of 'adhesive' contacts to move forward, the more classical idea, that growth cones turned because filopodia on one side adhered more strongly, is not consistent with more recent evidence. Instead, filopodia are thought to act as sensors and to signal in some way growth cone reorientation. Work by Goldberg and his colleagues on *Aplysia* growth cones (Goldberg et al., 1992; Goldberg and Wu, Ch. 8 this volume) showed that those filopodia and lamellipodia in contact with a more favorable substratum became preferentially filled by microtubules and other organelles from the core of the growth cone, and thus resulted in a change of direction. More recent observations on grasshopper neuron pathfinding in the embryo indicate that filopodial contact with a specific guidepost cell causes microtubules to selectively enter that filopodium (Sabry et al., 1991). This is preceded by a swelling of the base of that filopodium associated with accumulation of filamentous actin (O'Connor and Bentley, 1993), suggesting a critical role for actin in this process. This view is consistent with recent observations of cultured *Aplysia* neurons (Lin and Forscher, 1993). The role played by myosin in these processes is not yet clear.

Mechanisms and molecules involved in growth cone advance and guidance

Growth cones can advance and reorient to guidance cues fixed on the surfaces or extracellular matrix of neurons, glia, muscle, or other cells along their pathway. Alternatively, they can also orient via chemotaxis to gradients of diffusible substances. Several recent reviews discuss the evidence for these mechanisms and what is known of their molecular basis (Bixby and Harris, 1991; Goodman and Shatz, 1993).

A large number of fixed adhesion molecules have now been identified on growing axons. These can be divided into several major classes. The first contains Ca^{2+}-independent, immunoglobulin-like molecules that include L1, TAG-1/axonin-1, and NCAM (Fig. 1). These molecules can bind in a homophilic manner to the same molecule on another cell, and in some cases heterophilically to other ligands, to either cause a growth cone to fasciculate or to advance. Although they are capable of mediating adhesion, many recent observations indicate that they can also act by triggering intracellular signaling cascades (Doherty and Walsh, 1992). A second class of molecules are the Ca^{2+}-dependent cadherins which are present on many neurons and on muscle (Takeichi, 1991). Finally, a variety of heterodimeric integrins on the growth cone can interact with laminin and/or fibronectin in the extracellular matrix (Reichardt and Tomaselli, 1991). Many of these molecules exist in multiple isoforms which are developmentally regulated in both space and time, leading to the suggestion that the various isoforms may play somewhat different roles and pointing to the complexity of the situation at the molecular level.

Important advances in understanding how these molecules function have come from studying them in highly simplified systems; for example, a growth cone translocating on a substratum composed of a single molecule (Lemmon et al., 1992) or on cells transfected with a single adhesion molecule or isoform (Doherty et al., 1991). However, most growth cones have many of these molecules present at the same time; for example, dorsal root ganglion (DRG) sensory neurons have L1, NCAM, TAG-1/axonin-1, SC1/BEN/DM-GRASP, *N*-cadherin and integrin all present at the time of initial outgrowth. Thus it is also necessary to

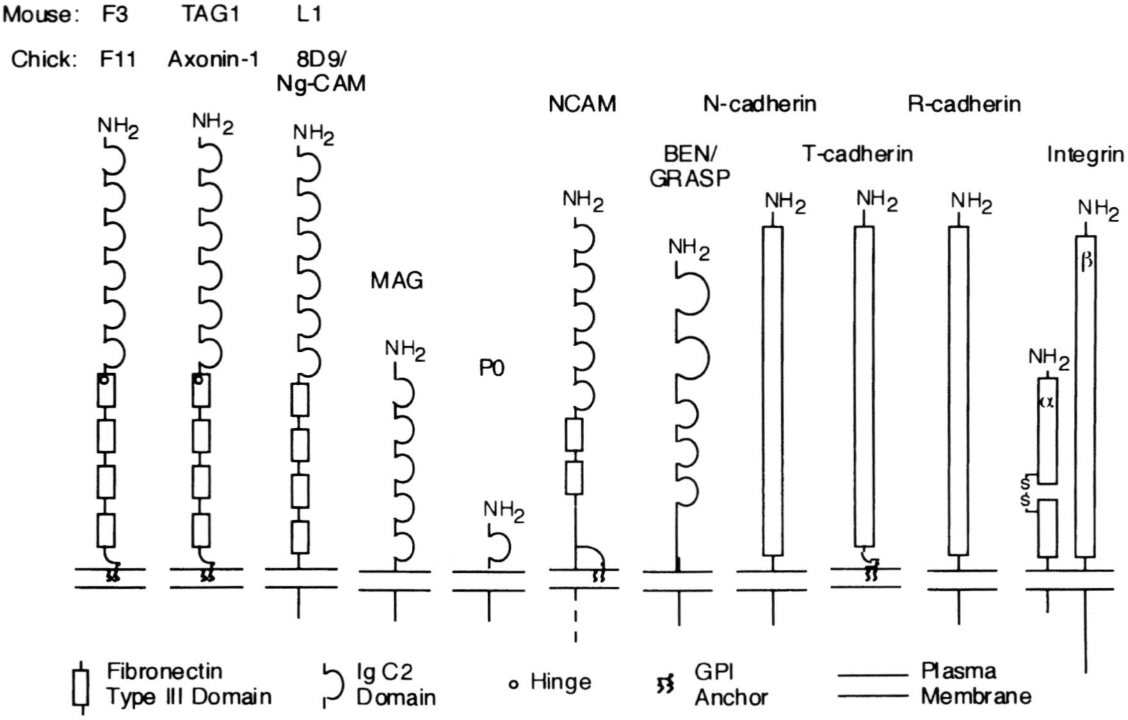

Fig. 1. Examples of the major classes of cell adhesion/recognition/signaling molecules of importance in neural development. Reproduced by courtesy of Vance Lemmon.

determine how these molecules act in the context of the intact organism, since they may interact with each other in complex and as yet unknown ways. The mere presence of a molecule on a growth cone does not mean that it is playing a role in growth cone advance, fasciculation or guidance. Therefore determining the effect of perturbing the function of such molecules in situ, either by antibodies (Landmesser et al., 1988, 1990; Tang et al., 1992), or by genetic means (Tomasiewicz et al., 1993), will remain important goals.

Growth cones can also orient via chemotaxis to gradients of diffusible factors. The first clear evidence of this in normal development was the demonstration that maxillary neurons could orient toward a factor coming from the jaw mesenchyme (Lumsden and Davies, 1986; see Lumsden, 1992 and Tessier-Lavigne, 1992 for reviews). Commissural spinal neurons have also been shown to exhibit chemotaxis toward the floorplate (Tessier-Lavigne et al., 1988), and a diffusible factor from the pons induces cortical-pontine neurons to sprout collaterals to innervate this target (Heffner et al., 1990). A recent report indicates that diffusible signals may also be inhibitory (Pini, 1993). Finally, cultured *Xenopus* motoneurons can be made to turn in response to a gradient of db-cAMP (Lohof et al., 1992). As indicated in Fig. 2, neither the receptors for these factors nor the way in which they transduce signals is known. Although the signals are normally thought to operate only over short distances (millimeters), it might be possible to induce specific regeneration over longer distances by depositing multiple point sources of such factors, once they have become

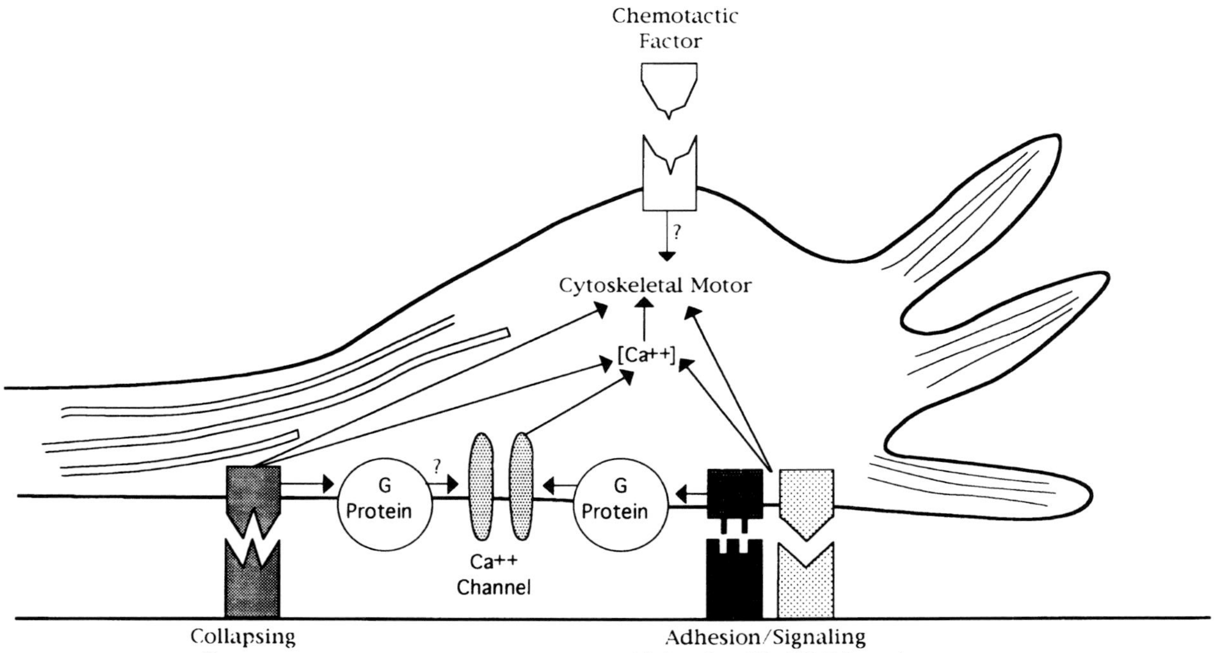

Fig. 2. A growth cone showing possible modes of signal transduction. Actin filaments are shown in the filopodia, and microtubles entering the base of the growth cone. Arrows indicate some of the different pathways through which growth and guidance molecules may affect the cytoskeleton. Since their precise mode of action on individual cytoskeletal components is unknown, they are shown acting on a generic cytoskeletal motor.

identified. Since these agents must, by their nature, act relatively specifically, this might be one way of inducing regrowth of specific groups of axons during regeneration.

Guidance cues may be negative as well as positive

For many years guidance was thought of as growth cones being guided by positive interactions with favorable substrata. However, it was also noticed that chick motoneurons growing in vivo appeared to actively avoid regions of pre-cartilage mesenchyme (Tosney and Landmesser, 1984, 1985), a finding more fully explored by Tosney and Oakley (1990). This tissue contains chondroitin sulphate proteoglycan and peanut agglutinin binding activity, both of which are known today to be repulsive to growth cones (the mechanism of action of the former is explored in the chapter by Letourneau et al., Ch. 9, this volume).

The first clear evidence for the cellular events that might result in active avoidance came from Raper and his colleagues, who found that when growth cones of certain types of neurons contacted neurites from certain other classes, they were caused to collapse with transient cessation of motility (Kapfhammer and Raper, 1987). Raper and his colleagues have recently purified a collapsing factor from chick brain (Luo et al., 1993) and have found that it has considerable homology to fasciclin IV from *Drosophila* (Kolodkin et al., 1992). Another collapsing factor has been isolated from posterior somites which are actively avoided by outgrowing spinal nerves (Davies et al., 1990). Finally, the well-defined preference of temporal retinal axons for anterior over posterior tectum has also been shown to be inhibitory in nature (Cox et al., 1990). Thus inhibitory cues seem to play major roles in guidance in several neural systems (see Schwab et al., 1993 for review).

Of more obvious relevance to CNS regeneration was the discovery by Schwab and his colleagues that DRG growth cones collapsed upon contact with mature oligodendrocytes (Bandtlow et al., 1990), and the subsequent isolation of several collapsing factors. One of these, NI-35 (Bandtlow et al., 1993), present on mature oligodendrocytes and central myelin, can be neutralized by specific antibodies both in culture (Bandtlow et al., 1990) and in the rat spinal cord, resulting in enhanced regeneration (Schnell and Schwab, 1990). These and similar molecules clearly contribute to making the CNS an inhospitable environment for axonal regeneration, and fuller characterization of these factors and ways of neutralizing their activity are important strategies for enhancing CNS regeneration (see also Steeves et al., Ch. 20, this volume).

Signal transduction of growth and guidance cues

Considerable effort is being focused on understanding how the signals from growth and guidance molecules are transduced to produce the appropriate cytoskeletal response (Doherty and Walsh, 1992). Doherty and his colleagues (Doherty et al., 1991) have shown that some signals from NCAM and *N*-cadherin are conveyed via activation of a G-protein and subsequent entry of Ca^{2+} from the outside. A recent report implicates G-proteins in the transduction of some inhibitory signals as well (Igarashi et al., 1993). However, as indicated by the multiple arrows in Fig. 2, it is too early to make any overall generalizations, and it is likely that signals may be transduced through a variety of different pathways. For example, Ca^{2+} may also be released from intracellular stores, or signaling may be via direct activation of different kinases (Goldberg and Wu, Ch. 8, this volume) in some cases independently of Ca^{2+}.

Recent evidence on how inhibitory or collapsing factors may act illustrates this diversity. Chondroitin sulphate proteoglycan appears to act by causing Ca^{2+} entry from the outside (Letourneau et al., Ch. 9, this volume), whereas NI-35 appears to trigger growth cone collapse by releasing Ca^{2+} primarily from intracellular stores (Bandtlow et al., 1993). In contrast, the brain-derived collapsing factor, collapsin, appears to trigger collapse without an elevation of intracellular Ca^{2+}, via a more direct effect on actin polymerization (Fan et al., 1993). However, Lankford and Letourneau (1989) have shown that actin stability in the growth cone can also be affected by Ca^{2+}.

Conclusions

Important progress has been made in understanding, at the molecular level, how general growth and guidance signals are transduced by the growth cone. Despite its considerable complexity, this fuller understanding of the growth cone's capabilities should allow strategies to be developed to bypass, by pharmacological or other means, specific steps and signals which might not occur following axotomy, but which are necessary for regeneration and restoration of function. Once the goal of regeneration of long fiber tracts is realized, attention must be paid to the reestablishment of specific circuits. Ongoing work to determine how specific circuits are formed during development (Goodman and Shatz, 1993), including the nature of specific recognition molecules (Johansen et al., Ch. 11, this volume), will be needed to judge better the extent to which this is likely to occur following regeneration and to devise means to enhance this process.

Acknowledgements

My laboratory was supported by NIH grant NS 19640 and NSF grant BNS 9109529. I thank Vance Lemmon for permission to reproduce Figure 1 and Gabriel Pilar for help with Figure 2.

References

Bandtlow, C.E., Zachleder, T. and Schwab, M. (1990) Oligodendrocytes arrest neurite growth by contact inhibition. *J. Neurosci.*, 10: 3837–3848.

Bandtlow, C.E., Schmidt, M.F., Hassinger, T.D., Schwab, M.E., and Kater, S.B. (1993) Role of intracellular calcium in NI-35 evoked collapse of neuronal growth cones. *Science*, 259: 80–83.

Bixby, J.L. and Harris, W.A. (1991) Molecular mechanisms of axon growth and guidance. *Annu. Rev. Cell Biol.*, 7: 117–159.

Bridgman, P.C. and Daily, M.E. (1989) The organization of myosin and actin in rapidly frozen nerve growth cones. *J. Cell Biol.*, 108: 95–109.

Burns, F.R., vonKannen, S., Guy, L., Raper, J.A., Kamholtz, J. and Chang, S. (1991) DM-GRASP, a novel immunoglobulin superfamily axonal surface protein that supports neurite extension. *Neuron*, 7: 209–220.

Carter, D.A., Bray, G. and Aguayo, A.J. (1994) Long-term growth and remodeling of regenerated retino-collicular connections in adult hamsters. *J. Neurosci.*, 14: 590–598.

Cox, E.C., Muller, B. and Bonhoeffer, F. (1990) Axonal guidance in the chick visual system: posterior tectal membranes induce collapse of growth cones from the temporal retina. *Neuron*, 4: 31–37.

Davies, J.A., Cook, G.M.W., Stern, C.D. and Keynes, R.J. (1990) Isolation from chick somites of a glycoprotein fraction that causes collapse of dorsal root ganglion growth cones. *Neuron*, 4: 11–20.

Dodd, J., Morton, S.B., Karagogeos, D., Yamamoto, M. and Jessell, T. (1988) Spatial regulation of axonal glycoprotein expression on subsets of embryonic spinal neurons. *Neuron*, 1: 105–116.

Doherty, P. and Walsh, F.S. (1992) Cell adhesion molecules, second messengers and axonal growth. *Curr. Opin. Neurobiol.*, 2: 595–601.

Doherty, P., Ashton, S.V., Moore, S.E. and Walsh, F.S. (1991) Morphoregulatory activities of NCAM and *N*-Cadherin can be accounted for by a G-protein- dependent activation of L- and N- type Ca^{++} Channels. *Cell*, 67: 21–33.

Fan, J., Mansfield, S.G., Redmond, T., Gordon-Weeks, P.R. and Raper, J.A. (1993) The organization of F-actin and microtubules in growth cones exposed to a brain-derived collapsing factor. *J. Cell Biol.*, 121: 867–878.

Goodman, C.S. and Shatz, C. (1993) Developmental mechanisms that generate precise patterns of neuronal connectivity. *Neuron*, 10 (Suppl.): 77–88.

Goldberg, D.J., Burmmeister, D.W. and Rivas, R.J. (1992) Video microscopic analysis of events in the growth cone underlying axon growth and the regulation of these events by substrate-bound proteins. In: P.C. Letourneau, S.B. Kater and R. Macagno (Eds.), *The Nerve Growth Cone*, Raven Press, New York, pp. 79–95.

Heffner, C.D., Lumsden, A.G.S. and O'Leary, D.M. (1990) Target control of collateral extension and directional axon growth in the mammalian brain. *Science*, 247: 217–220.

Igarashi, M., Strittmatter, S.M., Vartanian, T. and Fischman, M.C. (1993) Mediation by G-proteins of signals that cause collapse of growth cones. *Science*, 253: 77–79.

Ivins, J.K., Raper, J.A. and Pittman, R.N. (1991) Intracellular calcium levels do not change during contact-mediated collapse of chick DRG growth cone structure. *J. Neurosci.*, 11: 1597–1608.

Joshi, H.C. and Bass, P.W. (1993) A new perspective on microtubules and axon growth. *J. Cell Biol.*, 121: 1191–1196.

Kapfhammer, J.P. and Raper, J.A. (1987) Collapse of growth

cone structure on contact with specific neurites in culture. *J. Neurosci.*, 7: 201–212.

Kolodkin, A.L., Mathes, D.J., O'Connor, T.P., Patel, N.H., Admon, A., Bentley, D. and Goodman, C.S. (1992) Fasciclin IV: sequence, expression and function during growth cone guidance in the grasshopper embryo. *Neuron,* 9: 831–845.

Landmesser, L., Dahm, L. Schultz, K. and Rutishauser, U. (1988) Distinct roles for adhesion molecules during innervation of embryonic chick muscle. *Dev. Biol.*, 130: 645–670.

Landmesser, L., Dahm, L., Tang, J. and Rutishauser, U. (1990) Polysialic acid as a regulator of intramuscular nerve branching during embryonic development. *Neuron,* 4: 655–667.

Lankford, K.L. and Letourneau, P.C. (1989) Evidence that calcium may control neurite outgrowth by regulating the stability of actin filaments. *J. Cell Biol.,* 109: 1229–1243.

Lankford, K.L. and Letourneau, P.C. (1991) Roles of actin filaments and three second messenger systems in short term regulation of chick dorsal root ganglion neurite outgrowth. *Cell Motil. Cytoskel.*, 20: 7–29.

Lemmon, V., Burden, S., Payne, H.R., Elmslie, G.J. and Hlavin, M.L. (1992) Neurite growth on different substrates: permissive versus instructive influences and the role of adhesive strength. *J. Neurosci.*, 12: 818–826.

Letourneau, P.C., Shattuck, T.A. and Ressler, A.H. (1987) 'Pull' and 'push' in neurite elongation: observations on the effects of different concentrations of cytochalasin B and taxol. *Cell Motil. Cytoskel.,* 8: 193–209.

Lin, C-H. and Forscher, P. (1993) Cytoskeletal remodeling during growth cone-target interactions. *J. Cell Biol.,* 121: 1369–1383.

Lohof, A.M. , Quillam, M., Dan, Y. and Poo, M-m. (1992) Asymmetric modulation of cytosolic cAMP activity induces growth cone turning. *J. Neurosci.*, 12: 1253–1261.

Lumsden, A. (1992) Chemotaxis in the developing nervous system. In: P.C. Letourneau, S.B. Kater and R.E. Macagno (Eds.), *The Nerve Growth Cone*, Raven Press, New York, pp. 167–180.

Lumsden, A. and Davies, A.M. (1986) Chemotropic effect of specific target epithelium in the development of the mammalian nervous system. *Nature (Lond.),* 323: 538–539.

Luo, Y., Raible, D. and Raper, J. (1993) Collapsin: a protein in brain that induces the collapse and paralysis of neuronal growth cones. *Cell,* 75: 217–227.

O'Connor, T.P. and Bentley, D. (1993) Accumulation of actin in subsets of pioneer growth cone filopodia in response to neural and epithelial guidance cues in situ. *J. Cell Biol.*, 123: 935–948.

Pini, A. (1993) Chemorepulsion of axons in the developing mammalian central nervous system. *Science,* 261: 95–98.

Ramón y Cajal, S. (1890) A quelle epoque apparaissent les expansions des cellules nerveuses de la moelle epinere du poulet. *Anat. Anz.*, 5: 609–613.

Reichardt, L.F. and Tomaselli, K.J. (1991) Extracellular matrix molecules and their receptors: functions in neural development. *Annu. Rev. Neurosci.,* 14: 531–570.

Sabry, J.H., O'Connor, T.P., Evans, L., Toroian-Raymomd, A., Kirschner, M. and Bentley, D. (1991) Microtubule behavior during guidance of pioneer neuron growth cone in situ. *J. Cell Biol.,* 115: 381–395.

Schnell, L. and Schwab, M.E. (1990) Axonal regeneration in the rat spinal cord produced by an antibody against myelin-associated growth inhibitors. *Nature (Lond.),* 343: 269–272.

Schwab, M.E., Kapfhammer, J.P. and Bandtlow, C.E. (1993) Inhibitors of neurite growth. *Annu. Rev. Neurosci.*, 16: 565–595.

So, K.F. and Aguayo, A.J. (1985) Lengthy regrowth of cut axons from ganglion cells after peripheral nerve transplantation into the retina of adult rats. *Brain Res*., 328: 349–354.

Takeichi, M. (1991) Cadherin cell adhesion receptors as a morphogenetic regulator. *Science,* 251: 1451–1455.

Tanaka, H., Matsui, T., Agata, A., Tomura, M., Kubota, I., McFarland, K.C., Kohr, B., Lee, A., Phillips, H. and Shelton, D. (1991) Molecular cloning and expression of a novel adhesion molecule SC1. *Neuron,* 7: 535–545.

Tang, J., Landmesser, L. and Rutishauser, U. (1992) Polysialic acid influences specific pathfinding by avian motoneurons. *Neuron,* 8: 1031–1044.

Tessier-Lavigne, M. (1992) Axon guidance by molecular gradients. *Curr. Opin. Neurobiol.,* 2: 60–65.

Tessier-Lavigne, M., Placzek, M., Lumsden, A.G.S., Dodd, J. and Jessell, T.M. (1988) Chemotropic guidance of developing axons in the mammalian CNS. *Nature (Lond.),* 336: 755–778.

Tomasiewicz, H., Ono, K., Yee, D., Thompson, C., Goridis, C., Rutishauser, U. and Magnuson, T. (1993) Genetic deletion of a neural cell adhesion molecule variant (NCAM-180) produces distinct defects in the central nervous system. *Neuron,* 11: 1163–1174.

Tosney, K. and Landmesser, L. (1984) Pattern and specificity of axonal outgrowth following varying degrees of chick limb bud ablation. *J. Neurosci.,* 4: 2518–2527.

Tosney, K. and Landmesser, L. (1985) Development of the major pathways for neurite outgrowth in the chick hind limb. *Dev. Biol.,* 109: 193–214.

Tosney, K. and Oakley, R. (1990) The perinotochordal mesenchyme acts as a barrier to axon advance in the chick embryo: implications for a general mechanism of axon guidance. *Exp. Neurol.*, 109: 75–89.

F.J. Seil (Ed.)
Progress in Brain Research, Vol 103

CHAPTER 8

Regulation of events within the growth cone by extracellular cues: tyrosine phosphorylation

Daniel J. Goldberg and Da-Yu Wu

Department of Pharmacology and Center for Neurobiology and Behavior, Columbia University, 630 W. 168th St., New York, NY 10032, U.S.A.

Introduction

The growth cone is a critical site for the interactions with environmental cues that produce directed axonal growth during development and regeneration. The digitate filopodia that project tens of microns from the body of the growth cone to sample the environment are key sites for these interactions. Filopodia become more numerous when a growth cone reaches a region in which one of multiple potential pathways must be selected (Tosney and Landmesser, 1985; Bovolenta and Mason, 1987). In the developing grasshopper limb, contact of a filopodium of the first ingrowing axon with a critical landmark in such a region is responsible for turning of the axon onto the correct pathway (Caudy and Bentley, 1986; O'Connor et al., 1990). If the formation of filopodia is pharmacologically prevented in this 'pioneer' axon, its growth is wayward (Bentley and Toroian-Raymond, 1986). Intracellular mechanisms mediating the detection of cues by filopodia and their transduction into changes in growth cone behavior are not well understood.

In this article, we will discuss evidence implicating protein-tyrosine phosphorylation in the functioning of filopodia. Several findings suggest an involvement of tyrosine phosphorylation in axon growth. The *src* protein-tyrosine kinase (PTK) is particularly highly expressed during nervous system development and is enriched in the growth cone (Matten et al., 1990). Another PTK, *abl,* as well as certain protein-tyrosine phosphatases (PTPs), are transiently expressed in certain axonal tracts of the developing *Drosophila* nervous system (Elkins et al., 1990; Hariharan et al., 1991; Tian et al., 1991), and genetic deletion of the *abl* PTK contributes to wayward axonal growth (Elkins et al., 1990). Certain molecules capable of stimulating axonal growth cause rapid changes in protein-tyrosine phosphorylation in neurons or neuron-like cell lines (Maher, 1988; Atashi et al., 1992).

While suggesting the involvement of protein-tyrosine phosphorylation in axon growth, the foregoing results do not define specific roles. In fact, the only role that has so far been established for protein-tyrosine phosphorylation is at the beginning of the signaling pathway for nerve growth factor, whose receptor is a PTK which undergoes autophosphorylation (Loeb et al., 1991). A role in the filopodium would put protein-tyrosine phosphorylation in a key spot to mediate effects of environmental cues on axonal growth, particularly pathfinding.

Concentration of phosphotyrosine at tip of filopodium

The bulk of our studies have involved the use of

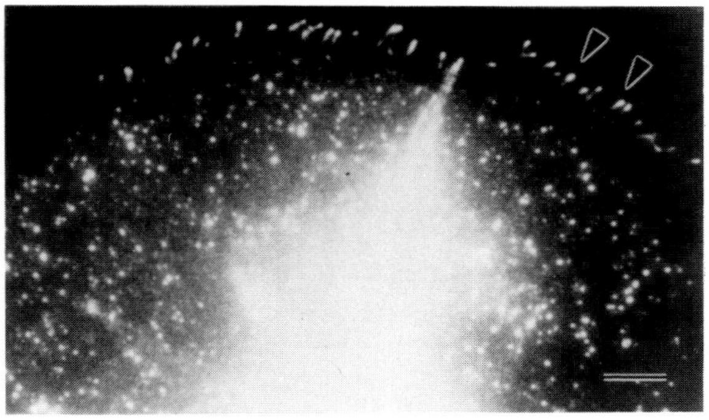

Fig. 1. Concentrated phosphotyrosine at the tips of the filopodia of an *Aplysia* growth cone. The neuron was cultured on a polylysine substrate in protein-free, defined medium and labeling with a monoclonal antibody to phosphotyrosine was visualized by indirect immunofluorescence. The growth cone was photographed with a 35-mm camera connected to the microscope. Arrowheads point to two of the many brightly stained filopodial tips. The filopodia are short in this growth cone. Bar, 10 μm.

isolated large neurons from the central nervous system (CNS) of the marine slug, *Aplysia,* displaying regenerative axon growth in culture. These neurons can produce growth cones which are especially suitable for the video microscopic techniques we employ. The axons grow quite slowly when cultured in protein-free medium on a substrate coated only with polylysine; growth is much faster when the substrate has also been pre-exposed to hemolymph from the animal, which contains a high molecular weight protein which promotes growth (Burmeister et al., 1991).

Fluorescent staining of *Aplysia* growth cones on the polylysine substrate with an antibody specific for phosphorylated tyrosine residues yields a striking pattern: the tips of most of the filopodia are intensely bright (Fig. 1). The pattern is especially impressive when viewed with video intensified fluorescence microscopy, with the image magnification increased several-fold (Fig. 2A). The bright staining is often associated with a swelling of the tip, but it is clear that the intensity of the staining results not simply from increased volume but from a concentration of phosphotyrosine at the tip. This is evident when the pattern of staining of phosphotyrosine (Fig. 2A) is compared with staining of the same growth cone with Texas Red (Fig. 2B), a fluorescent probe which indiscriminately stains cellular protein. The difference in intensity of staining between filopodial tip and shaft is much greater for phosphotyrosine than for Texas Red. We have also detected bright staining of filopodial tips of embryonic chick sympathetic and retinal ganglion neurons and neonatal rat hippocampal neurons cultured in serum-free medium on polylysine or polyornithine (Figs. 3 and 4A), though the fraction of filopodial tips that are brightly stained is substantially less than in the *Aplysia* cultures.

The role of the protein-tyrosine phosphorylation described here must be different from the single defined role, noted above, of initiating a signaling cascade in response to nerve growth factor (or analogous growth factors). This is clear because the *Aplysia* neurons are cultured in a protein-free medium on a protein-free substrate in the absence of substantial numbers of other neurons or non-neuronal cells. Yet, there are indications that the phosphorylation is involved in mediating interactions with environmental cues, as its location at the tips of filopodia would suggest. When *Aplysia* neurons are cultured on a substrate pre-exposed to hemolymph as well as polylysine, far fewer filopodial tips display intense staining with the anti-phosphotyrosine antibody (Wu and Goldberg, 1993). Phosphotyrosine disappears from tips within a few minutes of addition of hemolymph to neurons cultured on a polylysine substrate (Wu and Goldberg, 1993). In addition, we have found integrin to coconcentrate with phosphotyrosine in filopodial tips of cultured chick sympathetic neurons (Fig. 4). Integrin is the membrane receptor for the extracellular matrix proteins, laminin and collagen, which promote neurite growth in these cells.

Can the interaction of an individual filopodium with an environmental cue cause a change in the amount or distribution of phosphotyrosine in that filopodium? We do not yet know because, in the aforementioned experiments, the entire growth cone, not only the filopodium, is exposed to the growth promoting material of hemolymph. We are currently assessing the effects on phosphory-

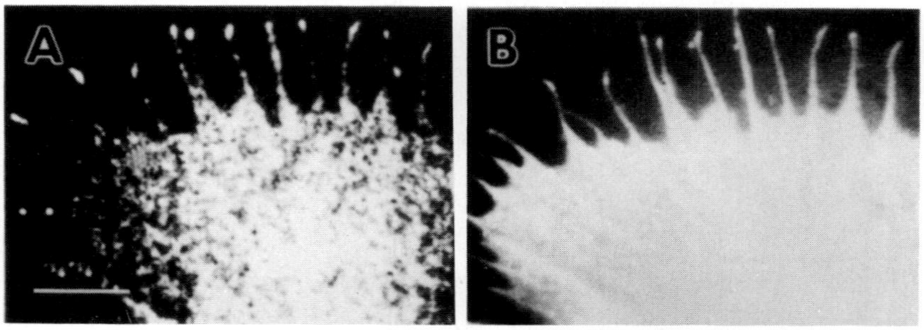

Fig. 2. Concentrated phosphotyrosine at the tips of the filopodia of an *Aplysia* growth cone, as recorded by video intensified fluorescence microscopy. Preparation was as described for Fig. 1, but the image was recorded with a SIT video camera connected to the microscope. This is a different growth cone from the one shown in Fig. 1. (B) This is the same growth cone as in panel A, showing the staining pattern obtained with Texas Red fluorophore, which indiscriminately stains proteins. Bar, 5 μm.

lation of exposure of filopodia alone to cues. It does appear that the machinery for dephosphorylation is present at the tip, since administration of an inhibitor of PTKs to a growth cone on polylysine results in dimming of the tip staining (Fig. 5).

Role of tyrosine phosphorylation in the filopodium

What is the role of the tyrosine phosphorylation in the filopodium? This question should be considered in the context of evidence that the phosphotyrosine associates or interacts with actin filaments. The core of the filopodium is a bundle of actin filaments (Fig. 6A); at the distal end of this bundle is the concentrated phosphotyrosine (Fig. 6B), though we do not know if there is a physical connection. We have recently shown that filopodia-like protrusions that have a core bundle of microtubules form for a short time after transection of *Aplysia* axons in culture (Goldberg and Burmeister, 1992). These microtubule based protrusions do not develop concentrations of phosphotyrosine at their tips, while conventional actin-based filopodia forming at the same time do (see Fig. 8B). In addition, one can cause the network of actin filaments in the peripheral region of the growth cone to rapidly withdraw into the central region by administering the actin-specific drug, cytochalasin (Fig. 7A). Phosphotyrosine withdraws from the tip in clumps, sometimes fragmenting or spreading (Fig. 7B). Thus, the concentration of phosphotyrosine in the filopodial tips depends on the presence of actin filaments. With this in mind, we will consider three possible roles for the tyrosine phosphorylation.

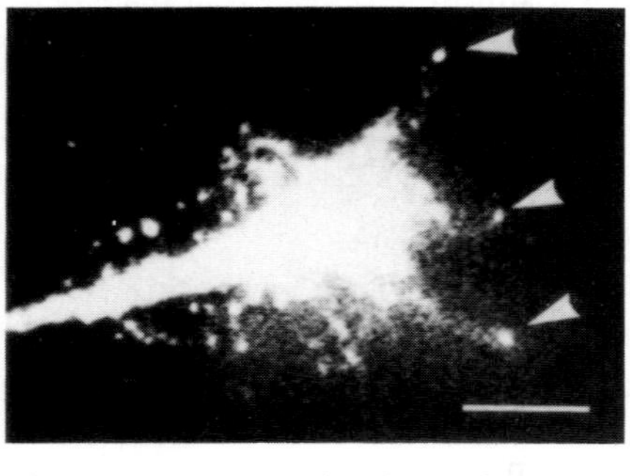

Fig. 3. Concentrated phosphotyrosine at the tips of filopodia of a neonatal rat hippocampal neuron. The neuron was cultured on a polylysine substrate in a defined, serum-free medium. Staining was as described in previous figures, and this and all subsequent fluorescent images were recorded with the SIT camera. Arrowheads point to the stained tips. The shafts of these short filopodia are so lightly stained that they are difficult to see in this view. Bar, 5 μm.

Formation of filopodia

The first is in the formation of filopodia. Non-neuronal motile cells, such as fibroblasts, have peripheral actin-rich regions similar to that found in the growth cone. The actin filament bundles underlying their microspikes (short filopodia) form

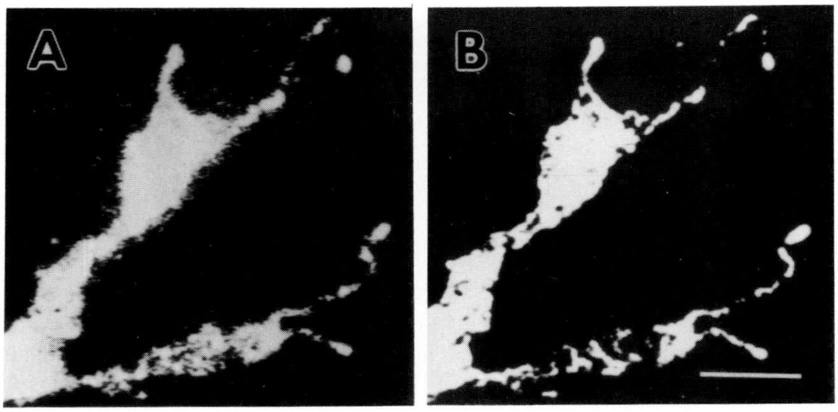

Fig. 4. Concentrated phosphotyrosine at the tips of filopodia of an embryonic chick sympathetic neuron. The neuron was cultured on a polyornithine substrate in a defined, serum-free medium. (B) The same growth cone was also labeled with a polyclonal antibody to the β_1 subunit of integrin, and visualized with a different fluorophore from that used for panel A. Concentrated integrin is present at the tips, which displayed concentrated phosphotyrosine. Bar, 5 μm.

by an initial coalescence of the distal ends of filaments, followed by a disto-proximal zippering of the filaments into a bundle (Izzard, 1988). The localization of phosphotyrosine at the distal end of the actin bundle in the growth cone filopodia suggests it could be involved in this coalescence. However, we think this is not the case. As mentioned above, axotomy causes massive numbers of filopodia to form within a short time and so is a convenient means for studying factors underlying their formation. Contrary to the expectation if tyrosine phosphorylation were involved in the initial stages of filopdial formation, bright tip staining is not present when the filopodium first forms but only develops later. Figure 8, which shows an axon 25 min after axotomy (actin based filopodia start to form about 10 min after axotomy), demonstrates that many of the filopodia have no discernible concentration of phosphotyrosine at their tips. Even for those filopodia that display tip staining, the concentrations of phosphotyrosine are more modest than many seen later after axotomy (Fig. 9).

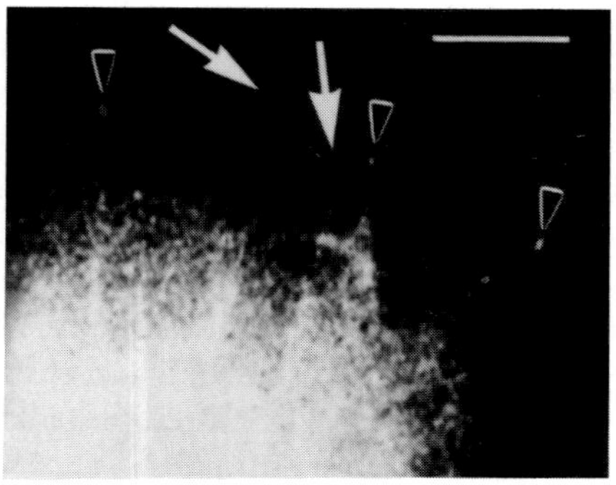

Fig. 5. Dimming of staining for phosphotyrosine at the tips of filopodia of an *Aplysia* growth cone which had been exposed for 10 min to 100 μM genistein, a broad-specificity inhibitor of PTKs. The arrowheads point to filopodia which have relatively dim staining, while the arrows point to the positions of filopodia which cannot be seen because they have lost all their staining. Bar, 5 μm.

Regulation of filopodial length

A second possible role is in regulating filopodial length by regulating the polymerization of the core bundle of actin filaments. This is once again suggested by the location of the concentrated phosphotyrosine at the distal end of the core bundle. Filopodia are dynamic structures, moving in and out between pauses. The distal end of the filaments is the preferred site for addition and loss of subunits; in fact, there is a continual addition of subunits at this end, regardless of

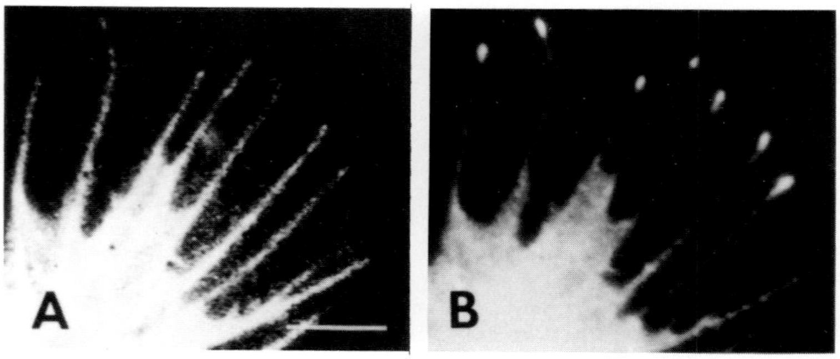

Fig. 6. Concentrated phosphotyrosine is adjacent to the distal ends of the bundles of actin filaments that comprise the cores of the filopodia. (A) This panel shows staining of an *Aplysia* growth cone with fluorescent phalloidin, which binds to filamentous actin. (B) The same growth cone is also stained with antibody to phosphotyrosine, visualized with a different fluorophore. Bar, 5 μm.

whether the axon is growing rapidly (Forscher and Smith, 1988; Okabe and Hirokawa, 1991). Thus, the distal tip of the filopodium should be a key site for the regulation of filopodial dynamics.

In support of the idea that the tip phosphorylation is involved in regulating filopodial dynamics are our findings that filopodia exposed acutely to inhibitors of PTKs (such as genistein) or to hemolymph not only lose phosphotyrosine from their tips but lengthen considerably as a result of a change in their dynamics (Fig. 10). Underlying the lengthening of the filopodium is a lengthening of the core bundle of actin filaments (Wu and Goldberg, 1993). While these results indicate an association between loss of tip phosphotyrosine and acute lengthening, we cannot assuredly say that the former causes the latter. Both the addition of PTK inhibitors and hemolymph have strong effects in the central region of the growth cone. These effects probably involve the release of large numbers of actin subunits, which could diffuse to the filopodial tips to drive actin polymerization

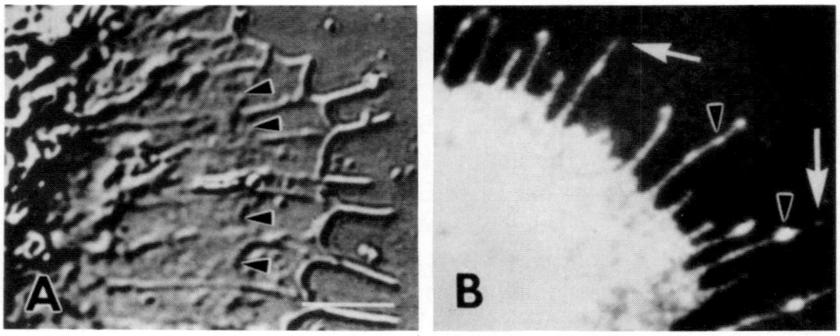

Fig. 7. Withdrawal of phosphotyrosine from the tips of filopodia when actin filaments are caused to withdraw by application of cytochalasin. (A) Video enhanced contrast-differential interference contrast (VEC-DIC) micrograph of an *Aplysia* growth cone 4 min after the application of 1 μM cytochalasin D. The arrowheads point to the distal border of the network of actin filaments as it withdraws from the margin of the growth cone. The area distal to the arrowheads appears flatter because of the withdrawal of the actin network. (B) Phosphotyrosine is visualized by indirect immunofluorescence in a different growth cone, also 4 min after the addition of cytochalasin. Arrows point to filopodial tips which are not stained and arrowheads point to clumps of tyrosine phosphorylated protein apparently in the process of moving proximally along the filopodia. Bar, 5 μm.

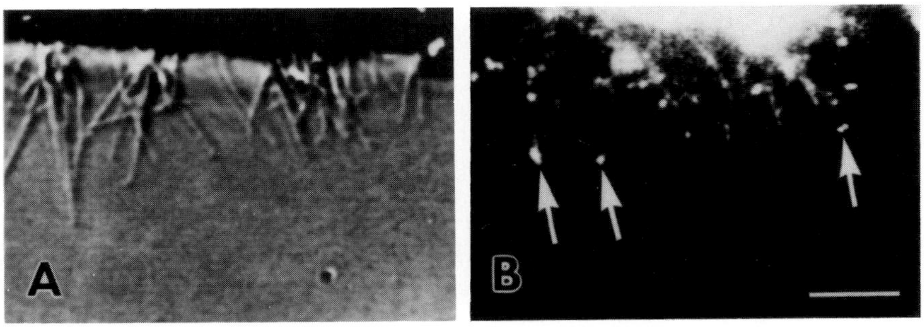

Fig. 8. Concentrated phosphotyrosine is not common in filopodial tips soon after formation of filopodia. (A) This VEC-DIC micrograph shows one side of a single *Aplysia* axon in culture which was transected 25 min previously. Numerous filopodia have grown from the side of the axon. (B) Only three of these filopodia (arrows) have marked concentrations of phosphotyrosine at their tips, as detected by indirect immunofluorescence. Bar, 5 μm.

and, thus, filopodial lengthening. So, additional data are needed to conclude that tip phosphorylation is involved in regulating filopodial dynamics. It should be useful, as noted above, to determine whether exposure of individual filopodia to PTK inhibitors or hemolymph (to avoid primary effects elsewhere in the growth cone which could secondarily influence the filopodia) affects filopodial dynamics. In addition, not all filopodia on a polylysine substrate have large concentrations of phosphotyrosine at their tips, nor are all of the

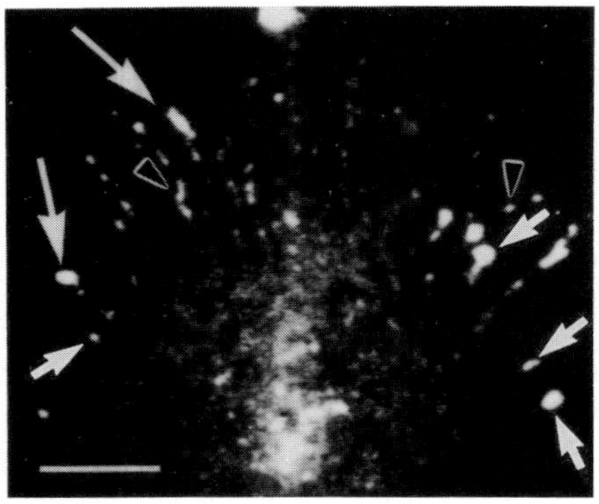

Fig. 9. Large tip concentrations of phosphotyrosine develop in filopodia after axotomy. This axon was fixed 45 min after transection. Several filopodial tips (arrows) have large concentrations of phosphotyrosine. Some others which have lesser concentrations have concentrations of phosphotyrosine more proximally along the shaft (arrowheads). Bar, 5 μm.

filopodia on a polylysine/hemolymph substrate lacking bright tip staining (Wu and Goldberg, 1993). So, we should be able to determine whether naturally occurring differences in tip phosphorylation among filopodia of individual growth cones correlate with differences in dynamics.

Attachment formation with cells or extracellular matrix

A last possible role to consider for tyrosine phosphorylation in the filopodium is in forming attachments with cells or extracellular matrix along the path of growth. Specialization of the tip of some filopodia for adhesion has been described (Tsui et al., 1985), and interactions of only the distal part of the filopodium with environmental cues seem sufficient to alter growth cone behavior (Hammarback and Letourneau, 1986; Bandtlow et al., 1990; O'Connor et al., 1990). The one site where phosphotyrosine has been found to be heavily concentrated in non-neuronal cells is at the adherens junction, either between cells or between a cell and the substrate (focal contact). The fact that the phosphotyrosine of an adherens junction is at the 'barbed' end of a bundle of polarized actin filaments, as in the filopodium, increases the appeal of this idea. In addition, we have preliminary evidence that, on a polylysine/hemolymph substrate where the majority of filopodial tips do not have concentrated

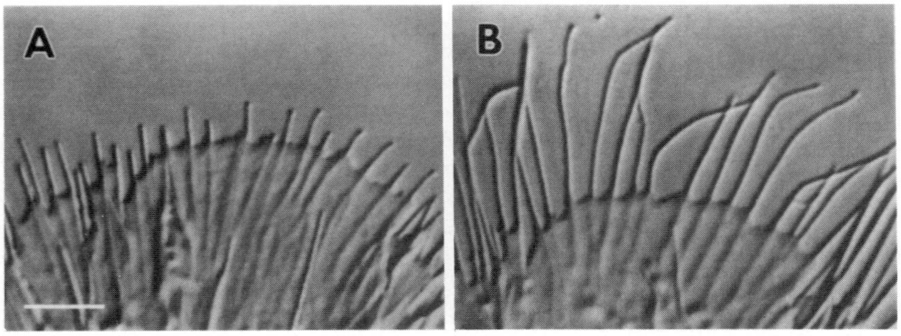

Fig. 10. Application of an inhibitor of PTKs causes filopodia to lengthen. VEC-DIC micrographs show an *Aplysia* growth cone immediately before (A) and 7 min after (B) application of 100 μm genistein. Bar, 5 μm.

phosphotyrosine, some sites of contact between filopodia show highly elevated levels of phosphotyrosine (Fig. 11).

However, it is clear that tyrosine phosphorylation in the filopodium need not be associated with attachments. The filopodial tips that display intense staining for phosphotyrosine on a polylysine substrate are quite mobile and can be seen by video microscopy to lift off the substrate frequently and move about (Wu and Goldberg, 1993).

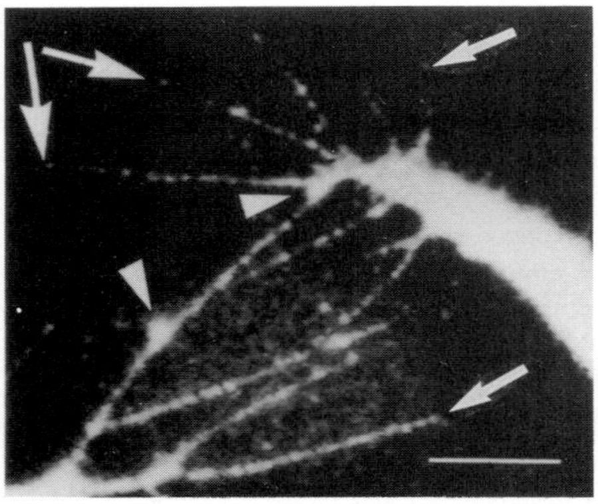

Fig. 11. Concentrated phosphotyrosine at filopodium-filopodium contacts. An *Aplysia* neuron was placed in culture on a substrate pre-exposed both to polylysine and to hemolymph. Arrows point to several filopodial tips which do not have marked concentrations of phosphotyrosine. Two sites of filopodium-filopodium contact display large concentrations of phosphotyrosine (arrowheads). Bar, 5 μm.

Assessment of the separation of these tips from the substrate by interference reflection microscopy confirms that these are not focal, or even close, contacts (Wu and Goldberg, 1993).

Thus, the accumulation of phosphotyrosine occurs independently of the formation of contacts. It has been suggested that protein tyrosine phosphorylation facilitates the formation of protein assemblies at the plasma membrane in response to growth-factor binding (Koch et al., 1991). Aggregates of non-organellar material have been described moving rapidly forward and rearward in growth cone filopodia (Sheetz et al., 1990). We find that high concentrations of phosphotyrosine at filopodial tips are often associated with swellings (Fig. 2; Wu and Goldberg, 1993) and that phosphotyrosine withdrawing from the tips of filopodia after cytochalasin treatment often moves back as a clump (Fig. 7B). We have also looked at the development of phosphotyrosine in newly formed filopodia after axotomy. Filopodia with intense tip staining tend to display bright staining only at the tip, whereas ones with dimmer tip staining, presumably earlier in development, have bright clumps along their shafts (Fig. 9B), suggesting that tyrosine phosphorylated protein moves in clumps towards the tip of the filopodium. Thus, protein tyrosine phosphorylation may facilitate formation of assemblies of proteins, such as integrin, or facilitate their association with actin filaments (or both), to promote their movement to and concentration in distal parts of the filopodium, where they would participate in pathfinding activities.

Conclusion

We have found tyrosine phosphorylated protein concentrated in the tips of some growth cone filopodia in culture. Its concentration there is acutely sensitive to the presence of growth promoting material on the substrate. These findings strongly suggest that one function of protein-tyrosine phosphorylation during axonal growth is in mediating or facilitating certain functions of filopodia, structures which detect and respond to environmental cues that guide axonal growth. Two possible specific roles for tyrosine phosphorylation are in regulating the dynamics, and thus the length, of filopodia and in facilitating the accumulation in the filopodium of membrane receptors for environmental cues with which the filopodium interacts. It will be important to identify the tyrosine phosphorylated proteins. It should also be illuminating to define the effects of well-defined, important environmental cues, such as identified growth promoting or inhibiting factors or synaptic target and non-target neurons on the amount and distribution of phosphotyrosine in individual filopodia.

Acknowledgements

This work was supported by NIH training grant MH15174, NIH fellowship NS09225, NIH research grant NS25161 and NIH program project GM32099.

References

Atashi, J.R., Klinz, S.G., Ingraham, C.A., Matten, W.T., Schachner, M. and Maness, P.F. (1992) Neural cell adhesion molecules modulate tyrosine phosphorylation of tubulin in nerve growth cone membranes. *Neuron,* 8: 831–842.

Bandtlow, C., Zachleder, T. and Schwab, M.E. (1990) Oligodendrocytes arrest neurite growth by contact inhibition. *J. Neurosci.,* 10: 3837–3848.

Bentley, D. and Toroian-Raymond, A. (1986) Disoriented pathfinding by pioneer neurone growth cones deprived of filopodia by cytochalasin treatment. *Nature (Lond.),* 323: 712–715.

Bovolenta, P. and Mason, C. (1987) Growth cone morphology varies with position in the developing mouse visual pathway from retina to first targets. J. *Neurosci.,* 7: 1447–1460.

Burmeister, D.W., Rivas, R.J. and Goldberg, D.J. (1991) Substrate-bound factors stimulate engorgement of growth cone lamellipodia during neurite elongation. *Cell Motil. Cytoskel.,* 19: 255–268.

Caudy, M. and Bentley, D. (1986) Pioneer growth cone steering along a series of neuronal and non-neuronal cues of different affinities. *J. Neurosci.,* 6: 1781–1795.

Elkins, T., Zinn, K., McAllister, L., Hoffmann, F.M. and Goodman, C.S. (1990) Genetic analysis of a Drosophila neural cell adhesion molecule: interaction of fasciclin I and Abelson tyrosine kinase mutations. *Cell,* 60: 565–575.

Forscher, P. and Smith, S.J. (1988) Actions of cytochalasins on the organization of actin filaments and microtubules in a neuronal growth cone. *J. Cell Biol.,* 107: 1505–1516.

Goldberg, D.J. and Burmeister, D.W. (1992) Microtubule-based filopodium-like protrusions form after axotomy. *J. Neurosci.,* 12: 4800–4807.

Hammarback, J.A. and Letourneau, P.C. (1986) Neurite extension across regions of low cell-substratum adhesivity: implications for the guidepost hypothesis of axonal pathfinding. *Dev. Biol.,* 117: 655–662.

Hariharan, I.K., Chuang, P.-T. and Rubin, G.M. (1991) Cloning and characterization of a receptor-class phosphotyrosine phosphatase gene expressed on central nervous system axons in *Drosophila* melanogaster. *Proc. Natl. Acad. Sci. USA,* 88: 11266–11270.

Izzard, C.S. (1988) A precursor of the focal contact in cultured fibroblasts. *Cell Motil. Cytoskel.,* 10: 137–142.

Koch, C.A., Anderson, D., Moran, M.F., Ellis, C. and Pawson, T. (1991) SH2 and SH3 domains: elements that control interactions of cytoplasmic signaling proteins. *Science,* 252: 668–674.

Loeb, D.M., Maragos, J., Martin-Zanca, D., Chao, M.V., Parada, L.F. and Greene, L.A. (1991) The *trk* proto-oncogene rescues NGF responsiveness in mutant NGF-nonresponsive PC12 cell lines. *Cell,* 66: 961–966.

Maher, P.A. (1988) Nerve growth factor induces protein-tyrosine phosphorylation. *Proc. Natl. Acad. Sci. USA,* 85: 6788–6791.

Matten, W.T., Aubry, M., West, J. and Maness, P.F. (1990) Tubulin is phosphorylated at tyrosine by $pp60^{c\text{-}src}$ in nerve growth cone membranes. *J. Cell Biol.,* 111: 1959–1970.

O'Connor, T.P., Duerr, J.S. and Bentley, D. (1990) Pioneer growth cone steering decisions mediated by single filopodial contacts in situ. *J. Neurosci.,* 10: 3935–3946.

Okabe, S. and Hirokawa, N. (1991) Actin dynamics in growth cones. *J. Neurosci.,* 11: 1918–1929.

Sheetz, M.P., Baumrind, N.L., Wayne, D.B. and Pearlman, A.L. (1990) Concentration of membrane antigens by forward transport and trapping in neuronal growth cones. *Cell,* 61: 231–241.

Tian, S.-S., Tsoulfas, P. and Zinn, K. (1991) Three receptor-linked protein-tyrosine phosphatases are selectively expressed on central nervous system axons in the Drosophila embryo. *Cell,* 67: 675–685.

Tosney, K.W. and Landmesser, L.T. (1985) Growth cone morphology and trajectory in the lumbosacral region of the chick embryo. *J. Neurosci.,* 5: 2345–2358.

Tsui, H.-C.T., Lankford, K.L. and Klein, W.L. (1985) Differentiation of neuronal growth cones: specialization of filopodial tips for adhesive interactions. *Proc. Natl. Acad. Sci. USA*, 82: 8256–8260.

Wu, D.-Y. and Goldberg, D.J. (1993) Regulated tyrosine phosphorylation at the tips of growth cone filopodia. *J. Cell Biol.*, 123: 653–664.

F.J. Seil (Ed.)
Progress in Brain Research, Vol 103

CHAPTER 9

Regulation of growth cone motility by substratum bound molecules and cytoplasmic [Ca^{2+}]

Paul C. Letourneau, Diane M. Snow and Timothy M. Gomez

Department of Cell Biology and Neuroanatomy, 4-135 Jackson Hall, University of Minnesota, Minneapolis, MN 55455, U.S.A.

Introduction

Neuronal circuits are formed through highly stereotyped patterns of axonal elongation. For example, axons extend directly from motor neurons in the spinal cord to the developing muscles of a limb, where topographically organized connections are made, such that neighboring muscle fibers are innervated by axons projected from neighboring motoneurons in the spinal cord (Tosney and Landmesser, 1985a,b; Goodman and Schatz, 1993). These highly characteristic patterns of axonal growth and connectivity are produced by the navigational behaviors of the motile tips of elongating neurites, first described and named growth cones by Ramón y Cajal (1890). The movements and advance of nerve growth cones are regulated by complex distributions of certain molecules in the local environments of the tissues through which growth cones penetrate. These molecules are bound to surfaces, such as cell membranes and extracellular matrices, or are soluble in the extracellular milieu. These molecules can act as either positive or negative cues in growth cone navigation, thereby promoting or inhibiting the migration of growth cones.

Growth cone motility involves the continuous extension and exploratory movements of sensory filopodial and lamellipodial protrusions, which are endowed with a variety of cell surface receptors (Fig. 1). Since filopodial protrusions can extend up to 100 μm from the neurite tip, individual growth cones can interact with a significant portion of their local environment.

By saying that extending growth cones navigate to their targets, we mean that the nerve growth cone is a sensory-effector system, involving the expression of cell surface receptors for environmental molecules that serve as cues or signals. Binding of such cues to their receptors prompts transmembrane signals that regulate the growth cone machinery to produce appropriate motility, including advance, retreat, turning, and branching (Fig. 2). Growth cones contain the machinery for operating several regulatory second messenger systems, including Ca^{2+} ion, cAMP, G proteins, and several protein kinases. A number of recent papers have discussed issues related to growth cone navigation or guidance (Bray and Hollenbeck, 1988; Lankford et al., 1990; Bixby and Harris, 1991; Letourneau et al., 1991; Baier and Bonhoeffer, 1992; Kapfhammer and Schwab, 1992).

In this chapter we present some of our investigations of this navigational hypothesis for growth cone behavior. We are analysing growth cone behaviors at boundaries between combinations of permissive and inhibitory substratum-bound

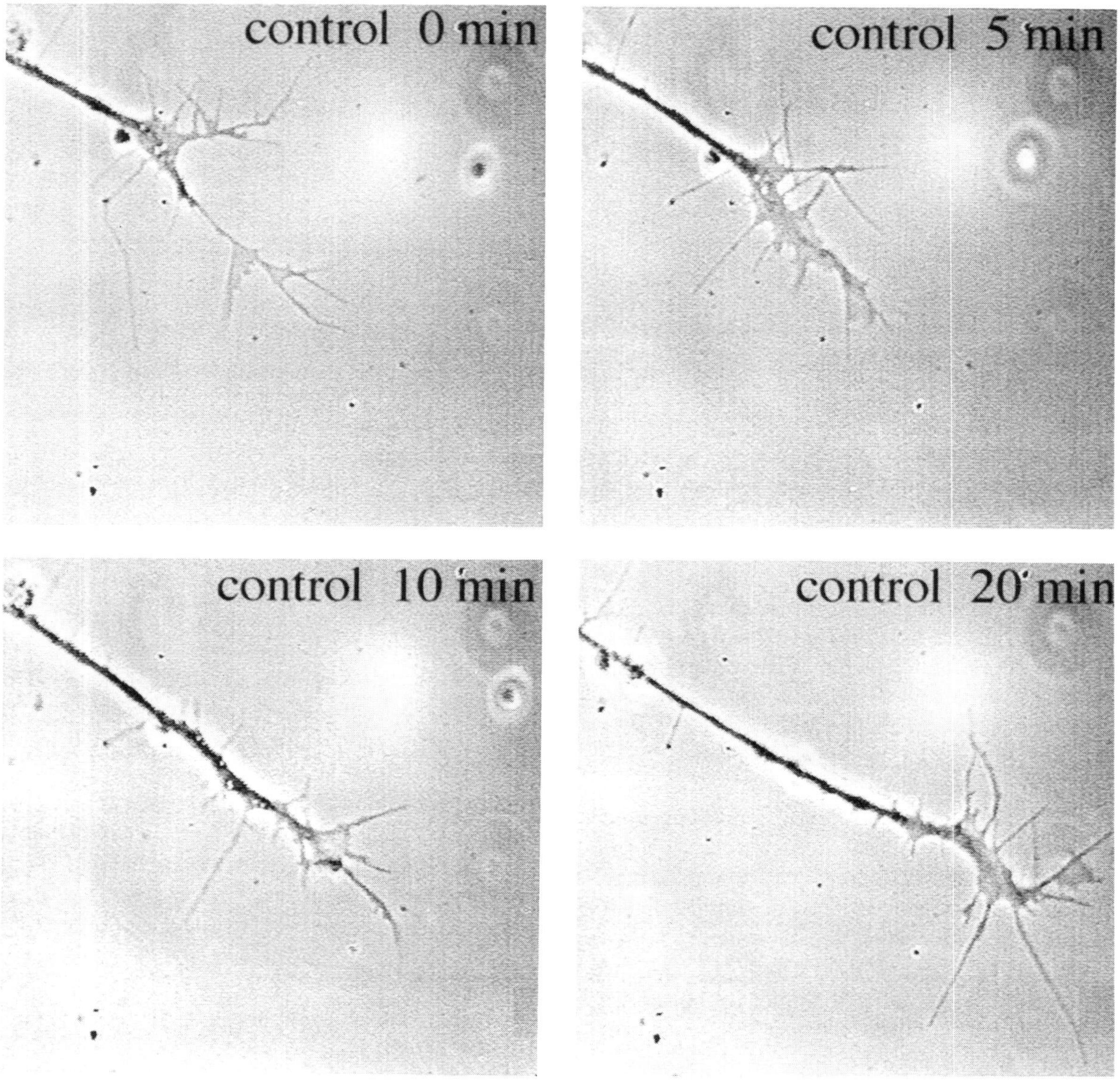

Fig. 1. Motility of a normal growth cone. This growth cone is migrating across an unpatterned laminin treated substratum. Protrusion of filopodia and lamellipodia create a constantly changing growth cone shape, and greatly expand the area of growth cone exploration.

molecules. In addition, we are investigating the involvement of one cytoplasmic regulatory factor, namely cytoplasmic [Ca^{2+}], in controlling growth cone behaviors. Our results suggest that: (1) growth cone behavior changes at boundaries between substratum adsorbed molecules, (2) interactions with surface bound molecules can trigger changes in growth cone [Ca^{2+}]$_i$, (3) recurrent spikes of cytoplasmic [Ca^{2+}] can be generated in growth cones, and (4) growth cones contain

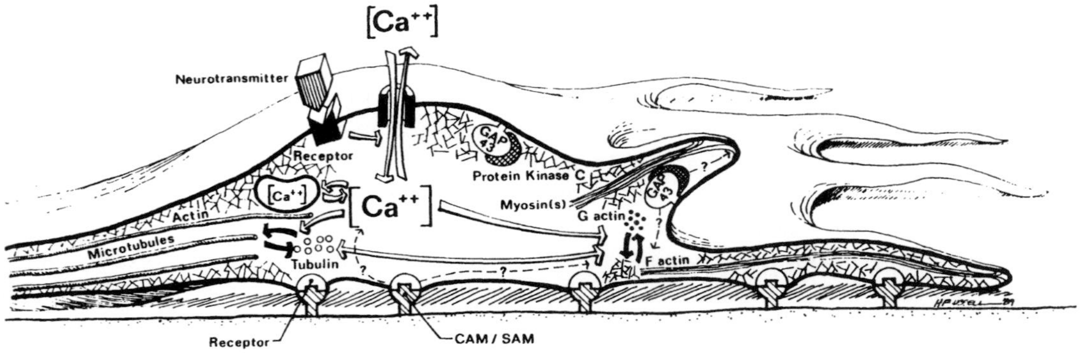

Fig. 2. A model of the sensory-effector machinery of growth cone navigation. To simplify the drawing, only the calcium second messenger system is shown. Open arrows are regulatory relationships between calcium extracellular signals, and cytoskeletal assembly. Changes in internal calcium ion levels regulate the assembly/disassembly of actin and tubulin. The movements of calcium ions between compartments are reversible and regulated. Possible relationships between binding of adhesion receptors to CAMs (cell adhesion molecules) and SAMs (substratum adhesion molecules) and intracellular calcium or the cytoskeleton are indicated with question marks.

Ca^{2+}-regulated proteins that may be important in controlling the organization and functions of actin filaments and microtubules.

These issues are relevant to nerve regeneration, as axons that are separated from their synaptic targets must re-express the activities necessary for growth cone migration and axonal elongation. Often, neurons with injured axons show a rapidly increased expression of the major cytoskeletal components of growing neurites, actin and tubulin. Perhaps increased expression of cell surface receptors for environmental cues and the cytoplasmic signaling systems that mediate regulation of growth cone motility are also required for successful axonal regeneration. Better understanding of these activities will contribute to strategies for promoting nerve regeneration and functional recovery.

Machinery of growth cone movement

The machinery that drives neurite elongation involves the two major cytoskeletal systems, microtubules and actin filaments. These cytoskeletal components are involved in the generation of distinct forces of 'push' and 'pull' that contribute to neurite elongation (Bray, 1987; Letourneau et al., 1987; Mitchison and Kirschner, 1988; Goldberg and Burmeister, 1989; Heidemann et al., 1990).

The 'push' for the neurite to advance is produced by microtubules, which have two roles: (1) as the major supportive components of neurites, and (2) as the tracks along which organelles and other components are transported. In a growing neurite, microtubules advance both via microtubule translocation and by tubulin polymerization onto the distally oriented plus ends of microtubules (Mitchison and Kirschner, 1988; Hollenbeck, 1989; Reinsch et al., 1991; Okabe and Hirokawa, 1992, 1993; Joshi and Baas, 1993). Since growth cones contain many plus-oriented microtubule ends, which are the sites of tubulin polymerization in neurites (Letourneau, 1983; Mitchison and Kirschner, 1988; Okabe and Hirokawa, 1988; Robson and Burgoyne, 1988; Joshi and Baas, 1993), they are an important site for regulating microtubule advance in growing neurites.

The 'pull' of growth cone migration is produced by activities that involve actin filaments (Letourneau, 1983; Smith, 1988; Bridgman and Dailey, 1989). Bundles and networks of actin filaments fill the transient filopodial and lamellipodial protrusions of the growth cone. These actin filaments are required for the protrusive motility of growth cones, as demonstrated by the inhibition of protrusive activity in the presence of the drug, cytochalasin B (Marsh and Letourneau, 1984; Letourneau et al., 1987). The interactions of actin filaments are diverse, dynamic, and central to growth cone motility. These include associations of actin filaments: (1) with the plasma membrane, where they are linked to adhesive molecules and transmit mechanical forces to points of adhesive contact, (2) with microtubules, which may influence the position of microtubules and, consequently, other neuritic components, and (3) with mechanochemical enzymes such as myosin(s), which produce the forces that move growth cone protrusions and pull the neurite forward (Letourneau, 1983; Bridgman and Dailey, 1989; Letourneau and Shattuck, 1989).

These 'push' and 'pull' activities generated by microtubules and actin filaments are the principal components that drive neurite elongation. Our proposal of growth cone navigation is based on the hypothesis that regulation of these two filament systems is a primary focus of transmembrane signals triggered by environmental cues.

Growth cone behavior at boundaries

Although neurite elongation can occur without actin filament-driven protrusion and motility (Marsh and Letourneau, 1984), growth cone navigation usually involves changes in growth cone position, movement, or direction that require the participation of filopodia (Raper et al., 1983; O'Connor et al., 1990). We have continued investigations of the navigational behavior of growth cones by analyses of growth cone behavior at boundaries between substrata coated with molecules that either promote or inhibit growth cone migration. We have been especially interested in the behaviors of growth cones that are in contact with one substratum, and are making filopodial contacts ahead of the body of the growth cone at the boundary with another substratum. Although the underlying mechanisms of filopodial signaling remain unclear, the results so far confirm our ideas about the regulatory roles of filopodia.

One experimental design that we have investigated involves growth cones that encounter surfaces coated with proteoglycans (PGs), many of which inhibit migration. It has been recently recognized that inhibitory cues are also very important in regulating growth cone migration (Kapfhammer and Raper, 1987; Patterson, 1988; Davies and Cook, 1991; Fishman and Strittmatter, 1993). In several regions of developing neural tissues, migrating growth cones do not enter spaces that are rich in extracellular PGs (Snow et al., 1990, 1991; Tosney and Oakley, 1990), such as chondroitin sulfate proteoglycan (CSPG). We therefore analysed the behavior of sensory and retinal neuronal growth cones that migrate on the

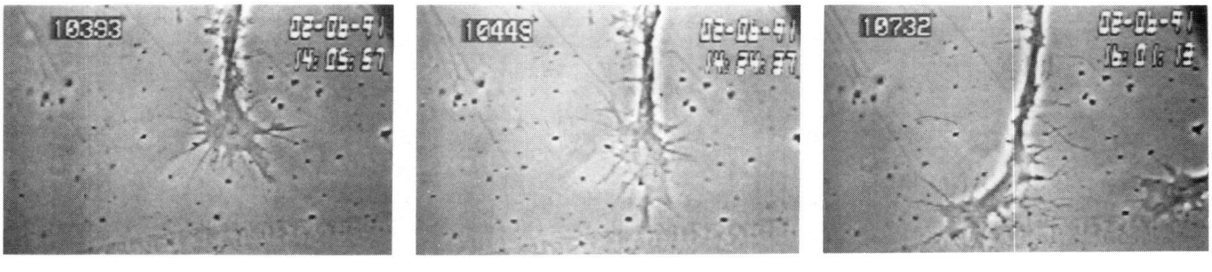

Fig. 3. Arrest of growth cone migration at a boundary with chondroitin sulfate proteoglycan (CSPG). A growth cone advances on a laminin (LM) substratum toward a boundary where CSPG is deposited over LM. In the middle figure, 20 min later, filopodial and lamellipodial extensions are seen contacting the CSPG, and in the right figure the growth cone has turned and is migrating along the boundary with CSPG.

adhesive glycoprotein, laminin (LM), and encounter a stripe of chondroitin sulfate deposited on LM. Growth cones stop or turn aside upon contact with CSPG mixed with LM, and then migrate along the LM/CSPG border (Fig. 3; Snow et al., 1991).

Although the arrest of growth cone migration at a boundary with CSPG depends on the concentration of CSPG deposited on the substratum, we also found an interesting modulation of the response to CSPG by growth cones on a step gradient of CSPG deposition (Snow and Letourneau, 1992). Retinal neuronal growth cones can cross onto a surface containing a higher concentration of CSPG if they first encounter a lower concentration of deposited CSPG (Fig. 4). That is to say, they can adapt to substratum-bound CSPG by prior exposure to low concentrations. It is still unclear how this adaptation occurs, whether by a decrease in an inhibitory signal produced by CSPG, or whether by an increase in the ability of growth cones to respond to the growth promoting LM substratum, e.g. by an up-regulation of integrin expression on the growth cone surface. Another possible mechanism of interaction with CSPG may involve regulation of cytoplasmic $[Ca^{2+}]$. In another section we present evidence for the modulation of growth cone $[Ca^{2+}]_i$ by CSPG.

Another experimental situation that we have investigated involves growth cones moving along substrata containing alternating stripes of LM and fibronectin (FN), two adhesive glycoproteins of extracellular matrices (ECM) that promote neurite elongation by chick sensory neurons (Rogers et al., 1983). Both these molecules have multiple domains that mediate interactions with neurons, while neurons, in turn, have multiple distinct surface components that recognize both FN and LM, including several integrin complexes that contain $\beta 1$ subunits (Bixby and Harris, 1991; Reichardt and Tomaselli, 1991; Letourneau et al., 1992). Sensory neurons initiate neurite growth on either FN or LM, so that behaviors of their growth cones can be observed on both FN and LM as they approach a boundary with the other ECM component.

We have found that most growth cones change their motile behavior in response to contact with the substratum component on the other side of the boundary, and, not surprisingly, these responses are initiated by filopodia that extend across the boundary and contact the alternate substratum. Some growth cones seem to choose to cross the boundary, since they accelerate and/or turn toward the boundary, whereas other growth cones choose to remain on their original substratum, turning and/or decelerating at the boundary. Both kinds of behavior are initiated by filopodial interactions, as these behavioral changes are observed several micrometers before the body of a growth cone touches the alternative substratum (Fig. 5). Surprisingly, these behaviors were exhibited equally by growth cones on both LM and FN. We do not know whether these results indicate that dorsal root ganglia (DRG) growth cones are a heterogeneous population, in which some prefer LM while others prefer FN, or alternatively, filopodial contact with a different substratum usually triggers changes in cytoplasmic second messenger levels that produce changes in motile behaviors.

As with the behavior of growth cones at a boundary with CSPG deposited on LM, the mechanisms of this modulation of growth cone behavior are unclear. We have examined the morphologies and distances of growth cone-substratum contacts, using the technique of interference reflection microscopy, and the results indicate that the choice to cross or turn at the boundary is not correlated with either maintaining or achieving a greater degree of contact with the substratum. This means that filopodia do not prompt changes in growth cone behaviors at boundaries simply by providing the best anchorage for pulling a growth cone in a particular direction. Given the multiplicity of receptors for FN and LM on sensory neurons, plus the potential for involvement of several cytoplasmic second messenger systems, it will be a formidable task unraveling the mechanisms of these changes in

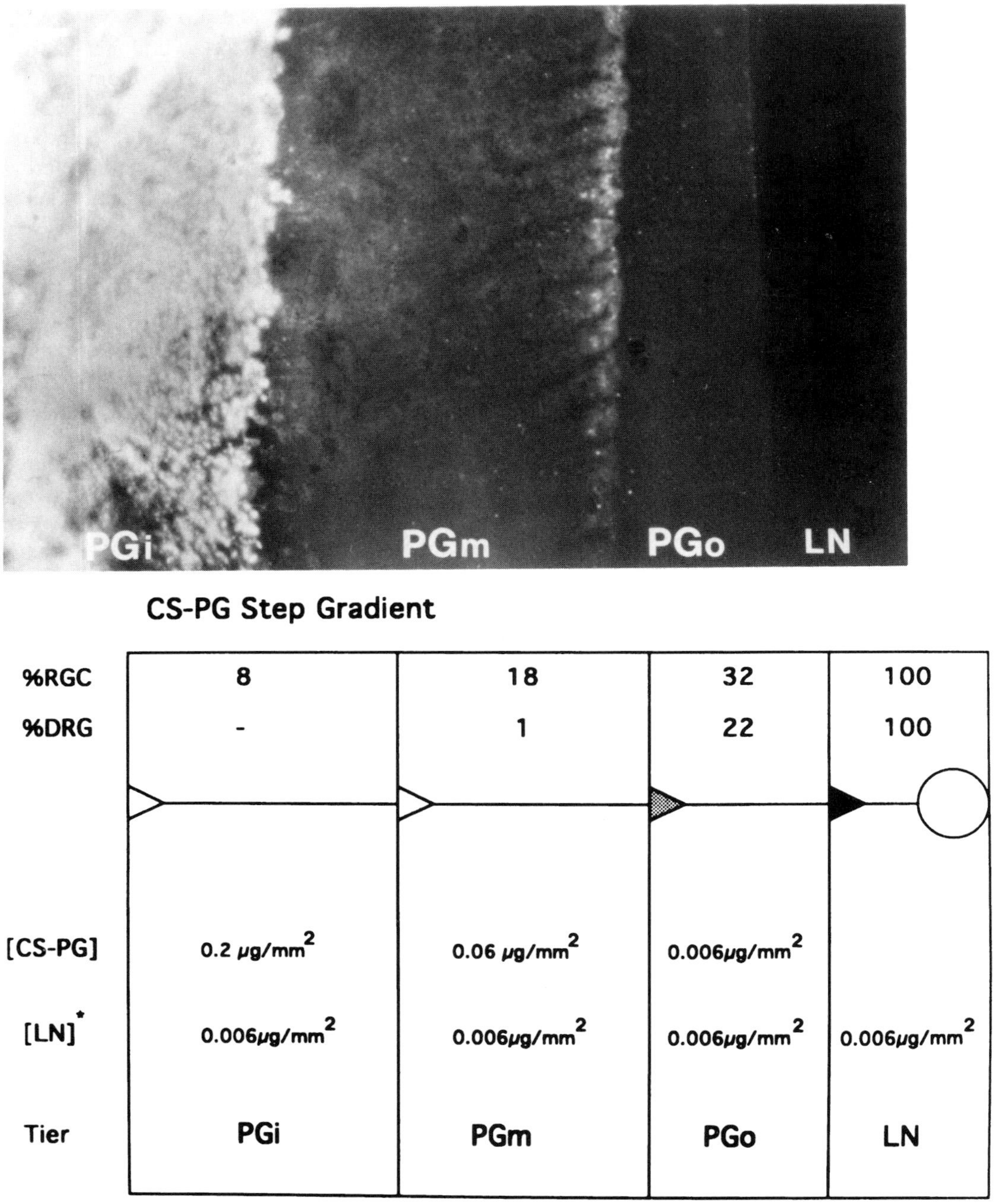

Fig. 4. Migration of dorsal root ganglia (DRG) and retinal growth cones on a step gradient of CSPG deposition. Immunofluorescence staining for CSPG in the photograph at the top shows the step gradient of CSPG deposition on LN. The figure at the bottom indicates the approximate concentrations of LN and CSPG deposition, as well as the percent of DRG and retinal growth cones that can cross from LN to successively higher concentrations of deposited CSPG. Growth cones are totally blocked by a single step of CSPG deposition of 0.02 $\mu g/mm^2$, but some of them can cross onto a substratum of 0.06 $\mu g/mm^2$ after first encountering a low level of CSPG.

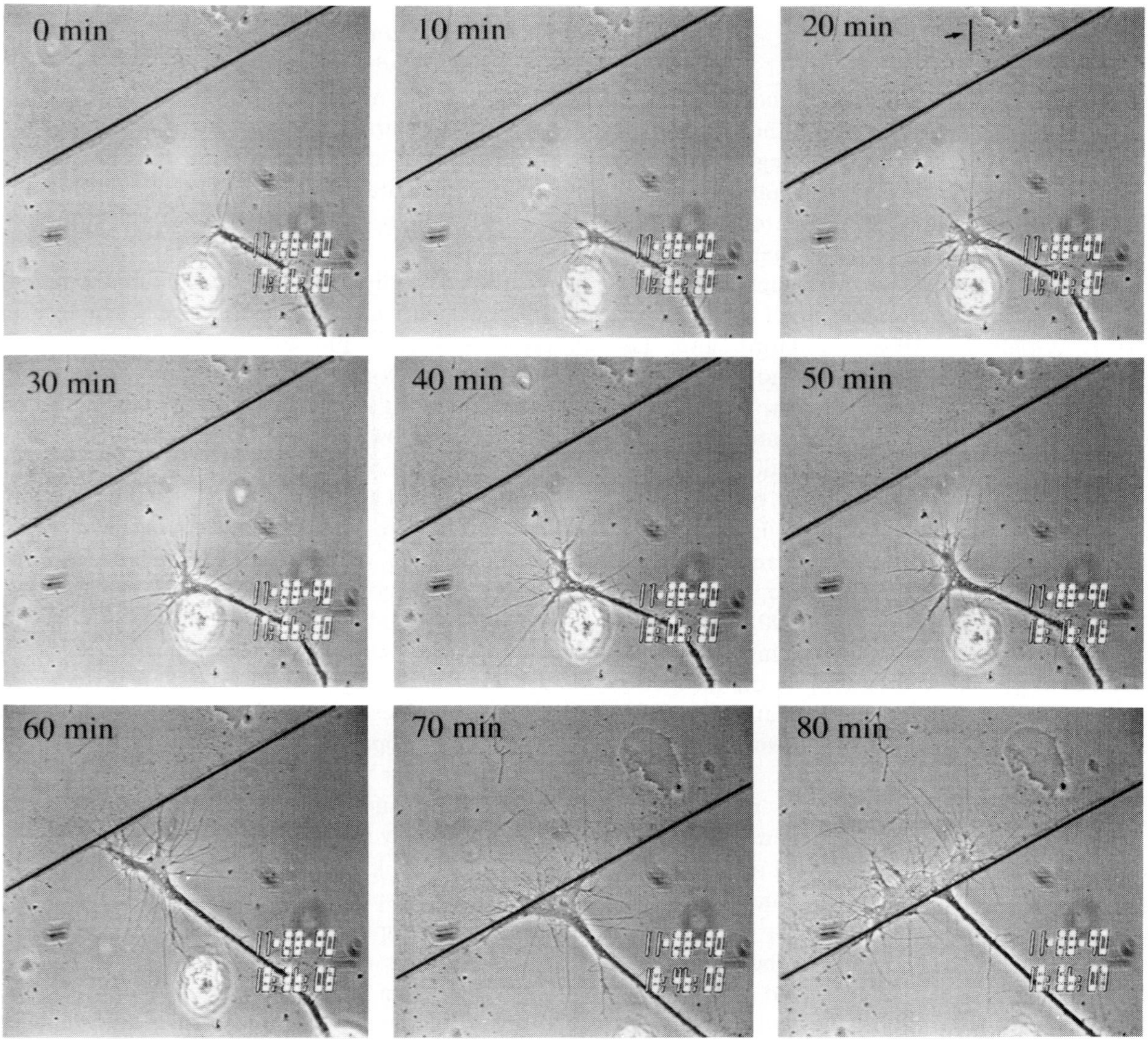

Fig. 5. Growth cone behavior at a boundary between fibronectin (FN) and LM. The growth cone is initially on FN and approaches the boundary with LM (indicated by a black line). At 20 min the tip of a single long filopodium has contacted the LM (arrow and line). In subsequent images the growth cone is seen to orient towards the LM surface. It accelerates and flattens dramatically after the body of the growth cone contacts the LM.

growth cone behavior, even in a simple in vitro system (Bixby and Harris, 1991; Reichardt and Tomaselli, 1991; Damsky and Werb, 1992; Doherty and Walsh, 1992; Hynes, 1992; Hynes and Lander, 1992; Letourneau et al., 1992; Rivas et al., 1992; Schweighoffer and Shaw, 1992; Fishman and Strittmatter, 1993). A factor that has been implicated in regulation of cell motility is cytoplasmic [Ca^{2+}], and in the next section we describe studies of cytoplasmic [Ca^{2+}] as a possible regulator of growth cone motility, as well as in responses to substratum bound molecules.

Cytoplasmic [Ca^{2+}] as a regulator of growth cone motility

Cytoplasmic [Ca^{2+}] is one of the most important second messengers involved in the short-term regulation of cell behaviors, including growth cone migration (Kater et al., 1988; Lankford et al., 1990; Kater and Mills, 1991; Letourneau and Cypher, 1991; Berridge, 1993). Changes both in growth cone behavior and cytoskeletal organization are associated with changes of growth cone [Ca^{2+}]$_i$ (Goldberg, 1988; Lankford and Letourneau, 1989, 1991; Davenport and Kater, 1992; Rehder and Kater, 1992; Bandtlow et al., 1993; Davenport et al., 1993). Experimental manipulations that produce sustained elevation of growth cone [Ca^{2+}]$_i$ lead to breakdown of actin filaments, while manipulations that lower growth cone [Ca^{2+}]$_i$ reduce the dynamic reorganization of actin filaments (Lankford and Letourneau, 1989, 1991; Lankford et al., 1990). We have, therefore, begun to investigate the involvement of dynamics of growth cone [Ca^{2+}]$_i$ in the navigational behaviors of growth cones at boundaries between different combinations of substratum associated ECM molecules.

Recall that growth cones do not cross a boundary from LM onto LM coated with a sufficient level of CSPG (Fig. 3; Snow et al., 1991). We have used the calcium sensitive fluorescent dye, Fura-2, to monitor cytoplasmic [Ca^{2+}] in growth cones that interact with surface-bound CSPG, either on a microbead or deposited on the substratum in a striped pattern. We find that contact of a growth cone body with CSPG leads to a rapid and significant elevation of growth cone [Ca^{2+}]$_i$ (Fig. 6; Snow et al., 1993). Use of Ca^{2+}-free media and Ca^{2+} channel blockers indicate that this elevation requires an influx of extracellular Ca^{2+}. We are not sure whether Ca^{2+} release from intracellular stores also contributes to the elevation of cytoplasmic [Ca^{2+}]. Enzymatic removal of the chondroitin sulfate glycosaminoglycan, which abolishes CSPG inhibition of neurite elongation, also abolishes the elevated [Ca^{2+}]$_i$ response, indicating that the glycosaminoglycan of the CSPG is the active component. The magnitude of the [Ca^{2+}]$_i$ elevation is consistent with a [Ca^{2+}]$_i$ increase that leads to breakdown of actin filaments in the leading margin of the growth cone (Lankford and Letourneau, 1989, 1991; Lankford et al., 1990). Such a disruption of the leading margin could contribute to mechanisms responsible for the arrest of growth cone migration at a boundary with CSPG.

In other studies, we are investigating the mechanisms underlying spontaneous rapid changes in cytoplasmic [Ca^{2+}] in sensory growth cones. As a result of monitoring cytoplasmic [Ca^{2+}] of growth cones migrating in normal culture media, we noted that some growth cones exhibit frequent Ca^{2+} transients, consisting of spikes of over 100 nM magnitude and approximately 10–20 sec duration. The spikes were usually confined to growth cones, as the [Ca^{2+}]$_i$ of neurites and cell bodies was substantially more stable. In order to study the mechanisms underlying these Ca^{2+} transients, we found that elevation of extracellular [Ca^{2+}] from the normal 2 mM level to 20 mM reliably triggers repetitive spikes of [Ca^{2+}]$_i$. These [Ca^{2+}]$_i$ spikes have been proposed as an important regulatory mechanism for cellular behaviors in many cell types (Tsien and Tsien, 1990). In growth cones they are usually initiated within 1 min of elevating external [Ca^{2+}], and spike duration is about 15 sec. Multiple spikes are common, and the intervals between spikes can be irregular. The mean spike height is about 200–300 nM, with [Ca^{2+}]$_i$ increasing from about 100 nM to 400 nM. Initiation and maintenance of these Ca^{2+} transients is not inhibited by drugs that block voltage-gated Ca^{2+} channels, but 1 mM La^{3+} blocks spikes or terminates spikes in the presence of 20 mM external Ca^{2+} (Figs. 7, 8). These Ca^{2+} transients seem to be locally regulated, since there is no correlation between the spiking behavior of different growth cones at the ends of several branches of a parent neurite. In addition, when a growth cone exhibits [Ca^{2+}]$_i$ spikes, the adjacent neurite and neuronal perikaryon usually do not show [Ca^{2+}]$_i$ transients.

We are continuing to characterize this dynamic

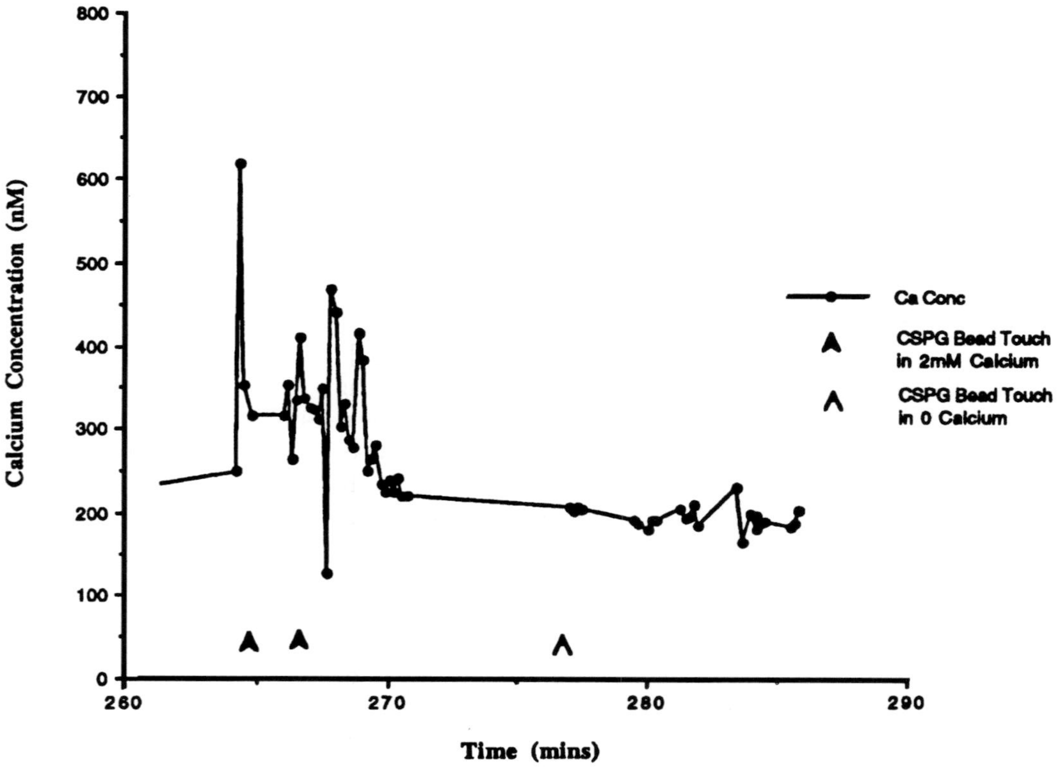

Fig. 6. Contact with a CSPG coated beads induces Ca^{2+} transients in a DRG neuron. A DRG neuron was touched with a CSPG coated polystyrene bead at the first arrowhead, inducing a large rise in $[Ca^{2+}]_i$. Another touch induces a similar response, but when the neuron was touched again after changing the bath to a Ca^{2+}-free medium, no rise in $[Ca^{2+}]_i$ occurred.

regulation of growth cone $[Ca^{2+}]_i$. Clearly, these Ca^{2+} transients in growth cones involve Ca^{2+} influx from extracellular spaces. It is unclear what the channels are that admit the Ca^{2+} ions, since our data indicate that voltage gated channels are not involved. It is not necessary to elevate external $[Ca^{2+}]$ to 20 mM in order to initiate spikes, since we have observed increased frequency of spiking after elevating external $[Ca^{2+}]$ from the normal level of 2 mM to just 3 mM. We are also unsure of the mechanisms responsible for the rapid decrease of cytoplasmic $[Ca^{2+}]$ at the end of a spike. This may result from both Ca^{2+} pumps in the plasma membrane and in cytoplasmic organelles, as well as inactivation of influx from the outside. Preliminary results with the drug ryanodine indicate that release of Ca^{2+} from cytoplasmic storage organelles contributes to spike generation. Our initial findings on responses to two inhibitors of the Ca^{2+} pump in the endoplasmic reticulum, thapsigargin and cyclopiazonic acid (Takemura et al., 1989), indicate that growth cones indeed contain membranous organelles that can remove Ca^{2+} from the cytoplasmic compartment. When these pumps are blocked by these drugs, spike frequency increases, and the baseline between spikes is higher (Fig. 9). These results indicate that a thapsigargin-sensi-

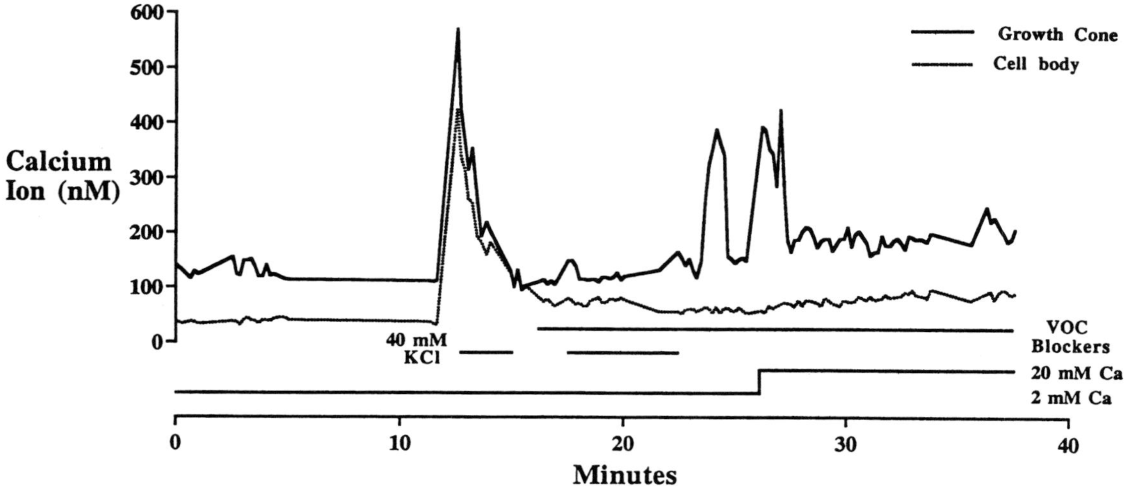

Fig. 7. The effects of voltage gated channel (VOC) blockers on the induction of Ca^{2+} spiking by exposure to 20 mM external $[Ca^{2+}]$. Initially, the neuron is depolarized with 40 mM KCl, which opens voltage gated Ca^{2+} channels and produces a Ca^{2+} spike in the growth cone. Then, a mixture of nifedipine and omega conotoxin (VOC blockers) are added to block N, L, and T Ca^{2+} channels. KCl is added again, but $[Ca^{2+}]_i$ does not rise because of the channel blockers. The external $[Ca^{2+}]$ was shifted from 2 mM to 20 mM, and spiking of cytoplasmic $[Ca^{2+}]$ began, despite the presence of the voltage gated channel blockers.

tive pump buffers $[Ca^{2+}]_i$ and may contribute to the down-slope of the spikes.

Thus, growth cones contain mechanisms for rapidly changing cytoplasmic $[Ca^{2+}]$ and producing complex signals consisting of Ca^{2+} spikes of varying height, duration and frequencies. There are many implications of these events for regulation of growth cone behavior. The regulatory actions of calcium ions are mediated and modulated by a rich diversity of kinases, actin associated proteins, and regulatory proteins in both a direct and an indirect manner (Tsien and Tsien, 1990). Ca^{2+} transients may permit selective regulation of Ca^{2+} sensitive processes, which is not possible

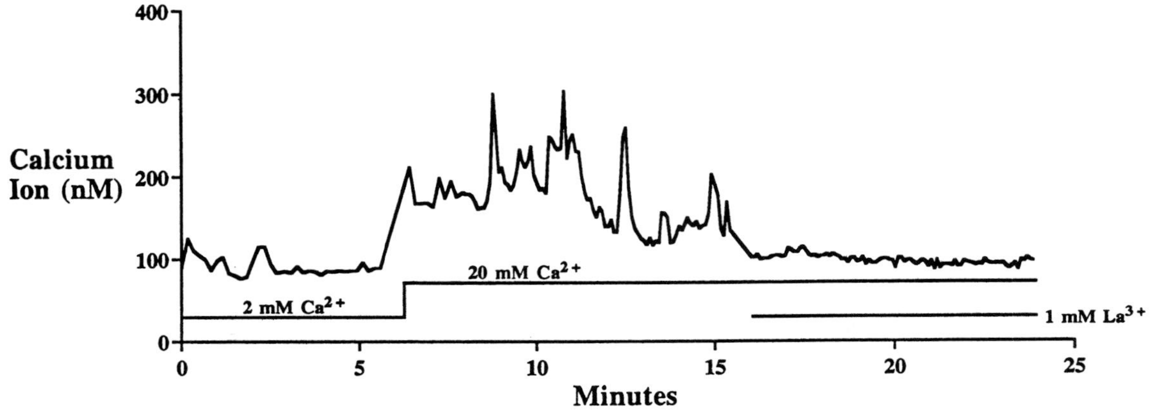

Fig. 8. The inhibition of growth cone $[Ca^{2+}]_i$ spiking by the global Ca^{2+} channel blocker, La^{3+}. $[Ca^{2+}]_i$ is initiated in a growth cone by elevation of $[Ca^{2+}]_o$ from 2 mM to 20mM. When 1 mM La^{3+} is perfused into the medium, growth cone $[Ca^{2+}]_i$ spiking stops immediately.

by elevation of $[Ca^{2+}]_i$ to a single higher plateau concentration. We have previously reported that sensory growth cones contain several cytoskeletal associated proteins that are regulated by $[Ca^{2+}]$ (Letourneau and Shattuck, 1989), and, recently, we have examined growth cones for the presence of several other Ca^{2+} regulated proteins that may regulate growth cone motility.

Ca^{2+} regulated proteins in growth cones

The organization of actin filaments is regulated by a variety of proteins that control actin polymerization, interactions of actin filaments with other filaments and organelles, and the integrity of filaments. Caldesmon, which is regulated by Ca^{2+}/calmodulin, may regulate interactions of actin filaments with other cytoskeletal components (Hartwig and Kwiatowski, 1991; Matsumura and Yamashiro, 1993). Figure 10 shows the immunofluorescence localization of caldesmon in growth cones. Gelsolin binds to actin filaments, and in the presence of $[Ca^{2+}] > 100$ nM, it severs actin filaments. This causes the breakdown of filament networks, but also creates new filament ends for actin repolymerization (Hartwig et al., 1989; Hartwig and Kwiatowski, 1991). Figure 10 shows an immunofluorescence demonstration of enriched localization of gelsolin in the leading margin and filopodia of growth cones. We have also demonstrated the presence of gelsolin and caldesmon by Western blot analysis of growth cone preparations from chick embryo brain.

The actions of $[Ca^{2+}]$ are modulated by many Ca^{2+}-binding regulatory proteins (Baimbridge et al., 1992). Figure 10 shows additional immunocytochemical evidence for the presence of two such proteins in growth cones: calmodulin, a ubiquitous regulator of protein kinases and other enzymes; and calcineurin, a Ca^{2+}- and calmodulin-dependent serine/threonine phosphoprotein phosphatase.

Conclusions

The model for the navigational machinery of growth cones proposed at the beginning of this article depends on cell surface receptors that respond to interactions with environmental cues by transmembrane signaling to cytoplasmic regulatory systems. The identification of these puta-

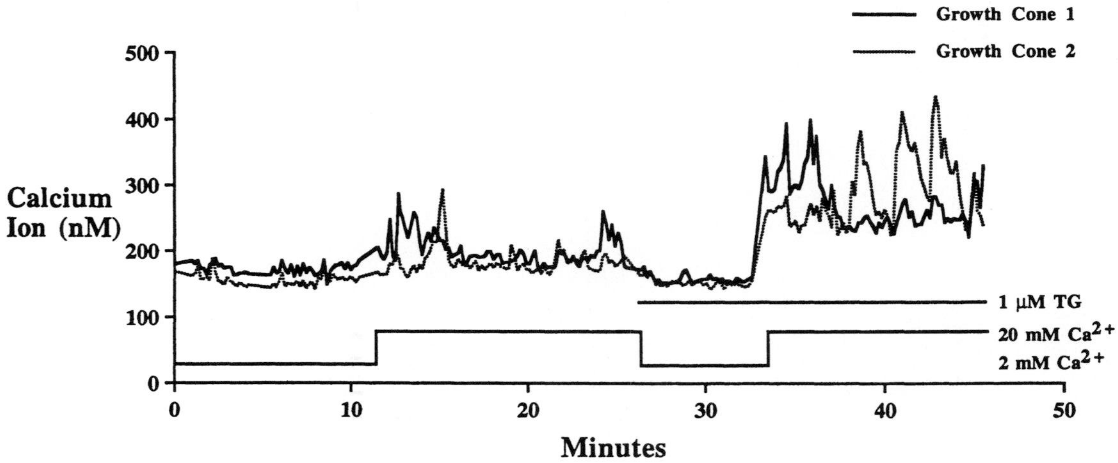

Fig. 9. The effects of 1 μM thapsigargin (TG) on induction of growth cone Ca^{2+} spiking. Ca^{2+} spiking is initiated in two growth cones by elevation of $[Ca^{2+}]_o$ from 2 mM to 20 mM. Return of $[Ca^{2+}]_o$ to 2 mM stops spiking. Then, 1 μM TG is added, and $[Ca^{2+}]_o$ is returned to 20 mM. Spiking of $[Ca^{2+}]_i$ is now more frequent and spikes are higher. This is interpreted to indicate that Ca^{2+} pumps in cytoplasmic organelles are involved in buffering growth cone $[Ca^{2+}]_i$.

tive receptors and the mode of their transmembrane signaling is the focus of research in many laboratories. We have focused our efforts on growth cone interactions with surface-bound environmental components, and we find that the inhibitory effects of PGs and glycosaminoglycans may be mediated in part by rapid elevation of growth cone cytoplasmic [Ca^{2+}]. We also are investigating how growth cones produce their calcium signals, perhaps via distinct plasma membrane channels, cytoplasmic Ca^{2+} storage organelles and Ca^{2+} pumps that are not yet completely identified or located. Growth cones contain a diversity of Ca^{2+} regulated proteins that could participate in the regulation of growth cone motility, and elucidation of the roles of all these molecules and metabolic events in growth cone navigation will continue to be a challenging and fertile ground for research. However, the knowledge gained by these efforts will hopefully aid in promoting recovery from spinal cord injuries.

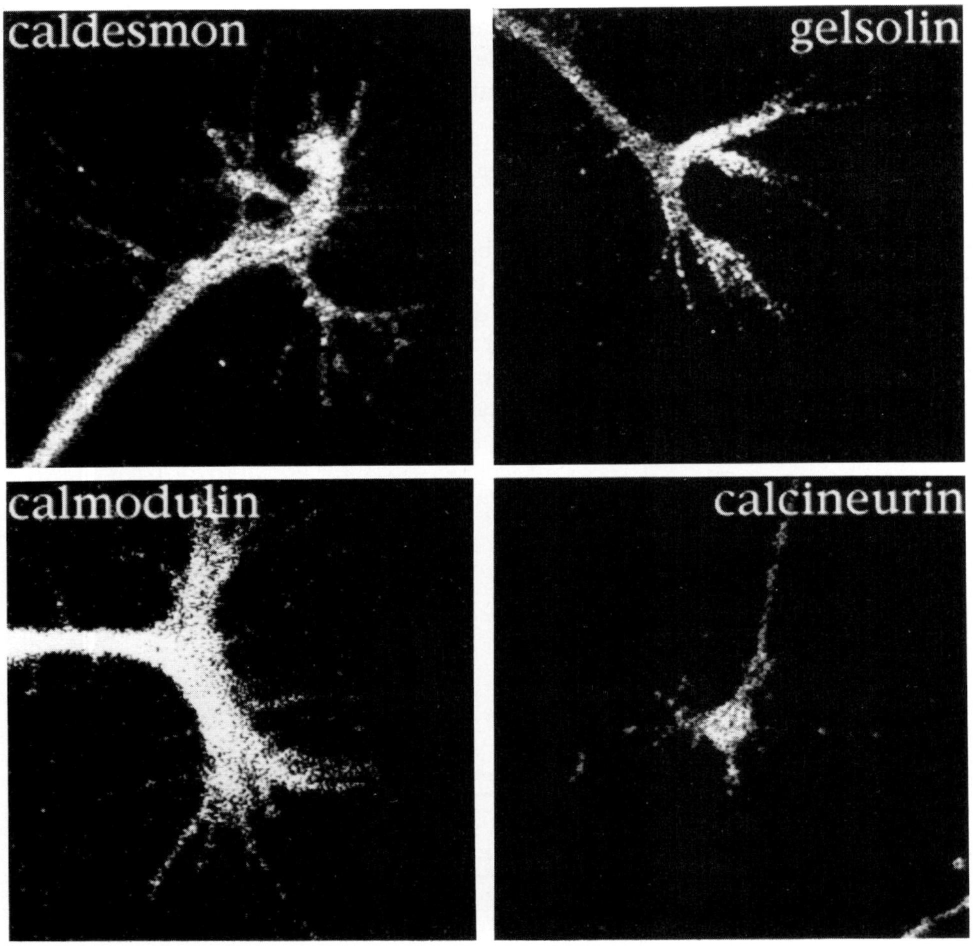

Fig. 10. Immunofluorescence localization using antibodies against four calcium regulated proteins in sensory neuronal growth cones. Caldesmon and gelsolin are actin binding proteins, calmodulin is a ubiquitous regulator of enzymes and other proteins, and calcineurin is a Ca^{2+} regulated protein phosphatase.

Acknowledgements

This research was supported by NIH research grants HD19950 and NS28807 to P.C.L., NIH NRSA EY06331 to D.M.S., and NIH grant EY07133 predoctoral traineeship to T.M.G. We thank Jerry Sedgewick for excellent assistance in producing the figures.

References

Baier, H. and Bonhoeffer, F. (1992) Axon guidance by gradients of a target-derived component. *Science*, 255: 472–475.

Baimbridge, K.G., Celio, M.R. and Rogers, J.H. (1992) Calcium-binding proteins in the nervous system. *Trends Neurosci.*, 8: 303–308.

Bandtlow, C.E., Schmidt, M.F., Hassinger, T.D., Schwab, M.E. and Kater, S.B. (1993) Role of intracellular calcium in NI-35-evoked collapse of neuronal growth cones. *Science*, 259: 80–83.

Berridge, M.J. (1993) Inositol triphosphate and calcium signaling. *Nature (London)*, 361: 315–325.

Bixby, J.L. and Harris, W.A. (1991) Molecular mechanisms of axon growth and guidance. *Annu. Rev. Cell Biol.*, 7: 117–159.

Bray, D. (1987) Growth cones: do they pull or are they pushed? *Trends Neurosci*, 10: 431–434.

Bray, D. and Hollenbeck, P.J. (1988) Growth cone motility and guidance. *Annu. Rev. Cell Biol.*, 4: 43–61.

Bridgman, P.C. and Dailey, M.E. (1989) The organization of myosin and actin in rapidly frozen nerve growth cones. *J. Cell Biol.*, 108: 95–109.

Damsky, C.H. and Werb, Z. (1992) Signal transduction by integrin receptors for extracellular matrix: cooperative processing of extracellular information. *Curr. Opin. Cell Biol.*, 4: 772–781.

Davenport, R.W. and Kater, S.B. (1992) Local increases in intracellular calcium elicit local filopodial responses in Helisoma neuronal growth cones. *Neuron*, 9: 405–416.

Davenport, R.W., Dou, P., Rehder, V. and Kater, S.B. (1993) A sensory role for neuronal growth cone filopodia. *Nature (London)*, 361: 721–724.

Davies, J.A. and Cook, G.M.W. (1991) Growth cone inhibition — an important mechanism in neural development? *BioEssays*, 13(1): 11–15.

Doherty, P. and Walsh, F.S. (1992) Cell adhesion molecules, second messengers and axonal growth. *Curr. Opin. Neurobiol.*, 2: 595–601.

Fishman, M.C. and Strittmatter, S.M. (1993) Detection and amplification of inhibitory signals at the neuronal growth cone. *Neurosci. Facts*, 4(6): 21–22.

Goldberg, D.J. (1988) Local role of Ca^{2+} in formation of veils in growth cones. *J. Neurosci.*, 8: 2596–2605.

Goldberg, D.J. and Burmeister, D.W. (1989) Looking into growth cones. *Trends Neurosci.*, 12: 503–506.

Goodman, C.S. and Schatz, C. (1993) Developmental mechanisms that generate precise patterns of neuronal connectivity. *Neuron*, 10 (Suppl.): 77–98.

Hartwig, J.H., Chambers, K.A. and Stossel, T.P. (1989) Association of gelsolin with actin filaments and cell membranes of macrophages and platelets. *J. Cell Biol.*, 108: 467–479.

Hartwig, J.H. and Kwiatowski, D.J. (1991) Actin-binding proteins. *Curr. Opin. Cell Biol.*, 3: 87–97.

Heidemann, S.R., Lamoureux, P. and Buxbaum, R.E. (1990) Growth cone behavior and production of traction force. *J. Cell Biol.*, 111: 1949–1957.

Hollenbeck, P.J. (1989) The transport and assembly of the axonal cytoskeleton. *J. Cell Biol.*, 108: 223–227.

Hynes, R.O. (1992) Integrins: versatility, modulation, and signaling in cell adhesion. *Cell*, 69: 11–25.

Hynes, R.O. and Lander, A.D. (1992) Contact and adhesive specificities in the associations, migrations, and targeting of cells and axons. *Cell*, 68: 302–322.

Joshi, H.C. and Baas, P.W. (1993) A new perspective on microtubules and axon growth. *J. Cell Biol.*, 121: 1191–1196.

Kapfhammer, J. and Raper, J. (1987) Collapse of growth cone structure on contact with specific neurites in culture. *J. Neurosci.*, 7(1): 201–212.

Kapfhammer, J.P. and Schwab, M.E. (1992) Modulators of neuronal migration and neurite growth. *Curr. Opin. Cell Biol.*, 4: 863–868.

Kater, S.B. and Mills, L.R. (1991) Regulation of growth cone behavior by calcium. *J. Neurosci.*, 11: 891–899.

Kater, S.B., Mattson, M.P., Cohan, C. and Connor, J. (1988) Calcium regulation of the neuronal growth cone. *Trends Neurosci.*, 11: 315–321.

Lankford, K.L. and Letourneau, P.C. (1989) Evidence that calcium may control neurite outgrowth by regulating the stability of actin filaments. *J. Cell Biol.*, 109: 1229–1243.

Lankford, K.L. and Letourneau, P.C. (1991) Roles of actin filaments and three second-messenger systems in short-term regulation of chick dorsal root ganglion neurite outgrowth. *Cell Motil. Cytoskel.*, 20: 7–29.

Lankford, K., Cypher, C. and Letourneau, P.C. (1990) Nerve growth cone motility. *Curr. Opin. Cell Biol.*, 2: 80–85.

Letourneau, P.C. (1983) Differences in the organization of actin in the growth cones compared with the neurite of cultured neurons from chick embryos. *J. Cell Biol.*, 97: 963–973.

Letourneau, P.C. and Cypher, C. (1991) Regulation of growth cone motility. *Cell Motil. Cytoskel.*, 20: 267–271.

Letourneau, P.C. and Shattuck, T.A. (1989) Distribution and possible interactions of actin-associated proteins and cell adhesion molecules of nerve growth cones. *Development*, 105: 505–519.

Letourneau, P.C., Shattuck, T.A. and Ressler, A.H. (1987) 'Pull' and 'push' in neurite elongation: observations on the effects of different concentrations of cytochalasin B and taxol. *Cell Motil. Cytoskel.*, 8: 193–209.

Letourneau, P.C., Kater, S.B. and Macagno, E.R. (Eds.) (1991) *The Nerve Growth Cone*, Raven Press, New York, 535 pp.

Letourneau, P.C., Condic, M.L. and Snow, D.M. (1992) Extracellular matrix and neurite outgrowth. *Curr. Opin. Gen. Devel.*, 2: 625–634.

Marsh, L. and Letourneau, P.C. (1984) Growth of neurites without filopodial or lamellipodial activity in the presence of cytochalasin B. *J. Cell Biol*, 99: 2041–2047.

Matsumura, F. and Yamashiro, S. (1993) Caldesmon. *Curr. Opin. Cell Biol.*, 5: 70–76.

Mitchison, T. and Kirschner, M. (1988) Cytoskeletal dynamics and nerve growth. *Neuron*, 1: 761–772.

O'Connor, T.P., Duerr, J.S. and Bentley, D. (1990) Pioneer growth cone steering decisions mediated by single filopodial contact in situ. *J. Neurosci.*, 10: 3935–3946.

Okabe, S. and Hirokawa, N. (1988) Microtubule dynamics in nerve cells: analysis using microinjection of biotinylated tubulin into PC12 cells. *J. Cell Biol.*, 107: 651–664.

Okabe, S. and Hirokawa, N. (1992) Differential behavior of photoactivated microtubules in growing axons of mouse and frog neurons. *J. Cell Biol.*, 117: 105–120.

Okabe, S. and Hirokawa, N. (1993) Do photobleached fluorescent microtubules move? Re-evaluation of fluorescent laser photobleaching both in vitro and in growing *Xenopus* axons. *J. Cell Biol.*, 120: 1177–1186.

Patterson, P.H. (1988) On the importance of being inhibited, or saying no to growth cones. *Neuron*, 1: 263–267.

Ramón y Cajal, S. (1890) Sur l'origine et les ramifications des fibres nerveuses de la moelle embryonalre. *Anat. Anz.*, 5: 609–613, 631–639.

Raper, J.A., Bastiani, M. and Goodman, C.S. (1983) Pathfinding by neuronal growth cones in grasshopper embryos. I. Divergent choices made by the growth cones of sibling neurons. *J. Neurosci.*, 3: 20–30.

Rehder, V. and Kater, S.B. (1992) Regulation of neuronal growth cone filopodia by intracellular calcium. *J. Neurosci*, 12: 3175–3186.

Reichardt, L.F. and Tomaselli, T.J. (1991) Extracellular matrix molecules and their receptors. *Annu. Rev. Neurosci.*, 14: 531–570.

Reinsch, S.S., Mitchison, T.J. and Kirschner, M.W. (1991) Microtubule polymer assembly and transport during axonal elongation. *J. Cell Biol.*, 115: 365–380.

Rivas, R.J., Burmeister, D.W. and Goldberg, D.J. (1992) Rapid effects of laminin on the growth cone. *Neuron*, 8: 107–115.

Robson, S.J. and Burgoyne, S.D. (1988) Differential levels of tyrosinated, detyrosinated, and acetylated alpha-tubulin in neurites and growth cones of dorsal root ganglion neurons. *Cell Motil. Cytoskel.*, 12: 273–282.

Rogers, S.L., Letourneau, P.C., Palm, S.L., McCarthy, J.B. and Furcht, L.T. (1983) Neurite extension by peripheral and central nervous system neurons in response to substratum-bound fibronectin and laminin. *Dev. Biol.*, 96: 212–220.

Schweighoffer, T. and Shaw, S. (1992) Adhesion cascades: diversity through combinatorial strategies. *Curr. Opin. Cell Biol.*, 4: 824–829.

Smith, S.J. (1988) Neuronal cytomechanics: the actin-based motility of growth cones. *Science*, 242: 708–715.

Snow, D.M. and Letourneau, P.C. (1992) Neurite outgrowth on a step gradient of chondroitin sulfate proteoglycan (CS-PG). *J. Neurobiol.*, 23(3): 322–336.

Snow, D.M., Steindler, D.A. and Silver, J. (1990) Molecular and cellular characterization of the glial roof plate of the spinal cord and optic tectum: a possible role for a proteoglycan in the development of an axon barrier. *Dev. Biol.*, 138: 359–376.

Snow, D., Watanabe, M., Letourneau, P.C. and Silver, J. (1991) A chondroitin sulfate proteoglycan may influence the direction of retinal ganglion cell outgrowth. *Development*, 113: 1473–1485.

Snow, D.M., Atkinson, P., Hassinger, T., Kater, S.B. and Letourneau, P.C. (1993) Growth cone intracellular calcium levels are elevated upon contact with sulfated proteoglycans. *Soc. Neurosci. Abstr.*, 19: 876.

Takemura, H., Hughes, A.R., Thastrup, O. and Putney, J.W. (1989) Activation of calcium entry by the tumor promoter thapsigargin in parotid acinar cells. *J. Biol. Chem.*, 264: 12266–12271.

Tosney, K.W. and Landmesser, L.T. (1985a) Development of the major pathways for neurite outgrowth in the chick hind limb. *Devel. Biol.*, 109: 193–214.

Tosney, K.W. and Landmesser, L.T. (1985b) Growth cone morphology and trajectory in the lumbrosacral region of the chick embryo. *J. Neurosci.*, 5: 2345–2358.

Tosney, K. and Oakley, R. (1990) The perinotochordal mesenchyme acts as a barrier to axon advance in the chick embryo: implications for a general mechanism of axonal guidance. *Exp. Neurol.*, 109: 75–89.

Tsien, R.W. and Tsien, R.Y. (1990) Calcium channels, stores, and oscillations. *Annu. Rev. Cell Biol.*, 6: 715–760.

F.J. Seil (Ed.)
Progress in Brain Research, Vol 103

CHAPTER 10

Contributions of multiple forms of myosin to nerve outgrowth

P.C. Bridgman, M.W. Rochlin, A.K. Lewis and L.L. Evans

Department of Anatomy and Neurobiology, Washington University School of Medicine, 660 S. Euclid Avenue, St. Louis, MO 63110, U.S.A.

Introduction

The specific pattern of neuronal connections that form during development or following recovery from nerve injury results from directed axonal outgrowth followed by synapse formation with specific targets. Directed outgrowth involves the coordination of two distinct processes: growth cone locomotion and axon assembly. Locomotion refers only to growth cone advance and entails continuous remodeling (protrusion and retraction) of the growth cone cytoplasm and the exertion of a rearward directed traction force upon the substratum. In contrast, axon assembly refers to the construction of a relatively quiescent non-motile cylinder of differentiated cytoplasm (Goldberg and Burmeister, 1986). Because the materials used for axon assembly are synthesized in the cell body, axonal transport of new materials toward the distal tip of the axon is a prerequisite for assembly. Each of the processes described above requires force production by molecular motors, and force production also appears to be involved in their coordination. There are a number of classes of molecular motors found in neurons, including the actin-based myosins and the microtubule-based dyneins and kinesins. We have focused on the role of myosins in growth cone locomotion, axon assembly and transport.

At least seven families of myosin have been identified in vertebrate cells (Cheney et al., 1993a). Although it has not yet been determined whether representatives from each of these families are expressed in nervous tissue, myosins I, II and V (Fig. 1) are abundant in neurons and therefore are likely to be involved in growth cone locomotion and axon assembly (Bridgman and Dailey, 1989; Bridgman and Kordyban, 1[illegible]; Miller et al., 1992; Espreafico et al., 1993; [illegible]idgman et al., unpublished results). Myosin II is the conventional, two-headed myosin that forms bipolar filaments with other myosin II molecules via interactions between their coiled-coil tail domains. Myosin I was originally characterized in the unicellular organism, *Acanthamoeba*. It is single-headed and has a short tail that does not form filaments (Pollard et al., 1991). Depending on the species (and on isoform within a species), myosin I tail domains may contain an ATP-independent actin binding site, a lipid binding site, calmodulin binding sites, or a combination of these domains. Myosin I isoforms have been purified and their ATPase activity characterized from *Acanthamoeba, Dictyostelium discoideum*, chick intestinal brush border cells and several mammalian tissues (Pollard et al., 1991), including, most recently, bovine brain (Barylko et al., 1992). Myosin I

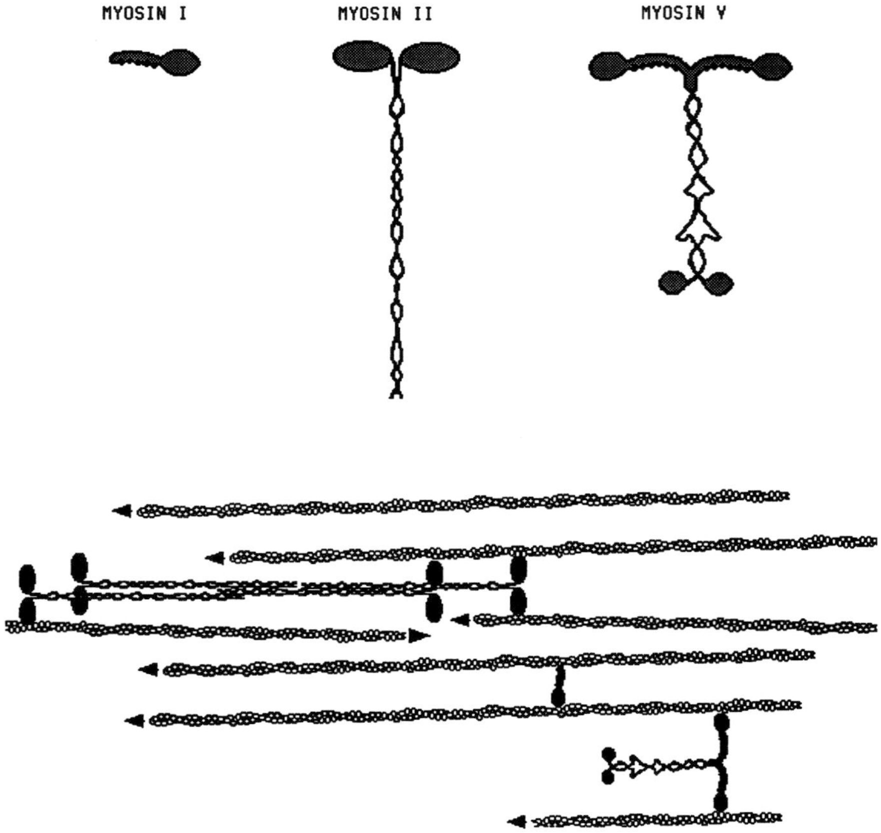

Fig. 1. Diagrammatic representation of myosin molecules from the three myosin families known to be present in mammalian neurons. The lower portion of the diagram shows potential actin filament cross-linking abilities of the different myosins. Arrowheads indicate the polarity of the actin filaments.

cDNAs have also recently been cloned from mouse and rat brain (Lewis and Bridgman, 1992a; Ruppert et al.,1993; Sherr et al., 1993). Another form of myosin, myosin V, is encoded by the murine dilute locus (Mercer et al., 1991); closely related molecules have also been identified in chicken and yeast (reviewed by Hammer, 1992). Myosin V is double-headed, with a unique tail comprised of a mixture of coiled-coil and globular domains (Espreafico et al., 1993). Myosin V forms dimers but does not form filaments (Cheney et al., 1993b). Homozygous myosin V deletion mutations in mice result in lethal convulsions indicating that myosin V could be crucial to nervous system function (Mercer et al., 1991). Our recent focus has been to elucidate the function of these three myosin families in neurons.

Growth cone locomotion

Growth cones advance by exerting a (traction) force on their environment (substratum) in the direction opposite to that of the advance: to move forward, they push rearward against the substratum. The direction and rate of this advance appear to be affected by protrusion and retraction of the growth cone periphery. How are the forces for traction and the activity of the periphery (protrusion and retraction) generated? We will discuss evidence that acto-myosin dynamics are involved in this force production.

Traction force

Two possible models for the generation of traction force have been suggested. Both models depend upon linkage between cortical actin filaments and the substratum via integral membrane proteins. Both are also contingent upon a rearward directed force exerted on actin filaments by molecular motors, probably myosins. The principal differences between the two models are the identity of the actin filament population involved and the location and type of the myosins involved. In one model, the proposition is that a rearward flowing actin filament network distributed throughout the periphery of the growth cone produces traction force. Such an actin network undergoing retrograde flow in growth cones was first suggested by Bray (1970), who applied particles to the upper surface of growth cones and observed that they moved rearward. The contribution of actin filaments to the retrograde flow was later documented by the work of Forscher and Smith (1988a). Cytochalasins, which block polymerization at the barbed end of f-actin, caused the distal edge of the cortical network to retract from the distal edge of the growth cone at the same rate as the bulk retrograde movement. The simplest interpretation is that actin polymerization normally replenishes the distalmost edge of the network as it is pulled centrally. The most likely candidates responsible for pulling the actin network are myosins, since these are the only known force producing proteins associated with actin. The en masse retraction of the actin network following cytochalasin treatment suggests that the myosins involved in causing the movement are distributed throughout the lamellipodia or in the more centrally located region immediately adjacent. Aminated polystyrene beads applied to the surface of growth cones move retrogradely at the same rate as the actin network, and their movement is stopped by cytochalasin treatment (Forscher and Smith, 1988b). This observation, in combination with the original observation by Bray (1970), supports the possibility that the actin network is linked to the exterior of the cell by proteins that span the lipid bilayer. If this linkage occurs on the ventral surface where attachment to the substratum can occur, then traction would result.

An alternative, but not exclusive model, is that filopodia contract, pulling the cone forward. This model was first proposed by Bray (1982) and is supported by the observation that filopodial shortening exerts tension on substrate associated objects, causing them to move. Filopodial shortening is associated with an increase in thickness, suggesting a contractile mechanism at work (Heidemann et al., 1990). Furthermore, filopodia that have been mechanically isolated from the growth cone can contract (Davenport et al., 1993). This model predicts that myosins involved in filopodial pulling are associated with the actin filament bundles that form the core of filopodia.

As indicated by these models, the organization and polarity of the actin filaments within the lamellipodia is important. We found that there are two populations of actin filaments within lamellipodia distinct from the filament bundles forming filopodia (Lewis and Bridgman, 1992a). One population consisted of small bundles of actin filaments that span the length of the lamellipodia and were oriented primarily with their barbed (rapid polymerizing) ends toward the leading edge. The second population consisted of shorter, branched filaments oriented randomly with respect to the leading edge. The bundles were primarily located ventrally, close to the membrane in contact with substratum, while the population of short, branched filaments was primarily dorsally located. The bundles of actin filaments that formed the core of filopodia were larger than the bundles found in lamellipodia. However, the proximal ends of these bundles often penetrated into the lamellipodia for varying distances. The different organization and location of these populations of filaments suggest that they may have distinct behaviors and functions. Because the bundled filaments were ventrally located and spanned the length of the lamellipodia or formed the core of filopodia, they appear to be the most likely to be involved in the generation of traction force. As will be discussed below, the local actin organization places constraints on which myosins can participate in traction force production.

Generation of traction force by myosin has two minimum requirements: a population of actin filaments that are oriented with their barbed ends toward the leading edge, and a means of anchoring the myosin molecules responsible for their movement. At least two methods for accomplishing this are possible. In a manner similar to skeletal muscle contraction, myosin could contract against anti-parallel actin filaments (Huxley, 1973). In this case the 'anchor' could be provided by actin filaments that are anti-parallel to the filaments oriented with barbed ends toward the leading edge. This mechanism is best suited for myosin II, which can form bipolar filaments. However, myosin I isoforms with an ATP-independent actin binding site could also potentially use this mechanism. Alternatively, myosin molecules that are anchored to other components of the cytoskeleton could pull appropriately oriented actin filaments rearward. This mechanism could be accommodated by any type of myosin. Thus, traction force may depend upon the types of myosin involved, and also upon the actin filament organization in regions in which the force is generated. Both models predict that the myosins involved in generating traction force bind to actin filaments that are or can become linked to integral membrane proteins on the ventral membrane surface.

Protrusion and retraction

During locomotion the growth cone maintains its basic shape and size as it moves across the substratum. Net protrusion at the leading edge is balanced by net retraction at the base of the cone. Transient alterations in growth cone shape often do occur, reflecting a change in the balance between protrusion and retraction. For example, if protrusion of the forward edges temporarily is greater than retraction at the rear edges, the surface area of the growth cone increases. Although protrusion entails forward extension of lamellipodia and filopodia, the observation that this extension typically occurs above the substratum suggests that protrusion does not require traction force. Protrusion could result exclusively from concerted localized actin polymerization (Cooper, 1991). While a polymerization based mechanism does not require myosin activity, myosin may modulate protrusive activity by altering cortical surface tension. Myosins could also be involved in retraction of lamellipodia and filopodia. By exerting tension on actin networks that are not well attached to the substratum, myosins could pull them toward networks which are more securely anchored.

The above focused on the contribution of the force generating capabilities of myosins. The f-actin cross-linking capability of many myosin isoforms can also have a role in locomotion. By cross-linking actin networks that are being pulled in different directions, myosins could serve as integrators of traction force, thereby influencing the net direction of these traction forces. Cross-linking of actin networks by myosins in the growth cone periphery could influence the size of lamellipodia and filopodia undergoing protrusion or retraction. The direction of net protrusion is thought to bias the outgrowth direction; myosins may influence navigation by this means. Clearly, both the force generating and f-actin cross-linking properties of myosins make them ideal candidates for regulators of the rate and direction of growth cone locomotion.

Evidence supporting a role of particular myosins in traction force and protrusion / retraction

Myosin II is the best studied family of myosin in cells, including nerve growth cones. Its distribution has been studied at both the light and electron microscope level of resolution (Bridgman and Dailey, 1989; Miller et al., 1992). Recently it has become clear that non-muscle myosin II exists in multiple isoforms (Miller et al., 1992). Therefore, we have reinvestigated the distribution of the myosin II in growth cones of cultured rat superior cervical ganglion (SCG) neurons using antibodies specific for the most abundant isoforms, myosin II A and B (Rochlin et al., 1992). The B isoform appears to be the most abundant isoform in brain as determined by immunoblot experiments; it is also the most abundant isoform in SCG neurons as determined by immunofluorescence. In rapidly advancing growth cones it is primarily located in a marginal zone between the thin actin rich peripheral region and the thicker, organelle rich central region. This location is consistent with a role of myosin II in the retrograde flow of actin observed in lamellipodia. The pointed ends of bundled actin filaments that span the lamellipodia (see below) overlap this concentration of myosin IIB. If myosin IIB forms bipolar filaments, it could interact with the pointed ends of these bundles while being anchored through interactions with larger bundles of actin that are seen to run through the marginal zone. However, because the growth cone increases in thickness in this area, it is necessary to use immunoelectron microscopy in combination with serial sections or whole-mounts viewed in stereo to precisely determine if myosin IIb is involved in such interactions.

Growth cone filopodia and lamellipodia sometimes make adhesive contacts with neighboring axons. This causes the contacted axon to be deflected toward the adherent growth cone. If the growth cone involved in the pulling is labeled for myosin IIB using immunofluorescence, it shows a periodic alignment of stain along actin filaments oriented lengthwise within the extended process contacting the axon (Rochlin et al., 1992). This staining pattern is reminiscent of that seen in fibroblast stress fibers, suggesting that the formation of the pattern occurs as a result of increased amounts of tension along the axis involved in the pulling. This would suggest that myosin IIB is involved in the development of tension that results from the pulling.

In order to determine the role of myosin II in growth cone motility, we have conducted experiments to inhibit its function. Myosin light chain kinases (MLCK) and CAM kinase II regulate acto-myosin interactions by phosphorylating the regulatory light chain of myosin II. We found that the actin-activated ATPase activity of fetal rat brain myosin II undergoes a 15-fold increase following phosphorylation (Rochlin and Bridgman, 1991). Given this sensitivity, we tested the influence of a MLCK and CAM kinase II inhibitor, KT5926, on axon growth. Three and 10 μM KT5926 slowed the radial growth from SCG explants in a dose-dependent manner to 78 and 63%, respectively, of control explants after either 7 or 15 h of treatment. KT5926 increased the number of varicosities on axons and decreased the size of lamellipodia. Differential interference contrast microscopy of growth cones treated with 10 μM KT5926 revealed a decrease in lamellipodial activity. K252b, a KT5926 analog with greater potency for inhibiting other kinases and lower potency for inhibiting MLCK, only slowed growth to 86% at 10 μM and did not induce morphological effects as pronounced as those consequent to treatment with KT5926. These results indicate that inhibition of myosin II function can have profound effects on growth cone shape and rate of axon outgrowth.

In the experiments described above, we are confident that we have inhibited myosin II function. However, inhibition of CAM kinase II activity is destined to produce effects on the nerve cell unrelated to myosin II activity. In order to produce a more specific knockout of myosin IIB function, we have recently isolated a cDNA clone to rat brain myosin IIB (Rochlin et al., unpublished results). We have used sequence information from the 5′ end of the transcript which spans the start codon to produce phosphorothioate-modified synthetic antisense oligonucleotides. Experiments are in progress using these oligonucleotides to treat cultured SCG neurons to suppress the synthesis of myosin IIB. The role of myosin IIB in traction force and maintenance of growth cone shape is supported both by the pattern of staining and the dramatic change in growth cone structure and the slowing of outgrowth that occurs in response to inhibition of its activity. Further experiments will provide a more specific assessment of the role of myosin IIB in these activities. However, because myosin II inhibition does not fully suppress growth cone motility, it appears likely that other myosins, such as myosin I and V, may also contribute to one or more of these activities. Consistent with this idea, myosins I and V are located throughout the growth cone, although they are more concentrated in the organelle rich central region (see below).

Myosins and axon assembly

Axon assembly involves the construction of new segments of the axon cylinder. This appears to involve two separate processes: constriction at the base of the growth cone to form the cylinder and mass addition to increase length. We will discuss the potential roles of myosins in both these processes.

Active constriction at the base of the growth cone is apparent from observations made on growth cones that have been severed from their axons (Bridgman, 1990). When the growth cone has been severed with minimal damage, it continues to move across the substratum without interruption. If the remaining stump of the axon attached to the growth cone is adherent to the substratum, it lengthens as the growth cone advances. Although the lengthening appears to result from stretching, the maintenance of the cylindrical shape of the axon stump implies that the base of the growth cone is being actively constricted. Immunofluorescence observations show that myosin IIB is concentrated along actin filaments at the concave surface of the constriction, as is typically observed in non-severed axons. This localization indicates that this form of myosin may be involved in the constriction process.

Elongation of the axon cylinder requires the continued transport and polymerization of the cytoskeletal elements necessary for new axon construction. The mechanism by which this is achieved has been controversial, although, recently, attempts have been made to reconcile different views (Joshi and Baas, 1993). In addition, new membrane must be added along with proteins that act as receptors for tropic factors and adhesion molecules. Because the proteins and lipids that are assembled into new axon segments are synthesized in the cell body, these materials must be transported down the axon.

Microtubule based motors such as kinesin and dynein are responsible for fast axonal transport of organelles in the anterograde and retrograde directions respectively. However, recent observations of organelle movement in dissociated squid axoplasm suggest that actin-based motors may also contribute to organelle transport (Kuznetsov et al., 1992). The motors responsible for actin-based transport appear to reside on the same vesicles as the microtubule-based motors. Thus, moving organelles can switch between microtubules and actin based motors. One intriguing possibility is that microtubule motors are used for long distance axial transport (the highway system) while actin based motors are required for local radial transport (local street system) and for access to the plasma membrane. Therefore, myosins may be necessary for delivery of material required for axon assembly. Preliminary experiments suggest that two unconventional myosins (myosin I and V) may be involved in organelle transport in cultured neurons.

Myosin I has been implicated in organelle transport in non-vertebrate systems (Adams and Pollard, 1986). Organelles coated with purified myosin I move on actin filaments. The recent cloning of myosin I cDNAs from brain libraries and the localization of myosin I transcripts in brain nerve cells by in situ hybridization (Lewis and Bridgman, 1992a; Ruppert et al., 1993; Sherr et al., 1993) support the notion that this family of myosin may also be important for organelle transport in nerve cells. We have isolated, from a rat brain library, a myosin I cDNA clone that is most similar to brush border myosin I (Hoshimaru and Nakanishi, 1987). This clone corresponds to the recently isolated myr 1a clone from rat (Ruppert et al., 1993) and myosin Iα clone from mouse (Sherr et al., 1993). In situ hybridization results indicate that this myosin I is found in brain nerve cells (Sherr et al., 1993) and in SCG neurons (Lewis and Bridgman, 1992a). Immunofluorescence studies using antibodies made to a myosin I fusion protein show that myosin I is located in both growth cones and axons of SCG neurons (Lewis and Bridgman, unpublished results). In contrast, antibodies made to myosin I purified from bovine adrenal gland (Barylko et al., 1992) do not stain SCG neurons (Bridgman et al., unpublished observations). Myosin I is widely distributed throughout the growth cone in a finely punctate pattern but is most concentrated in the thick central region. The concentration of myosin I may result from association with organelles, many of which are attached to or closely associated with microtubules in the central region. However, organelle transport may not be the only function of myosin I, since its staining is also located in growth cone regions devoid of organelles. To determine the function of this myosin I, we have begun knockout experiments using application of myosin I antisense oligonucleotides to cultured SCG neurons.

Another myosin which may be involved in organelle movement is myosin V. Similar to myosin I, myosin V has been shown to bind phospholipids (Cheney et al., 1993b). The importance of myosin V for normal nerve function is underscored by the consequences of myosin V deletion mutations in mice that show lethal neurological defects either prenatally or at about 10–14 days postnatal (Rinchik et al., 1985). Although it is not clear whether myosin V is essential for initial outgrowth, it must become important for normal nerve function later in development. Myosin V has been shown to be expressed in nerve cells and is concentrated both in the Golgi region of the cell body and in growth cones (Espreafico et al., 1993; Evans and Bridgman, unpublished results). Although the function of myosin V in nerve cells is not yet known, in non-neuronal cells, such as melanocytes, there is evidence to suggest that this family of myosin is involved in organelle transport. In melanocytes from dilute mice that lack myosin V, transport of melanosomes to the tips of dendritic processes is disrupted (Rinchik et al., 1985).

Recently, we isolated cDNA clones to mouse and rat brain myosin V (Hammer and Bridgman, unpublished results). We have produced antibodies to myosin V fusion proteins and have used affinity purified fractions of these antibodies for immunolocalization of myosin V in cultured SCG neurons. Our results indicate that while myosin V partially colocalizes with areas containing numerous microtubules and membranous organelles, it is also often located in organelle free regions of the cytoplasm (Evans and Bridgman, unpublished results). Using immunoelectron microscopy, we have found that myosin V label is sometimes closely associated with microtubules in the central region of the growth cone (Evans and Bridgman, unpublished results). Because the labeling procedures involve partial solubilization of membranes, it is difficult to determine if this label is also associated with small membrane bound organelles. Further work, including knockout experiments as described above for myosin I and II, should clarify this point.

Influence of growth cone locomotion on axon assembly

Although the average axon assembly rate must equal the average growth cone locomotion rate for normal outgrowth to occur, locomotory rates can temporarily exceed estimated axon assembly rates, as indicated by the apparent elastic stretching of the axon during growth cone advance (Dennerll et al., 1989; Lamoureux et al., 1989). Could the tension exerted on the axon influence the rate of axon assembly? Three lines of evidence indicate that it does: (1) tension applied externally to growth cones or nascent axons is capable of reorienting or accelerating axon assembly (Bray, 1984; Dennerll et al., 1988); (2) although tension is not necessary for growth cone advance, as indicated by the ability of growth cones to advance after they have been severed from their axons (Bridgman, 1990), axon assembly will not proceed unless axon tension exceeds a threshold (Zheng et al., 1991); and (3) tension has been measured in axons, and it is positively correlated with the axon outgrowth rate (Lamoureux et al., 1989). Together, these observations imply that tension may be sufficient and necessary for axon assembly, and that it varies predictably in freely growing axons.

As already indicated, elastic stretching of the axon is one mechanism that may contribute to tension development in axons (Dennerll et al., 1989; Lamoureux et al., 1989; Zheng et al., 1991). The axon itself may also produce tension by contraction of acto-myosin networks distributed along its length. We suspect that elastic stretching has a more significant role in regulating axon tension, especially in vivo, because it is clear that the advance rate of growth cones varies in response to environmental cues. Support for the second mechanism is less direct. In one study, axon tension increased in the absence of growth cone advance if axons were first slackened, but not if they were kept taut (Dennerll et al., 1989). Thus, axons may be capable of contracting, but this ability is only revealed by slackening. Although this observation does not address whether mechanoenzymes within the axon contribute to its elastic properties, it argues against axons having a role in varying their tension. Thus, we propose that functionally significant regulation of tension is exercised primarily by growth cones. Since myosins are implicated in growth cone advance, they also have at least an indirect role in regulating axon assembly. Myosins may also have a direct role in tension transmission and/or tension restoration following slackening. Actin filaments run the length of axons in close association with the plasma membrane. Myosin IIB is distributed in a punctate manner along the entire length of the axon (Rochlin et al., 1992). Myosin IIB may therefore act as an actin cross-linker that supports tension throughout an actin network that is continuous between growth cone and axon. When slackening of the axon occurs, myosin IIB could then act to restore this tension.

Growth cone locomotion not only influences the rate of outgrowth but also the direction. As the growth cone changes its direction of movement, it pulls the distal portion of the trailing axon from side to side. If the axon is adherent along its length, the changes in direction are reflected by bends in the axon at points of adherence. Non-adherent axons are straight because their only point of adherence is at branch points or the cell body. Therefore, in vitro and presumably in vivo, it is the locomotory behavior of the growth cone that determines the final path of the axon.

Conclusion

Coordination of the activities of the growth cone that lead to locomotion and to assembly of the axon undoubtedly requires the orchestration of hundreds of molecules, including receptors, messengers, and effectors. Our focus is on the effectors of locomotion and transport: the actin cytoskeleton and the family of mechanoenzymes that move actin, the myosins. Myosins appear likely to have multiple functional roles in neurons. It is important to understand these roles and the results of their interactions in living cells to fully explain the mechanisms that underlie growth cone locomotion and axonal assembly. An understanding of the mechanisms underlying axon growth will help guide the development of strategies designed to facilitate axonal regeneration following nerve injury.

References

Adams, R.J. and Pollard, T.D. (1986) Propulsion of organelles isolated from Acanthamoeba along actin filaments by myosin-I. *Nature (Lond.)*, 322: 754–756.

Barylko, B., Wagner, M.C., Reizes, O. and Albanesi, J.P. (1992) Purification and characterization of a mammalian myosin I. *Proc. Natl. Acad. Sci. USA*, 89: 490–494.

Bray, D. (1970) Surface movements during the growth of single explanted neurons. *Proc. Natl. Acad. Sci. USA*, 65: 905–909.

Bray, D. (1982) Filopodial contraction and growth cone guidance. In: R. Bekkair, A. Curtis and G. Dunn (Eds.), *Cell Behavior,* Cambridge University Press, Cambridge, pp. 299–319.

Bray, D. (1984) Axonal growth in response to experimentally applied tension. *Dev. Biol.*, 102: 379–389.

Bridgman, P.C. (1990) Amputated growth cones can form neurites. *J. Cell Biol.*, 111: 490a.

Bridgman, P.C. and Dailey, M.E. (1989) The organization of myosin and actin in rapid frozen nerve growth cones. *J. Cell Biol.,* 108: 95–109.

Bridgman, P.C. and Kordyban, M.A. (1989) Detection of myosin I like immunoreactivity in vertebrate brain and nerve. *J. Cell Biol.*, 109(4): 84a.

Cheney, R.E., Riley, M.A. and Mooseker, M.S. (1993a) Phylogenetic analysis of the myosin superfamily. *Cell Motil. Cytoskel.*, 24: 215–223.

Cheney, R.E., O'Shea, M.K., Heuser, J.E., Coelho, M.V., Wolenski, J.S., Espreafico, E.M., Forscher, P., Larson, R.E. and Mooseker, M.S. (1993b) Brain myosin-V is a two headed unconventional myosin with motor activity. *Cell,* 75: 13–23.

Cooper, J. A. (1991) The role of actin polymerization in cell motility. *Annu. Rev. Physiol.*, 53: 585–605.

Davenport, R.W., Dou, P., Rehder, V. and Kater, S.B. (1993) A sensory role for neuronal growth cone filopodia. Nature (Lond.), 361: 721–724.

Dennerll, T.J., Joshi, H.C., Steel, V.L., Buxbaum, R.E. and Heidemann, S.R. (1988) Tension and compression in the cytoskeleton: II. Quantitative measurements. *J. Cell Biol.*, 107: 665–674.

Dennerll, T.J., Lamoureux, P., Buxbaum, R.E. and Heidemann, S.R. (1989) The cytomechanics of axonal elongation and retraction. *J. Cell Biol.*, 109: 3073–3083.

Espreafico, E.M., Cheney, R.E., Matteoli, M., Nascimento, A.A.C., De Camilli, P.V., Larson, R.E. and Mooseker, M.S. (1993) Primary structure and cellular localization of chicken brain myosin-V (p190), an unconventional myosin with calmodulin light chains. *J. Cell Biol.*, 119: 1541–1558.

Forscher, P. and Smith, S.J. (1988a) Actions of cytochalasins on the organization of actin filaments and microtubules in a neuronal growth cone. *J. Cell Biol.*, 107: 1505–1516.

Forscher, P. and Smith, S.J. (1988b) Membrane surface marker flow is coupled to retrograde flow of f-actin in neuronal growth cones. *J. Cell Biol.*, 107: 219a.

Goldberg, D.J. and Burmeister, D.W. (1986) Stages in axon formation: observation of growth of *Aplysia* axons in culture using video-enhanced contrast-differential interference contrast microscopy. *J. Cell Biol.*, 103: 1921–1931.

Hammer, J.A. (1992) Novel myosins. *Trends Cell Biol.*, 1: 50–56.

Heidemann, S.R., Lamoureux, P. and Buxbaum, R.E. (1990) Growth cone behavior and production of traction force. *J. Cell Biol.*, 111: 1949–1957.

Honer, B., Chi, S., Kendrick-Jones, J. and Jockusch, B.M. (1988) Modulation of cellular morphology and locomotory activity by antibodies against myosin. *J. Cell Biol.*, 107: 2181–2189.

Hoshimaru, M. and Nakanishi, S. (1987) Identification of a new type of mammalian myosin heavy chain by molecular cloning: overlap of its mRNA with preprotachykinin B mRNA. *J. Biol. Chem.,* 262: 14625–14632.

Huxley, H.E. (1973) Muscular contraction and cell motility. *Nature (Lond.),* 243: 445–449.

Knecht, D.A. and Loomis, W.F. (1987) Antisense RNA inactivation of myosin heavy chain gene expression in *Dictyostelium discoideum. Science,* 236: 1081–1085.

Kolodney, M.S. and Wysolmerski, R.B. (1992) Isometric contraction by fibroblasts and endothelial cells in tissue culture: a quantitative study. *J. Cell Biol.*, 117: 73–82.

Kuznetsov, S.A., Langford, G.M. and Weiss, D.G. (1992) Actin-dependent organelle movement in squid axoplasm. *Nature (Lond.),* 356: 722–725.

Lamoureux, P., Buxbaum, R.E. and Heidemann, S.R. (1989) Direct evidence that growth cones pull. *Nature (Lond.),* 340: 159–162.

Lewis, A.K. and Bridgman, P.C. (1992a) Isolation of a rat brain cDNA clone that may encode a myosin I. *Mol. Biol. Cell,* 3: 157a.

Lewis, A.K. and Bridgman, P.C. (1992b) Nerve growth cone lamellipodia contain two populations of actin filaments that differ in organization and polarity. *J. Cell Biol.*, 119: 1219–1243.

Mercer, J.A., Seperack, P.K., Strobel, M.C., Copeland, N.G. and Jenkins, N.A. (1991) Novel myosin heavy chain encoded by murine dilute coat color locus. *Nature (Lond.),* 349: 709–713.

Miller, M., Bwer, E., Levitt, P., Li, D. and Chantler, P.D. (1992) Myosin II distribution in neurons is consistent with a role in growth cone motility but not synaptic vesicle mobilization. *Neuron,* 8: 25–44.

Pollard, T.D., Doberstein, S.K. and Zot, H.G. (1991) Myosin-I. *Annu. Rev. Physiol.*, 53: 653–681.

Rinchik, E.M., Russel, L.B., Copeland, N.G. and Jenkins, N.A. (1985) The dilute-short ear (d-se) complex of the mouse: lessons from a fancy mutation. *Trends Genet.*, 1: 170–176.

Rochlin, M.W. and Bridgman, P.C. (1991) Neurite outgrowth is reduced by a potent myosin light chain kinase inhibitor. *J. Cell Biol.*, 115: 29a.

Rochlin, M.W., Phillips, C.L., Yamakawa, K., Adelstein, R.S. and Bridgman, P.C. (1992) The distribution of myosin II A & B isoforms in growth cones. Mol. Biol. Cell, 3: 160a.

Sherr, E.H., Joyce, M.P. and Greene, L.A. (1993) Mammalian myosin Iα, Iβ, and Iχ: new widely expressed genes of the myosin I family. J. Cell Biol., 120: 1405–1416.

Ruppert, C. Kroschewski, R. and Bahler, M. (1993) Identification, characterization and cloning of myr 1, a mammalian myosin-I. J. Cell Biol., 120: 1393–1403.

Zheng, J., Lamoureux, P., Santiago, V., Dennerll, T., Buxbaum, R.E. and Heidemann, S.R. (1991) Tensile regulation of axonal elongation and initiation. J. Neurosci., 11: 1117–1125.

F.J. Seil (Ed.)
Progress in Brain Research, Vol 103

CHAPTER 11

Hierarchical guidance cues and selective axon pathway formation

Jørgen Johansen[1], Kristen M. Johansen[1], Kristen K. Briggs[1], Diane M. Kopp[2] and John Jellies[2]

[1]Department of Zoology and Genetics, 3156 Molecular Biology Building, Iowa State University, Ames, IA 50011, U.S.A. and [2]Neurobiology Research Center / Department of Physiology and Biophysics, University of Alabama, Birmingham, AL 35294, U.S.A.

Introduction

During nervous system formation, nerve cells extend axons in order to form precise patterns of neuronal connectivity. These connections are often established after the neuronal growth cones have pioneered or navigated through complex pathways to their target area both within the central nervous system (CNS) and to and from the periphery. Recent studies have provided evidence that the process of specific pathway formation may rely on a number of molecular guidance mechanisms such as selective adhesion, growth cone avoidance, epithelial gradients, guidepost cells and chemotropism (reviewed in Dodd and Jessell, 1988; Jessell, 1988; Goodman and Schatz, 1993). Different combinations of these pathfinding strategies forming a hierarchy of guidance cues are likely to be employed in different developmental systems and contexts. Molecular analysis of some of the potential guidance proteins identified so far has revealed that they often possess striking common structural features defining distinct multigene families. For example, L1, TAG-1, N-CAM, contactin, and fasciclin II have all been shown to belong to the immunoglobulin supergene family and to contain multiple Ig-like domains (Dodd and Jessell, 1988; Harrelson and Goodman, 1988; Furley et al., 1990). Thus, common structural motifs in many functionally related molecules have been conserved in both invertebrates and vertebrates. Important questions are how these molecules interact to mediate growth cone navigation and formation of specific axon pathways and how many different molecules and gene families involved in these events may exist.

The leech is an excellent model system in which to study developmental mechanisms of neuronal connectivity due to its relatively simple, segmentally iterated nervous system and accessibility to functional perturbation experiments (Jellies and Kristan, 1988, 1991; Zipser et al., 1989). In leech, the central projections of peripheral sensory neurons (Fig. 1A) segregate into four specific axonal tracts (Fig. 1B), which are distinguished by differential expression of antigens recognized by the monoclonal antibodies lan 3-2, lan 4-2, and lan 3-6 (Fig. 2) (Zipser and McKay, 1981; McKay et al., 1983; Johansen et al., 1985, 1992; Briggs et al., 1993). We have characterized and analysed the navigation and pathway formation of the sensory neuron growth cones in the periphery and CNS during early development by using the antibodies as markers, by intracellular dye injection of single

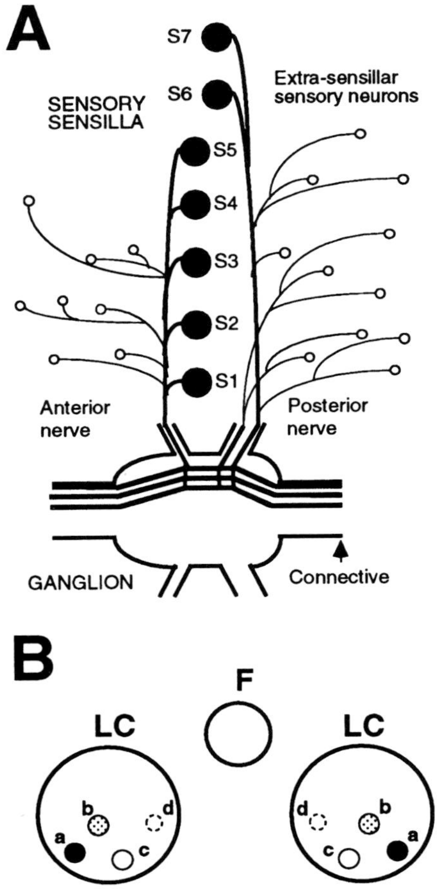

Fig. 1. Diagram of peripheral neurons that form specific axonal tracts in the CNS. One hemisegment is shown. There are seven groups of sensory neurons constituting the sensilla, which are labeled S1–S7. The axons from S1–S5 enter the ganglion through the anterior nerve; the axons from S6 and S7 enter through the posterior nerve. In addition to the sensillar neurons, various unidentified extrasensillar neurons scattered in the body wall (open circles) also contribute antibody-positive axons to the tracts. These neurons, in contrast to the sensillar neurons, appear late in embryogenesis. (B) Diagram of a cross section of a connective (see A) illustrating the stereotyped position of the four axonal tracts (a, b, c, and d) formed by the projections from the peripheral neurons. The 'd' fascicle arises later in development (E11–12) than the first three, which are formed at approximately the same time (E8–10). The interganglionic connective is composed of a pair of lateral nerves (LC) and an unpaired medial nerve, Faivre's nerve (F).

peripheral neurons, and by surgical manipulation of the CNS. The results derived from these studies all imply the existence of a hierarchy of CNS-derived guidance cues which mediate the specific tract formation and segregation of axons in this system.

Development of peripheral sensilla and axon fascicles

In leech the formation of both the central and peripheral nervous system proceeds in a rostro-caudal sequence (Stent et al., 1982). Generally, each posterior segment is approximately 2.5 h later in development than the more anterior one (Jellies and Kristan, 1991). Consequently, since there are 32 segments, an embryo exhibits segments in different stages of development spanning a period of about 2–3 days (Fig. 3), which greatly facilitates the analysis of axonal outgrowth (Johansen et al., 1992). The first peripheral neurons to differentiate, as revealed by lan 3-2 antibody labeling, are the sensillar neurons, which are clusters of mixed sensory neurons composed of chemoreceptors, photoreceptors and mechanoreceptors found on the central annulus of each segment (Fig. 1A) (Muller et al., 1981; Philips and Friesen, 1982; Johansen et al., 1992). The sensilla are termed S1–S7, with the most ventral sensillum closest to the CNS in each hemisegment designated S1. S1–S5 sensillar neurons send their axons toward the CNS through the anterior nerve root, whereas S6 and S7 neurons extend their axons through the posterior nerve root (Fig. 1A). In addition to the rostro-caudal progression, each sensillum arises within a given segment in a distinct pattern that does not, however, follow a simple sequence (Johansen et al., 1992). The first sensillar primordium to appear at embryonic day 7–8 (E7–8) is that of the middle sensillum, S3, followed by the neurons in S6 and S7. Subsequently, sensillar neurons in S1, S2, S4 and S5 differentiate. When the growing axons of the sensillar neurons reach the ganglionic CNS, they execute a 90° change of direction and segregate both anteriorly and posteriorly into three distinct tracts, fascicles 'a', 'b', and 'c' (Fig. 1B). The three tracts are bilaterally symmetrical and stereotypically positioned in the lateral connectives linking

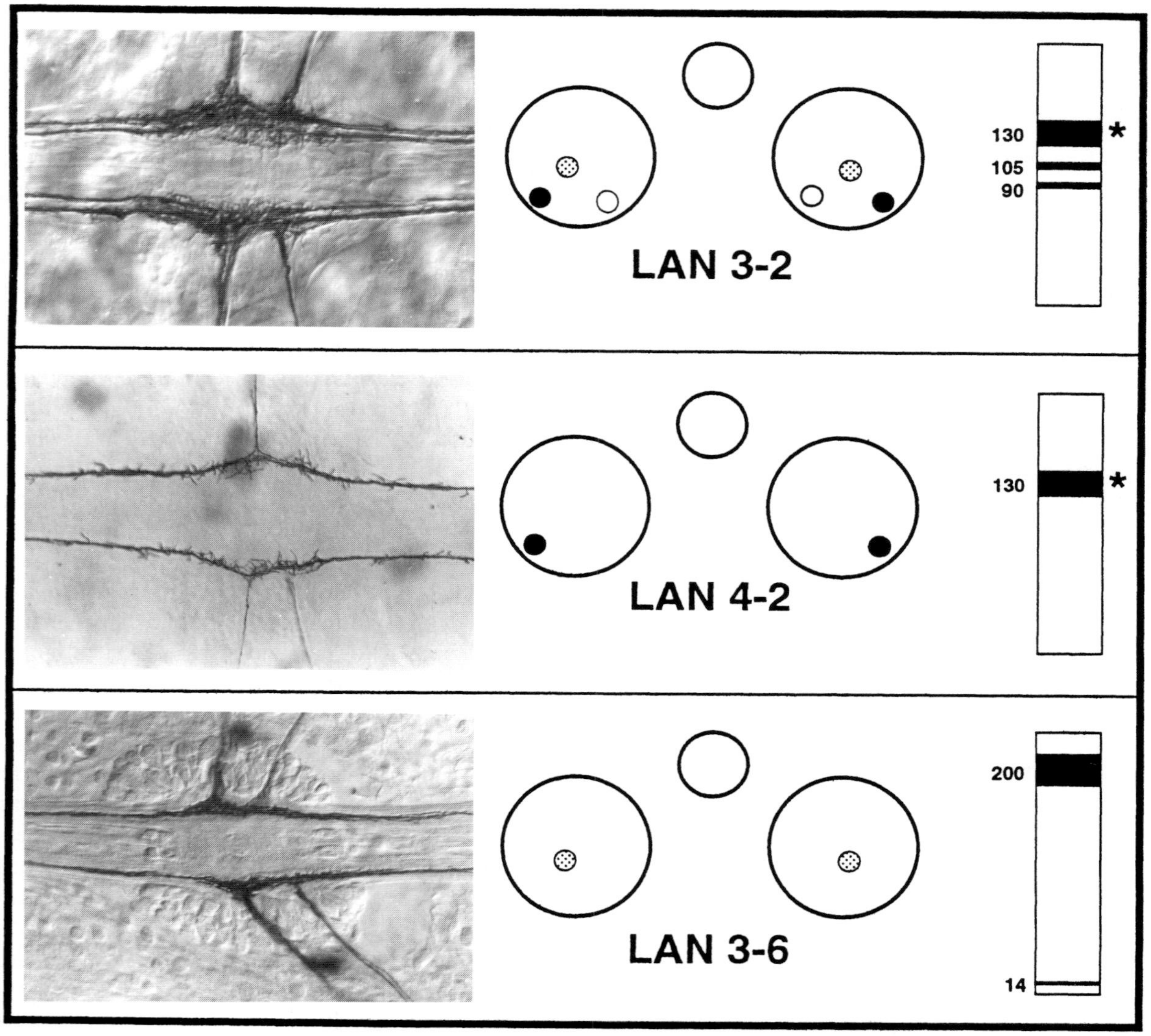

Fig. 2. Comparison of the properties of the three monoclonal antibodies, lan 3-2, lan 4-2 and lan 3-6, which label specific groups of peripheral neurons and axon tracts in leech embryos. The left panel shows micrographs of axon fascicles in the CNS labeled by the three antibodies at E10 at comparable stages of development. The middle panel indicates the position in the connective of the labeled fascicles. Lan 3-2 labels all the tracts formed by peripheral neurons present at this stage in development, whereas lan 4-2 and lan 3-6 label only single but different tracts. The right panel summarizes what is known about the molecular nature of the antigens in adult *Haemopis* CNS-derived from immuno- and Northern blots, as well as from immunoprecipitation experiments. Lan 3-2 recognizes three glycosylated protein bands of 130, 105, and 90 kDa, respectively. Lan 4-2 recognizes only a single glycosylated 130-kDa protein band. The lan 3-2 and lan 4-2 130-kDa antigens are molecularly interrelated (asterisks). Lan 3-6 may recognize a protein complex consisting of a 14-kDa and a 200-kDa protein, as deduced from immunoprecipitation with the antibody and Northern analysis with the cloned lan 3-6 gene.

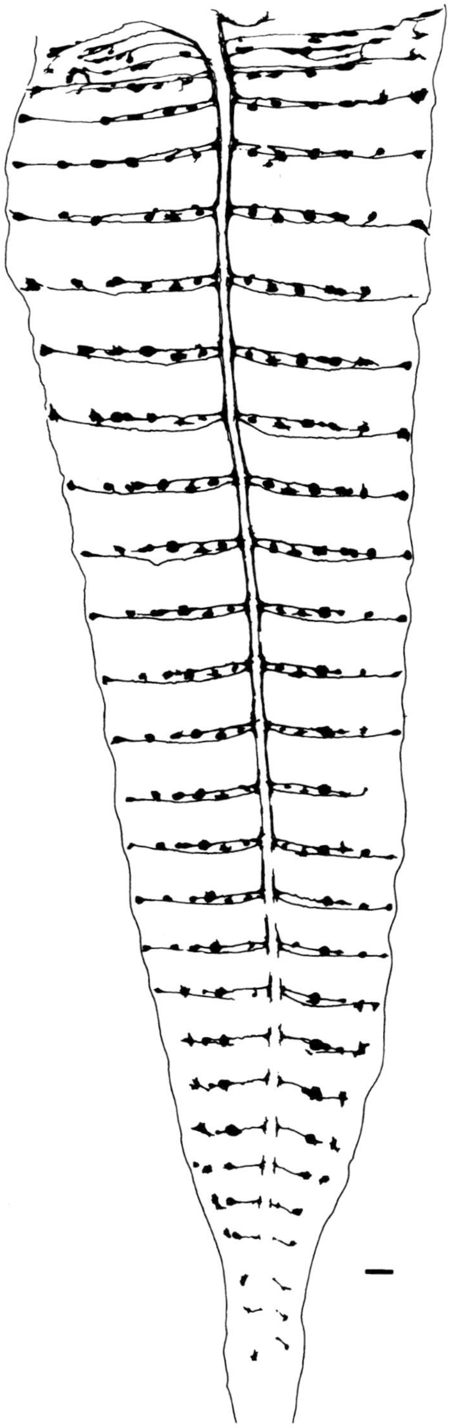

the ganglia. However, with a considerable delay a fourth fascicle, 'd', also arises at E11–12 (Fig. 1B) (Johansen et al., 1992). After axogenesis and the initial fascicle formation is completed, the axons are wrapped by process invaginations from a single glial cell in each connective (Morrissey and McGlade-McCulloh, 1988). Although sensillar neurons are the first peripheral sensory neurons to differentiate and extend axons into specific fascicles in the CNS, an entirely different population of extrasensillar peripheral neurons scattered throughout the skin differentiates much later, around E16–25 (Fig. 1A) (Johansen et al., 1992). All of these neurons, which are of unknown function, also extend axons toward the CNS, where they selectively fasciculate with the sensillar neuronal tracts pioneered earlier (Johansen et al., 1992; Briggs et al., 1993).

The process outgrowth of the peripheral sensory neurons in leech provides an accessible and well-defined system in which to study mechanisms of neuronal guidance and its molecular components. We have used a combination of anatomical, biochemical and molecular approaches to analyse three peripheral neuron antigens recognized by the monoclonal antibodies lan 3-2, lan 4-2, and lan 3-6, respectively, which are strong candidates for being molecules involved in selective axon fasciculation.

The lan 3-2 and lan 4-2 antigens

The lan 3-2 and lan 4-2 antigens have been the most extensively studied since it has been demonstrated that Fab fragments of lan 3-2 antibody can perturb normal fascicle formation in cultured embryos (Zipser et al., 1989), directly implicating a functional role for this antigen in pathway for-

Fig. 3. Camera lucida drawing of an E10 *Hirudo* embryo labeled by lan 3-2 showing the differentiation of the sensilla and the formation of the axon fascicles. The expression of the antigen proceeds in a clear rostrocaudal gradient exhibiting segments in different stages of development. The head ganglia are at the top and the tail ganglia at the bottom of the figure. Scale bar: 100 μm

mation. Immunocytochemistry and light and electron microscopy in *Hirudo* (Johansen et al., 1992) demonstrate that the lan 3-2 antigen is likely to be expressed by all of the developing peripheral neurons, and that at E10 the central projections of their axons segregate into three separate axon fascicles (Fig. 2). Figure 4 provides a three-dimensional view of the spatial relationship in a whole-mount preparation between the lan 3-2-positive fascicles and the growth cones of incoming axons in the CNS using high definition stereo light microscopy (Greenberg and Boyde, 1993). In contrast, the lan 4-2 antibody at this stage recognizes only a few peripheral neurons that also send axons to the CNS; however, their projections are confined to extend along only one of the lan 3-2-positive axon fascicles (Fig. 2). This has been directly demonstrated using double labeling with the lan 3-2 and lan 4-2 antibodies (Johansen et al., 1992).

Both the lan 3-2 and lan 4-2 antibodies were originally made toward adult *Haemopis* CNS but cross-react with sensory axon fascicles in all leech species examined, representing two different orders (Johansen et al., 1992). This conservation of both epitopes over a phylogenetically broad spec-

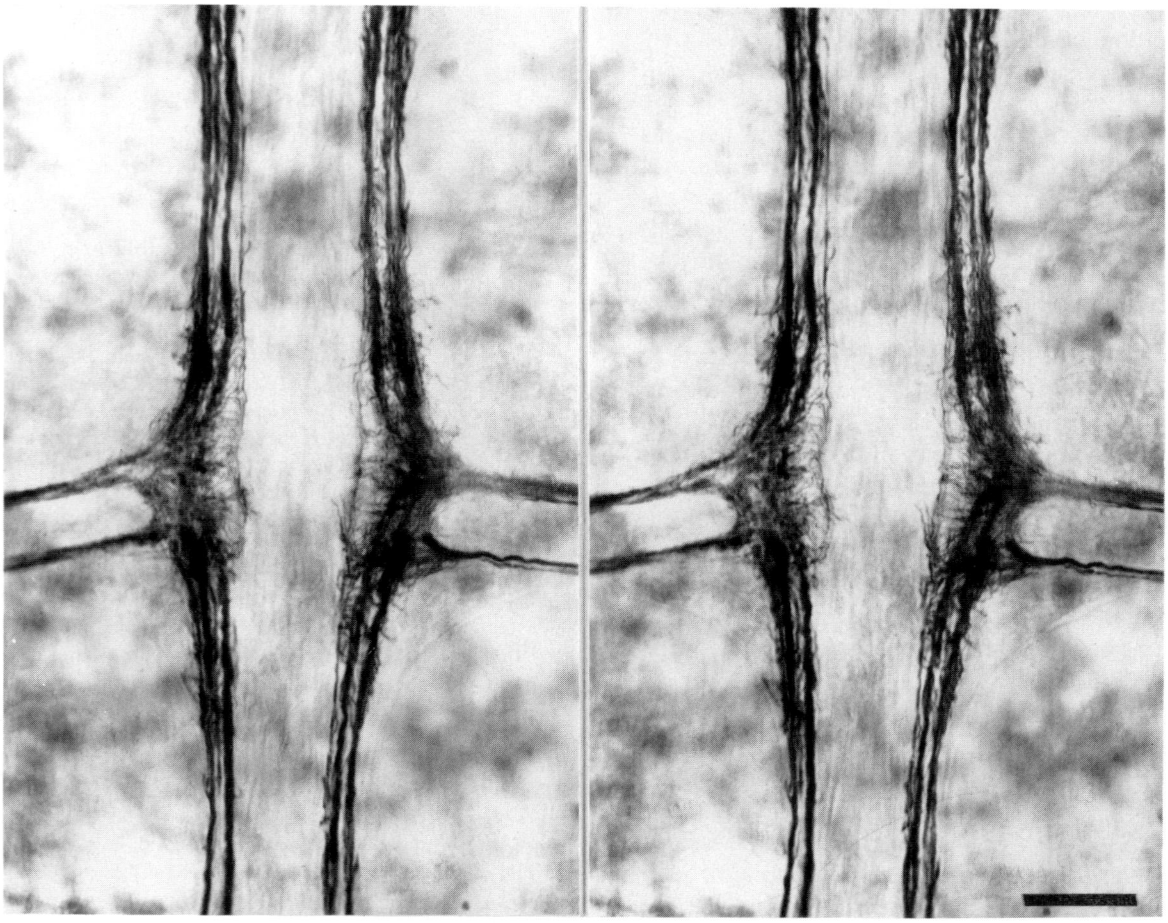

Fig. 4. High definition stereo image of lan 3-2 labeled axon fascicles and growth cones demonstrating their spatial relationship in the CNS of an E10 embryo. Anterior is at the top. Scale bar: 20 μm. (Micrographs courtesy of Edge Scientific.)

trum further suggests that they are functionally important. The antigens are surface glycoproteins and on immunoblots of adult CNS extract from *Haemopis* (McKay et al., 1983), lan 3-2 recognizes three protein bands with molecular masses of 130, 105, and 90 kDa respectively, whereas lan 4-2 recognizes only a 130-kDa band (Figs. 2 and 5). However, the significance of the two lower bands recognized by lan 3-2 is presently unclear, since immunoblots of embryonic CNS suggest that in E8–10 embryos, when the lan 3-2-positive fascicles are being formed, only the 130-kDa version of the antigens is expressed (McGlade-McCulloh et al., 1990). Thus, these experiments suggest that the 130-kDa protein may be the key molecular form of the lan 3-2 antigens involved in the formation of the axon fascicles, being the only form expressed when the fascicles are first pioneered.

Given that lan 4-2-positive peripheral neurons represent a subset of the lan 3-2-positive neurons, and that both antibodies recognize epitopes expressed on 130-kDa glycoproteins, we investigated the biochemical relationship of the antigens and their epitopes (Johansen et al., 1992). Immunoprecipitation experiments with lan 3-2 and lan 4-2 (Fig. 5) demonstrated that the antigens of these antibodies are closely molecularly interrelated, suggesting that the lan 4-2 epitope may also function in fascicle formation. Lan 4-2 recognizes the 130-kDa protein immunoprecipitated by lan 3-2 but does not recognize the two lower molecular weight proteins (Fig. 5). In the reverse experiment, lan 3-2 labels the 130-kDa protein immunoprecipitated by lan 4-2. There are two ways to account for the observed relationship between the lan 3-2 and lan 4-2 antigens (Johansen et al., 1992). One possibility is that the lan 3-2 and lan 4-2 epitopes are expressed on separate 130-kDa proteins which coprecipitate due to strong mutual adhesion; the other possibility is that the lan 3-2 and lan 4-2 epitopes are expressed on the same molecule. In this case, all of the peripheral neurons express a 130-kDa protein carrying the lan 3-2 epitope, whereas only a subset of these neurons express a 130-kDa version of the protein which carries both the lan 3-2 and the lan 4-2

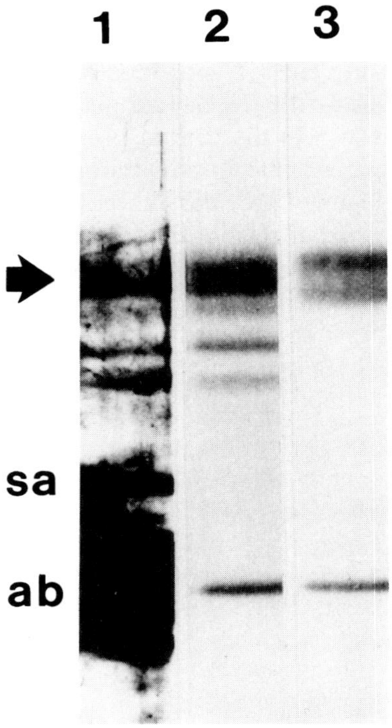

Fig. 5. Lan 3-2 immuno-affinity purified antigen from *Haemopis* separated by SDS-PAGE and analysed on immunoblots by lan 3-2 and lan 4-2. Lane 1: lan 3-2 immuno-affinity purified antigens from the equivalent of 5 nerve cords which were separated by SDS-PAGE and silver stained. The three lan 3-2-positive protein bands are clearly visible, including the 130-kDa protein (arrow). No protein bands corresponding to other proteins than those revealed by the lan 3-2 antibody (lane 2) can be detected in this region of the gel. However, material due to serum albumin (sa) from the hybridoma supernatant and the primary antibody (ab) are present in the lower part of the gel. Lanes 2 and 3: immunoblots of samples of the same material as in lane 1 stained with lan 3-2 (lane 2) and lan 4-2 (lane 3), respectively. The lan 3-2 immunoreactive bands correspond closely to the lan 3-2 immuno-affinity purified bands seen on the silver stained gel in lane 1, whereas lan 4-2 labels only the 130 kDa-antigen. A lower protein band corresponding to the primary antibody (ab) is also labeled in these lanes. The greater extension of the ab band on the silver stained gel is due to the much greater amount of material loaded on the gel in this lane compared with the immunoblot lanes. Because of the swelling during fixation of the silver stained gel, prints of the three lanes were photographically adjusted to match each other as closely as possible.

epitopes. While our combined biochemical and immunocytochemical data show that not all 130-

kDa lan 3-2-positive proteins would coexpress the lan 4-2 epitope, the lan 4-2 epitope may always be coexpressed with the lan 3-2 epitope. Thus, the 130-kDa protein may be composed of a core protein that, either by differential mRNA splicing or by differential glycosylation, expresses different epitopes involved in selective fascicle formation. An example of the latter mechanism has been described in the chick embryo, where dynamically regulated levels of polysialylation of N-CAM affect nerve branching and axon fasciculation (Landmesser et al., 1990; Rutishauser and Landmesser, 1991). In either event, the experiments clearly demonstrate that the lan 3-2 and lan 4- 2 epitopes are differentially expressed, both on subsets of axonal tracts and on molecules which are closely interrelated, presenting an opportunity to study the molecular nature of this interaction.

The lan 3-6 antigen

Another candidate molecule for being involved in hierarchical fascicle formation in the leech CNS is the lan 3-6 antigen (Briggs et al., 1993). By immunocytochemistry and double labeling with lan 3-2, it was demonstrated that, like the lan 4-2 epitope, the lan 3-6 epitope is expressed only by a small subgroup of the peripheral neurons in hirudinid leeches. The axons of these neurons selectively fasciculate in the CNS, but only in one of the three lan 3-2-positive tracts, 'b', which is different from the tract 'a' chosen by the lan 4-2-positive subpopulation (Fig. 2). The first lan 3-6-positive pathway is initially constituted by a single neuron in S3. Together with additional lan 3-6-positive peripheral neurons growing into the CNS, this neuron forms primordial axon tracts in the ganglia. Growth cones of these neurons are subsequently extended from each segmental ganglion into both the anterior and posterior connectives (Fig. 6A, B). The growth cones from rostrally and caudally located ganglia meet in the connective in perfect register without any apparent realignment (Fig. 6 A, B, arrowheads). This suggests that the pathway followed by the lan 3-6-positive axons may already have been established before the outgrowth of these axons. Subsequently, this

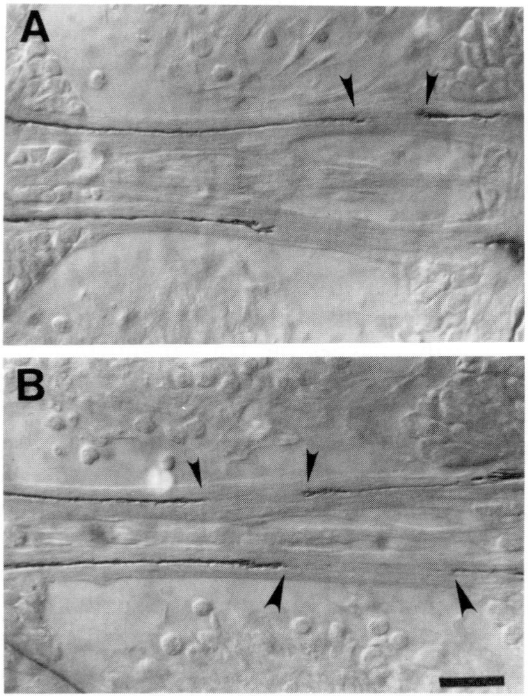

Fig. 6. The growth cones of lan 3-6-positive axons appear to follow preformed pathways in the connectives. A and B show examples of the extension of anteriorly and posteriorly directed axons in the interganglionic connectives. The growth cones meet in the middle of the connectives (arrowheads) in perfect register without any apparent realignment to form a single tract. Anterior is to the left. Scale bar: 20 μm.

embryologically established axon tract may serve as a navigational guide for the entire population of later differentiating lan 3-6-positive neurons which preferentially fasciculate with the first lan 3-6-positive axons establishing the pathway.

The very restricted expression of the lan 3-6 antigen to a subset of peripheral neurons which specifically fasciculate together into a single tract during development raises the possibility that the antigen may play a role in this process. However, since the lan 3-6 antibody does not recognize the denatured antigen on immunoblots, its biochemical nature has been difficult to study, and since the lan 3-6 epitope is intracellular (Briggs et al., 1993), antibody perturbation studies assessing function cannot be performed with the lan 3-6 antibody. Therefore, we initiated a biochemical and molecular characterization of the antigen with the aim of generating future probes for performing such an analysis (Briggs et al., 1992). Preliminary data from a partial clone obtained by screening a leech expression vector library suggests that the antigen is a novel protein possessing two EF-hand Ca^{2+} binding domains (Briggs et al., 1992). That the clone corresponds to the lan 3-6 antigen has been verified by in situ hybridizations with the clone to embryos, the labeling of which exactly matches the lan 3-6 antibody pattern (Briggs et al., unpublished data). Northern analysis suggests that translation of the lan 3-6 message would yield a protein with a molecular weight of about 14 kDa (Briggs et al., unpublished data). However, immunoaffinity purification with the lan 3-6 antibody followed by SDS-PAGE and analysis of the gels by silver staining also yields a prominent protein band of approximately 200 kDa which is being selectively affinity purified by this procedure (Briggs et al., 1993). Broad protein bands of this nature are frequently characteristic of glycoproteins, as is the case for the lan 3-2 and lan 4-2 antigens (Johansen et al., 1992). Thus the possibility exists that the lan 3-6 antigen is a small Ca^{2+} binding protein which is associated with and regulates a larger 200-kDa glycosylated protein.

Late differentiating extrasensillar neurons expressing the antigens

Why do the peripheral neurons fasciculate in specific tracts and why do the antigens continue to be expressed throughout development as well as in the adult leech? The answers to these questions may derive from the fact that extrasensillar sensory neurons expressing the antigens continue to differentiate late in development and that their numbers increase as the animal grows (Peinado et al., 1990). This observation was obtained by axon counts on electron micrographs of nerve sections from juvenile and adult leeches of different sizes, which showed that total axon number (including sensory afferents) increases with leech size (Peinado et al., 1990). A rationale for why these peripheral neurons travel together in distinct fascicles could be that the increasing numbers of peripheral neurons recruited with the growth of the leech are likely to be sensory neurons (Peinado et al., 1990) which may make synaptic contacts with common targets in the CNS. Throughout embryonic development and postembryonic maturation, guidance cues on the existing fascicles, which were pioneered when distances were short, would be critical for the correct navigation in the CNS of the axons of the peripheral neurons. Direct support for the notion that the peripheral neuron axon fascicles indeed carry some form of label that can direct fasciculation and neuronal recognition comes from regeneration experiments (Peinado et al., 1987). If the nerve roots are crushed, almost all of the regenerating axons from neurons in the peripheral sensilla were found within the lan 3-2-positive tracts in the nerve roots and not elsewhere (Peinado et al., 1987). This clearly indicates that the regenerating peripheral axons are preferentially guided to grow along specific tracts. The fact that the antigens continue to be expressed throughout the lifespan of the leech correlates with a role in this process.

Specific pathway selection by single sensillar neurons

Although the previously described results from antibody labeling studies suggest that individual sensory afferents express a distinct complement of glycoproteins correlated with the selection of particular central fascicles, these studies involved antibody labeling of multiple cells and could not resolve the pathway choices of single afferents. To address this, we combined intracellular dye filling of single sensillar neurons using Lucifer Yellow with lan 3-2 antibody labeling (Fig. 7) to produce doubly labeled preparations of *Hirudo* embryos at early stages (E9–11) (Jellies and Johansen, 1993). In this way, the projections of individual sensillar neurons can be assessed with respect to the fascicles they choose. We have obtained 68 such dye-filled sensory neurons in the third sensillum (S3 is the first to differentiate).

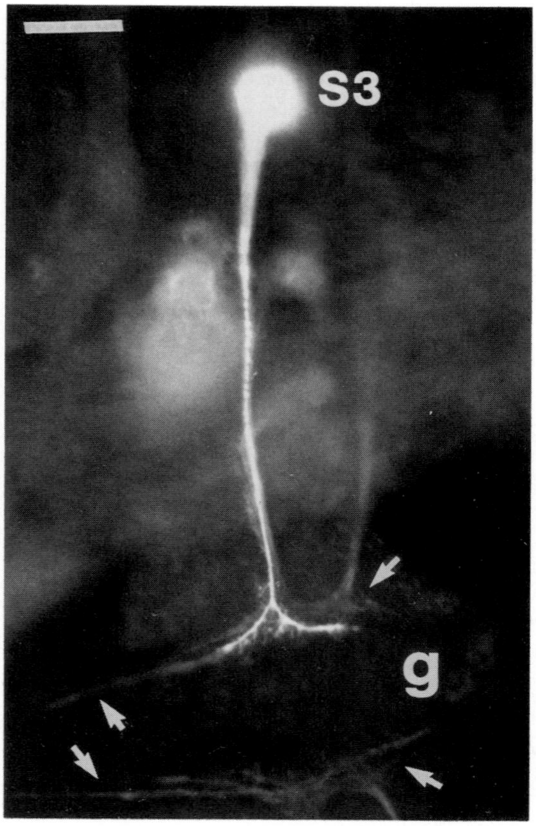

Fig. 7. Single Lucifer Yellow injected sensillar neuron in S3. The preparation was double labeled with lan 3-2 antibody and visualized with rhodamine conjugated second antibody. The rhodamine fluorescence appears gray (arrowheads) in this black and white micrograph whereas the Lucifer Yellow fluorescence is bright white. The injected neuron bifurcates when reaching the ganglion (g), choosing a single lan 3-2 labeled fascicle. Note the numerous filopodia branching off the bifurcated axon. Anterior is to the left. Scale bar: 50 μm.

None of these neurons branched into more than one central fascicle; rostrally and caudally directed branches of single sensory neurons in all cases examined chose the same fascicle, indicating a specific choice of a distinct labeled pathway. Furthermore, examples of neurons selecting each of the three possible fascicles were found in the third sensillum, approximately 13% choosing the 'a', 12% choosing the 'b', and 75% choosing the 'c' fascicle. Thus, these results suggest that each sensillum may contain mixed subpopulations of sensory cells which segregate into specific tracts according to their sensory modality. The experiments seem to rule out the possibility that the segregation is based on sensillar number and identity.

The role of CNS-derived guidance cues in peripheral sensory neuron navigation

A question we wanted to address was the source of the guidance cues in response to which peripheral neurons navigate in both the periphery and in the CNS. While it had been suggested that the posterior nerve is pioneered by the centrally located dorsal pressure (P) mechanosensory neuron (Kuwada, 1985), this study did not directly address the possible contribution of peripheral neurons. By dye filling dorsal P-cells early in development and double labeling with lan 3-2 antibody, we have confirmed that at least the posterior nerve is indeed pioneered by the P-cell rather than the peripheral neurons (Jellies et al., unpublished data). In addition, it has recently been demonstrated that the correct branching and extension of axons to the periphery of other central neurons is dependent on the dorsal P-cell (Gan et al., 1993). Thus it appears that critical guidance cues are provided by pioneer CNS neurons. We therefore decided to investigate the effect of CNS removal on the navigation of peripheral sensory neurons. Part of the nervous cord was surgically removed from E9–10 embryos which were then allowed to develop to either E12 or E16 before dissection and labeling with lan 3-2 antibody. Unoperated animals served as controls. Figure 8 shows the results of such an experiment where the CNS was removed from an E10 embryo which was later examined at E16. In the control (Fig. 8A), the nerves have formed normally and numerous extrasensillar neurons have differentiated and extended axons toward the CNS, forming orderly nerve branches. In contrast, when the CNS has been removed (Fig. 8B), the sensory neurons appear to lose direction and the axons of the sensillar neurons grow toward the nephridiopore, where they fasciculate upon one another, in many cases forming a circular path (Fig. 8B, large arrowhead). This result was consistent and was found in all 110 peripheral hemisegments examined in 15 experimental embryos. Note that the direction of growth of the S1 axons have even been reversed. The extrasensillar neurons still differentiate (Fig. 8B, small arrowheads) but their axonal outgrowth is stunted, without apparent direction and, at best, small local bundles of axons are formed. In some cases axons from the dorsal sensilla S6 and S7, which form the posterior nerve, joined the anterior sensillar fascicles (Jellies and Johansen, unpublished data). The two nerves under normal conditions are strictly separated in the periphery. These experiments seem to indicate that CNS-derived guidance cues are necessary for correct

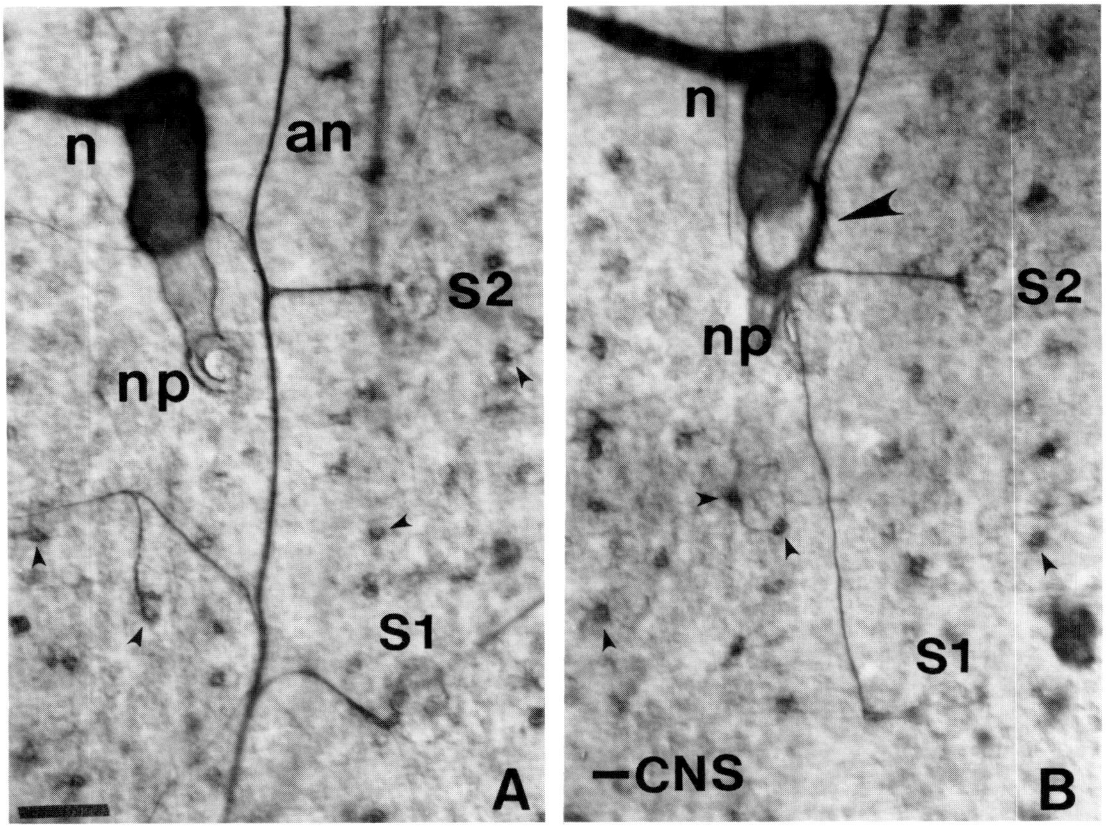

Fig. 8. Perturbation of peripheral neuron pathway formation by CNS removal. (A) Micrograph of peripheral neurons labeled by lan 3-2 extending axons to the CNS at E16 through the anterior nerve (an). The nerve receives orderly projected axons from S1 and S2 as well as from extrasensillar neurons (small arrowheads) which differentiate late in development. (B) Micrograph from a corresponding segment to the one shown in A but from a preparation where the CNS was surgically removed at E10 and the embryo allowed to develop to E16 before dissection and labeling with lan 3-2 antibody. Without the CNS present, the extrasensillar neurons (small arrowheads) still differentiate but do not form orderly projections as in A. Axons from the sensillar neurons congregate close to the nephridia (n) and the nephridiopore (np), where they fasciculate with each other, often forming circular paths (large arrowhead). Note that the direction of the projections from S1 is reversed. Anterior is to the left and dorsal is up. Scale bar: 50 μm.

navigation of the peripheral neurons and that in the absence of these guidance cues, the default option for at least the sensillar neurons is to fasciculate with each other. The results furthermore make it unlikely that these neurons respond to epithelial gradients or proximately located guidepost cells, in contrast to the guidance mechanisms operating for pioneer neurons in the grasshopper limb bud (Caudy and Bentley, 1987; Kolodkin et al., 1992).

Conclusion

We have explored developmental mechanisms of navigation and selective fasciculation of peripheral sensory neurons in the embryo of the leech. We have shown that CNS-derived guidance cues are necessary for correct pathway formation of these neurons into the CNS. In the absence of these cues, the growing axons lose their orientation and default to fasciculation onto each other, often forming circular paths. In normal development, when the peripheral neurons reach the CNS, they segregate into four well-defined axonal tracts. We have demonstrated that at least two antigenically distinct subpopulations of peripheral neurons can be defined which have selective affinity for two different pathways. These results provide compelling evidence for the existence of a hierarchy of guidance cues mediating specific tract formation in this system. The guidance cues for the segregation are likely to be provided by the CNS, since rostrally and caudally directed peripheral neuron growth cones in the CNS often meet in the middle of the connectives in perfect register without any apparent realignment, indicating that they are tracking preformed pathways. Thus these results, combined with the CNS perturbation studies, suggest that all peripheral neurons express a molecule which, in the absence of other cues, will mediate the fasciculation of the axons of these neurons. We further propose that different subsets of peripheral neurons differentially express other molecules or epitopes which can interact with CNS-derived guidance cues, possibly through heterophilic mechanisms and signal transduction events. These interactions override the common fasciculation and mediate selective segregation and tract formation.

The expression of the lan 3-2 antigen by all peripheral neurons suggests that it is a prime candidate for mediating the common fasciculation exhibited by these neurons in the absence of CNS cues. In this scenario, the lan 3-2 antigen functions as a homophilic adhesion molecule that promotes growth cone extension along common pathways by neurons mutually expressing the antigen. That lan 3-2 does serve some function in the fasciculation process has been corroborated by perturbation experiments (Zipser et al., 1989), although the exact mechanism has yet to be determined. In contrast, the biochemical and molecular properties and the highly specific localization to single fascicles of the lan 4-2 and lan 3-6 epitopes make them strong candidates for being molecules which could mediate specific axon tract selection by interaction with CNS derived guidance cues.

Our long range goal in analysing and cloning these antigens is to obtain probes which can test these hypotheses in order to gain a basic understanding of the functional significance of these molecules, their possible hierarchical organization, and their developmental regulation of expression. As our results demonstrate, the relatively simple and accessible system of the leech embryo promises to be very useful for investigating developmental mechanisms mediating axonal pathway formation.

Acknowledgements

We wish to thank Edge Scientific Instrument Corporation for graciously providing us access to their newly developed high definition real-time 3D microscope and for help in making the stereomicrographs. This work was supported by NIH grant NS 28857 (J. Johansen), by NSF grant 9209237 (J. Jellies), by Iowa State University and Iowa State Biotechnology grants (J. Johansen), and by a NSF training grant DIR 9113595 graduate fellowship (K.K. Briggs). J. Jellies is a Fellow of the Sloan Foundation.

References

Briggs, K.K., Johansen, K.M. and Johansen, J. (1992) Hierarchical guidance cues and the formation of molecularly distinct axonal tracts during leech development. *Soc. Neurosci. Abstr.*, 18: 1273.

Briggs, K.K., Johansen, K.M. and Johansen, J. (1993) Selective pathway choice of a single central axonal fascicle by a subset of peripheral neurons during leech development. *Dev. Biol.*, 158: 380–389.

Caudy, M. and Bentley, D. (1987) Pioneer growth cone behavior at a differentiating limb segment boundary in the grasshopper embryo. *Dev. Biol.*, 119: 454–465.

Dodd, J. and Jessell, T.M. (1988) Axon guidance and the patterning of neuronal projections in vertebrates. *Science*, 242: 692–699.

Furley, A.J., Morton, S.B., Manalo, D., Karagogeos, D., Dodd, J. and Jessell, T.M. (1990) The axonal glycoprotein TAG-1 is an immunoglobulin superfamily member with neurite outgrowth-promoting activity. *Cell*, 61: 157–170.

Gan, W.B., Wolszon, L.R. and Macagno, E.R. (1993) The development of the peripheral terminal fields of AP and dorsal T neurons depends on pioneer dorsal P neurons. *Soc. Neurosci. Abstr.*, 19: 1085.

Goodman, C.S. and Shatz, C.J. (1993) Developmental mechanisms that generate precise patterns of neuronal connectivity. *Cell*, 72 (Suppl.): 77–98.

Greenberg, G. and Boyde, A. (1993) Novel method for stereo imaging in light microscopy at high magnifications. *Neuroimage*, 1: 121–128.

Harrelson, A.L. and Goodman, C.S. (1988) Growth cone guidance in insects: fasciclin II is a member of the immunoglobulin superfamily. *Science*, 242: 700–708.

Jellies, J. and Johansen, J. (1993) Specific pathway selection by the early projections of individual peripheral sensory neurons in the embryonic medicinal leech. *Soc. Neurosci. Abstr.*, 19: 40.

Jellies, J. and Kristan, W.B. (1988) An identified cell is required for the formation of a major nerve during embryogenesis in the leech. *J. Neurobiol.*, 19: 153–165.

Jellies, J. and Kristan, W.B. (1991) The oblique muscle organizer in *Hirudo medicinalis*, an identified embryonic cell projecting multiple parallel growth cones in an orderly array. *Dev. Biol.*, 148: 334–354.

Jessell, T.M. (1988) Adhesion molecules and the hierarchy of neural development. *Neuron*, 1: 3–13.

Johansen, J., Thompson, I., Stewart, R.R. and McKay, R.D.G. (1985) Expression of surface antigens recognized by the monoclonal antibody lan 3-2 during embryonic development in the leech. *Brain Res.*, 343: 1–7.

Johansen, K.M., Kopp, D.M., Jellies, J. and Johansen, J. (1992) Tract formation and axon fasciculation of molecularly distinct peripheral neuron subpopulations during leech embryogenesis. *Neuron*, 8: 559–572.

Kolodkin, A.L., Matthes, D.J., O'Conner, T.P., Patel, N.H., Admon, A., Bentley, D. and Goodman, C.S. (1992) Fasciclin IV: sequence, expression, and function during growth cone guidance in the grasshopper embryo. *Neuron*, 9: 831–845.

Kuwada, J.Y. (1985) Pioneering and pathfinding by an identified neuron in the embryonic leech. *J. Embryol. Exp. Morphol.*, 86: 155–167.

Landmesser, L., Dahm, L., Tang, J. and Rutishauser, U. (1990) Polysialic acid as a regulator of intramuscular nerve branching during embryonic development. *Neuron*, 4: 655–667.

McGlade-McCulloh, E., Muller, K.J. and Zipser, B. (1990) Expression of surface glycoproteins early in leech neural development. *J. Comp. Neurol.*, 299: 123–131.

McKay, R.D.G., Hockfield, S., Johansen, J., Thompson, I. and Frederiksen, K. (1983) Surface molecules identify groups of growing axons. *Science*, 222: 788–794.

Morrissey, A.M. and McGlade-McCulloh, E. (1988) Development of identified glia that ensheath axons in *Hirudo medicinalis*. *J. Neurosci. Res.*, 21: 513–520.

Muller, K.J., Nicholls, J.G. and Stent, G.S. (1981) *Neurobiology of the Leech*, Cold Spring Harbor Laboratory, Cold Spring Harbor, NY.

Peinado, A., Zipser, B. and Macagno, E.R. (1987) Regeneration of afferent axons into discrete tracts within peripheral nerves in the leech. *Brain Res.*, 410: 330–334.

Peinado, A., Zipser, B. and Macagno, E.R. (1990) Segregation of afferent projections in the central nervous system of the leech Hirudo medicinalis. *J. Comp. Neurol.*, 301: 232–242.

Phillips, C.E. and Friesen, W.O. (1982). Ultrastructure of the water-movement-sensitive sensilla in the medicinal leech. *J. Neurobiol.*, 13: 473–486.

Rutishauser, U. and Landmesser, L. (1991) Polysialic acid on the surface of axons regulates patterns of normal and activity-dependent innervation. *Trends Neurosci.*, 14: 528–532.

Stent, G.S., Weisblat, D.A., Blair, S.S. and Zackson, S.L. (1982) Cell lineage in the development of the leech nervous system. In: N.C. Spitzer (Ed.), *Neuronal Development*, Plenum Press, New York, pp. 1–44.

Zipser, B. and McKay, R. (1981) Monoclonal antibodies distinguish identifiable neurons in the leech. *Nature (London)*, 289: 549–554.

Zipser, B., Morell, R.J. and Bajt, M.L. (1989) Defasciculation as a neuronal pathfinding strategy: involvement of a specific glycoprotein. *Neuron*, 3: 621–630.

SECTION III

Calcium and Gene Expression

F.J. Seil (Ed.)
Progress in Brain Research, Vol 103

CHAPTER 12

Calcium and gene expression

Nicholas C. Spitzer

Department of Biology and Center for Molecular Genetics, University of California, San Diego, La Jolla, CA 92093, U.S.A.

Introduction

Neuronal differentiation and regeneration are regulated by diverse and complex processes. At early stages of development, during embryogenesis, maternally derived intracellular components and products of intracellular metabolism combine with those generated by the genetic program to contribute to the signaling cascades that drive differention. Overlapping with these factors are environmental cues that increase in importance as the complexity of the exterior milieu increases, both in terms of the heterogeneity of cell types and the ability of the embryo to transduce stimuli from the external world. Later, when the nervous system faces the challenge of regeneration, both intracellular and extracellular cues appear to be important in promoting regrowth of processes and rewiring of connections, and some of the mechanisms that are apparent during development are reutilized.

Given such complexity, identification of simplifying underlying principles becomes an urgent goal. In all of these instances, stimuli either from the outside or the inside of the cell must activate second messenger systems that can lead to changes in gene expression and cytoskeletal reorganization. A striking observation has been that both during development and regeneration, transient elevations of intracellular calcium serve to direct these critical functions in many systems. Sustained shifts in steady-state levels of intracellular calcium are not prominent, perhaps because they would lead to inactivation or accommodation of responses. Calcium transients appear to satisfy the necessary requirement for second messenger machinery. The mechanisms by which they are generated are turning out to be familiar in some cases, but seem to be quite novel in others.

In many cases, calcium transients are produced by calcium influx achieved by developmentally regulated function of voltage-dependent calcium channels and neurotransmitter receptors (Spitzer et al., 1994). Although the action of ion channels in generating action potentials and postsynaptic potentials in the time domain of milliseconds is familiar, developmentally and potentially regeneratively relevant signals appear to be somewhat longer in duration, operating over the time scale of minutes to hours. While more rapid than the time domain of action of many trophic factors, which act over weeks to months, this is still three orders of magnitude slower than rapid electrical signaling of the adult nervous system.

The control of differentiation with ion channels is beneficially parsimonious, since these molecules are already expressed as components of differentiating and regenerating neurons. An unfortunate downside, however, is the exceptional vulnerability of the immature or regenerating nervous system to seizure activity. Specializations that promote calcium influx, stimulate calcium release from stores, and reduce calcium buffering capability can all contribute to abnormal neurotransmitter release, bursts of action potentials and excitotoxicity.

Spontaneous calcium transients are generated in multiple regions of the nervous system, including spinal and cortical neurons and cerebellar Purkinje cells (Holliday and Spitzer, 1990; Sorimachi et al., 1990; Yuste et al., 1992). They were first characterized with respect to their role in hormonal release from endocrine cells (Schlegel et al., 1987), and are also observed in astrocytic glia (Fatatis and Russell, 1992). A particular benefit of investigating spontaneous activity is the assurance that relevant signal parameters, such as frequency, kinetics, amplitude and duration, are characterized (Hamburger, 1966).

Questions

These observations raise a number of issues. First, one would like to know how many variations or forms of calcium transients, characterized on the basis of their amplitude, duration and kinetics, are generated spontaneously by neurons in their standard environments as they are differentiating or regenerating. Second, it would be helpful to determine how they are regulated spatially and temporally. Are they restricted to particular regions of a neuron or propagated through its entirety? Do they appear and disappear at different times during the process of development or regrowth? Third, it is essential to understand the mechanism by which they are generated, not only for the insight this provides, but for the implicit opportunity for control that may be beneficial in stimulating regeneration. Fourth, it is important to define the functions exerted by different calcium transients, and to understand the code by which they are effective. In principle, information could be transmitted in their amplitude, duration, kinetics or frequency.

Assessment of the kinds of spontaneously generated calcium transients and their regulation can be pursued by direct examination of differentiating and regenerating systems. The mechanisms by which transients are produced as well as the functions they implement can also be studied in this way. However, questions of mechanism of generation and functional effect are addressed more rapidly by direct application of exogenous stimuli, directed to differentiating or regenerating systems in vivo or in culture. This has proven to be a useful approach, since it allows greater experimental control and clarity of interpretation.

Almost all studies of calcium transients make use of one or more of three major tools. Of particular value are the probes of free intracellular calcium ions, with fluorescence properties that allow specific detection of nM changes from steady-state. Also essential is the pharmacological tool kit, replete with agents that affect channels and transporters of surface and internal membrane compartments. Finally, immunocytochemical reagents allow visualization of arrays of cytoskeletal proteins or newly expressed gene products, and probes for in situ hybridization identify directly the products of transcription generated as the consequence of patterns of calcium transient activity.

Answers

Developmental studies

The mechanisms and functions of several types of spontaneous fluctuations in intracellular calcium have been investigated in *Xenopus* spinal neurons (Holliday and Spitzer, 1990; Holliday et al., 1991; Gu and Spitzer, 1993; Gu et al., 1994). Transient, repeated elevations of calcium have been recorded over periods of 1 h in vitro and in vivo, confocally imaging fluo-3 loaded cells at 5 sec intervals. Calcium spikes and calcium waves are found both in neurons in culture and in the intact spinal cord (Fig. 1). Spikes rise rapidly to ~ 400% of baseline fluorescence and have a characteristic double exponential decay, while waves rise slowly to ~ 200% of baseline fluorescence and decay slowly as well. Imaging of fura-2 loaded neurons indicates that intracellular calcium increases from 50 to 500 nM during spikes. Both spikes and waves are abolished by removal of extracellular calcium. Developmentally, the incidence and frequency of spikes decrease while the incidence and frequency of waves are constant. In contrast, the incidence and frequency of waves are spatially regulated, occurring at a higher level in growth cones than in the cell body.

Spikes are generated by spontaneous calcium-dependent action potentials that can be triggered by low threshold T-type calcium current; they are eliminated by agents that block voltage dependent calcium channels. They can be elicited by depolarization, are generated in an all-or-none manner, and are rapidly and bidirectionally propagated. Spikes also utilize intracellular calcium stores, since blocking release from stores substantially reduces their amplitude. Waves are not elicited by depolarization or by activation of glutamate receptors, and are propagated at a rate consistent with diffusion of calcium. Waves are blocked by Ni^{2+} at a higher concentration than required to block classical voltage-dependent calcium channels. Spontaneous spikes appear to be required for developmentally regulated expression of the transmitter, GABA, and for potassium channel modulation. Naturally generated waves in growth cones are likely to regulate neurite extension.

In the first of the three chapters which follow, Douglas Fields (chapter 13) describes the effects of imposing particular frequencies of action potentials on cultured fetal mouse dorsal root ganglion neurons. The effects on growth cone motility and expression of immediate early genes, c-*fos* and *nur/77*, are correlated with stimulus-induced calcium flux. It is clear that calcium plays important developmental roles in regulating these aspects of neuronal differentiation. Significantly, this includes mechanisms that regulate the ability of calcium to exert these regulatory effects. Thus the response of neurons to patterns of electrical activity and calcium elevation depends not only on the stage of differentiation but on the recent history of activity.

Regeneration studies

Jeffery Kocsis and his colleagues (chapter 14)

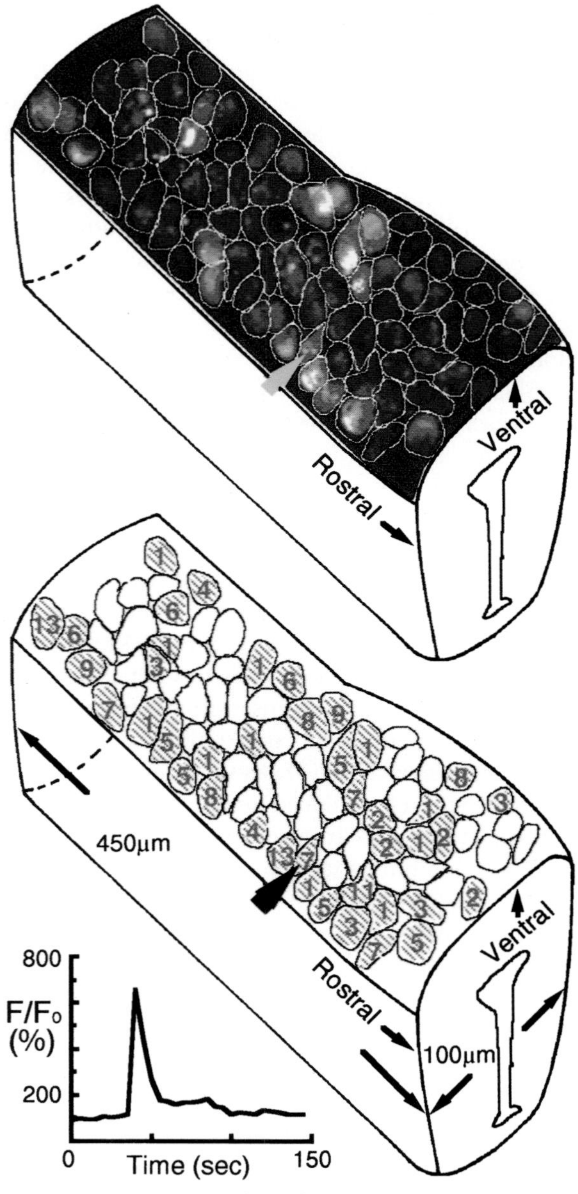

Fig. 1. Spontaneous transient elevations of intracellular calcium in the intact *Xenopus* embryonic spinal cord (Nieuwkoop and Faber stage 19), imaged at 0.2 Hz for 1 h. Top, single image displays 84 cells visualized on the ventral aspect of the cord, 41 of which exhibited spikes during a 10-min period. Middle, aggregate spontaneous activity; cells are represented by circles and the number in each indicates the spikes produced in that cell (1–13). Bottom, time course of a calcium spike in the active cell indicated by the arrow, digitized at 0.2 Hz; rapid rate of rise and double exponential decay of fluorescence identify it as a neuron. Scale, 25 μm. (From Gu et al., 1994.)

next describe aspects of calcium handling during early stages of regeneration of rat dorsal root ganglion neurons in vitro. The levels of calcium in the cytoplasm and nucleus are strongly influenced by calcium-induced release of calcium, not only in culture but in intact isolated embryonic ganglia as well. Interestingly, these signals are not observed in adult neurons in situ. They are also reduced in embryonic cultured neurons following outgrowth of processes, and depletion of these stores at earlier stages reduces neurite outgrowth. Elevation of calcium in the nucleus is suggested to stimulate immediate early gene expression as part of a cascade promoting neurite outgrowth.

Thomas Herdegen and Manfred Zimmermann (chapter 15) then review the activation of immediate early genes following a variety of stimuli. Transection of either peripheral or central nerve fibers causes selective induction of c-Jun and Jun D, with suppression of CREB, the calcium/cAMP response element binding protein. These observations raise the hypothesis that the appearance of the first two of these transcription factors is involved in the initiation and maintenance of the cell body response that leads to axonal outgrowth. Several lines of evidence implicate retrogradely transported signals from the innervated target as normally inhibitory factors, the absence of which leads to the induction of c-Jun and Jun D.

Future work will define the mechanisms by which calcium transients encode information more clearly and define the molecular basis of downstream events. Immediate early genes have been shown to be involved in the regulation of expression of nerve growth factor, proenkephalin and prodynorphin (Sonnenberg et al., 1989; Hengerer et al., 1990; Naranjo et al., 1991), and could regulate expression of cytoskeletal proteins as well. Calcium transients are one of many factors that appear to be involved in promoting regeneration. Nonetheless the ability to impose them deliberately on regenerating axons may afford the prospect of enhancing this important process.

Acknowledgements

I thank my colleagues in the laboratory for their insights and critical thinking. My work is supported by NS15918 and NS25916 from the NIH.

References

Fatatis, A. and Russell, J.T. (1992) Spontaneous changes in intracellular calcium concentration in type I astrocytes from rat cerebral cortex in primary culture. *Glia*, 5: 95–104.

Gu, X. and Spitzer, N.C. (1993) Low-threshold Ca^{2+} current and its role in spontaneous elevations of intracellular Ca^{2+} in developing *Xenopus* neurons. *J. Neurosci.*, 13: 4936–4948.

Gu, X., Olson, E.C. and Spitzer, N.C. (1994) Spontaneous neuronal calcium spikes and waves during early differentiation. *J. Neurosci.* (in press).

Hamburger, V., Wenger, E. and Oppenheim, R. (1966) Motility in the chick embryo in the absence of sensory input. *J. Exp. Zool.*, 162: 133–160.

Hengerer, B., Lindholm, D., Heumann, R., Rüther, U., Wagner, E. and Thoenen, H. (1990) Lesion-induced increase in nerve growth factor mRNA is mediated by c-*fos*. *Proc. Nat. Acad. Sci. USA*, 87: 3899–3903.

Holliday, J. and Spitzer, N.C. (1990) Spontaneous calcium influx and its roles in differentiation of spinal neurons in culture. *Dev. Biol.*, 141: 13–23.

Holliday, J., Adams, R. J., Sejnowski, T.J. and Spitzer, N.C. (1991) Calcium-induced release of calcium regulates differentiation of spinal neurons. *Neuron*, 7: 787–796.

Naranjo, J.R., Mellstrøm, B., Achaval, M., Lucas, J.J., Del Rio, J. and Sassone-Corsi, P. (1991) Co-induction of JUN-B and c-FOS in a subset of neurons in the spinal cord. *Oncogene*, 6: 223–227.

Schlegel, W., Winiger, B.P., Mollard, P., Vacher, P., Wuarin, F., Zahnd, G.R., Wollheim, C.B. and Dufy, B. (1987) Oscillations of cytosolic Ca^{2+} in pituitary cells due to action potentials. *Nature (London)*, 329: 719–721.

Sonnenberg, J.L., Rauscher, F.J. III, Morgan, J.I. and Curran, T. (1989) Regulation of proenkephalin by Fos and Jun. *Science*, 246: 1622–1625.

Sorimachi , M., Morita, Y. and Nakamura, H. (1990) Possible regulation of the cytosolic-free calcium concentration by Na^{+} spikes in immature cerebellar Purkinje cells. *Neurosci. Lett.*, 111: 333–338.

Spitzer, N.C., Gu, X. and Olson, E.C. (1994) Action potentials, calcium transients and the control of differentiation of excitable cells. *Curr. Opin. Neurobiol.*, 4: 70–77.

Yuste, R., Peinado, A. and Katz, L.C. (1992) Neuronal domains in developing neocortex. *Science*, 257: 665–669.

F.J. Seil (Ed.)
Progress in Brain Research, Vol 103

CHAPTER 13

Regulation of neurite outgrowth and immediate early gene expression by patterned electrical stimulation

R. Douglas Fields

Laboratory of Developmental Neurobiology, Bldg. 49, Room 5A-38, National Institute of Child Health and Human Development, National Institutes of Health, Bethesda, MD 02892, U.S.A.

Introduction

The formation, modification and repair of synaptic connections is guided by neuronal activity flowing within the brain as it processes information (for review see Shatz, 1990; Fields and Nelson, 1992). Electrical activity may act by strengthening, weakening or breaking synaptic connections, or regulating growth cone motility to affect neurite outgrowth and synaptogenesis. Without sensitivity to the functional operation of neural networks, genetic programs could not provide sufficient instruction to specify the wiring and rewiring of individual synaptic connections with adequate precision in complex nervous systems. Genetic sensitivity to environmental input is provided by a class of genes, termed immediate early (IE) genes, that are rapidly transcribed in response to a rich variety of external stimuli (Morgan and Curran, 1989, 1991; Ginty et al., 1992). These genes encode transcription factors, which in turn regulate the transcription of secondary genes, to produce appropriate structural and functional alterations in neurons. Given that information is coded in the temporal pattern of nervous impulses, it follows that gene transcription and neurite outgrowth must display sensitivity to particular patterns of impulses to produce appropriate responses. Nerve impulses are transduced into intracellular signals by calcium ions entering the cell through voltage sensitive calcium channels. Both motility of growth cones and transcription of IE genes can be influenced by calcium fluxes, but the cellular mechanisms responsible for this stimulus pattern sensitivity are obscure at the present time.

Effect of action potentials on growth cone motility

Action potentials can have a profound effect on growth cone behavior. Within minutes of firing action potentials in a mouse dorsal root ganglion (DRG) neuron in culture, growth cones cease motility, the lamellipodium withdraws, and filopodia consolidate (Fields et al., 1990). This response has been called 'growth cone collapse', a behavior that can also be elicited by diffusible or substrate bound factors (reviewed by Schwab et al., 1993; Fields and Nelson, 1994a). The biological significance of growth cone collapse is not well understood. It has been suggested that this represents the initial steps in the transformation of a growth cone into a synaptic ending (Forscher et al., 1987), a means of terminating neurite outgrowth once the neuron enters a functionally effective circuit (Cohan and Kater, 1986), or of pruning collaterals from neurite branches that have failed to form synaptic connections at the time the cell becomes electrically active (Cohan and Kater 1986; Fields et al., 1990). Alternatively, it may represent an artificial response observed only in cell culture, which may only regulate the steering or other activities of growth cones in vivo (Walter et al., 1990). Nevertheless, experiments with electrical stimulation demonstrate graphically the extent to which action potentials can impact the cellular machinery subserving growth cone motility and structural integrity. The basis for this interaction is believed to be related to the calcium levels which rise sharply upon stimulating neurites (Cohan et al., 1987; Mattson and Kater, 1987).

Experiments on the subject published before 1990 tended to indicate that extension of neurites should not be possible during development once neurons became electrically active, nor should electrically active neurons be capable of repair after injury. A non-invasive method of electrical stimulation enabled more extensive observations (Fig. 1), which showed that growth cones can recover eventually from the inhibitory effects of electrical stimulation, and resume normal morphology and rates of outgrowth (Fields et al., 1988, 1990). It is suggested that a slow process of recovery permits outgrowth after a transient period of activity-dependent growth cone collapse that may be necessary for specifying the development of functionally appropriate connections. This

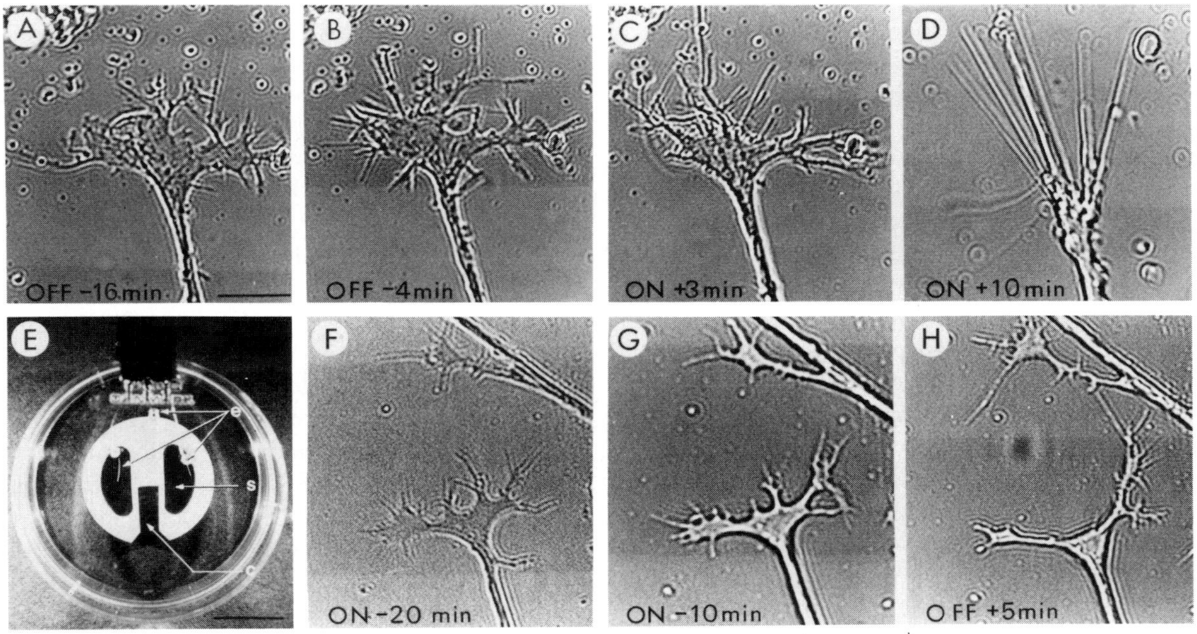

Fig. 1. Collapse and recovery of mouse DRG growth cones in response to electrical stimulation. Sensory neurons were dissociated from dorsal root ganglia of fetal mice and plated into the side compartments (s) of a Teflon insert attached to a 35-mm culture dish. After 1 week, neurites grow under the barrier allowing stimulation through electrodes (e) placed on opposite sides of the barrier. Responses to electrical stimulation and changes in intercellular calcium were observed in growth cones in the central compartment (c). The time sequence (A–D) shows the collapse of a growth cone upon electrical stimulation. The stimulus (ON or OFF) and time relative to change in stimulus condition are shown at the bottom of each panel. As the neurite retracted, the microscopic field was repositioned 15 μm proximally in D. After > 24 h of electrical stimulation, many growth cones have recovered motility and they do not collapse when the stimulus is stopped or reapplied (F–H). Scale bars = 10 μm and 10 mm. (From Fields et al., 1993.)

recovery process proceeds slowly during continuous electrical stimulation, with a half-time of about 3 h (Fields et al., 1993). By 24 h all growth cones appear to be fully accommodated to the inhibitory effects of electrical stimulation. Moreover, outgrowth is unimpeded by turning off the stimulus, and outgrowth proceeds normally once stimulation is resumed.

Studies of the cellular basis for this accommodation have forced a re-examination of the fundamental theory of how Ca^{2+} regulates growth cone motility. Considerable evidence has been compiled which supports the 'calcium optimum' theory, that growth cone motility is a function of the intracellular Ca^{2+} concentration (Kater et al., 1988; Mattson et al., 1988; Lankford and Letourneau, 1989; Lipton and Kater 1989). Concentrations of Ca^{2+} that are greater or less than the permissive range will lead to collapse of the growth cone. One attraction of this theory is that multiple stimuli impinging on the neuron affect the concentration of $[Ca^{2+}]_i$, and the net calcium concentration resulting from all such influences could serve as an effective means of integrating the numerous signals influencing growth cone behavior and thereby lead to a single appropriate response. Exceptions to this theory have challenged this concept, however. Some growth cones can experience large calcium transients and maintain outgrowth (Garyantes and Regeher, 1992), and others will grow without impairment in medium lacking external calcium (Campenot and Draker, 1989). Exceptions such as these and others have been explained by the failure to document the actual perturbation of intracellular calcium produced by the intervention, or failing to consider the possibility that intracellular calcium may adapt during continuous stimulation to levels conducive to normal outgrowth (Kater and Mills, 1991).

Evidence for adaptation of intracellular calcium concentration during maintained electrical stimulation was provided in mouse DRG neurons subjected to prolonged 10 Hz stimulation (Fields et al., 1993). Calcium concentrations rise rapidly following single exponential kinetics with a time constant of about 1.4 sec. (These kinetics refer to the rate of change in ratio of fura-2 fluorescence excited at 340 and 380 nm. This treatment of the data avoids uncertainties introduced by calibration procedures used to convert fluorescence ratio to $[Ca^{2+}]_i$. In general, the changes in $[Ca^{2+}]_i$ would reach a peak concentration more rapidly than the single exponential response of the ratio changes [see Fields et al., 1993].) The concentration then lowers slowly (time constant of 90 sec) to a level that is only moderately elevated from resting by 15 min of stimulation. Interestingly, this places the intracellular calcium concentration back within what must be near the permissive range for outgrowth at the time the growth cone is in the final stages of collapse. Therefore, only a brief period of high intracellular calcium must be necessary to activate the processes leading to this dramatic collapsing behavior. Also, the growth cone does not recover immediately after calcium has adapted to continuous stimulation by recovering to moderately elevated levels. A period of 1 to several hours is required for the growth cone to recover normal morphology and resume outgrowth (Fields et al., 1990, 1993). The discontinuity between the resumption of near normal calcium concentration, and the time it takes for growth cones to resume normal outgrowth may be explained by slower kinetics for reassembly of growth cone cytoskeletal structure and motility following growth cone collapse and homeostasis of $[Ca^{2+}]_i$.

These experiments on adaptation provided evidence for a modification of the calcium optimum hypothesis, which was termed the 'calcium set-point' hypothesis (Kater and Mills 1991). That is, homeostatic mechanisms may act to restore calcium to a normal range (the set-point) following perturbation. Clearly, failure to consider that calcium could recover to normal levels during a stimulus could explain some of the apparent discrepancies of the calcium hypothesis that have been reported in the literature, if the concentration of calcium was not measured in the growth cone, or if it was measured too long after the stimulus.

While applicable to a wide set of situations, the calcium set-point hypothesis ultimately failed to fully account for the recovery of mouse DRG growth cones after chronic electrical stimulation (Fields et al., 1993). It was observed that after 24 h or more of continuous stimulation, calcium had once again risen in the growth cones significantly beyond the moderately elevated levels that had been achieved after 15 min of stimulation. Although stopping the stimulus allowed the $[Ca^{2+}]_i$ to lower in chronically stimulated growth cones to levels that were indistinguishable from unstimulated growth cones, a test stimulus caused the $[Ca^{2+}]_i$ to reach peak concentrations that were just as high as those that were associated with collapse of naive growth cones (Fig. 2). This observation is incompatible with the simplest version of the calcium hypothesis of growth cone motility and with the set-point hypothesis. It suggests that changes in the cytoskeletal structure of the growth cone, or adjustments of the biochemical reactions maintaining growth cone motility, may develop after prolonged electrical stimulation to render the growth cones insensitive to high levels of intracellular calcium. Given the large number of cellular processes in which calcium acts as a second messenger, this accommodation could have broader implications for developing neuronal circuits. Neurons would presumably respond differently to calcium-mediated stimuli, depending on the prior state of electrical activity of the neuron. This discrimination of neuronal responses on the basis of activity-dependent influences could be important during the extensive remodeling seen during development and regeneration of neural circuits.

Quantitative comparisons of the kinetics of electrically evoked calcium transients in naive and accommodated growth cones revealed differences that may contribute to the resistance of these growth cones to electrically-induced collapse, and these observations may lead to a further refinement of the calcium hypothesis of growth cone collapse. After a chronic period of

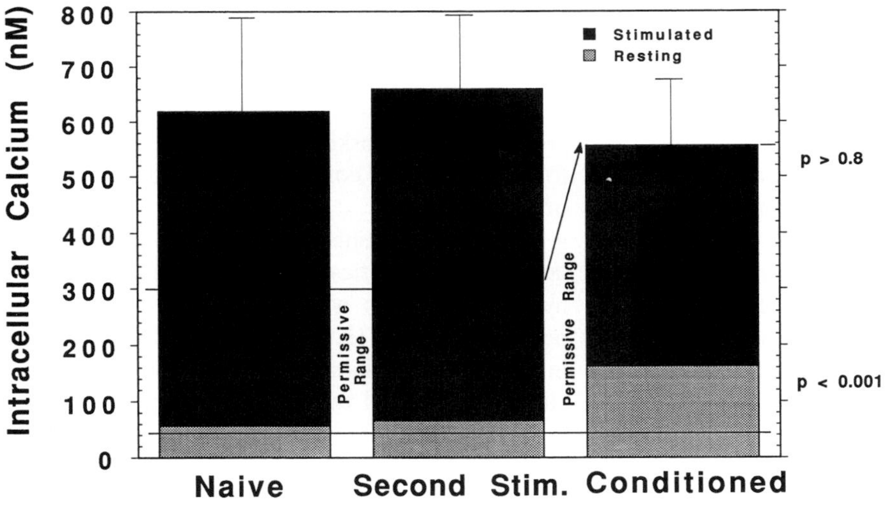

Fig. 2. Although high levels of intracellular calcium have been associated with growth cone collapse (i.e., higher than the permissive range of Ca^{2+} for neurite outgrowth), growth cones that are rendered insensitive to electrically-induced collapse by prolonged electrical stimulation still exhibit large increases in $[Ca^{2+}]_i$. The peak concentration of $[Ca^{2+}]_i$ in growth cones is not significantly different in response to the first or second stimulation of naive growth cones or the electrically induced increase in growth cones conditioned by > 24 h of stimulation. The resting levels of $[Ca^{2+}]_i$ (i.e., concentration in the absence of stimulation) was significantly elevated in chronically stimulated growth cones (stippled bar). (From Fields and Nelson, 1994a.)

electrical stimulation (> 24 h), intracellular calcium increases much more slowly in response to 10 Hz stimulation than in naive growth cones ($\tau = 6$ sec compared with 1.4 sec in naive growth cones) (Fig. 3). Interestingly, the kinetics of calcium increase are not altered measurably after a brief (i.e., 15 min) period of stimulation, allowing the possibility that regulation of transcription could contribute to the reduced rate of calcium increase. No differences in adaptation rates (i.e., recovery of $[Ca^{2+}]_i$ during 15-min stimulus trains), or rates of removal of residual calcium after terminating the stimulus were detected between naive and accommodated growth cones, suggesting that the homeostatic processes that restore calcium during these periods are not altered by chronic activity. A comparison of rates of radioactive calcium efflux in accommodated and naive neurons also supports this conclusion. This suggests that a rapidly acting calcium homeostatic mechanism, which could operate during the initial period of calcium increase, could act to slow the rise in $[Ca^{2+}]_i$. Alternatively, the rate of electrically evoked calcium influx into the cytoplasm could be reduced after chronic electrical stimulation. This may involve reduction in calcium influx through voltage sensitive calcium channels, or diminished release of Ca^{2+} from any internal stores that may contribute to the electrically evoked rise in intracellular calcium. This regulation must be based on the prolonged period of electrical activation, rather than a regulatory mechanism mediated by the concentration of calcium in the cytoplasm, because no correlation between the kinetics of calcium rise and resting calcium concentration could be detected.

It is possible that the slower rate of increase in intracellular calcium may allow sufficient time for compensatory responses that help maintain growth cone integrity and motility. The calcium threshold concept for growth cone collapse fails to account for the insensitivity of growth cones to electrically-induced collapse, but the rate of increase in calcium does correlate with growth cone behavior. It would appear from these experiments that rates of Ca^{2+} increase that are faster than 2 sec (time constant for the fura-2 fluorescence ratio change) are associated with growth cone

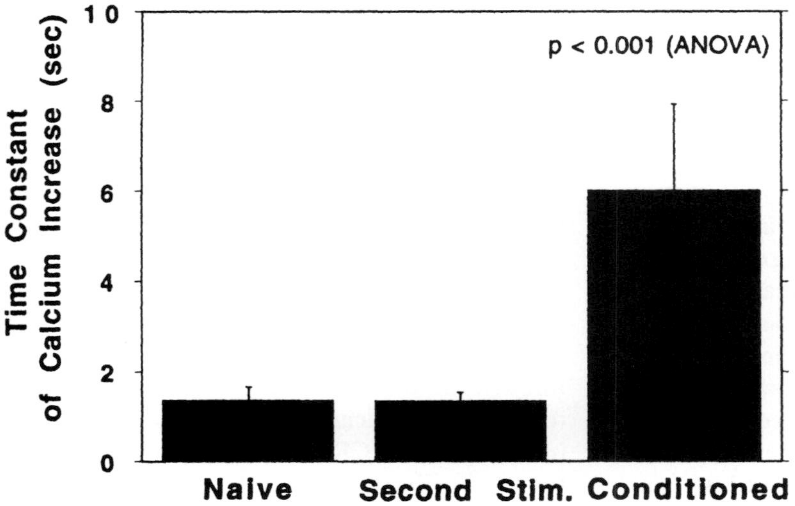

Fig. 3. The mean time constant for the increase in $[Ca^{2+}]_i$ is significantly slowed in growth cones accommodated to electrical stimulation (conditioned). No difference was evident between the first (naive) and replicate (second stimulation) test of responses to stimulation. This indicates that the change in kinetics requires prolonged stimulation. There was no correlation between the time constant of calcium increase and resting level of calcium in the growth cone (means and S.D.). (From Fields and Nelson, 1994b.)

collapse. Further experiments to test this hypothesis could lead to a new understanding that the kinetics of calcium increase in growth cones are essential in determining growth cone behavior in response to this important second messenger. Additional evidence that the kinetics of Ca^{2+} increase are important in growth cone collapse is provided by experiments comparing growth cone collapse in response to different frequencies and patterns of electrical stimulation. These experiments showed that repeated bursts of stimuli are more effective in affecting growth cone motility than constant frequency stimulation (Fields et al., 1990).

Activation of immediate early genes by patterned stimulation

Immediate early genes respond to a wide variety of external stimuli. The diversity of these stimuli make it less clear how IE gene activation could be linked to a stimulus-specific response. Moreover, if these genes are to regulate long-term changes in neurons according to the functional characteristics of a neuronal circuit, their transcription must be specific not only in terms of the mode and intensity of stimulation, but also with respect to the particular temporal pattern of action potentials.

Levels of mRNA for the IE genes c-*fos* and *nur/77* can be assessed using reverse transcription and semiquantitative polymerase chain reaction (PCR) of mouse DRG neurons subjected to patterned electrical stimulation in a multicompartment cell culture chamber (Sheng et al., 1993). Expression of the IE gene c-*fos* increases after 30 min of constant frequency stimulation. It reaches a maximum at about 1 h, and declines to basal levels by 6 h. The expression of this gene is directly proportional to stimulus frequency. Stimulation at 0.01 Hz produces no detectable increase in c-*fos* expression after 30 min of stimulation, but levels increase significantly with 0.1 Hz, to reach a maximum at 1–10 Hz stimulation.

Expression of IE genes in these neurons is dependent on the pattern of stimulation, and different IE genes display different pattern sensitivities. If the 180 action potentials that are delivered to DRG neurons during a 30-min stimulus period at a frequency of 0.1 Hz are, instead, grouped into short bursts of 6 action potentials (at 10 Hz) delivered every minute for 30 min, c-*fos* mRNA is expressed in higher amounts than after 0.1-Hz stimulation. The greater efficacy of repeated bursts of stimuli as compared with constant frequency stimulation parallels results with respect to growth cone motility, where 4 times as many action potentials at a constant frequency were required to elicit the same response seen after repeated bursts of stimuli (Fields et al., 1990). However, the same number of action potentials grouped into a different pattern of bursts (12 action potentials (10 Hz) delivered every 2 min) was completely ineffective in elevating c-*fos* expression above unstimulated levels (Fig. 4A). A different IE gene, *nur/77*, displayed a different pattern sensitivity, with levels of expression increased significantly by both patterns of stimulus bursts (i.e., 12 impulses every 2 min, and 6 impulses every 1 min) (Fig. 4B). Thus, transcription of IE genes is activated by specific patterns of electrical stimuli, not simply the number of action potentials delivered in a given period; and different IE genes display sensitivities to different patterns of electrical activation. This implies that stimulus/transcription coupling could activate specific genetic programs in response to particular patterns of neural circuit activity arising from spontaneous network activity and input to the nervous system from the environment. The cellular basis for this pattern sensitivity is an intriguing problem.

It is well known that the calcium signal transduction cascade leads to transcription of IE genes through the phosphorylation of transcription factors such as calcium/cAMP response element binding protein (CREB) and serum response factor (SRF) (Bartel et al., 1989; Morgan and Curran, 1989, 1991; Murphy et al., 1991; Sheng et al., 1991; Ginty et al., 1992; Bading et al., 1993). The stimulus pattern sensitivity of IE gene transcription is not consistent with some of the hypotheti-

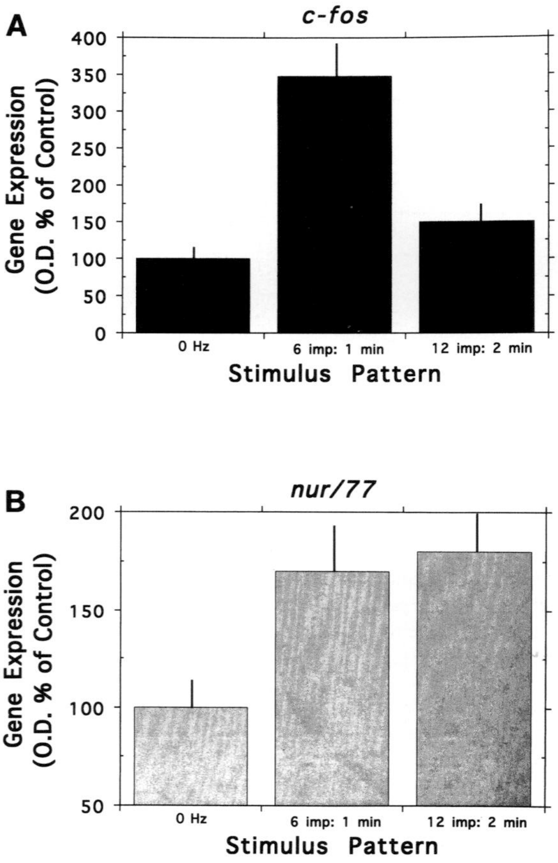

Fig. 4. Different patterns of electrical stimulation regulate transcription of different IE genes. In contrast to c-*fos* (A), transcription of the IE gene *nur/77* (B) was increased significantly by both stimulation patterns comprising 6-impulse bursts delivered at 1-min intervals (6 imp: 1 min), and 12-impulse bursts delivered at 2-min intervals (12: 2 min). (From Sheng et al., 1993.)

cal mechanisms by which different patterns of action potentials could be encoded by intracellular calcium levels. A simple means of explaining the pattern specificity in terms of intracellular calcium responses would be that the different patterns of stimulation differ in the peak calcium rise that is produced in the cytoplasm, because of differences in the degree to which pulses of calcium sum upon one another when delivered at different intervals. Specifically, bursts of calcium influx separated by intervals of 1 min might sum upon the residual calcium sustaining from the previous burst, but bursts of calcium influx separated by 2 min would fail to raise calcium beyond a threshold required to activate the gene. Previous experiments in which the kinetics of calcium influx and clearing were quantified following electrical activation in these neurons (discussed above) would not support this interpretation. A direct test of this hypothesis rejected the $[Ca^{2+}]_i$ summation mechanism (Fig. 5). No residual calcium was produced by either the stimulus pattern comprising a 6-impulse burst every minute or the 12-impulse burst every 2 min. Secondly, the peak calcium concentration reached with the 12-impulse burst was greater than that reached by a 6-impulse burst, but the stimulus producing the highest peak calcium was completely ineffective in activating c-*fos*. Thus, the pattern discrimination evident in gene expression following these two patterns of stimulation cannot be explained by differences in peak or residual calcium produced by either pattern. This suggests that the time-dependent aspects of the calcium fluxes must be taken into consideration in an effort to understand the stimulus pattern-specific aspects of stimulus/transcription coupling, not merely the steady-state changes in calcium concentration produced by the stimuli.

One possible measure of calcium flux that better incorporates time-dependent aspects is the total net calcium rise produced during the 30-min stimulus period. This represents the area under the calcium concentration curve (Fig. 5) produced with bursts of stimulation at different patterns integrated over the entire 30-min period of stimulation (Fig. 6). The net calcium increase was significantly higher in the stimulus pattern that was effective in increasing c-*fos* expression (6 impulses every 1 min), compared with the ineffective stimulus pattern (12 impulses every 2 min). However, by this measure the net calcium influx produced by the 0.1-Hz stimulus was significantly greater than either burst pattern, yet this constant frequency stimulus was the least effective means of increasing c-*fos* expression.

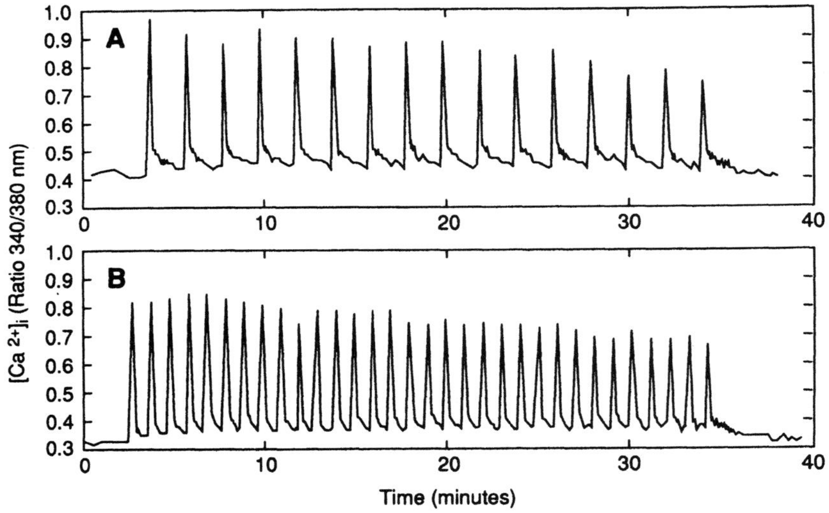

Fig. 5. The intracellular calcium transients in the soma of DRG neurons produced by the two patterns of stimulation were recorded with fura-2 during 30 min periods with (A) 12 impulse bursts delivered every 2 min, and (B) 6 impulse bursts delivered every min. The pattern in (A) was ineffective in stimulating c-fos expression, even though higher peak concentrations of $[Ca^{2+}]_i$ are produced by the 12 action potential bursts. No increase in residual calcium was produced by either pattern of stimulation, eliminating this possible explanation for the stimulus-specific IE gene transcription. (From Sheng et al., 1993.)

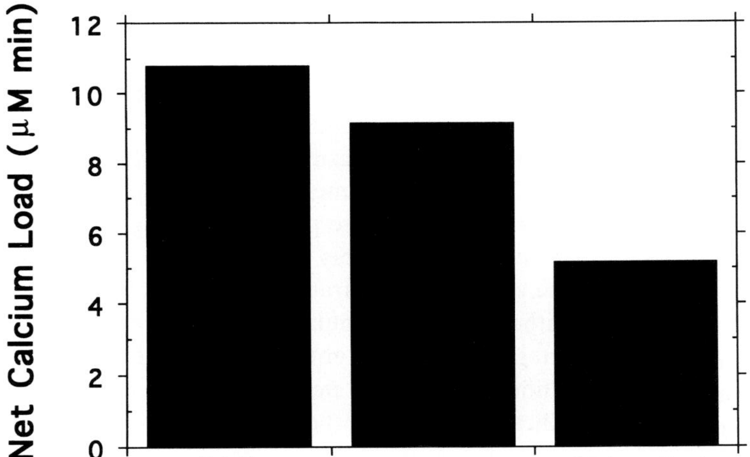

Fig. 6. The stimulus pattern producing the least net calcium load (i.e., the integrated area under the calcium transients (Fig. 5)), failed to increase transcription of c-*fos*. This stimulus consists of 12 impulses (10 Hz) delivered every 2 min (12 imp: 2 min). However, the greatest net calcium increase was observed for the 0.1-Hz stimulus, which produced lower levels of c-*fos* mRNA compared with the 6-impulse burst (10 Hz) delivered every min (6 imp: 1 min). (From Fields and Nelson, 1994b.)

The results suggest that while the time-dependent aspect of calcium fluxes must be taken into consideration in understanding the pattern-specific activation of IE genes, the net calcium flux does not fully capture the basis for this pattern specificity. This has lead to the theory of 'resonant signal transduction', which posits that different temporal patterns of activation will activate selectively different intracellular processes, even though these different intracellular processes may share elements of the same signal transduction cascade (Fields and Nelson, 1994b). This pattern sensitivity would arise by virtue of differences in the activation and inactivation kinetics of the sequential elements comprising the signal transduction cascade. This would include the rates of calcium increase and removal, as well as the concentration dynamics of downstream reactions that comprise the signal transduction cascade. The theory would predict that stimuli of different temporal patterns could selectively activate different cellular responses even if the two stimuli produced the same total increase in calcium (or other downstream reactant), provided that the time-dependent concentration dynamics of the relevant second messenger was different for the two stimuli. While steady-state concentration levels of second messengers may be adequate for regulating stimulus responses in other tissues, resonant signal transduction could be particularly important in nervous tissue where information is carried in the temporal pattern of activation.

Discussion

A summary of current research suggests that growth cones display a sensitivity to intracellular calcium concentration, but the dynamics of intracellular calcium responses to stimulation must be considered more closely. These dynamics are regulated by the state of activity of the neuron; furthermore, the sensitivities of cellular mechanisms maintaining growth cone motility appear to be regulated by chronic electrical activation. The dynamics of Ca^{2+} concentration changes, in contrast to steady-state levels, are an equally important consideration for understanding activation of IE gene expression by patterned stimulation. Neither a large increase in $[Ca^{2+}]_i$, nor a prolonged increase in residual $[Ca^{2+}]_i$ are required to activate IE gene transcription, and discrimination between different patterns of electrical activity cannot be explained on this basis. The significant increase in c-*fos* expression produced by delivering one action potential every 10 sec for 30 min shows that large or sustained increases in $[Ca^{2+}]_i$ are not required for inducing IE gene transcription. This modest stimulus produces only a transient rise of about 20 nM $[Ca^{2+}]_i$, and no significant increase in residual calcium. Activation of different IE genes by different patterns of stimulation seems to reflect resonant properties that may depend on the rates of generation and decay of sequential elements in the signal transduction cascades that link electrical depolarization to gene transcription.

Clearly the subjects considered here continue to be areas of intensive research, and undoubtedly our understanding will change a great deal as data accumulates. Examination of these issues is central to understanding how, during periods of development and repair, neurons can extend connections to form appropriate networks, and remodel them according to how well the networks operate in a given environment.

Acknowledgements

It is my pleasure to acknowledge and thank Dr Phillip Nelson and Dr Hui Sheng of the Laboratory of Developmental Neurobiology. Much of the research summarized in the present review derives from studies that we have pursued and published jointly.

References

Bading, H., Ginty, D.D. and Greenberg, M.E. (1993) Regulation of gene expression in hippocampal neurons by distinct calcium signaling pathways. *Science*, 260: 181–186.

Bartel, D.P., Sheng, M., Lau, L.F. and Greenberg, M.E. (1989) Growth factors and membrane depolarization activate distinct programs of early response gene expression: dissociation of fos and jun induction. *Genes Dev.*, 3: 304–313.

Campenot, R.B. and Draker, D.D. (1989) Growth of sympathetic nerve fibers in culture does not require extracellular calcium. *Neuron*, 3: 733–743.

Cohan, C.S. and Kater, S.B. (1986) Suppression of neurite elongation and growth cone motility by electrical activity. *Science*, 232: 1638–1640.

Cohan, C.S., Connor, J.A. and Kater, S.B. (1987) Electrically and chemically mediated increases in intracellular calcium in neuronal growth cones. *J. Neurosci.*, 7: 3588–3599.

Fields, R.D. and Nelson, P.G. (1992) Activity-dependent development of the vertebrate nervous system. *Int. Rev. Neurobiol.*, 34: 133–214.

Fields, R.D. and Nelson, P.G. (1994a) Growth cone collapse in response to electrical activity, cell contact and diffusible factors. *Physiol. Chem. Phys. Med. NMR*, 26: (in press).

Fields, R. D. and Nelson, P.G. (1994b) Resonant activation of calcium signal transduction in neurons. *J. Neurobiol.*, 25: 281–293.

Fields, R.D., Neale, E.A. and Nelson, P.G. (1988) Effects of electrical activity on outgrowth of neurites from mouse sensory neurons in vitro. *J. Cell Biol.*, 107: 729a.

Fields, R.D., Neale, E.A. and Nelson, P.G. (1990) Effects of patterned electrical activity on neurite outgrowth from mouse sensory neurons. *J. Neurosci.*, 10: 2950–2964.

Fields, R.D., Guthrie, P.B., Russell, J.T., Kater, S.B., Malhotra, B.S. and Nelson, P.G. (1993) Accommodation of mouse DRG growth cones to electrically induced collapse: kinetic analysis of calcium transients and set-point theory. *J. Neurobiol.*, 24: 1080–1089.

Forscher, P., Kaczmarek, L.K., Buchanan, J. and Smith, S.J. (1987) Cyclic AMP changes in distribution and transport of organelles within growth cones of Aplysia bag cell neurons. *J. Neurosci.*, 7: 3600–3611.

Garyantes, T.K. and Regehr, W.G. (1992) Electrical activity increases growth cone calcium but fails to inhibit neurite outgrowth. *J. Neurosci.*, 12: 96–103.

Ginty, D.D., Bading, H. and Greenberg, M.E. (1992) Trans-synaptic regulation of gene expression. *Curr. Opin. Neurobiol.*, 2: 312–316.

Kater, S.B. and Mills, L.R. (1991) Regulation of growth cone behavior by calcium. *J. Neurosci.*, 11: 891–899.

Kater, S.B., Mattson, M.P., Cohan, C. and Connor, J. (1988) Calcium regulation of neuronal growth cone. *Trends Neurosci.*, 11: 315–321.

Lankford, K.L. and Letourneau, P.C. (1989) Evidence that calcium may control neurite outgrowth by regulating the stability of actin filaments. *J. Cell Biol.*, 109: 1229–1243.

Lipton, S.A. and Kater, S.B. (1989) Neurotransmitter regulation of neuronal outgrowth, plasticity and survival. *Trends Neurosci.*, 12: 265–270.

Mattson, M.P. and Kater, S.B. (1987) Calcium regulation of neurite elongation and growth cone motility. *J. Neurosci.*, 7: 4034–4043.

Mattson, M.P., Guthrie, P.B. and Kater, S.B. (1988) Components of neurite outgrowth that determine neuronal cytoarchitecture: influence of calcium and the growth substrate. *J. Neurosci. Res.*, 20: 331–345.

Morgan, J.I. and Curran, T. (1989) Stimulus-transcription coupling in neurons: role of cellular immediate-early genes. *Trends Neurosci.*, 12: 459–462.

Morgan, J.I. and Curran, T. (1991) Stimulus-transcription coupling in the nervous system: involvement of the inducible proto-oncogenes *fos* and *jun*. *Annu. Rev. Neurosci.*, 14: 421–451.

Murphy, T.H., Worley, P.F. and Baraban, J.M. (1991) L-Type voltage-sensitive calcium channels mediate synaptic activation of immediate early genes. *Neuron*, 7: 625–635.

Schwab, M.E., Kapfhammer J.P. and Bandtlow, C.E. (1993) Inhibitors of neurite growth. *Annu. Rev. Neurosci.*, 16: 565–595.

Shatz, C.J. (1990) Impulse activity and the patterning of connections during CNS development. *Neuron*, 5: 745–756.

Sheng, M., Thompson, M.A. and Greenberg, M.E. (1991) CREB: A Ca^{++}-regulated transcription factor phosphorylated by calmodulin-dependent kinases. *Science*, 252: 1427–1430.

Sheng, H.Z., Fields, R.D. and Nelson, P.G. (1993) Specific regulation of immediate early genes by patterned neuronal activity. *J. Neurosci. Res.*, 35: 459–467.

Walter, J., Allsopp, T.E. and Bonhoeffer, F. (1990) A common denominator of growth cone guidance and collapse? *Trends Neurosci.*, 11: 447–452.

F.J. Seil (Ed.)
Progress in Brain Research, Vol 103

CHAPTER 14

Nuclear calcium elevation may initiate neurite outgrowth in mammalian neurons

Jeffery D. Kocsis, Mark N. Rand, Karen Lankford and Stephen G. Waxman

Department of Neurology, Yale University School of Medicine and Neuroscience and Regeneration Research Center, Veterans Affairs Medical Center, West Haven, CT 06516, USA

Introduction

Calcium is an important second messenger and has a role in a variety of cellular functions (Rasmussen, 1990; Ferris and Snyder, 1992; Berridge, 1989). Recent confocal imaging studies using Ca^{2+} sensitive dyes reveal a heterogeneous distribution of Ca^{2+} signals in the nuclear and cytoplasmic compartments of neurons (Hernandez-Cruz et al., 1990; Holliday and Spitzer, 1990; Holliday et al., 1991; Pryzwara et al., 1991; Birch et al., 1992), with signals in the nucleus often being several times larger than in the cytoplasm. Since increases in intracellular Ca^{2+} can trigger events associated with gene expression (Greenberg et al., 1986; Sheng et al., 1990, 1991; Morgan and Curran, 1991), it has been suggested that large depolarization-induced nuclear Ca^{2+} signals may play a role in controlling neuronal development and regeneration.

Stimulus-induced nuclear Ca^{2+} signals are prominent both in embryonic (Holliday et al., 1991; Kocsis et al., 1993a; Segal and Manor, 1992; Utszschneider et al., 1994) and adult (Birch et al., 1992) dorsal root ganglion (DRG) neurons at early times in culture and decline in both cytoplasm and nucleus at later stages of development (Holliday et al., 1991; Utzschneider et al., 1994) or after later times in culture (Birch et al., 1992). We recently proposed that mobilization of Ca^{2+} from intracellular stores during this time plays an important role in generating these signals (Kocsis et al., 1993b, 1994) and have tested this idea by depleting intracellular Ca^{2+} stores and studying the time course and extent of neurite outgrowth of adult rat DRG cells in culture (Lankford et al., 1993; Kocsis et al., 1994).

In this chapter we provide evidence that the majority of the Ca^{2+} signals observed in both nucleus and cytoplasm of adult DRG neurons are derived from calcium-induced calcium release (CICR) and that depletion of intracellular Ca^{2+} stores reduces neurite outgrowth. These results give rise to the proposal that membrane depolarization may elicit CICR, which in turn may be important for gene expression necessary for neurite outgrowth. These results emphasize the importance of CICR and intracellular Ca^{2+} mobilization as a potential intermediate linking depolarization to gene expression essential for neurite outgrowth.

Methods

Cell culture

Female Wistar rats (180–200 g) were exsanguinated by carotid section following anesthesia with sodium pentobarbital (i.p., 60 mg/kg). L4 and L5 DRG were carefully excised and placed in cold, Ca^{2+}-free normal electrolyte solution (NS, see below), containing 100 units/ml each of penicillin and streptomycin. The ganglia were placed in collagenase (1 mg/ml NS, with 1.5 mM $CaCl_2$, 0.5 mM EDTA and 0.2 mg/ml cysteine) for 25 min at 40°C, and then in NS containing 20–30 units/ml papain and 1 mg/ml collagenase for 25 min, and were triturated in culture solution consisting of 45% Dulbecco's modified Eagle's medium (DMEM), 45% Ham's F12 medium, and 10% fetal calf serum (FCS), with added trypsin inhibitor and bovine serum albumin (BSA) (1.5 mg/ml each). Cell suspensions were produced via trituration through a fire polished siliconized Pasteur pipette. Neurons were plated (approx. 250 neurons/mm^2) on UV-irradiated glass coverslips coated with polyornithine (0.1 mg/ml) and laminin (9 μg/coverslip), and incubated at 37°C in culture solution (as described above). After plating, adherent neurons were spherical and either lacked neurites or had a single short axon stump; nonneuronal cells were relatively sparse at this time.

Confocal scanning laser microscopy and dye loading

Neurons were dye loaded by incubation in NS containing 5 μM fluo-3AM (Molecular Probes, Eugene, OR) for 35 min at 37°C (Kao et al., 1989). Neuron bearing coverslips were placed in a low volume (200–400 μl) perfusion chamber and irrigated with NS for 5–10 min. The chamber was perfused at a rate of 2–3 ml/min. Solutions were saturated with 95% O_2/5% CO_2 and maintained at room temperature (20–24°C). The DRG neurons were imaged with a Bio-Rad MRC-500 confocal system and Nikon Diaphot inverted microscope, using a 40 × 1.3 N.A. Olympus D Apo UV objective. Fluorescence was elicited with the 488 nm line of an argon ion laser. The optical section sampled was approx. 1.5 μm thick.

Solutions and experimental procedures

Normal electrolyte solution (NS) consisted of (in mM): 124 NaCl, 3.0 KCl, 2.0 $MgCl_2$, 1.3 NaH_2PO_4, 26 $NaHCO_3$, 2 $CaCl_2$, and 10 dextrose, saturated with 95% O_2/5% CO_2. Neurons were depolarized by perfusing the chamber with NS containing 60 mM K^+ substituted for an equivalent amount of Na^+ (high-K^+ solution). In order to deplete intracellular Ca^{2+} stores, thapsigargin (200 nM) or ethanol vehicle for controls was applied to neurons in the perfusion bath for 20 min prior to depolarization in high K^+ solution. Caffeine (20 mM) was applied to individual neurons via pressure ejection from a micropipette. Trypan Blue (0.4%) in the micropipette solution facilitated visualization of applied solution to and around the neurons. In some experiments the effect of extracellular Ca^{2+} was examined by changing the bath from NS with 2 mM Ca^{2+} to NS with 200 μM EGTA and no Ca^{2+} (Ca^{2+}-free solution).

Image measurement and analysis

Confocal image files (8-bit resolution) were transferred to a Macintosh Quadra 700 and analyzed using Image (W. Rasband, NIH). Fluo-3 fluorescence in the nucleus and cytoplasm was measured before and after drug treatment or depolarization, and for purposes of statistical comparison it was assumed that the fluorescence output over the range of $[Ca^{2+}]_i$ was approximately linear and that it effectively paralleled changes in $[Ca^{2+}]_i$. The cytoplasm and nucleus were outlined and the average pixel values were obtained. A small proportion of neurons (approx. 5%) displayed much higher resting fluorescence ($\geq$ 4-times the remainder of the population) and were excluded from the analysis. Overall population fluorescence levels in NS were relatively homogeneous. For some statistical analyses we partially corrected for differences in dye loading by using the ratio of stimulation to prestimulation fluorescence values for each neuron (Minta et al., 1989). Experimental and control groups were compared using a 2-tailed, between-subjects Student's *t*-test; fluorescence values of a neuron's cytoplasm vs. its nucleus, or effects of different treatment solutions applied to the same neuron, were also compared using a 2-tailed, within-subjects Student's t-test. The n consisted of the number of cells measured; standard errors of the means are reported.

Analysis of thapsigargin effects on neurite outgrowth

Neurons were placed in culture for 3–4 h and then normal culture medium was removed and replaced for 20 min with media containing 200 nM thapsigargin, an irreversible endoplasmic reticulum Ca^{2+} ATPase inhibitor (Research Biochemicals Incorporated, Natick MA) or ethanol vehicle alone (0.02% final concentration). The cultures were washed three times in normal culture media and cultured as described above. After 3 days in culture, cell bearing coverslips were fixed with paraformaldehyde, permeablized with Triton X-100, and blocked with BSA and normal goat serum. Identification of neurons was confirmed by staining with the monoclonal antibody SMI 32 directed against nonphosphorylated rat neurofilament proteins and secondary and tertiary antibodies 501 and 405 (Sternberger Monoclonals Incorporated, Baltimore, MD) and visualized using standard immunocytochemical procedures described by Sternberger et al. (1970).

Neurofilament stained coverslips were examined with a 40 × objective on a Nikon Microphot. Images were acquired with a CCD video camera and analyzed using Image 1 imaging processing software. In order to eliminate axon stumps retained after dissociation as a confounding variable in assessing neurite outgrowth, we scored neurofilament-positive cells as positive for long neurites if they possessed one or more processes whose length was at least twice the cell body diameter. Cell bodies were measured and scored for outgrowth in all neurofilament-positive cells with reasonably intact cell bodies that were sufficiently separated from other cells to identify the source of neurites. Less than 5% of neurofilament-positive cells on a given coverslip could not be scored as a result of cell clumping or poor morphology. The percentages of neurons with long neurites were calculated from the numbers of neurofilament-positive cells meeting the outgrowth criteria divided by the total number of scored neurons.

Results

Subcellular distribution of Ca^{2+} in DRG neurons during the first day in culture

Confocal image of fluo-3 fluorescence revealed different calcium signals in the nucleus, nucleolus and cytoplasm of 1 day in vitro adult DRG cultures. A DRG neuron loaded with the Ca^{2+} indicator, fluo-3, and imaged with confocal microscopy after 1 day in culture is shown in Fig. 1A. The resting fluorescence level is relatively low, but sufficient fluorescence signal is present to distinguish the nucleus and nucleolus within the cytoplasm. At early times in culture, Ca^{2+} signals in the nucleus were consistently lower than those in the cytoplasm before stimulation. However, when the neurons were depolarized by bath application of 60 mM KCl, large increases were observed in both cytoplasmic and nuclear Ca^{2+} signals (Fig. 1 B). The nuclear Ca^{2+} signals increased about 8-fold, whereas the cytoplasmic signals increased about 3-fold. Figure 1C is a subtracted image (depolarized minus control) in the vicinity of the nucleus. Comparison with the matching brightfield (Hoffman modulation contrast optics) image in Fig. 1D shows that the region of highest fluorescence within the nucleus in Fig. 1C is the nucleolus. This pattern, characterized by depolarization-induced Ca^{2+} signals that were highest in the nucleolus and next highest in the nucleus, was typical of neurons in culture for 1 day.

Large nuclear Ca^{2+} signals occur in intact ganglia

In addition to being present in cultured cells, differential nuclear and cytoplasmic Ca^{2+} signals were also observed in intact embryonic DRGs, indicating that the large nuclear Ca^{2+} signals are not the result of tissue culture conditions (Utzschneider et al., 1994). Figure 2 shows high resolution confocal images obtained from isolated

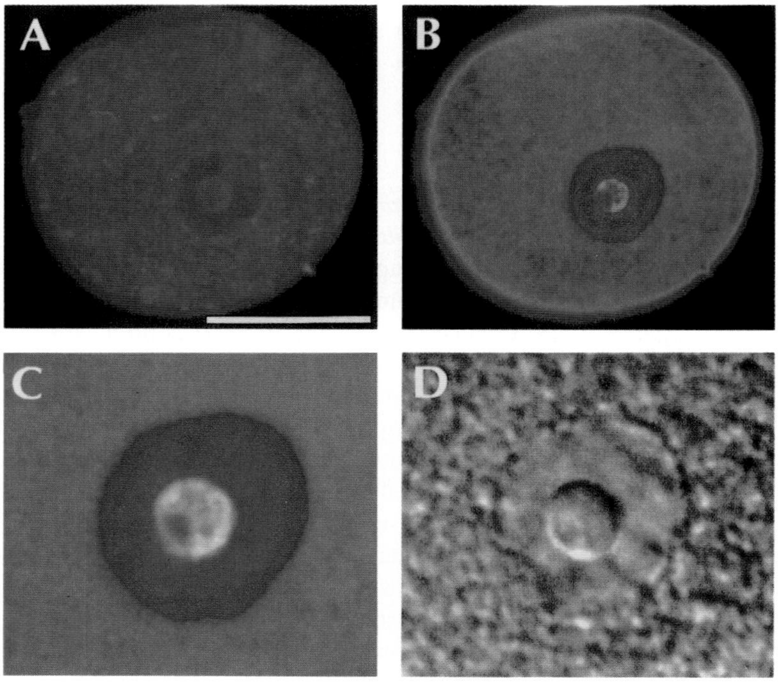

Fig. 1. (A) Confocal image of an adult rat DRG neuron in culture for one day and loaded with the Ca^{2+} fluorescent indicator dye, fluo-3, shown before depolarization. The basal fluorescence signal allows identification of the nuclear region in the resting state. The nuclear fluorescence level is decreased relative to that of the surrounding cytoplasm. Scale bar $= 25\ \mu m$. (B) Stimulation with 60 mM K^+-Krebs solution depolarized the neuron and triggered increased fluorescence signals in the cytoplasm, nucleus and nucleolus. The expanded nuclear region in C is a subtraction of the resting from the depolarized signals shown in A and B. The highest fluorescence is located in the nucleolus, as confirmed with Hoffman optics (D). Scale bar $= 10\ \mu m$. (Modified from Kocsis et al., 1994.)

intact embryonic and neonatal DRGs. Figure 2A shows a DRG from an E18 embryo in normal solution. There is clear variability in fluorescence intensity among the neurons. In some neurons the Ca^{2+} signals in the nuclei are considerably higher than in the cytoplasm. Figure 2B shows the same field of neurons after stimulation with high K^+. Approximately 50% of the neurons increased their fluorescence levels more than 2-fold. A higher magnification of the neurons before and after stimulation is shown in Fig. 2C and D, respectively.

Electrical stimulation at physiological frequencies also leads to elevation in intracellular Ca^{2+} in embryonic DRG neurons (Fig. 2E, F). The line scan of Fig. 2H shows that a clearly detectable nuclear Ca^{2+} signal can be generated following even a single electrical stimulus (top arrow), and that a prolonged nuclear signal occurs after a brief stimulus train at relatively low frequencies. These Ca^{2+} signals are observed in embryonic DRG but are not observed in adult excised DRG neurons and are considerably attenuated even within a few days after birth.

Intracellular Ca^{2+} mobilization as a source of the Ca^{2+} signals

The depolarization-induced Ca^{2+} transients in the DRG neurons at early times in culture required the presence of extracellular Ca^{2+} (Birch

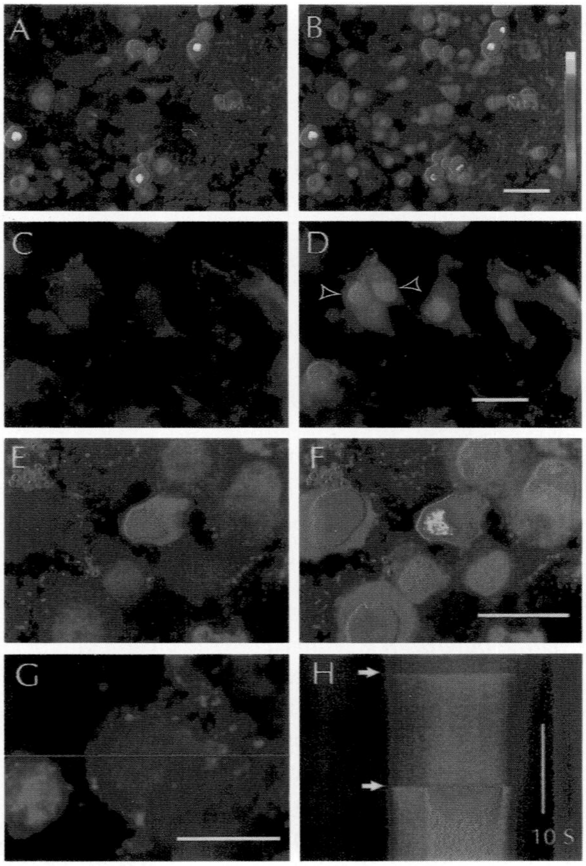

Fig. 2. (A, B) Confocal images showing Ca^{2+} signals in embryonic (E18) DRG neurons before (A) and after (B) depolarization with high K^+. Approximately 50% of the neurons in the optical section of the intact ganglion displayed more than a 2-fold increase in their resting nuclear or cytoplasmic Ca^{2+} signals following depolarization with K^+. A smaller proportion of neurons had relatively large ambient Ca^{2+} signals prior to depolarization with high K^+. (C, D) Ca^{2+} signals in an intact embryonic DRG imaged at a higher resolution before (C) and after (D) depolarization with high K^+ showed that a subset of the DRG neurons had nuclear Ca^{2+} signals greater than their cytoplasmic signals (arrowheads). (E, F) Electrical stimulation of the embryonic DRG increased cytoplasmic and nuclear Ca^{2+} signals. An embryonic (E18) ganglion prior to (E) and immediately following (F) a 2.5 sec, 20 Hz stimulus train. (G, H) Nuclear Ca^{2+} signals evoked by a single electrical stimulus. A line scan through the center of the neuron seen in G (red line) shows increased Ca^{2+} signals after a single electrical stimulus (top arrow in H), and a prolonged Ca^{2+} transient lasting 250 msec (lower arrow). Scale bars are 40 μm (A, B), 25 μm (C, D), 20 μm (E, F) and 15 μm (G, H). The color scale shown in B represents absolute fluorescence values of 0–255 and applies to A–H. (Modified from Utzschneider et al., 1994.)

et al., 1992). Depletion of intracellular Ca^{2+} stores by blockade of the Ca^{2+} ATPase associated with the endoplasmic reticulum resulted in a prominent reduction of the depolarization-induced Ca^{2+} signals (Kocsis et al., 1994). Depolarization-induced Ca^{2+} signals in the DRG neurons are substantially reduced following exposure to the Ca^{2+} ATPase inhibitor, thapsigargin, as shown in Fig. 3, indicating that the large depolarized-induced Ca^{2+} signals require intact intracellular Ca^{2+} stores.

The elevation of intracellular calcium levels following caffeine application provides additional evidence for a large, releasable intracellular pool of Ca^{2+} (Rand et al., 1993). Caffeine has been shown to potentiate intracellular Ca^{2+} release (Endo, 1975), possibly by acting at the ryanodine receptor (Pessah et al., 1987; McPherson et al., 1991). Microapplication of caffeine to the neurons resulted in large intracellular Ca^{2+} signals, presumably as a result of release of Ca^{2+} from intracellular stores. This is illustrated in Fig. 4, which shows a neuron that was stimulated with caffeine, with and without Ca^{2+} in the bath, using a micropipette containing 20 mM caffeine which was positioned within 20 μm of the neuron. Microapplication of caffeine to the neuron, both with and without Ca^{2+} in the bath, resulted in cytoplasmic and nuclear Ca^{2+} signals similar to those observed with depolarization. The similar amplitude of the signals with and without Ca^{2+} in the bath suggests that release of Ca^{2+} from intracellular stores is sufficient to induce the large nuclear and cytoplasmic Ca^{2+} signals, and supports the idea that CICR is important in the generation of the intracellular Ca^{2+} signals in these neurons. CICR may serve not only as an amplification mechanism for intracellular Ca^{2+}, but also as a means to propagate a Ca^{2+} signal from the cell membrane to the nucleus, and thus may be important in the signal transduction pathway for depolarization-induced gene expression (see Discussion). Note that in Fig. 4 a propagated wave of Ca^{2+} travels through the cytoplasm and nucleus.

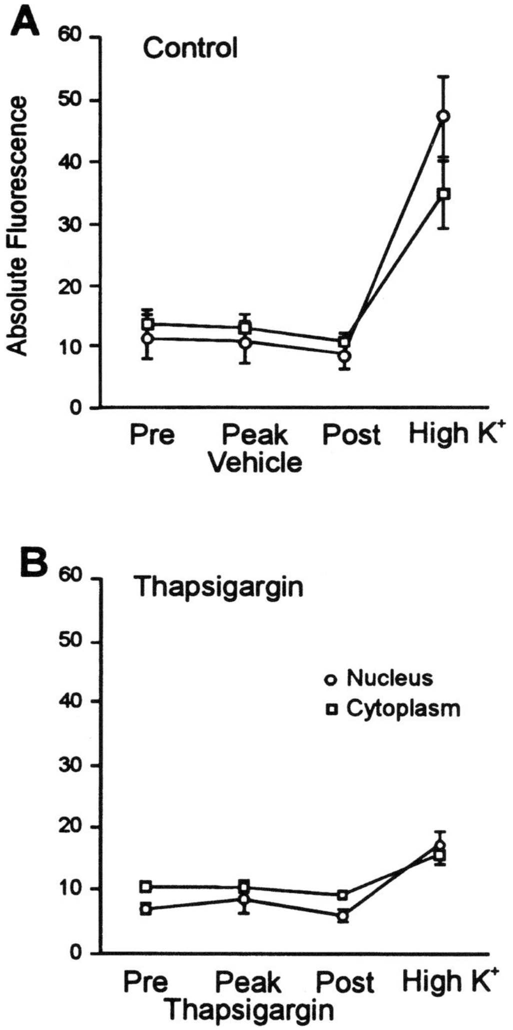

Fig. 3. Thapsigargin reduces the cytoplasmic and nuclear Ca^{2+} signals evoked by depolarization. The graph shows relative Ca^{2+} fluorescence for control (A, ethanol vehicle alone) and thapsigargin treated neurons (B) before and after depolarization with high K^+. (Modified from Kocsis et al., 1994.)

Nuclear Ca^{2+} signals are reduced after neurite outgrowth

The adult DRG neurons were initially spherical and virtually aneuritic at the time of plating (Fig. 5A), but within 3 days in culture neuritic outgrowth was more robust (Fig. 5B). At 6 days in culture, neuritic outgrowth was extensive and the depolarization-induced Ca^{2+} signals were appreciably attenuated, with the nuclear signals no longer exceeding those of the cytoplasm (Fig. 5C,D). Absolute depolarization-induced fluorescence changes in cytoplasm, nucleus and nucleolus are illustrated in Fig. 6, which shows a large increase in all three subcellular compartments at day 1 in culture (Fig. 6A), but much smaller Ca^{2+} signals at day 6 (Fig. 6B). The nuclear Ca^{2+} signals induced by depolarization at day 6 in culture exceeded the cytoplasmic signals.

Neurite outgrowth is reduced after depletion of intracellular calcium stores with thapsigargin

In order to examine the hypothesis that intact intracellular Ca^{2+} stores are a prerequisite for neuritogenesis, DRG cultures were transiently exposed to thapsigargin shortly after cell attachment and examined for neurite outgrowth after 3 days in culture (Lankford et al., 1993). These experiments revealed a striking decrease in neurite initiation in thapsigargin treated neurons. In control cultures, 71 ± 10% of neurofilament-positive cells had neurites at least twice as long as their cell bodies, but only 33 ± 19% of neurons exposed to 200 nM thapsigargin bore neurites which met the length criterion after 3 days in culture (Fig. 7C). The reduction in numbers of neurons initiating neurites in thapsigargin treated cultures was not due to increased cell death or selective loss of a particular population of neurons, as both the total number of neurons and the size distribution of cells were not statistically different between control and thapsigargin treated cultures, and neurite outgrowth from neurons of all sizes was inhibited by thapsigargin to roughly the same extent (Fig. 7D). Both thapsigargin and

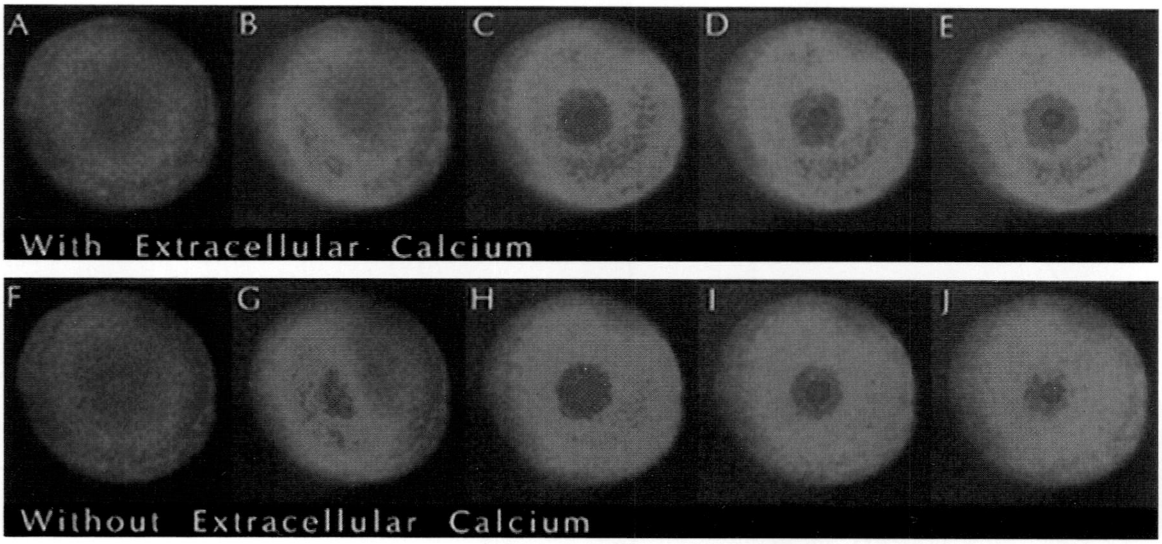

Fig. 4. Microapplication of caffeine with and without Ca^{2+} in the bath elicits large cytoplasmic and nuclear Ca^{2+} signals in DRG neurons in culture. A brief puff of caffeine (20 mM) was focally applied to the neuron through a micropipette. A propagated wave of Ca^{2+} travels through the cytoplasm and nucleus (A–E and F–J). The Ca^{2+} signals in the cytoplasm and nucleus were similar to those observed following depolarization. (Modified from Kocsis et al., 1994.)

control treated neurons appeared healthy and excluded Trypan Blue. These results indicate that depletion of intracellular calcium stores can inhibit neurite outgrowth, and suggest that calcium mobilization may be required for neurite initiation.

Discussion

Intracellular Ca^{2+} transients are important in a variety of neuronal functions, including transmitter release and secretion (Katz and Miledi, 1967; Llinas et al., 1981; Augustine et al., 1987), regulation of growth cone behavior (Kater and Mills, 1991) and gene activation (Greenberg et al., 1986; Milbrandt, 1987; Kennedy, 1989; Sheng et al., 1990; Morgan and Curran, 1991). Confocal microscopy studies using Ca^{2+} sensitive dyes have demonstrated that depolarization can generate large Ca^{2+} signals in the neuronal nucleus (Hernandez-Cruz et al., 1990; Pryzwara et al., 1991; Birch et al., 1992). These studies implicate Ca^{2+} influx and CICR as potential sources for the nuclear Ca^{2+} transients. Although Ca^{2+} can be released from endoplasmic reticulum (ER) stores via 1,4,5-inositol trisphosphate (IP3) stimulation as well as CICR, depolarization-induced Ca^{2+} signals of adult rat DRG neurons require both extracellular Ca^{2+} and intact intracellular Ca^{2+} stores, suggesting that the signals are derived from CICR.

Depolarization-induced Ca^{2+} influx via voltage-gated Ca^{2+} channels and amplification of this initial signal via CICR both contribute to elevations of Ca^{2+} within DRG neurons. Depletion of ER Ca^{2+} stores with thapsigargin substantially reduced the induction of intracellular Ca^{2+} signals, and eliminated differences between nuclear and cytoplasmic signals. Calcium signals are also reduced when DRG neurons are treated with 2,5-di(tert-butyl)-1,4-benzohydroquinone (DTBHQ), a compound which is chemically unre-

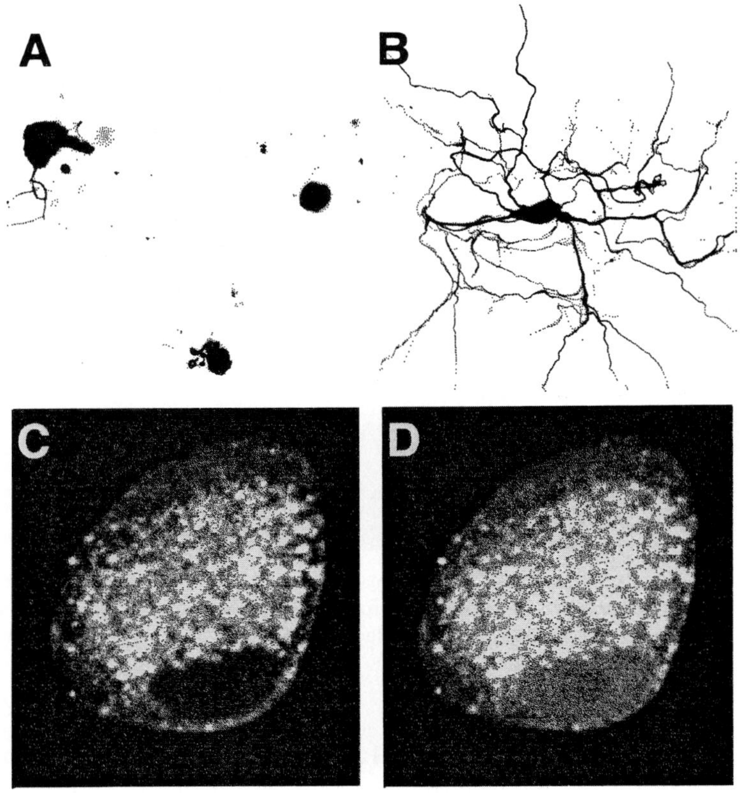

Fig. 5. Neurons grown in culture for 1 day (A) have fewer neurites than those grown in culture for 6 days (B) as indicated by neurofilament staining. Scale bar = 50 μm. Confocal images of fluo-3 fluorescence in a DRG neuron after 6 days in culture are shown before (C) and after (D) depolarization with 60 mM K^+. Scale bar = 25 μm. This neuron was imaged through the region of the nucleus, and the neuritic arbor was out of the confocal plane. Since the resting and stimulated fluorescence levels in day 6 neurons were low compared to those in day 1 neurons, the displayed gain has been augmented. Notice that the cytoplasmic fluorescence pattern was granular and the nuclear level was lower than the cytoplasmic level in day 1 neurons (C). Following K^+-induced depolarization (60 mM), there was a small increase in cytoplasmic and nuclear Ca^{2+}, but the nuclear fluorescence level never exceeded the cytoplasmic fluorescence level. Thus there are markedly different Ca^{2+} transients in response to K^+ depolarization in 1 day cultured neurons (Fig. 1) compared to day 6 neurons. (Modified from Birch et al., 1992.)

lated to thapsigargin but also depletes intracellular Ca^{2+} stores by blocking the ER associated Ca^{2+} ATPase (Rand, Kocsis and Waxman, unpublished observations). These results indicate that intact intracellular Ca^{2+} stores are a prerequisite for the induction of the large nuclear Ca^{2+} signals, and that the stores comprise the major source of Ca^{2+} required for the generation of the intracellular signals. Since micropipette application of caffeine can produce comparable elevations in nuclear Ca^{2+} signals with or without the presence of extracellular Ca^{2+}, we conclude that the signals are generated primarily by intracellular Ca^{2+} release. The Ca^{2+} signals induced by caffeine, which stimulates the release of intracellular stores, were similar in magnitude to those induced by depolarization. These results indicate that CICR is the primary source of the elevated signals observed upon depolarization of DRG neurons at early times in culture when neuritogenesis is occurring.

CICR may act both as a mechanism for Ca^{2+}

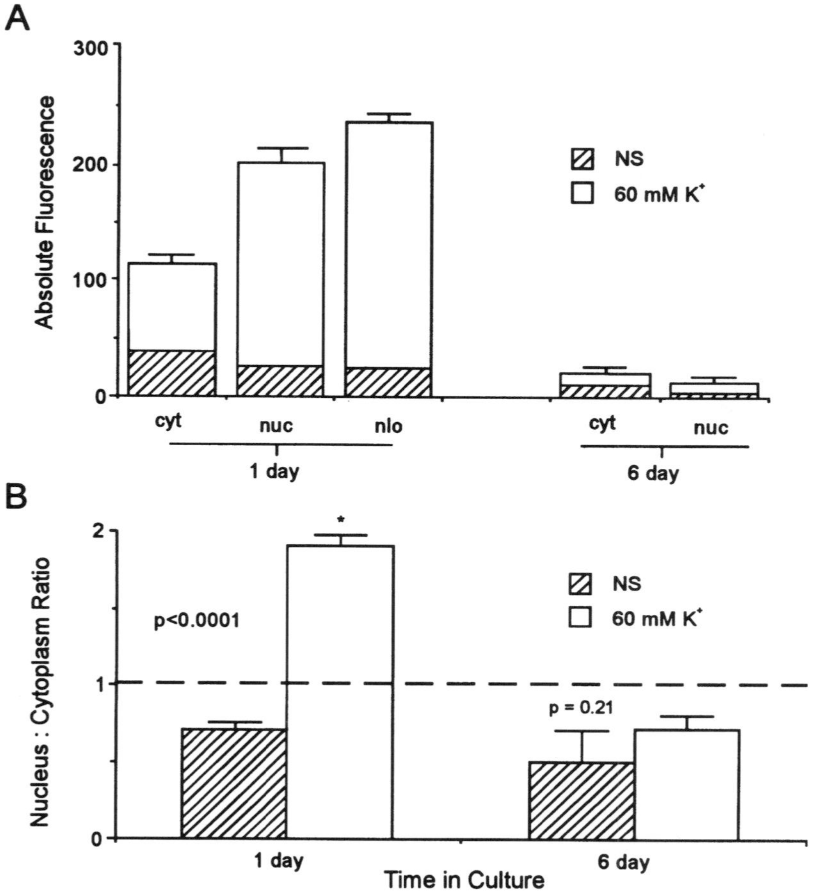

Fig. 6. (A) Fluorescence intensity was plotted for day 1 and day 6 nuclear and cytoplasmic regions both prior to and following K^+-induced depolarization. The resting nuclear fluorescence is lower than resting cytoplasmic fluorescence in both day 1 and day 6 DRG neurons. At 1 day, depolarization elicited the largest increase in fluorescence in the nucleolus, and the next largest increase in the nucleus. At day 6, the cytoplasmic fluorescence due to K^+ stimulation of the cytoplasmic region was larger than the nuclear fluorescence increase. (B) Nuclear/cytoplasmic fluorescence ratios were obtained for 1-day and 6-day cultured neurons before and after stimulation. Both 1-day and 6-day neurons show resting fluorescence ratios of less than 1.0, but following stimulation, day 1 nuclear fluorescence ratios increased to approximately 2.0, whereas the ratio remains below 1.0 for the 6-day cultured neurons. (Modified from Birch et al., 1992.)

signal amplification and as a mechanism for moving the Ca^{2+} signal from cell membrane to the nucleus. Since Ca^{2+} buffering systems in the neuron restrict the range of Ca^{2+} action (Albritton et al., 1992), CICR could extend the range of action of Ca^{2+} by propagating a wave of Ca^{2+} release from consecutive layers of ER as indicated in the model shown in Fig. 8. In this model, Ca^{2+} influx through voltage-gated Ca^{2+} channels initiates Ca^{2+} release from outer layers of ER via ryanodine receptor activation. The release of Ca^{2+} from the outer ER layer then elicits release from deeper layers of ER and thus initiates a self-propagating centripetal wave of Ca^{2+}. Given that the nuclear envelope is contiguous with the ER, this mechanism could also lead to release of

Ca^{2+} from the nuclear envelope into the nucleus. Indeed, we have observed propagating waves of Ca^{2+} sweeping across the cytoplasm and into and through the nucleus (Rand et al., 1993). The propagation of Ca^{2+} waves from the cell membrane to the nucleus could provide a rapid signal transduction pathway whereby depolarization induces changes in nuclear Ca^{2+} levels.

Elevated nuclear Ca^{2+} signals can persist for tens of minutes in rat DRG neurons following chronic depolarization (Thayer and Miller, 1990; Birch et al., 1992), but it is not known clear

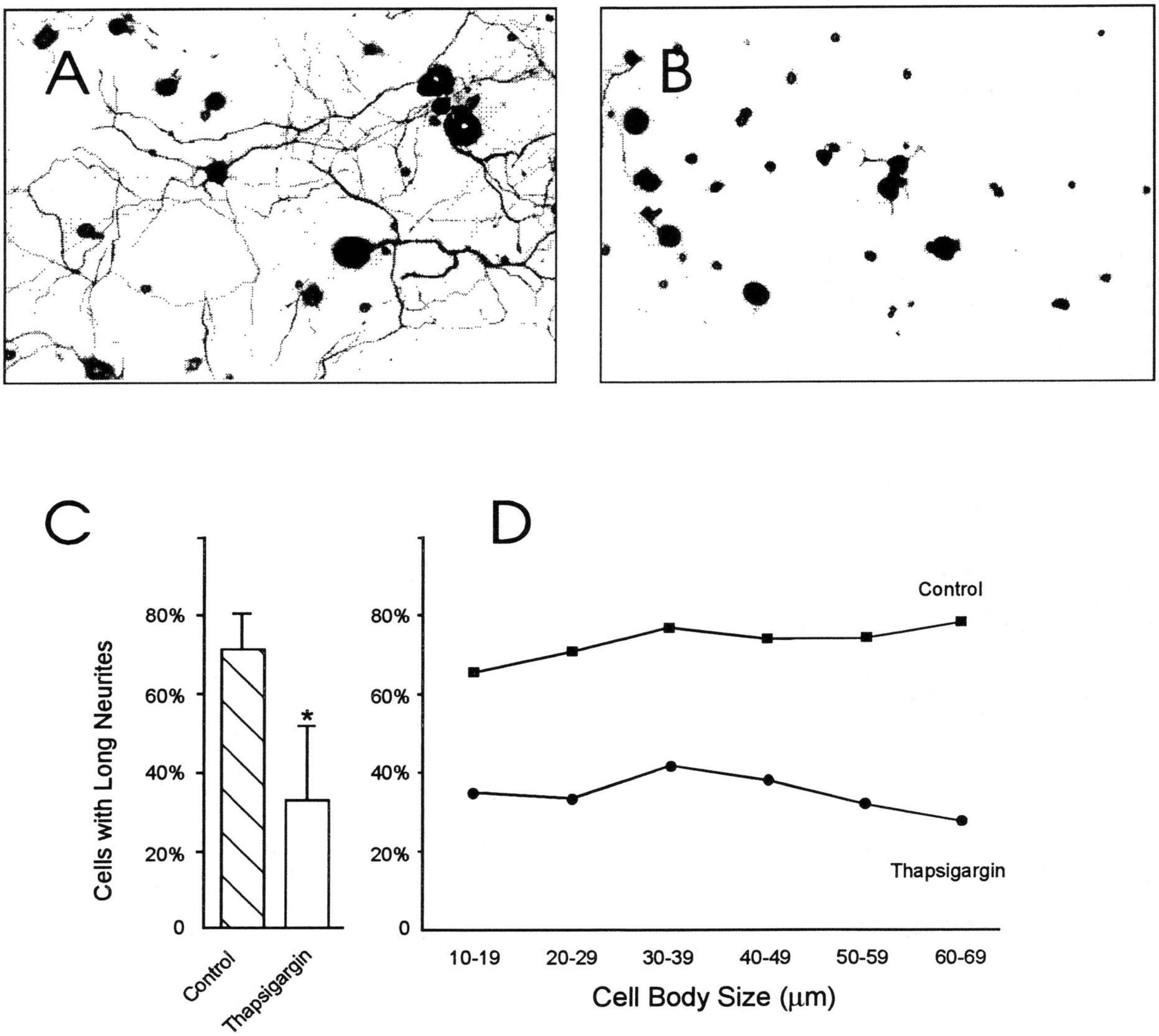

Fig. 7. Neuritic outgrowth of adult DRG neurons in culture is reduced by exposure to thapsagargin. Neurofilament stained neurons maintained in culture for 3 days are shown after treatment with vehicle alone (A) or thapsigargin (B) for 20 min 3 h after plating. The number of neurons with long neurites was considerably reduced ($P < 0.05$) in the thapsigargin treated group (C). Reduced neurite outgrowth following exposure to thapsigargin occurred for all cell sizes (D). (Modified from Kocsis et al., 1994.)

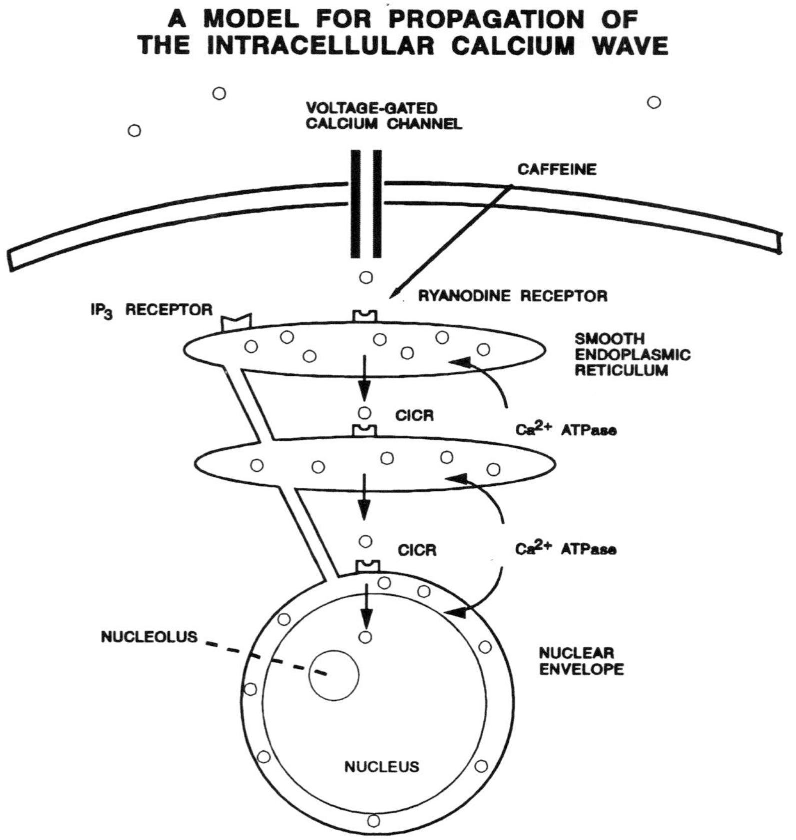

Fig. 8. A mechanism by which CICR could elicit a wave of Ca^{2+} which propagates from the cell membrane to the nucleus. Depolarization leads to a relatively small amount of Ca^{2+} influx due to activation of voltage-gated Ca^{2+} channels. The local increase in $[Ca^{2+}]$ near the cell membrane would then lead to release of Ca^{2+} from intracellular stores by activation of ryanodine receptors in the ER membrane. This process of Ca^{2+} release and activation of additional Ca^{2+} mobilization from intracellular stores would create a centripetal wave of Ca^{2+} travelling toward the nucleus.

whether Ca^{2+} levels are actually higher in the nucleus than in the cytoplasm. It has been suggested that an elevated nuclear Ca^{2+} gradient may be produced by pumping or other active processes (Pryzwara et al., 1991; Himpens et al., 1992; Segal and Manor, 1992), or by selective Ca^{2+} release in the nucleus (Hernandez-Cruz et al., 1990, 1991). The large nuclear Ca^{2+} signals suggests that the nuclear envelope imposes a barrier to the diffusion of Ca^{2+} ions. However, it has been argued that nuclear pores provide no barrier to ions (Newport and Forbes, 1987; Agutter, 1991), and a recent study has been interpreted as providing no evidence for selective permeability of ions across the nuclear envelope (Al Mohanna et al., 1994). These apparently disparate observations could be reconciled if the permeability of the nuclear pore channel varied with different physiological or developmental conditions of the neuron. For example, nuclear pore permeability to Ca^{2+} might be reduced at early times in culture. It would be interesting if nuclear pore permeability were reduced during intense transport of RNA and proteins, as might be expected during development or regeneration.

The presence of large depolarization-induced

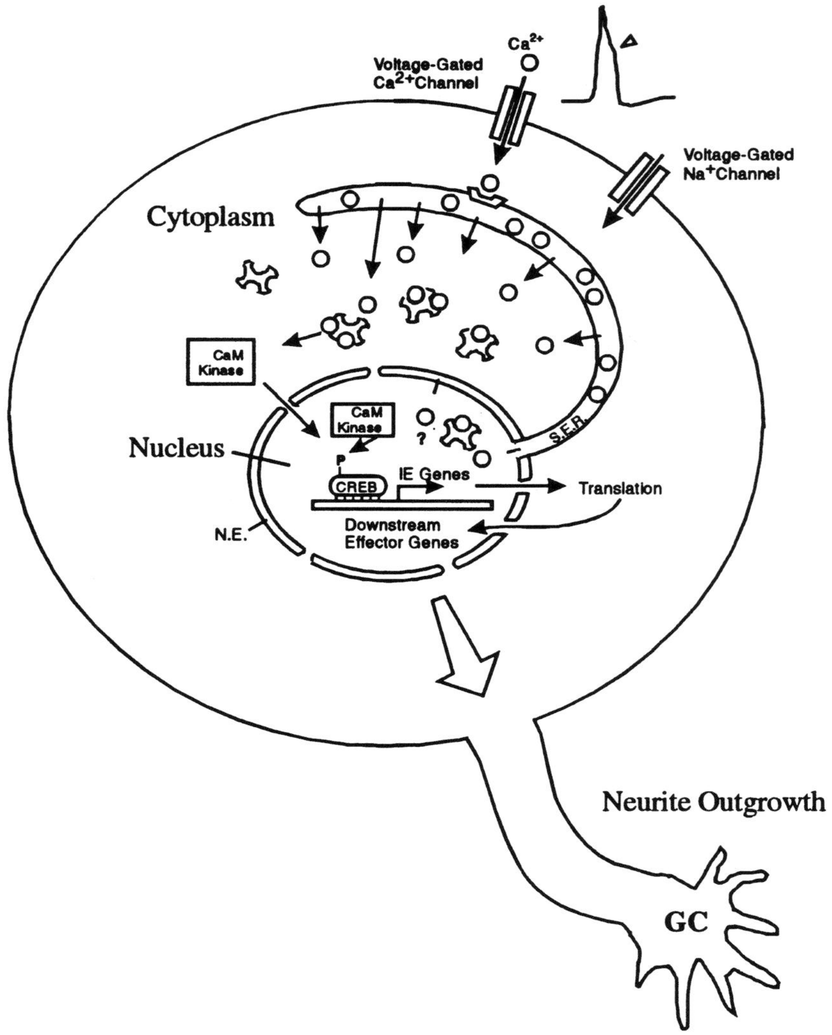

Fig. 9. A model illustrating possible pathways for gene induction secondary to neuronal depolarization. Depolarization leads to activation of voltage-gated Ca^{2+} channels which permit Ca^{2+} entry into the neuron. Intracellular Ca^{2+} concentrations are amplified via CICR from the endoplasmic reticulum and possibly the nuclear envelope. CaM kinase may be activated by Ca^{2+}/calmodulin complexes and phosphorylate transcription factors such as the calcium response element binding protein (CREB). Phosphorylation of CREB, or a comparable element, may facilitate transcription for immediate early (IE) genes whose products could activate downstream effector genes responsible for neurite outgrowth and regeneration. (Modified from Kocsis et al., 1993b.)

Ca^{2+} transients in the nucleus is correlated with the maturational state of embryonic *Xenopus* neurons in culture (Holliday et al., 1991); this is also the case in regenerating adult rat DRG neurons (Birch et al., 1992). In both of these systems, confocal microscopy with Ca^{2+} sensitive dyes demonstrated that the nuclear Ca^{2+} response was reduced following neurite extension. Such observations have led to the hypothesis that increases in nuclear Ca^{2+} levels may be involved in gene expression associated with cell differentiation or activation of regenerative processes. The mechanisms underlying the reduction in nuclear Ca^{2+} signalling at later times in culture, after the period of neuritogenesis, are not known but may involve developmental changes in Ca^{2+} conductances or in intracellular Ca^{2+} buffering, sequestration, or pumping (Holliday et al., 1991; Birch et al., 1992). It might be expected that Ca^{2+} mobilization capacity would be greatest just prior to cell differentiation if activity-dependent Ca^{2+} changes are important in gene activation. Determining the mechanisms which control the capacity of the cells to mobilize Ca^{2+} during development and following injury will therefore be important.

Figure 9 shows one hypothetical pathway for gene modulation secondary to electrical activity in neurons. In this model, depolarization triggers the activation of voltage dependent Ca^{2+} channels, which allow Ca^{2+} to enter the neuron. The initial Ca^{2+} influx is then amplified via CICR release from intracellular stores (e.g., ER and the nuclear envelope). We propose that increases in Ca^{2+}, particularly in the nucleus, in turn influence gene expression. In other cell types, Ca^{2+} entry secondary to membrane depolarization has been shown to induce *c-fos* transcription via phosphorylation of the calcium regulatory binding protein, CREB (Sheng et al., 1990). It has also been proposed that the formation of Ca^{2+}/calmodulin complexes activates Ca^{2+}/calmodulin dependent kinases (CaM kinases) which enter the nucleus and phosphorylate CREB, leading to induction of immediate early genes such as *c-fos* (Sheng et al., 1990). CREB phosphorylation can also occur via cAMP dependent kinases or CaM kinases, which can also be activated by depolarization and activation of voltage-gated Ca^{2+} channels (Sheng et al., 1990; Dash et al., 1991). CaM kinase II and CREB immunostaining are present in the nucleus of adult DRG neurons at early times in culture (Herdegen et al., 1993; Kocsis et al., 1994). Phosphorylation of CREB is known to enhance the transcription of immediate early genes (Sheng et al., 1991), and after immediate early gene transcription their protein products may enter the nucleus and activate downstream effector genes important for cell differentiation. CICR amplification of depolarization-induced Ca^{2+} entry may be important for directing gene expression in neurons in response to increased action potential activity occurring after injury or during the course of normal development.

Changes in Ca^{2+} sequestration, buffering and pumping may account for attenuation of the depolarization-induced nuclear Ca^{2+} responses during maturation and neurite extension. If the Ca^{2+} transients of regenerating DRG neurons prove to be necessary, as we have proposed, for the activation of enzymes associated with gene expression, then the processes which control Ca^{2+} availability in the nucleus may be important in neuronal repair and axonal regeneration. Moreover, the hyperexcitability and increased action potential activity associated with nerve injury-triggered nuclear Ca^{2+} transients might provide a stimulus for promoting gene expression appropriate for nerve repair or regeneration (Birch et al., 1992). According to this idea, reduction in the depolarization-induced nuclear and cytoplasmic Ca^{2+} signals in mature neurons would be important in limiting neurite outgrowth and controlling further cell differentiation. Action potential activity in normal mature sensory neurons would then serve the physiological role of transducing information about the external environment rather than the regulatory role of modulating mechanisms related to gene expression. Our data suggest that CICR may play an important role in triggering this new gene expression.

Acknowledgements

This work was supported in part by the NIH (NS10174) and the Medical Research Service of the Department of Veterans Affairs.

References

Agutter, P.S. (1991) *Between Nucleus and Cytoplasm*, Chapman and Hall, London, 148 pp.

Allbritton, N.L., Meyer, T. and Stryer, L. (1992) Range of messenger action of calcium ion and inositol 1,4,5-trisphosphate. *Science*, 258: 1812–1815.

Augustine, G.J., Charlton, M.P. and Smith, S.J. (1987) Calcium action in synaptic transmitter release. *Annu. Rev. Neurosci.*, 10: 633–693.

Berridge, M.J. (1989) Inositol trisphosphates and cell signalling. *Nature (Lond.)*, 361: 315–325.

Birch, B.D., Eng, D.L. and Kocsis, J.D. (1992) Intranuclear Ca^{2+} transients during neurite regeneration of an adult mammalian neuron. *Proc. Natl. Acad. Sci. USA*, 89: 7978–7982.

Dash, P.K., Karl, K.A., Colicos, M.A., Prywes, R. and Kandel, E.R. (1991) cAMP response element-binding protein is activated by Ca^{2+}/calmodulin- as well as cAMP-dependent protein kinase. *Proc. Natl. Acad. Sci. USA*, 88: 5061–5065.

Endo, M. (1975) Mechanism of action of caffeine on the sarcoplasmic reticulum of skeletal muscle. *Proc. Japan Acad.*, 51: 479–484.

Ferris, C.D. and Snyder, S.H. (1992) Inositol phosphate receptors and calcium disposition in the brain. *J. Neurosci.*, 12: 1567–1574.

Greenberg, M.E., Ziff, E.B. and Greene, L.A. (1986) Stimulation of neuronal acetylcholine receptors induces rapid gene transcription. *Science*, 234: 80–83.

Herdegen, T., Bravo, R., Waxman, S.G. and Kocsis, J.D. (1993) Jun, Fos, KROX and CREB protein expression is different in adult dorsal root ganglion neurons studied in vivo and in vitro. *Soc. Neurosci. Abstr.*, 19: 1729.

Hernandez-Cruz, A., Sala, F. and Adams, P.R. (1990) Subcellular calcium transients visualized by confocal microscopy in a voltage-clamped vertebrate neuron. *Science*, 247: 858–862.

Hernandez-Cruz, A., Sala, F. and Connor, J.A. (1991) Stimulus-induced nuclear Ca^{2+} signals in fura-2-loaded amphibian neurons. *Ann. N.Y. Acad. Sci.*, 635: 416–420.

Himpens, B., De Smedt, H., Droogmans, G. and Casteels, R. (1992) Differences in regulation between nuclear and cytoplasmic Ca^{2+} in cultured smooth muscle cells. *Am. J. Physiol.*, 263: 95–105.

Holliday, J. and Spitzer, N.C. (1990) Spontaneous calcium influx and its roles in differentiation of spinal neurons in culture. *Dev. Biol.*, 141: 13–23.

Holliday, J., Adams, R.J., Sejnowski, T.J. and Spitzer, N.C. (1991) Calcium-induced release of calcium regulates differentiation of cultured spinal neurons. *Neuron*, 7: 787–796.

Kao, J.P.Y., Harootunian, A.T. and Tsien, R.Y. (1989) Photochemically generated cytosolic calcium pulses and their detection by fluo-3. *J. Biol. Chem.*, 264: 8179–8184.

Kater, S.B. and Mills, L.R. (1991) Regulation of growth cone behavior by calcium. *J. Neurosci.*, 11: 891-899.

Katz, B. and Miledi, R. (1967) A study of synaptic transmission in the absence of nerve impulses. *J. Physiol. (Lond.)*, 192: 407–436.

Kennedy, M.B. (1989) Regulation of neuronal function by calcium. *Trends Neurosci.*, 12: 417- 420.

Kocsis, J.D., Rand, M.N., Chen, B., Waxman, S.G. and Pourcho, R. (1993a) Kainate elicits elevated nuclear calcium signals in retinal neurons via calcium-induced calcium release. *Brain Res.*, 616: 273–292.

Kocsis, J.D., Rand, M.N. and Eng, D.L. (1993b) Intracellular calcium mobilization in adult rat dorsal root ganglion neurons: cytoplasmic and nuclear signals. In: A. Scriabine, R. Janis and D.J. Triggle (Eds.), *Calcium Antagonists in the CNS: Drugs in Review 1993*, Neva Press, Branford, CT, pp. 457–470.

Kocsis, J.D., Rand, M.N., Lankford, K. and Waxman, S.G. (1994) Intracellular calcium mobilization and neurite outgrowth in mammalian neurons. *J. Neurobiol.*, in press.

Lankford, K.L., Rand, M.N., Waxman, S.G. and Kocsis, J.D. (1993) Blocking Ca^{2+} mobilization with thapsigargin reduces neurite initiation in cultured adult rat DRG cells. *Soc. Neurosci. Abstr.*, 19: 876.

Llinas, R., Steinberg, I.Z. and Walton, K. (1981) Relationship between presynaptic calcium current and postsynaptic potential in squid giant synapse. *Biophys. J.*, 33: 323–351.

McPherson, P.S., Kim, Y.-K., Valdivia, H., Knudson, C.M., Takekura, H., Franzini-Armstrong, C., Coronado, R. and Campbell, K.P. (1991) The brain ryanodine receptor: a caffeine-sensitive calcium release channel. *Neuron*, 7: 17–25.

Milbrandt, J. (1987) A nerve growth factor-induced gene encodes a possible transcriptional regulatory factor. *Science*, 238: 797–799.

Minta, A., Kao, J.P.Y. and Tsien, R.Y. (1989) Fluorescent indicators for cytosolic calcium based on rhodamine and fluorescein chromophores. *J. Biol. Chem.*, 264: 8171–8178.

Morgan, J.I. and Curran, T. (1991) Stimulus-transcription coupling in the nervous system: involvement of the inducible proto-oncogenes fos and jun. *Annu. Rev. Neurosci.*, 14: 421–451.

Newport, J.W. and Forbes, D.J. (1987) The nucleus: structure, function and dynamics. *Annu. Rev. Biochem.*, 56: 535–563.

Pessah, I.N., Stambuk, R.A. and Casida, J.E. (1987) Ca^{2+}-activated ryanodine binding: mechanisms of sensitivity and intensity modulation by Mg^{2+}, caffeine, and adenine nucleotides. *Molec. Pharmacol.*, 31: 232–238.

Przywara, D.A., Bhave, S.V., Bhave, A., Wakade, T.D. and Wakade, A.R. (1991) Stimulated rise in neuronal calcium is faster and greater in the nucleus than in the cytosol. *FASEB J.*, 5: 217–222.

Rand, M.N., Waxman, S.G. and Kocsis, J.D. (1993) Intracellular calcium waves induced in adult mammalian neurons by caffeine. Soc. *Neurosci. Abstr.*, 19: 1178.

Rasmussen, H. (1990) The complexities of intracellular Ca^{2+} signalling. *Biol. Chem.*, 371: 191- 206.

Segal, M. and Manor, D. (1992) Confocal microscopic imaging of $[Ca^{2+}]_i$ in cultured rat hippocampal neurons following exposure to *N*-methyl-D-aspartate. *J. Physiol. (Lond.)*, 448: 655–676.

Sheng, M., McFadden, G. and Greenberg, M.E. (1990) Membrane depolarization and calcium induce *c-fos* transcription via phosphorylation of transcription factor CREB. *Neuron*, 4: 571–582.

Sheng, M., Thompson, M.A. and Greenberg, M.E. (1991) CREB: a Ca^{2+}-regulated transcription factor phosphorylated by calmodulin-dependent kinases. *Science*, 252: 1427–1430.

Thayer, S.A. and Miller, R.J. (1990) Regulation of the intracellular free calcium concentration in single rat dorsal root ganglion neurones in vitro. *J. Physiol. (Lond.)*, 425: 85–115.

Utzschneider, D.A., Rand, M.N., Waxman, S.G. and Kocsis, J.D. (1994) Nuclear and cytoplasmic Ca^{2+} signals in developing rat dorsal root ganglion neurons studied in excised tissue. *Brain Res.*, 635: 231–237.

F.J. Seil (Ed.)
Progress in Brain Research, Vol 103

CHAPTER 15

Expression of c-Jun and JunD transcription factors represent specific changes in neuronal gene expression following axotomy

Thomas Herdegen and Manfred Zimmermann

II Institute of Physiology, University of Heidelberg, Im Neuenheimer Feld 326, 69120 Heidelberg, Germany

Introduction

It has been well established since Cajal's pioneer work that nerve transection induces lasting morphological, biochemical and physiological reactions in the cell body of axotomized neurons. The early findings included the observation of chromatolysis, and the involvement of the nucleus in the pathophysiological process following axonal transection, but the mechanisms behind these phenomena remained unexplained. The cellular response to axotomy ranges from successful reinnervation of the target organ to death of the axotomized neuron. Apart from the extraneuronal environment and age, intrinsic properties of the damaged neurons contribute to the postaxotomy neuronal reaction. Here, we will assess these intrinsic properties at the level of gene control.

Recently, the discovery of inducible genes encoding for transcription factor proteins provided new tools to assess nuclear processes underlying the reactive alterations in gene expression. At present, about 20 of these genes are known which can be rapidly induced in neurons and glial cells of the adult mammalian nervous system in vivo (Hunt et al., 1987; Morgan et al., 1987; Sagar et al., 1988; Wisden et al., 1990; Herdegen et al., 1991a, 1993d). These inducible genes belong to a major group generally designated as immediate early genes (IEGs) (reviewed by Bravo, 1990; Angel and Karin, 1991; Sheng and Greenberg, 1990; Herschman, 1991; Morgan and Curran, 1991). Noxious stimuli and nerve lesions are particularly powerful in activating IEGs. Therefore, the question naturally arises as to whether IEG activation might be a clue to the understanding of the long-lasting changes in the nervous system that are seen in these conditions.

In this article we review the general functions of IEGs in the nervous system and in particular examine their potential roles in adaptive gene expression following neuronal trauma.

Functions of immediate early genes encoding for transcription factor proteins

IEGs become rapidly activated when a eukaryotic cell is exposed to a stimulus such as serum, growth hormones or ion channel activators (Krujier et al., 1984; Lau and Nathans, 1985; Bravo et al., 1987; Almendral et al., 1988; Bartel et al., 1989). IEGs are involved in the regulation of normal growth, mitosis and differentiation of cells and encode for secretory proteins, enzymes, membrane-bound receptors and for transcription factors (reviewed by Bravo, 1990; Sheng and Greenberg, 1990; Angel and Karin, 1991; Herschman, 1991). In this chapter we focus on the inducible transcription factor proteins of the *jun*, *fos* and *krox* families. Jun (c-Jun, JunB, JunD), Fos (c-Fos, FosB) and Krox (Krox-20, also called Egr-2; Krox-24, also called NGFI-A, Egr-1, Zif/268, Tis 8) proteins bind to specific regulatory nucleotide sequences in the promotor and enhancer sites of genes. By binding to the DNA elements and by interaction with the nuclear enzyme complex, mRNA polymerase II, these proteins *trans*-activate the transcription of their target genes, and can also *cis*-activate their own promotors. The special feature of IEG encoded transcription factors is their induction by external stimuli. In contrast, the constitutively expressed transcription factors such as CREB (calcium/cAMP response element binding protein) and SRF (serum response factor) are mainly activated by transient posttranslational modifications such as phosphorylation (Montminy and Bilezikjian, 1987; Gonzalez et al., 1989; Treisman, 1990; Ginty et al., 1993).

In vitro studies on the activation of *c-fos* in nonneuronal and neuronal cells by external stimuli have provided a basic understanding of the induction of IEGs (Krujier et al., 1984; Bravo et al., 1987; Bartel et al., 1989). For example, the cellular surface receptor for a growth hormone activates second messengers such as Ca^{2+} or cAMP, which in turn induce phosphorylation of the constitutively expressed transcription factor, CREB. The CREB protein binds to the CRE (calcium/cAMP response element) in the promotor sites of IEGs such as *c-jun*, *junB*, *c-fos* and *krox-24*. Phosphorylation of the *trans*-activation domain of CREB results in the activation of mRNA polymerase II, with subsequent initiation of IEG transcription (Gonzalez et al., 1989; Sheng et al., 1990; Bading et al., 1993; Ginty et al., 1993).

The transcription promoting capability of Fos proteins becomes significant only after association with other nuclear proteins such as c-Jun or its related proteins, JunB and JunD (Halazonetis et al., 1988; Nakabeppu et al., 1988; Rauscher et al., 1988; Ryseck and Bravo, 1991). The Fos and Jun proteins can form a heterodimer by binding to each other at a series of leucine sites named the 'leucine zipper' (Gentz et al., 1988; Halazonetis et al., 1988; Landschulz et al., 1988). The Fos:Jun dimers, called AP-1 (activator protein-1) complex, bind to their response elements, the AP-1 binding site (Rauscher et al., 1988). Because many genes contain AP-1 sites, Fos and Jun proteins form a superordinate 'master switch' that controls gene transcription subsequent to transmembranous surface stimulation of the cell.

Variable composition of Jun- and Fos-containing complexes differ in their transcriptional properties

Jun and Fos proteins differ in their binding affinities to the regulatory DNA consensus sequences and in their activation potential (Nakabeppu et al., 1988; Ryseck and Bravo, 1991). Moreover, at least some of the transcription factor proteins can act as suppressors of gene expression, as has been reported for JunB and FosB (Chiu et al., 1989; Schütte et al., 1989b; Lazo et al., 1991; Nakabeppu and Nathans, 1991; Deng and Karin, 1993). Thus, the late and persistent appearance of FosB following transsynaptic pathophysiological stimuli (Herdegen et al., 1991a,d, 1993e, 1994b; Gass et al., 1992a,b) might suppress the transcriptional operations that have been initiated by the c-Fos protein. JunB counteracts the transcriptional potency of c-Jun, and the absence of JunB in axotomized neurons could contribute to a particular transcriptional potency of c-Jun. Finally, different secondary messenger pathways interact on IEG proteins and modulate their transcriptional activities, e.g., selective phosphorylation can increase or decrease the transcriptional activity of c-Jun protein (Pulverer et al., 1991).

Target genes of IEG encoded transcription factors

The research into the possible target genes of IEGs in the nervous system is still at an early stage. Thus, it is well established that AP-1 proteins are involved in the gene expression of the nerve growth factor (NGF) following neuronal lesions (Hengerer et al., 1990), in the expression of proenkephalin and prodynorphin following noxious stimulation (Draisci and Iadarola, 1989;

Sonnenberg et al., 1989; Noguchi et al., 1990; Naranjo et al., 1991b) and in the expression of tyrosine hydroxylase (Gisang-Ginsberg et al., 1989). Following axotomy, a close temporo-spatial covariation of c-Jun with galanin, calcitonin gene related peptide (CGRP), nitric oxide synthase and tyrosine hydroxylase was recently observed and is described in detail below.

Immediate early genes in the nervous system: expression following transsynaptic neuronal stimulation

IEGs were associated with developmental growth and differentiation of the nervous system (Ingraham et al., 1989; Wilkinson et al., 1989; Gubits et al., 1993; reviewed by He and Rosenfeld, 1991; Rose, 1991), and IEG encoded proteins such as c-Jun, JunD, Krox-20 and Krox-24 are present in the adult nervous system in the absence of any intentional stimuli (Mack et al., 1990; Herdegen et al., 1991c, 1993d,e; Gass et al., 1992a, 1993a). These IEG encoded transcription factors can be rapidly activated by a variety of neuronal stimuli under physiological and pathological conditions. The processes of IEG expression with subsequent transcription of target genes following extraneuronal stimuli are now subsumed under the concept of 'stimulation-transcription coupling' (Morgan and Curran, 1991).

The members of the *jun*, *fos* and *krox* gene families show extensive homologies, but in vivo their functions and individual behaviors show distinct differences. Each of these IEGs are expressed on different chromosomes (reviewed by Bravo, 1990), which explains the individual pattern of expression underlying the finely tuned formation of transcription complexes.

Dramatic upregulation of IEGs and appearance of their protein products is the first response at the gene level in spinal and supraspinal neurons following various stimuli, including noxious afferent stimulation, changes in blood pressure, epileptic seizures, ischemia, cortical spreading depression and long-term potentiation (Morgan et al., 1987; Sagar et al., 1988; Cole et al., 1989; Dragunow et al., 1989; Sonnenberg et al., 1989; Wisden et al., 1990; Herdegen et al., 1991a, 1993e, 1994b; Naranjo et al., 1991a; Sharp et al., 1991; Gass et al., 1992a,b, 1993a,b; Lanteri-Minet et al., 1993; Tölle et al., 1994). In spite of the difference of the applied stimuli, the temporo-spatial expression patterns of each IEG protein show an individual behavior that determines the formation of transcriptional complexes and thus the expression of effector genes. Within 2 h following the onset of stimulation, c-Fos, c-Jun, JunB and Krox-24 proteins reach their maximal expression, whereas JunD and FosB are on their maximal levels after 5 h. The persistence of the proteins depends on the intensity and duration of the stimulus. In the spinal cord, for example, a few minutes of electrical sciatic nerve stimulation at C fiber strength induces a rather transient expression between 8 h (c-Fos, JunB, c-Jun, Krox-24) and 24 h (FosB, JunD) (Herdegen et al., 1991a), whereas an experimental monoarthritis with subsequent chronic inflammation of the ankle evokes a persistent expression for up to 2–15 weeks (predominantly c-Fos and JunD) (Lanteri-Minet et al., 1993). In the cortex and the hippocampus, IEG proteins are detectable up to 72 h following kainate-induced epileptic seizures, whereas they disappear between 8 h (c-Fos, c-Jun, JunB, Krox-24) and 24 h (JunD, FosB) following bicuculline-induced seizures (Gass et al., 1992a, 1993a).

IEGs are expressed in a distinct and dissociated topographical distribution. Following noxious peripheral input from the hindpaw, for example, all investigated IEG proteins are present in spinal neurons of the superficial dorsal horn that are presumably activated by monosynaptic input. In contrast, neurons of the deep dorsal horn that are predominantly activated by polysynaptic input are devoid of c-Jun, JunB and FosB, while c-Fos, JunD and Krox-24 are fairly prominent (Herdegen et al., 1991a,d, 1994b; Tölle et al., 1994). c-Jun and FosB, which have the highest DNA binding affinity and transcriptional activity in vitro (Ryseck and Bravo, 1991), are expressed in a fairly low number of neurons in vivo. Following various experimental protocols with transynaptic neuronal activation, the number of neurons immunoreactive for c-Fos and JunB exceeds that of c-Jun.

The most pronounced dissociation between IEGs is the induction of c-Fos and JunB without substantial upregulation of c-Jun by membrane depolarization following application of KCl in vitro and cortical spreading depression in vivo (Fig. 1) (Bartel et al., 1988; Herdegen et al., 1993e). Thus, transsynaptic neuronal stimulation evokes transcriptional operations dominated by the c-Fos protein.

The expression of IEGs is characteristic for those neuronal populations that alter their cellular program by specific variation of de novo protein synthesis. Provided that changes in protein synthesis are a major concomitant mechanism of plasticity, IEGs can be used to visualize those neurons reacting to exogenous and endogenous stimulation with functional plasticity depending on altered gene expression. During development, c-Jun expression is distinctly related to processes of learning and memory formation (reviewed by Rose, 1992). The observation may be clinically relevant that following noxious inflammatory processes, the expression of IEGs covaries with the animal behavioral signs of disease (Abbadie and Besson, 1993; Lanteri-Minet et al., 1993).

Neurons can change their ability to react by IEG expression to external stimuli depending on the pathophysiological situation. On one hand, repeated seizure activity loses its ability to reinduce c-Fos in the cortex (Winston et al., 1990); on the other hand, spinal neurons can express c-Fos

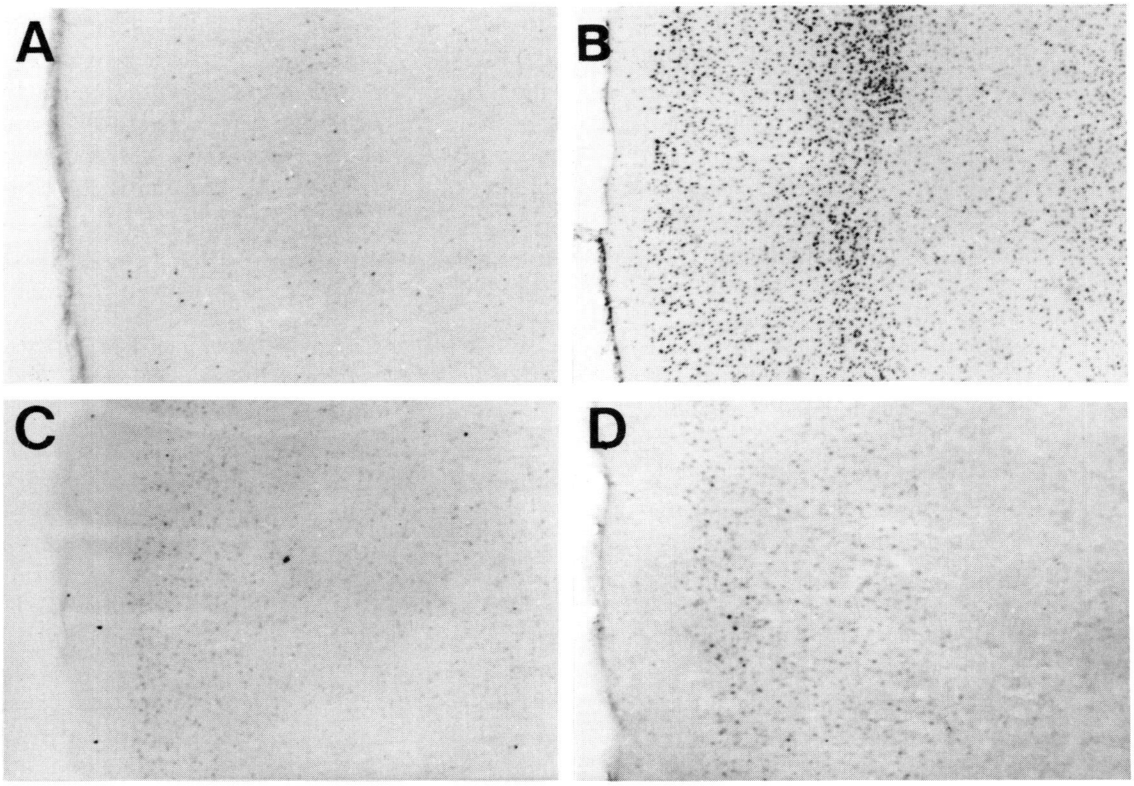

Fig. 1. c-Fos (A, B) and c-Jun (C, D) in the parietal cortex of untreated rats (A, C) and 2 h following KCl-induced cortical spreading depression (B,D). In contrast to c-Fos, c-Jun is only weakly induced over basal levels. (From Herdegen et al., 1993e.)

following non-noxious afferent stimulation when they have been conditioned by ongoing pathophysiological input due to nerve transection (Molander et al., 1992) and acute contralateral noxious stimulation (Leah et al., 1992). These examples demonstrate that the inducibility of IEG expression is not an invariable property of adult neurons but rather reflects the past and current pathophysiological 'experience'. Thus, we hypothesize that nerve cells can switch between plasticity and stability at the level of transcriptional control, depending on the context of events.

Induction of c-Jun and JunD and suppression of CREB after transection of peripheral and central axons

Transection of peripheral and central axons induces a selective expression of c-Jun and JunD, and, restricted to central intrinsic neurons, of Krox-24 in the axotomized neurons, whereas Fos proteins are not induced at all. Expression of these inducible transcription factors occurs coincident with the cell body response and is among the earliest responses at the level of gene expression. After successful regeneration of the axon, c-Jun returns to its basal level, whereas inhibition of target reinnervation provokes a long-lasting expression up to 15 months. Induction of c-Jun precedes the activation of several regeneration associated genes (RAGs) such as GAP-43, tubulins and cytoskeletal proteins (Mikucki and Oblinger, 1991; Tetzlaff et al., 1991). There is strong evidence that the presence of c-Jun reflects the endogenous regenerative potency or propensity of neurons, and that the suppression of c-Jun precedes neuronal cell death.

Transection of peripheral nerve fibers

Transection of nerve fibers evokes long-lasting alterations in the metabolism, morphology and gene expression of the injured parent cell body that start between a few hours and 24 h, depending on the distance from the lesion site. The information transfer that signals the injury and that drives the regenerative efforts occurs via axonal transport (reviewed by Lieberman, 1971; Grafstein, 1986; Stürmer et al., 1992). Thus, axotomy evokes a pathophysiological neuronal reaction that is much different from neuronal responses to transsynaptically conducted information transfer.

Transection of somatosensory spinal and cranial nerve fibers, as well as of sympathetic nerve fibers, induces c-Jun and JunD proteins in axotomized neurons such as primary afferent neurons, motoneurons and pre- and postganglionic sympathetic neurons, whereas JunB, c-Fos, FosB, Krox-20 and Krox-24 proteins are not expressed (Fig. 2) (Sagar et al., 1989; Herdegen et al., 1990, 1991b, 1992, 1993d; Jenkins and Hunt, 1991; Jones et al., 1991; Leah et al., 1991; Rutherford et al., 1992; Haas et al., 1993; Jenkins et al., 1993b; Koistinaho et al., 1993b; Gunkel et al., 1994). The issue of increased junB mRNA in axotomized neurons without increase in *JunB* protein is addressed below.

Following sciatic nerve cut, c-Jun immunoreactivity (IR) begins to increase over basal levels in both primary afferent neurons and motoneurons after 10 h and 15 h, respectively, and reaches its maximal expression (both number of labeled neurons and intensity of IR) between 48 h and 72 h. JunD shows the same distribution as c-Jun, with a delay in onset of a few hours. However, increase in JunD-IR over basal (constitutive) levels is less pronounced than that of c-Jun-IR. The persistence of both Jun proteins is related to the success of regeneration: after reestablishment of the neuron-target connection, Jun proteins return to basal levels between 30 and 50 days.

In contrast, elevated levels of c-Jun are visible in small diameter neurons of dorsal root ganglia (DRG) up to 15 months if successful regeneration is prevented by ligation of the proximal nerve stump; in large diameter DRG neurons, c-Jun returns to basal levels within 2 months (Leah et al., 1991; Herdegen et al., 1992a, 1993c; Jenkins et al., 1993b). The increased level of c-Jun protein is due to persistent transcription of the *c-jun* gene as demonstrated by in situ hybridization (Jenkins et al., 1991; Rutherford et al., 1992),

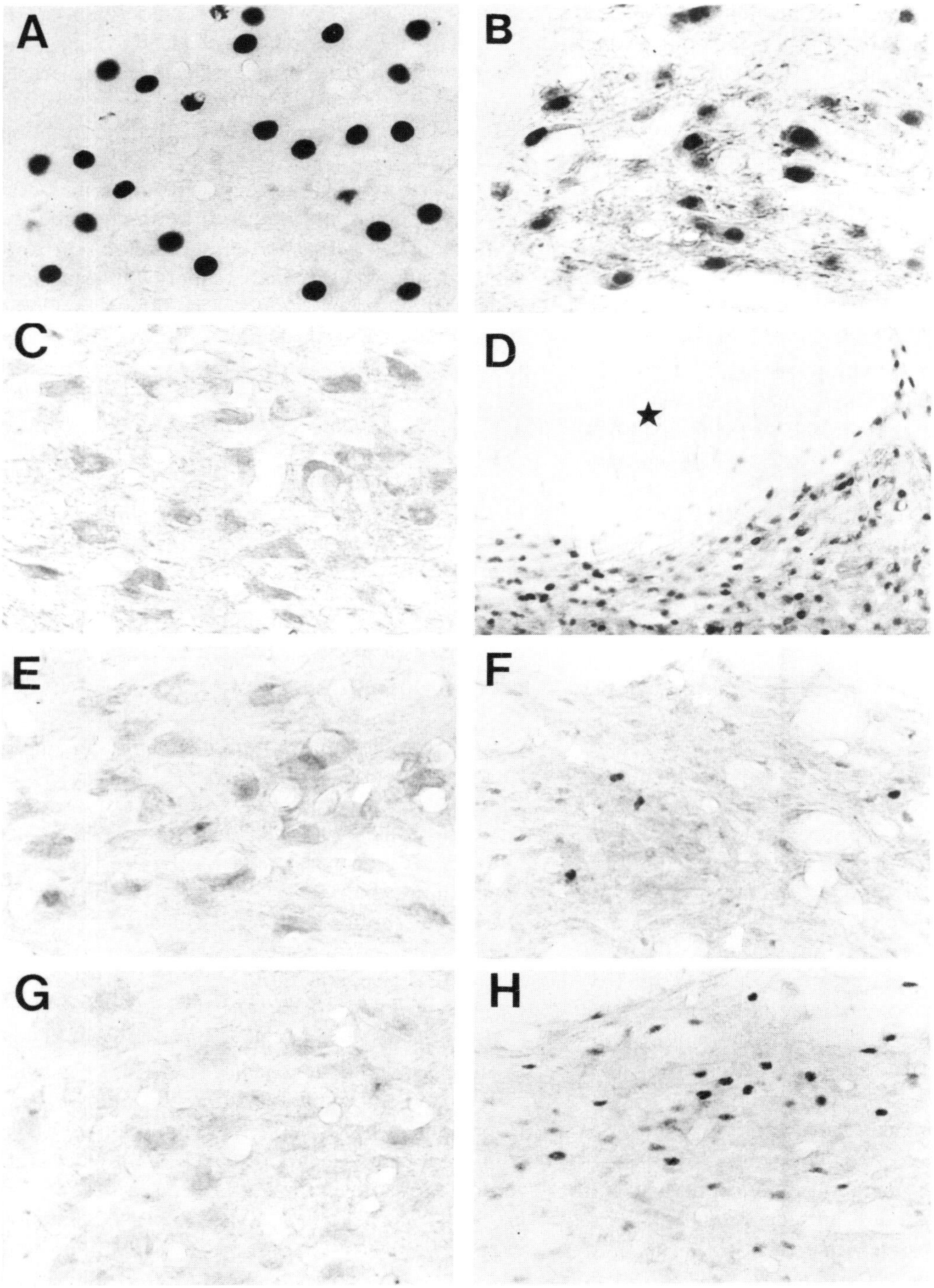

Fig. 2. c-Jun (A) and JunD (B) are rapidly induced in axotomized hypoglosal motoneurons 24 h following transection of hypoglossal nerve, whereas immunoreactivities of c-Fos (C), JunB (E) and Krox-24 (G) are not changed compared to the contralateral untreated side. Adjacent areas, however, show a distinct nuclear immunoreactivity (due to the experimental procedure) that proves the specific reaction of the applied antibodies: c-Fos in the inferior olivary complex (* marks the pyramidal tract) (D); JunB (F) and Krox-24 (H) in the superficial layers of the spinal trigeminal nucleus, interpolar part. (From Gunkel et al., 1994.)

Northern blotting (Jones et al., 1991; Haas et al., 1993; Koistinaho et al., 1993) and polymerase chain reaction (Herdegen et al., 1994a).

Tracing experiments using the retrograde tracers Fast Blue, HRG-coupled gold or FluoroGold have demonstrated that c-Jun is virtually expressed in axotomized neurons following transection of sciatic nerve (Fig. 3) (Leah et al., 1991), rubrospinal tract (Jenkins et al., 1993a), medial forebrain bundle (Brecht et al., 1994) and optic nerve (Hüll and Bähr, 1994; Robinson, 1994).

Transection of central nerve fibers

Following axotomy of mammalian intrinsic central neurons, the elongation of the proximal fiber sprout is impeded by the extracellular matrix, including the synthesis of inhibitory proteins and reactive gliosis (David and Aguayo, 1981; Schnell and Schwab, 1990; reviewed by Reier and Houle, 1988). Yet, local sprouting up to the glial scar and the elongation into grafts of peripheral nerves have demonstrated that the axotomized central nervous system (CNS) neurons have the endogenous potential to regenerate or at least to elongate their axons (David and Aguayo, 1981; Schnell and Schwab, 1990; Houle, 1992a,b). Furthermore, it has been suggested that the ability to regenerate is different depending on the type of neurons and area in the CNS (Björklund et al., 1973; Benfey et al., 1985; Fawcett, 1992). Axotomy of central intrinsic neurons in the adult rat evokes the expression of c-Jun and JunD, and, to

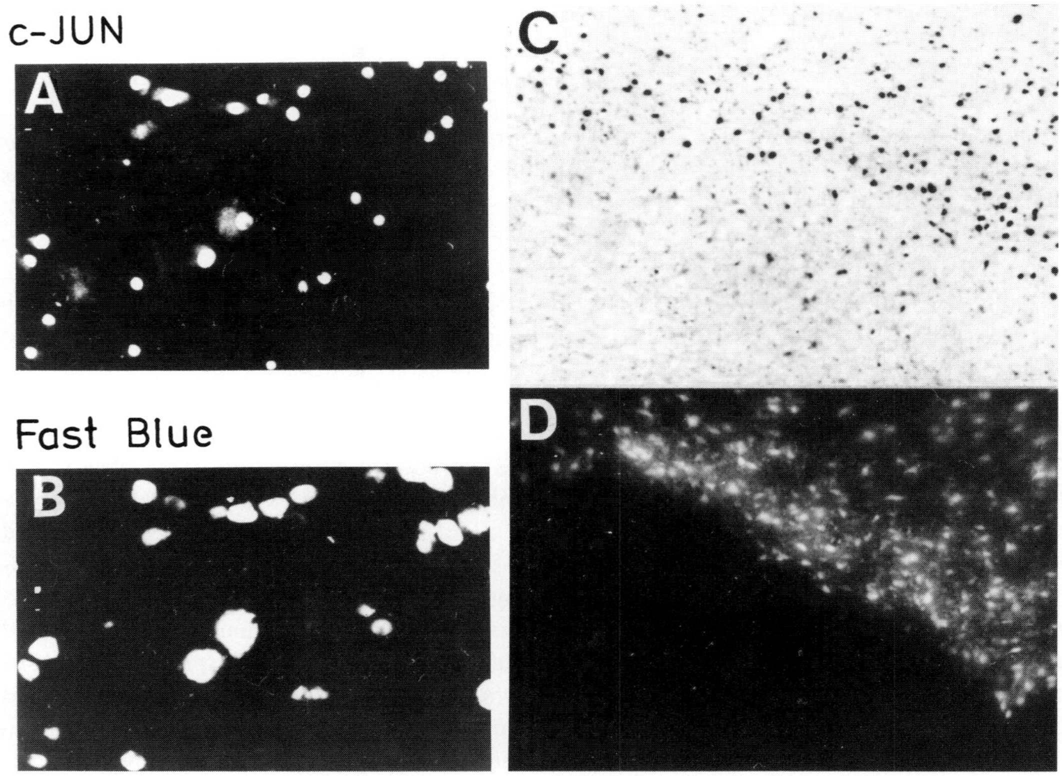

Fig. 3. c-Jun (A, C) is expressed in axotomized neurons of the lumbar dorsal root ganglia (A) and the substantia nigra compacta (C) 3 days following transection of the sciatic nerve (A) and the medial forebrain bundle (C). Axotomized neurons were visualized by application of the retrograde marker, Fast Blue, into the nerve stump of sciatic nerve (B) and into the medial forebrain bundle (D). Neurons that expressed c-Jun were also labeled by Fast Blue. (From Leah et al., 1991.)

a lesser extent, that of Krox-24. We have shown that the time courses of Jun and Krox-24 expression show clear differences between the axotomized neuronal populations and we hypothesize that the strength and persistence of IEG expression reflects the endogenous neuronal propensity for regeneration, irrespective of the inhibitory microenvironment.

In a comparative study we have investigated the expression of Jun, Fos, Krox and CREB in axotomized retinal ganglion cells (RGCs) following optic nerve crush in goldfish and optic nerve cut in rat (Herdegen et al., 1993a). In the goldfish, Jun-IR appeared in RGCs within 24 h postaxotomy and declined after 4 weeks, when the optic nerve fibers had successfully reinnervated the tectum (Stürmer et al., 1992). In the rat, c-Jun, JunD and, to a lesser extent, also Krox-24 were expressed within 24 h and reached maximal levels between 2 and 5 days, when the RGCs showed a transient sprouting. However, in contrast to goldfish, Jun and Krox expression declined between 5 and 8 days, and this decrease parallels the beginning of dramatic death of axotomized rat RGC neurons (Bähr et al., 1991; Villegas-Perez et al., 1993).

Peripheral nerve grafts implanted between the optic nerve stump and the tectum allows a successful axonal elongation of RGC neurons that reinnervate their target (David and Aguayo, 1981). Importantly, RGC neurons that grow into the graft continuously express the c-Jun protein over weeks during the regeneration process (Hüll and Bähr, 1994; Robinson, 1994).

c-Jun, JunD and Krox-24 were expressed in axotomized neurons following transection of the medial forebrain bundle (MFB) and the mammillo-thalamic tract (MT) in the rat, whereas c-Fos and JunB remained absent (Figs. 3C and 4) (Herdegen et al., 1993b; Leah et al., 1993). The onset of IEG expression was rather uniform between 24 and 36 h, but the time courses of expression were very different in the three neuronal populations: c-Jun, Jun D and Krox-24 declined after 10 days in substantia nigra pars compacta, after 30 days in the ventral tegmentum, and after 75 days in the parafascicular thalamic nucleus, whereas the proteins were detectable in many neurons of the mammillary nucleus even after 150 days, the end of the observation period. The majority of dopaminergic neurons of substantia nigra compacta die within a few weeks, and neuronal cell death starts in the second week postaxotomy when expression of c-Jun is also reduced. This early decrease of Jun expression in the dopaminergic neurons of substantia nigra and ventral tegmentum corroborates the finding of a restricted potency for axonal sprouting in vitro (Björklund et al., 1973).

Transection of fornix-fimbria induces a long-lasting expression of c-Jun and JunD in the axotomized medial septal nuclei (Dragunow, 1992; Brecht and Herdegen, unpublished observations).

Early and transient expression of IEGs following nerve transection can be related to transsynaptic impulse discharge

JunB, c-Fos, FosB and Krox-20 were not induced in axotomized intrinsic central neurons (Herdegen et al., 1993a,b; Leah et al., 1993; Weiser et al., 1993). However, following transection of the MFB, a transient expression of all Jun, Fos and Krox-24 proteins appeared within 2 h in the pars reticularis of substantia nigra close to the axotomized neurons of the pars compacta (Herdegen et al., 1993b; Weiser et al., 1993), most likely due to transsynaptic excitatory input evoked by the stereotaxic transection. This observation convincingly demonstrates that neurons of substantia nigra are capable of expressing JunB and c-Fos transcription factors after some stimuli, including transsynaptic excitation, but not after axotomy. In this context, it remains to be elucidated whether the early transient expression of c-Fos following transection of the rubrospinal tract is evoked by axotomy or by transmembranous stimulation (Jenkins et al., 1993a). Early and transient expression of IEG encoded proteins induced by spontaneous impulse discharge from damaged nerve fibers can also be observed in second-order

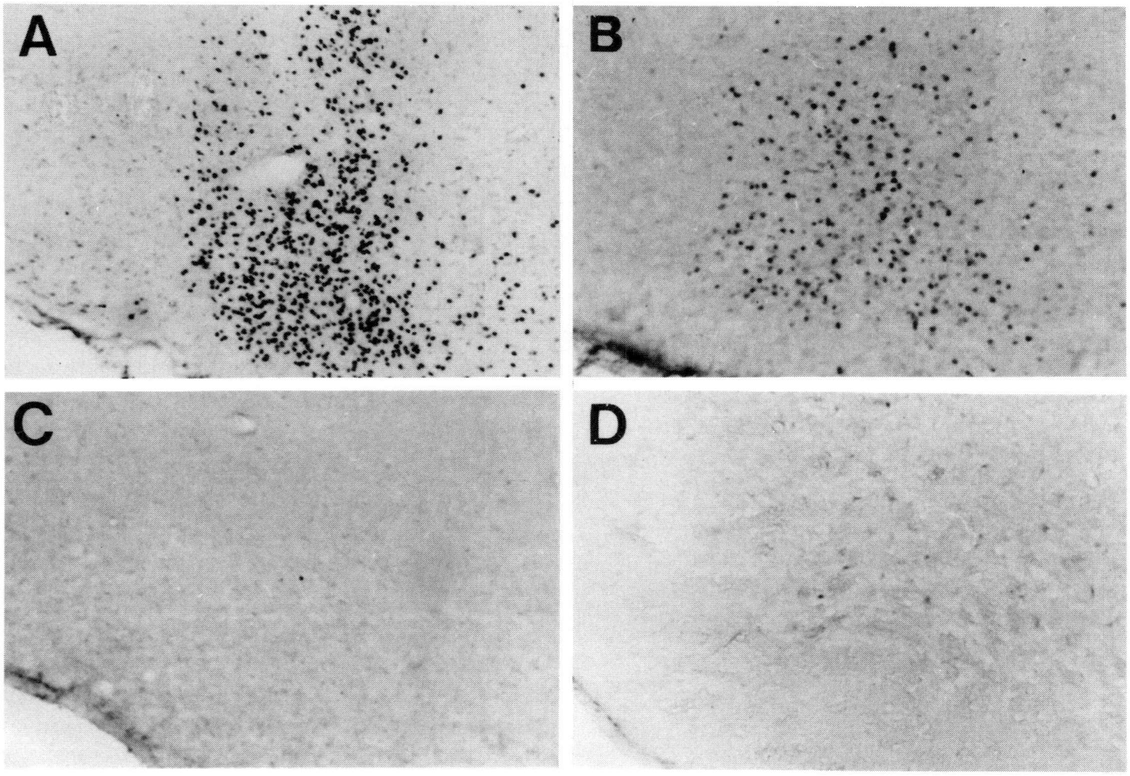

Fig. 4. c-Jun (A) and Krox-24 (B) expressed in axotomixed neurons of the mammillary body 5 days following transection of the mammillothalamic tract, whereas c-Fos (C) and JunB (D) remain absent. (From Herdegen et al., 1993b).

neurons following transection of sciatic nerve, trigeminal and vagal nerve fibers (Sharp et al., 1989; Herdegen et al., 1991b; Leah et al., 1991).

Increase in junB mRNA and absence of JunB protein after axotomy: block of translation?

Transection of the facial nerve results in a transient induction of *junB* mRNA in the axotomized facial motoneurons (Haas et al., 1993), whereas changes in nuclear JunB-IR could not be detected (Gunkel et al., 1994; Haas and Herdegen, unpublished observations). Nuclear JunB-IR was also absent in axotomized motoneurons following transection of vagal, hypoglossal and sciatic nerves, whereas JunB protein appeared in proximity to the axotomized neurons by transection-evoked transsynaptic input (Herdegen et al., 1991b, 1992). The absence of JunB protein following axotomy suggests a block of *junB* mRNA translation. This has important implications for the transcriptional activity of c-Jun, because JunB can counteract the transcriptional actions of c-Jun, including the positive autoregulatory effect of c-Jun on its own transcription (Chiu et al., 1989; Schütte et al., 1989b; Deng and Karin, 1993). Therefore, we consider that the absence of JunB is meaningful in the regeneration associated nuclear changes and contributes to the dominant role of c-Jun. The dissociation between c-Jun and JunB translation is presumably part of the specific intraneuronal signal pathways (Lord et al., 1990) activated by axotomy. Dissociation in the basal expression of *c-jun* and *junB* mRNAs was shown in the untreated adult rat brain (Schlingensiepen et al., 1994). Functional diversity of the Jun proteins was demonstrated in PC-12 cells and hippocampal neurons: inhibition of JunB expression reduced morphological differentiation whereas inhibition of c-Jun expression reduced proliferation and enhanced morphological differentiation (Schlingensiepen et al., 1993).

Our findings of the absence of JunB in axotomized neurons has been confirmed in axotomized rat RGCs (Robinson, 1994). A high basal expression of *junB* mRNA was reported in the nervous system of rats and mice (Hirai et al., 1989; Wisden et al., 1990; Mellström et al., 1991; Schlingensiepen et al., 1994) whereas JunB protein is almost absent (Gass et al., 1992a, 1993a; Herdegen et al., 1993c; Pertovaara et al., 1993). It remains to be elucidated whether this discrepancy is due to the antibody against JunB that was used (Kovary and Bravo, 1990) or due to inhibition of *junB* translation.

CREB is not phosphorylated at Ser^{133} and is suppressed in axotomized neurons

The transcription factor, CREB, holds a superior position in the transcription hierarchy because of its constitutive expression and its transcriptional control of both effector genes and inducible transcription factors (Montminy and Bilezikjian, 1987; Goodman et al., 1990). As noted earlier, CREB binds to the CRE sequences in the promotors of *c-jun*, *junB*, *c-fos* and *krox-24* genes. Activity of CREB is regulated on its posttranslational level by phosphorylation (Gonzalez et al., 1989; Dwarki et al., 1990; Sheng et al., 1991; Ginty et al., 1993; Peunova and Enikopolov, 1993), whereas even intense transsynaptic stimulation evokes, if at all, only a weak increase in CREB mRNA and protein levels (Guitart et al., 1992; Ginty et al., 1993; Herdegen et al., 1993e).

In view of the function of CREB as a transcriptional 'master switch', it is an important finding that axotomy evokes a suppression of CREB protein. Following sciatic, hypoglossal, facial and optic nerve section, CREB-IR decreased within 3 days in the axotomized neurons (Fig. 5A,B) and returned to its basal level after about 3–5 weeks (Herdegen et al., 1992, 1993a; Gunkel et al., 1994). This time course is approximately inverse to that of the c-Jun protein. In the axotomized RGCs of goldfish, the recoveries of elevated c-Jun and suppressed CREB between 30 and 50 days postaxotomy are associated in time with the reinnervation of the optic nerve into the tectum.

However, CREB continuously decreased and became absent in those neuronal populations that died following axotomy, such as RGCs and dopaminergic neurons of substantia nigra compacta of the rat (Herdegen et al., 1993a; Brecht et al., 1994). These observations suggest that the cascade of events induced by axotomy also includes constitutive transcription factors such as CREB. The fate of CREB might regulate the differential induction of c-Jun and, thus, contribute to the endogenous capability of neuronal survival and regeneration.

Phosphorylation of the amino acid serine at position 133 (Ser^{133}) activates the transcriptional function of CREB (Gonzalez et al., 1989; Ginty et al., 1993). Recent investigations have shown that CREB is not phosphorylated at Ser^{133} in axotomized neurons (Fig. 5C) (Herdegen et al., 1994c). The nonphosphorylated CREB can prevent the induction of c-Jun (Lamph et al., 1990) and, subsequently, the absence of CREB might relieve the permanent upregulation of c-Jun expression following axotomy. In contrast, transsynaptic stimulation rapidly activates CREB by phosphorylation at Ser^{133} followed by a strong and rapid induction of *c-fos*, whereas expression of *c-jun* was almost not affected (Ginty et al., 1993; Peunova and Enikopolov, 1993). These findings reveal that (1) transcriptional operations via activation of CREB are probably not part of the molecular genetic alterations induced by axotomy, and (2) phosphorylation of CREB might be a supercoordinate mechanism that determines the induction of major different genetic programs (Fig. 6).

The suppression of CREB itself might be harmful for cells. Functional inactivation of the

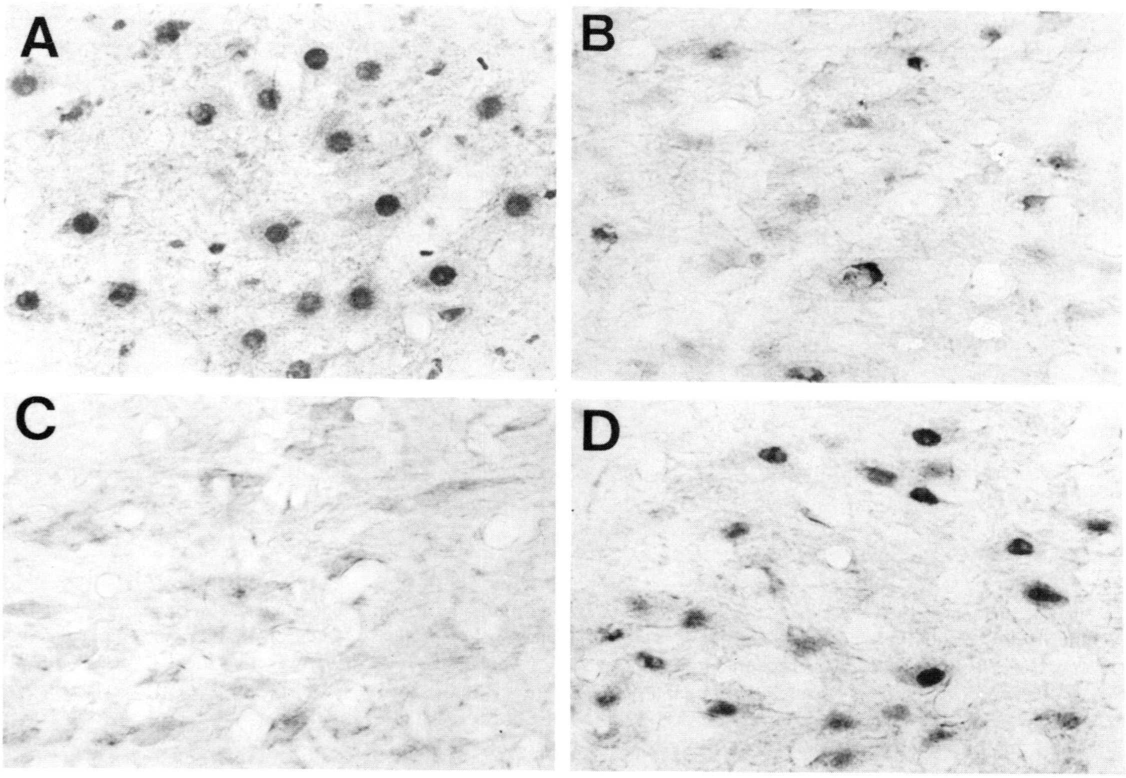

Fig. 5. Compared to the intact untreated side (A), CREB expression is suppressed after 4 days (B) in axotomized hypoglossal motoneurons. Between 15 and 24 h, CREB was not phosphorylated (C) as determined by reaction with specific antisera against the phosphorylated amino acid, serine, at position 133 of the CREB protein (Ginty et al., 1993; Hummler et al., 1994). In contrast to CREB, expression of CREM (D) increased after 48 h in the axotomized hypoglossal neurons.

CREB protein in mice by deletion of its phosphorylation site severely damages the affected neurons (Struthers et al., 1992). On the other hand, homozygous null mutants of CREB in transgenic mice do not produce obvious disturbances because the absence of CREB is compensated by an increase in the structurally and functionally related transcription factor, calcium response element modulator (CREM) protein (Foulkes et al., 1991; Hummler et al., 1994). At present we are investigating whether CREM is expressed in axotomized neurons following transection not only of peripheral but also of central nerve fibers (Fig. 5D).

Signal(s) mediating c-Jun expression following axotomy

It has yet to be clarified which signal(s) starts the cell body response provoked by axotomy and maintains the regenerative propensity of neurons. It is our prediction that the elucidation of those mechanisms mediating the selective induction of c-Jun without c-Fos are also responsible for the initiation and maintenance of the cell body response. Transcriptional operations and induction of c-Jun following axotomy can be initiated by positive signals such as the synthesis of lesion associated molecules from the denervated targets and/or electrical impulse discharge. On the other

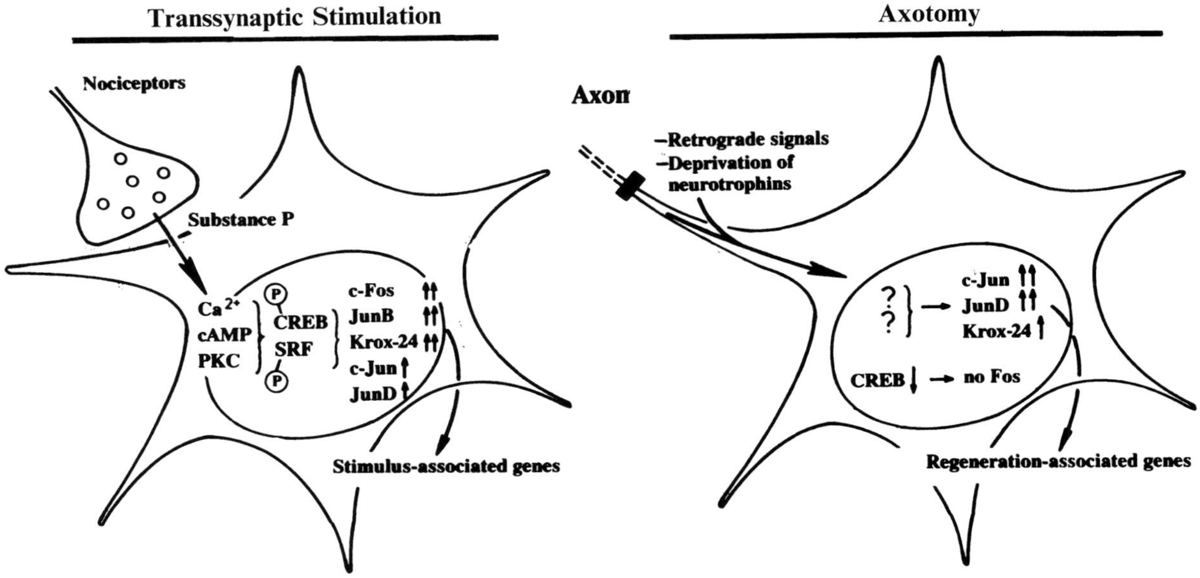

Fig. 6. Immediate early gene (IEG) encoded transcription factors are differentially regulated depending upon the applied stimulus. Left side: Transsynaptic stimulation , e.g., by activation of cutaneous nociceptors and release of neurotransmitters such as substance P, activates second messenger systems with subsequent phosphorylation of constitutive transcription factors such as CREB and SRF that, in turn, initiate the transcription of IEGs predominantly of c-Fos, JunB and Krox-24. Right side: Axotomy induces selective expression of c-Jun, JunD and, in intrinsic central neurons, Krox-24, probably mediated by deprivation of retrogradely transported substances such as neurotrophic factors. In contrast to transsynaptic stimulation, activation of CREB does not play a major role in IEG induction following axotomy.

hand, absence of information transfer (negative signals), e.g., by deprivation of retrogradely transported target derived proteins, could mediate the molecular genetic alterations during the cell body response.

Positive signals. Transection of peripheral nerves evokes de novo synthesis of various neurotrophic proteins. These proteins derive from three major sources: (i) target organs such as skin and muscle, (ii) Schwann cells surrounding the transected nerve fibers and the axotomized neurons, and (iii) the axotomized neurons themselves. If these factors are responsible for the induction of c-Jun, they have to be rapidly synthetized, released and/or activated. For example, *c-jun* mRNA is induced within 5 h after axotomy of facial motoneurons (Haas et al., 1993). Moreover, the intensity of expression of c-Jun increases with the shortness of the proximal nerve stump (Fig. 7, Table 1) (Jenkins et al., 1993a; Herdegen et al., 1994b; Robinson, 1994). These observations rather exclude the possibility that the onset of c-Jun expression is the consequence of positive de novo synthesized signals. Block of electrical impulse discharge by local anesthetics prior to transection does not interfere with c-Jun induction (Herdegen et al., 1991b; Leah et al., 1991). In addition to the length of the nerve stump, only a complete axotomy induced c-Jun, whereas transection of axon collaterals is not effective (Fig. 8) (Leah et al., 1993).

Although positive signals are unlikely to initiate c-Jun expression, they might control its maintenance and suppression. Application of NGF for 7 days, but not for 3 days, reduces c-Jun expression in sciatic DRG neurons (Gold et al., 1993; Herdegen et al., 1994a).

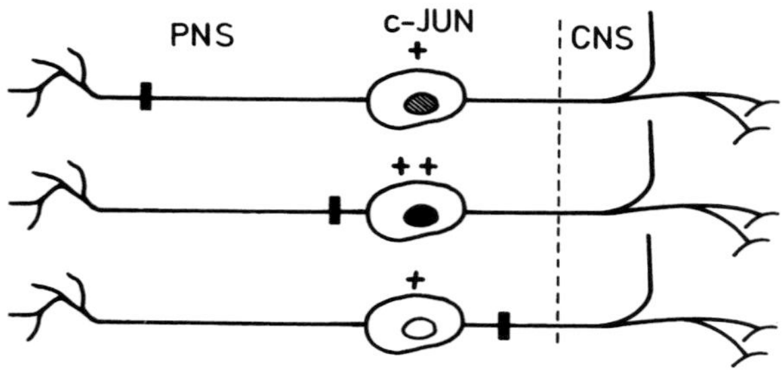

Fig. 7. The expression of c-Jun is increased in neurons of dorsal root ganglia following proximal sciatic nerve cut (+ +) compared to a more distal nerve cut (+). Transection of the dorsal roots induces a minor c-Jun expression compared to proximal nerve transection (Jenkins et al., 1993b; Herdegen et al., 1994a).

Negative signals. Molecules retrogradely conveyed with axonal transport and continuously released by target organs might provide information to the nucleus about the intactness of the neuron-target connection. Transection of nerve fibers interrupts this flow of information, and the ensuing deprivation of the target derived molecules could mediate expression of Jun proteins. This concept has been strongly supported by the finding that application of low doses of colchicine or vinblastine on the intact sciatic or vagal nerve provoked c-Jun and JunD expression in the corresponding primary afferent neurons and motoneurons (Herdegen et al., 1991b; Leah et al., 1991). Similarily, injection of colchicine and vinblastine into the striatum evoked c-Jun, JunD and Krox-24 expression but not c-Fos, JunB and Krox-20 around the injection site (Leah et al., 1993), and injection of colchicine into the rat eye resulted in the expression of c-Jun in ipsilateral RGCs (Koistinaho et al., 1993a).

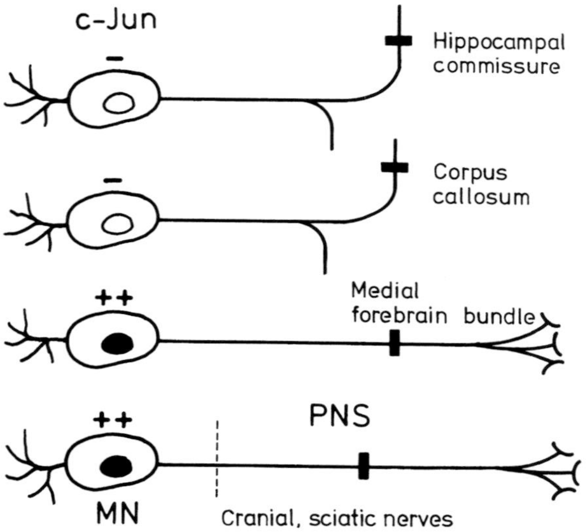

Fig. 8. Transection of axon collaterals of cortical or hippocampal neurons does not induce c-Jun expression (Leah et al., 1993). Complete axotomy of medial forebrain bundle, cranial and peripheral nerve fibers evokes a dramatic upregulation of c-Jun in the axotomized neurons, such as substantia nigra compacta neurons and motoneurons (MN).

Successful regeneration of sciatic, vagal and optic nerve fibers suppresses c-Jun (Herdegen et al., 1991b, 1993a; Jenkins et al., 1993b), indicating that target derived suppressors (positive signals) prevent the induction of c-Jun and that their ommission due to nerve fiber transection (negative signals) contributes to the upregulation of inducible transcription factors.

The function of Jun proteins in the neuronal cell body response after axotomy

The expression of c-Jun and JunD proteins is an early constituent of the neuronal cell body response. This conclusion is supported by the observation that only those protocols of axonal transection induce Jun proteins that also evoke the cell body response. Transection of axon collaterals, e.g., of hippocampal and cortical neurons, do not induce c-Jun (Fig. 8) (Leah et al., 1993; Tetzlaff, 1994), and transection of dorsal roots is also less effective compared to peripheral nerve transection (Fig. 7) (Jenkins et al., 1993b). Expression of c-Jun and RAGs (Tetzlaff Ch. 12, this volume) such as GAP-43 or Tα1-tubulin (Table 1) depend on the distance between the perikaryon and the site of axonal lesion. Thus, the presence of Jun proteins might be an intrinsic molecular genetic prerequisite for the known RAGs that underlie successful regeneration (Mickuki and Oblinger, 1991; Tetzlaff et al., 1991), suggesting that RAGs

TABLE 1

c-Jun and regeneration associated genes (RAGs) are concomitantly expressed in axotomized neurons dependent on the site of axonal transection

Transected nerve fibers	Site of transection for effective induction	Site of transection without induction	Ref.
Optic nerve	Intraorbital	Intracranial	Hüll and Bähr, 1994; Robinson, 1994
Cortical neurons	Axon stump < 200 μm	Axon stump < 200 μm	Leah et al., 1993; Tetzlaff et al., this volume 1994
Rubrospinal tract	Cervical spinal cord	Thoracic spinal cord	Jenkins et al., 1993a; Tetzlaff et al., this volume 1994

are target genes for c-Jun, JunD and/or Krox-24.

We have compiled evidence to support the hypothesis that Jun proteins are the transcription factors that control the change of effector gene encoded proteins associated with axonal elongation and synaptic remodeling. The c-Jun protein precedes other known changes in gene expression following axotomy, indicating that the c-Jun has commander function in this process. Following sciatic nerve cut, c-Jun precedes and covaries with the expression of nitric oxide synthase and galanin in DRG neurons and with CGRP in motoneurons (Fiallos-Estrada et al., 1993; Herdegen et al., 1993c). In axotomized neurons of substania nigra, c-Jun covaries with the residual synthesis of tyrosine hydroxylase (Brecht et al., 1994). Because tyrosine hydroxylase has AP-1 and CRE binding sites for the c-Jun protein in its promoter regions (Lewis et al., 1987; Gizang-Ginsberg and Ziff, 1990), the covariation of c-Jun suggests its involvement in *TH* gene expression.

In mammalian cells, the mere persistence of c-Jun can evoke neoplastic transformation (Schütte et al., 1989a). Following nerve fiber transection, the prolonged presence of c-Jun suggests a controlled overexpression that endows the nerve cells with a high potential for regenerative growth. This case of physiological overexpression is reversible, in contrast to the process of neoplastic transformation.

Acknowledgement

This work was supported by the Deutsche Forschungsgemeinschaft, grant Zi 110/22-2.

References

Abbadie, C. and Besson, J.M. (1993) Effects of morphine and naloxone on basal and evoked Fos-like immunoreactivity in lumbar spinal cord neurons of arthritic rats. *Pain*, 52: 29–39.

Almendral, J.M., Sommer, D., MacDonald-Bravo, H., Burckhardt, J., Perera, J. and Bravo R. (1988) Complexity of the early genetic response to growth factors in mouse fibroblasts. *Mol. Cell. Biol.*, 8: 2140–2148.

Angel, P. and Karin, M. (1991) The role of Jun, Fos and the AP-1 complex in cell-proliferation and transformation. *Biochim. Biophys. Acta*, 1072: 129–157.

Angel, P., Allegretto, E.A., Okino, S.T., Hattori, K., Boyle, W.J., Hunter T. and Karin, M. (1988) Oncogene jun encodes a sequence-specific *trans*-activator similar to AP-1. *Nature (Lond.)*, 332:166–171.

Bading, H., Ginty, D.D. and Greenberg, M.E. (1993) Regulation of gene expression in hippocampal neurons by distinct calcium signaling pathways. *Science*, 260: 181–186.

Bähr, M. (1991) Adult rat retinal glia in vitro: effects of in vivo crush-activation on glia proliferation and permissiveness for regenerating retinal ganglion cell axons. *Exp. Neurol.*, 111: 64–73.

Bartel, D.P., Sheng, M., Lau, L.F. and Greenberg, M.E. (1989) Growth factors and membrane depolarization activate distinct programs of early response gene expression: dissociation of *fos* and *jun* induction. *Genes Dev.*, 3: 304–313.

Benfey, M., Bünger, U.R., Vidal-Sanz, M. and Bray, G.M. (1985) Axon regeneration from GABAergic neurons in the adult rat thalamus. *J. Neurocytol.*, 14: 279–296.

Björklund, A., Nobin, A. and Stenevi, U. (1973) Regeneration of central serotonin neurons after axonal degeneration induced by 5,6-dihydrotryptamine. *Brain Res.*, 50: 214–220.

Bravo, R. (1990) Growth factor inducible genes in fibroblasts. In: A. Herschman (Ed.), *Growth Factors, Differentiation Factors and Cytokines*, Springer-Verlag, Heidelberg, pp. 324–343.

Bravo, R., MacDonald-Bravo, H., Müller, R., Hübsch, D. and Almendral, J.M. (1987) Bombesin induces *c-fos* and *c-myc* expression in quiescent swiss 3T3 cells. *Exp. Cell Res.*, 170: 103–115.

Brecht, S., Gass, P., Anton, F., Bravo, R., Zimmermann, M. and Herdegen, T (1994) Induction of c-Jun and suppression of CREB transcription factors in axotomized neurons of substantia nigra, and covariation with tyrosine-hydroxylase. *Mol. Cell. Neurosci.*, in press.

Chiu, R., Angel, P. and Karin, M. (1989) JUN B differs in its biological properties from, and is a negative regulator of, c-JUN. *Cell*, 59: 979–986.

Cole, A.J., Saffen, D.W., Baraban, J.M. and Worley, P.F. (1989) Rapid increase of an immediate early gene messenger RNA in hippocampal neurons by synaptic NMDA receptor activation. *Nature (Lond.)*, 340: 474–476.

David, S. and Aguayo, A. (1981) Axonal elongation into peripheral nervous system bridges after central nervous system injury in adult rats. *Science*, 214: 931–933.

Deng, T. and Karin, M. (1993) Jun B differs from c-Jun in its DNA- binding and dimerization domains, and represses c-Jun by formation of inactive heterodimers. *Genes Dev.*, 7: 479–490.

Dragunow, M. (1992) Axotomized medial septal-diagonal band neurons express Jun-like immunoreactivity. *Mol. Brain Res.*, 15: 141–144.

Dragunow, M., Abraham, W.C., Goulding, M., Mason, S.E., Robertson, H.A. and Faull, R.L.M. (1989) Long-term potentiation and the induction of *c-fos* mRNA and proteins in the dentate gyrus of unanaesthetized rats. *Neurosci. Lett.*, 101: 274–280.

Draisci, G. and Iadarola, M.J. (1989) Temporal analysis of increases in *c-fos*, preprodynorphin and preproenkephalin mRNAs in rat spinal cord. *Mol. Brain Res.*, 6: 31–37.

Dwarki, V.J., Montminy, M. and Verma, I. (1990) Both the basic region and the leucine zipper domain of the cyclic AMP response element binding (CREB) protein are essential for transcriptional activation. *EMBO J.*, 9: 225–232.

Fawcett, J.W. (1992) Intrinsic neuronal determinants of regeneration. *Trends Neurosci.*, 15: 5–8.

Fiallos-Estrada, C.E., Kummer, W., Mayer, W., Bravo, R., Zimmermann, M. and Herdegen, T. (1993) Long-lasting increase of nitric oxide synthase immunoreactivcity and NADPH-diaphorase reaction, and co-expression with the nuclear c-JUN protein in rat dorsal root ganglion neurons following sciatic nerve transection. *Neurosci. Lett.*, 150: 169–173.

Foulkes, N.S., Borelli, E. and Sassone-Corsi, P. (1991) CREM gene: use of alternative DNA-binding domains generates multiple antagonists of cAMP-induced transcription. *Cell*, 64: 739–749.

Gass, P., Herdegen, T., Bravo, R. and Kiessling, M. (1992a) Induction of immediate early gene encoded proteins in the rat hippocampus after bicuculline-induced seizures: differential expression of KROX-24, FOS and JUN proteins. *Neuroscience*, 48: 315–324.

Gass, P., Spranger, M., Herdegen, T., Köck, P., Bravo, R., Hacke, W. and Kiessling, M. (1992b) Induction of FOS and JUN proteins after focal ischemia in the rat: differential effect of the *N*-methyl-D-aspartate receptor antagonist MK-801. *Acta Neuropathol.*, 84: 545–553.

Gass, P., Herdegen, T., Bravo, R. and Kiessling, M. (1993a) Induction and suppression of immediate early genes (IEGs) in specific rat brain regions by the non-competitive NMDA receptor antagonist MK-801. *Neuroscience*, 53: 749–758.

Gass, P., Herdegen, T., Bravo, R. and Kiessling, M. (1993b) Induction of six immediate-early gene encoded proteins in the rat brain after kainic acid induced limbic seizures: effects of NMDA receptor antagonist MK-801. *Eur. J. Neurosci.*, 5: 933–943.

Gentz, R., Rauscher, F.J., Abate, C. and Curran, T. (1989) Parallel association of Fos and Jun leucine zippers juxtaposes DNA binding domains. *Science*, 243: 1695–1699.

Ginty, D.D., Kornhauser, J.M., Thompson, M.A., Bading, H., Mayo, K.E., Takahashi, J.S. and Greenberg, M.E. (1993) Regulation of CREB phosphorylation in suprachiasmatic nucleus by light and a circadian clock. *Science*, 260: 238–241.

Gizang-Ginsberg, E. and Ziff, E.B. (1990) Nerve growth factor regulates tyrosine hydroxylase gene transcription through a nucleoprotein complex that contains c-Fos. *Genes Dev.*, 4: 477–491.

Gold, B.G., Storm-Dickerson, T. and Austin, D.R. (1993) Regulation of the transcription factor c-JUN by nerve growth factor in adult sensory neurons. *Neurosci. Lett.*, 154:129–133.

Gonzalez, G.A., Yamamoto, K.Y., Fisher, W.H., Karr, D., Menzel, P., Biggs, W.I., Vale, W.W. and Montminy, M.R. (1989) A cluster of phosphorylation sites on the cyclic AMP-regulated nuclear factor CREB predicted by its sequence. *Nature (Lond.)*, 337: 749–752.

Goodman, R.H. (1990) Regulation of neuropeptide gene expression. Annu. *Rev. Neurosci.*, 13: 111–127.

Grafstein, B. (1986) The retina as a regeneration organ. In R. Sadler and D. Farber (Eds.), *The Retina: A Model for Cell Biology Studies*, Academic Press, New York, pp. 275–335.

Gubits, R.M., Yu, H., Casey, G., Munell, F. and Vitek, M.P. (1992) Altered genetic response to β-adrenergic receptor activation in late passage C6 glioma cells. *J. Neurosci. Res.*, 33: 297–305.

Gunkel, A., Herdegen, T., Angelov, D.N., Guntnias-Lichius, O., Schmid, W., Zimmermann, M., Stennert, E. and Neiss, W.F. (1994) Expression of inducible (Jun, Fos) and constitutive (CREB, CREM, SRF) transcription factor proteins in axotomized neurons following hypoglossal-facial anastomosis. *Eur. J. Neurosci.*, Suppl. 7, in press.

Haas, C.A, Donath, C. and Kreutzberg, G.W. (1993) Differential expression of immediate early genes after transection of the facial nerve. *Neuroscience*, 53: 91–99.

Halazonetis, T.D., Georgopoulos, K., Greenberg, M.E. and Leder, P. (1988) c-Jun dimerizes with itself and with c-Fos, forming complexes of different DNA binding affinities. *Cell*, 55: 917–924.

Hanley, M.R. (1988) Proto-oncogenes in the nervous system. *Neuron*, 1: 175–182.

He, X. and Rosenfeld, M.G. (1991) Mechanisms of complex transcriptional regulation: implications for brain development. *Neuron*, 7: 183–196.

Hengerer, B., Lindholm, D., Heumann, R., Rüther, U., Wagner, E. and Thoenen, H. (1990) Lesion-induced increase in nerve growth factor mRNA is mediated by *c-fos*. *Proc. Natl. Acad. Sci. USA*, 87: 3899–3903.

Herdegen, T., Leah, J. and Bravo, R. (1990) Different expression of JUN, FOS and KROX-24 proteins in adult CNS: dependence on neurobiological events. *J. Cell Biochem.*, Suppl 14F: 310.

Herdegen, T., Kovary, K., Leah, J.D. and Bravo, R. (1991a) Specific temporal and spatial distribution of JUN, FOS and KROX-24 proteins in spinal neurons following noxious transynaptic stimulation. *J. Comp. Neurol.*, 313: 178–191.

Herdegen, T., Kummer, W., Fiallos-Estrada, C.E., Leah, J.D. and Bravo, R. (1991b) Expression of c-JUN, JUN B and JUN D in the rat nervous system following transection of the vagus nerve and cervical sympathetic trunk. *Neuroscience*, 45: 413–422.

Herdegen, T., Leah, J.D., Manisali, A., Bravo, R. and Zimmermann, M. (1991c) c-Jun-like immunoreactivity in the CNS of the adult rat: basal and transynaptically induced expression of an immediate-early gene. *Neuroscience*, 41: 643–654.

Herdegen, T., Tölle, T., Bravo, R., Zieglgänsberger, W. and Zimmermann, M. (1991d) Sequential expression of JUN B, JUN D and FOS B proteins in rat spinal neurons: cascade of transcriptional operations during nociception. *Neurosci. Lett.*, 129: 221–224.

Herdegen, T., Fiallos-Estrada, C.E., Schmid, W., Bravo, R. and Zimmermann, M. (1992) Transcription factors c-JUN, JUN D and CREB, but not FOS and KROX-24, are differentially regulated in neurons following axotomy of rat sciatic nerve. *Mol. Brain Res.*, 14: 155–165.

Herdegen, T., Bastmeyer, M., Bähr, M., Bravo, R., Stürmer, C.A.O. and Zimmermann, M. (1993a) Expression of JUN, KROX and CREB transcription factors in goldfish and rat ganglion cells following optic nerve lesions is related to axonal sprouting. *J. Neurobiol.*, 24: 528–543.

Herdegen, T., Brecht, S., Kummer, W., Mayer, B., Leah, J., Bravo, R. and Zimmermann, M. (1993b) Persisting expression of JUN and KROX transcription factors and nitric oxide synthase in rat central neurons following axotomy. *J. Neurosci.*, 13: 4130–4145.

Herdegen, T., Fiallos-Estrada, C.E., Bravo, R. and Zimmermann, M. (1993c) Colocalisation and covariation of the nuclear c-JUN protein with galanin in primary afferent neurons and with CGRP in spinal motoneurons following transection of rat sciatic nerve. *Mol. Brain Res.*, 17: 147–154.

Herdegen, T., Kiessling, M., Bravo, R., Zimmermann, M. and Gass, P. (1993d) The KROX-20 transcription factor in the adult brain: novel expression pattern of an immediate-early gene encoded protein. *Neuroscience*, 57: 42–53.

Herdegen, T., Sandkühler, J., Gass, P., Kiessling, M., Bravo, R. and Zimmermann, M. (1993e) JUN, FOS, KROX and CREB transcription factor proteins in the rat cortex: basal expression and induction by spreading depression and epileptic seizures. *J. Comp. Neurol.*, 333: 271–288.

Herdegen, T., Brecht, S., Fiallos-Estrada, C.E., Wickert, H., Gillardon, F., Voss, S. and Bravo, R. (1994a) A novel face of immediate-early genes: transcriptional operations dominated by c-Jun and JunD proteins in neurons following axotomy and during regenerative efforts. In: T. Tölle and W. Zieglgänsberger (Eds.), *Immediate-early Genes in the CNS: More than Activity Markers*, Springer-Verlag, Heidelberg/Berlin, in press.

Herdegen, T., Rüdiger, S., Mayer, B., Bravo, R. and Zimmermann, M. (1994b) Increase in nitric oxide synthase and colocalization with Jun, Fos and Krox proteins in spinal neurons following noxious peripheral stimulation. *Mol. Brain Res.*, 22: 245–258.

Herdegen, T., Brecht, S., Neiss, W.F., Schmid, W. and Gass, P. (1994c) The transcription factor CREB is not phosphorylated at serine 133 in axotomized neurons: implications for the expression of AP-1 proteins. *Mol. Brain Res.*, in press.

Herschman, H.R. (1991) Primary response genes induced by growth factors and tumor promoters. *Annu. Rev. Biochem.*, 60: 281–319.

Hirai, S.I., Ryseck, R.P., Mechta, F., Bravo, R. and Yaniv, M. (1989) Characterization of junD: a new member of the jun proto-oncogene family. *EMBO J.*, 8: 1433–1439.

Houle, J.D. (1992a) Regeneration of dorsal root axons is related to specific non-neuronal cells lining NGF-treated intraspinal nitrocellulose implants. *Exp. Neurol.*, 118: 133–142.

Houle, J.D. (1992b) The structural integrity of glial scar tissue associated with a chronic spinal cord lesion can be altered by transplanted fetal spinal cord tissue. *J. Neurosci. Res.*, 31: 120–130.

Hüll, M. and Bähr, M. (1994) Regulation of immediate-early gene expression in rat retinal ganglion cells after axotomy and during regeneration through a peripheral nerve graft. *J. Neurobiol.*, 25: 92–105.

Hummler, E., Cole, J.A., Blendy, J.A., Ganss, R., Aguzzi, A., Schmid, W. and Schütz, G. (1994) Targeted mutation of the CREB gene: compensation within the CREB/ATF family of transcription factors. *Proc. Natl. Acad. Sci. USA.,* in press.

Hunt, S.P., Pini, A. and Evan, G. (1987) Induction of *c-fos*-like protein in spinal cord neurons following sensory stimulation. *Nature (Lond.)*, 328: 632–634.

Ingraham, C.A., Cox, M.E., Ward, D.C., Fults, D.W. and Maness, P.F. (1989) C-src and other proto-oncogenes implicated in neuronal differentiation. *Mol. Chem. Neuropathol.*, 10: 1–14.

Jenkins, R. and Hunt, S.P. (1991) Long-term increase in the levels of c-jun mRNA and Jun protein-like immunoreactivity in motor and sensory neurons following axon damage. *Neurosci. Lett.*, 129: 107–110.

Jenkins, R., Tetzlaff, W. and Hunt, S.P. (1993a) Differential expression of immediate early genes in rubrospinal neurons following axotomy in rat. *Eur. J. Neurosci.*, 5: 203–209.

Jenkins, R., McMahon, S.B., Bond, A.B. and Hunt, S. (1993b) Expression of c-Jun as a response to dorsal root and peripheral nerve section in damaged and adjacent intact primary sensory neurons in the rat. *Eur. J. Neurosci.*, 5: 751–759.

Jones, K.J. and Evinger, C. (1991) Differential neuronal expression of *c-fos* proto-oncogene following peripheral nerve injury or chemically-induced seizure. *J. Neurosci. Res.*, 28: 291–298.

Koistinaho, J., Hicks, K.J., and Sagar, S.M.(1993a) Long-term induction of c-jun mRNA and Jun protein in rabbit retinal ganglion cells following axotomy or colchicine treatment. *J. Neurosci. Res.*, 34: 250–255.

Koistinaho, J., Pelto-Huikko, Sagar, S.M., Dagerlind, A., Roivainen, R. and Hökfelt, T. (1993b) Injury-induced long-term expression of immediate early genes in the rat superior cervical ganglion. *NeuroReport*, 4: 37–40.

Kruijer, W., Cooper, J.A., Hunter, T. and Verma, I.M. (1984) Platelet-derived growth factor induces rapid but transient expression of the *c-fos* gene and protein. *Nature* (*Lond.*), 312: 711–716.

Lamph, W.W., Dwarki, V.J., Ofir, R., Montminy, M. and Verma, I.M. (1990) Negative and positive regulation by transcription factor cAMP response element-binding protein is modulated by phosphorylation. *Proc. Natl. Acad. Sci USA*, 87: 4320–4324.

Landschulz, W.H., Johnson P.F. and McKnight, S.L. (1988) The leucine zipper: a hypothetical structure common to a new class of DNA binding proteins. *Science*, 240: 1759–1764.

Lanteri-Minet, M., de Pommery, J., Herdegen, T., Weil-Fugazza, J., Bravo, R. and Menetrey, D. (1993) Differential time-course and spatial expression of Fos, Jun and Krox-24 proteins in spinal cord of rats undergoing subacute or chronic somatic inflammation. *J. Comp. Neurol.*, 333: 223–235.

Lau, L.F. and Nathans, D. (1985) Identification of a set of genes expressed during the G0/G1 transition of cultured mouse cells. *EMBO J.*, 4: 3145–3151.

Lazo, P.S., Dorfman, K., Noguchi, T., Mattei, M.G. and Bravo, R. (1991) Structure and mapping of the fosB gene. FosB downregulates the activity of the fosB promoter. *Nucleic Acids Res.*, 20: 343–350.

Leah, J.D., Herdegen, T., Kovary, K. and Bravo, R. (1991) Selective expression of JUN proteins following peripheral axotomy and axonal transport block in the rat: evidence for a role in the regeneration process. *Brain Res.*, 566: 198–207.

Leah, J.D., Sandkühler, J., Herdegen, T., Murashov, A. and Zimmermann, M. (1992) Potentiated expression of FOS protein in the rat spinal cord following bilateral noxious cutaneous stimulation. *Neuroscience*, 48: 315–324.

Leah, J.D., Herdegen, T., Murashov, A., Dragunow, M. and Bravo, R. (1993) Expression of immediate-early gene proteins following axotomy and inhibition of axonal transport in the rat CNS. *Neuroscience*, 57: 53–66.

Liebermann, A.R. (1971) The axon reaction: a review of the principal features of perikaryal response to axon injury. *Int. Rev. Neurobiol.*, 14: 49–124.

Lord, K.A., Hoffmann-Liebermann, B. and Liebermann, D.A. (1990) Complexity of the immediate early response of myeloid cells to terminal differentiation and growth arrest includes ICAM-1, JUN-B and histone variants. *Oncogene*, 5: 387–396.

Mack, K., Day, M., Milbrandt, J. and Gottlieb, D.I. (1990) Localization of the NGFI-A protein in the rat brain. *Mol. Brain Res.*, 8: 177–180.

Mellström, B., Achaval, M., Montero, D., Naranjo, J.R. and Sassone-Corsi, P. (1991) Differential expression of the jun family members in rat brain. *Oncogene*, 6: 1959–1964.

Mikucki, S.A. and Oblinger, M.M. (1991) Corticospinal neurons exhibit a novel pattern of cytoskeletal gene expression after injury. *J. Neurosci. Res.*, 30: 213–225.

Molander, C., Hongpaisan, J. and Grant, G. (1992) Changing pattern of *c-fos* expression in spinal cord neurons after electrical stimulation of the chronically injured sciatic nerve in the rat. *Neuroscience*, 50: 223–236.

Montminy, M.R. and Bilezikjian, L.M. (1987) Binding of a nuclear protein to the cyclic-AMP response element of the somatostatin gene. *Nature (Lond.)*, 328: 175–178.

Morgan, J.I. and Curran, T. (1991) Stimulus-transcription coupling in the nervous system: involvement of the inducible proto-oncogenes fos and jun. *Annu. Rev. Neurosci.*, 14: 421–451.

Morgan, J.I., Cohen, D.R., Hempstead, J.L. and Curran, T. (1987) Mapping patterns of *c-fos* expression in the central nervous system after seizure. *Science*, 237: 192–196.

Nakabeppu, Y. and Nathans, D. (1991) A naturally occurring

truncated form of FosB that inhibits Fos/Jun transcriptional activity. *Cell*, 64: 751–759.

Nakabeppu, Y., Ryder, K. and Nathans, D. (1988) DNA binding activities of three different jun proteins: stimulation by Fos. *Cell*, 55: 907–915.

Naranjo, J.R., Mellström, B., Achaval, M., Lucas, J.J., Del Rio, J. and Sassone-Corsi, P. (1991a) Co-induction of JUN-B and c-FOS in a subset of neurons in the spinal cord. *Oncogene*, 6: 223–227.

Naranjo, J.R., Mellström, B., Achaval, M. and Sassone-Corsi, P. (1991b) Molecular pathways of pain: fos/jun-mediated activation of a noncanonical AP-1 site in the prodynorphin gene. *Neuron*, 6: 607–617.

Neiss, W.F., Lichius, O.G., Angelov, D.N., Gunkel, A. and Stennert, E. (1992) The hypoglossal-facial anastomosis as model of neuronal plasticity in the rat. *Ann. Anat.*, 174: 419–433.

Noguchi, K., Dubner, R. and Ruda, M.A. (1992) Preproenkephalin mRNA in spinal dorsal horn neurons is induced by peripheral inflammation and is co-localized with Fos and Fos-related proteins. *Neuroscience*, 46: 561–570.

Pertovaara, A., Bravo, R. and Herdegen, T. (1993) Induction and suppression of immediate-early genes by selective alpha-2-adrenoceptor agonist and antagonist in the rat brain following noxious peripheral stimulation. *Neuroscience*, 54: 117–126.

Peunova, N. and Enikolopov, G. (1993) Amplification of calcium-induced gene transcription by nitric oxide in neuronal cells. *Nature (Lond.)*, 364: 450–453.

Presley, R.W., Menetrey, D., Levine, J.D. and Basbaum, A.I. (1990) Systemic morphine suppresses noxious stimulus-evoked Fos protein-like immunoreactivity in the rat spinal cord. *J. Neurosci.*, 10: 323–335.

Pulverer, B.J., Kyriakis, J.M., Avruch, J., Nikolakaki, E. and Woodgett, J.R. (1991) Phosphorylation of c-jun mediated by MAP kinases. *Nature (Lond.)*, 353: 670–674.

Rauscher, F.J.,III, Voulaslas, P.J., Franza, B.R., Jr. and Curran, T. (1988) Fos and jun bind cooperatively to the AP-1 site: reconstitution in vitro. *Genes Dev.*, 2: 1687–1699.

Reier, P. and Houle, J. (1988) The glial scar: its bearing on axonal elongation and transplantation approaches to CNS repair. In: S. Waxman (Ed.), *Functional Recovery in Neurological Disease, Advances in Neurology*, Vol. 47, Raven Press, New York, pp. 87–138.

Robinson, G.A. (1994) Immediate early gene expression in axotomized and regenerating retinal ganglion cells of the adult rat. *Mol. Brain Res.*, in press.

Rose, S.P.R. (1991) How chicks make memories: the cellular cascade from *c-fos* to dentritic remodeling. *Trends Neurosci.*, 14: 390–397.

Ruda, M.A., Iadarola, M.J., Cohen, L.V. and Young, W.S. (1988) In-situ hybridization histochemistry and immunohistochemistry reveal an increase in spinal cord dynorphin biosynthesis in a rat model of peripheral inflammation and hyperalgesia. *Proc. Natl. Acad. Sci. USA*, 85: 622–626.

Rutherford, S.D., Louis, W.J. and Gundlach, A.L. (1992) Induction of c-jun expression in vagal motoneurons following axotomy. *NeuroReport*, 3: 465–468.

Ryseck, P. and Bravo, R. (1991) c-JUN, JUN B, and JUN D differ in their binding affinities to AP-1 and CRE consensus sequences: effect of FOS proteins. *Oncogene*, 6: 533–542.

Sagar, S.M., Sharp, F.R. and Curran, T. (1988) Expression of *c-fos* proteins in brain: metabolic mapping at the cellular level. *Science*, 240: 1328–1331.

Schlingensiepen, K.H., Schlingensiepen, R., Kunst, M., Klinger, I., Gerdes, W., Seifert, W. and Brysch, W. (1993) Opposite functions of jun-B and c-jun in growth regulation and neuronal differentiation. *Dev. Genetics*, 14: 305–312.

Schlingensiepen, K.H., Kunst, M. Gerdes, W. and Brysch, W. (1994) Complementary expression patterns of c-jun and jun-B in rat brain and analysis of their function with antisense oligonucleotides. In: T. Tölle and W. Zieglgènsberger (Eds.), *Immediate-early Genes in the CNS: More than Activity Markers*, Springer-Verlag, Heidelberg/Berlin, in press.

Schnell, L. and Schwab, M.E. (1990) Axonal regeneration in the rat spinal cord produced by antibody against myelin-associated neurite growth inhibitors. *Nature (Lond.)*, 343: 269–272.

Schütte, J., Minna, J. and Birrer, M. (1989a) Deregulated expression of human c-jun transforms primary rat embryo cells in cooperation with an activated c-Ha-ras gene and transforms rate-1a as a single gene. *Proc. Natl. Acad. Sci. USA,* 86: 2257-2261.

Schütte, J., Viallet, J., Nau, M., Segal, S., Fedorko, J. and Minna, J. (1989b) Jun-B inhibits and c-FOS stimulates the transforming and transactivating activities of c-jun. *Cell*, 59: 987–997.

Sharp, F.R., Griffith, J., Gonzalez, M.F. and Sagar, S.M. (1989) Trigeminal nerve section induces Fos-like immunoreactivity (FLI) in brainstem and decreases FLI in sensory cortex. *Mol. Brain Res.*, 6: 217–220.

Sharp, F.R., Sagar, S.M., Hicks, K., Lowenstein, D. and Hisanaga, K. (1991) *c-fos* mRNA, Fos, and Fos-related antigen induction by hypertonic saline and stress. *J. Neurosci.*, 11: 2321–2331.

Sheng, M. and Greenberg, E. (1990) The regulation and function of *c-fos* and other immediate early genes in the nervous system. *Neuron*, 4: 477–485.

Sheng, M., Thompson, S.A. and Greenberg, M. (1991) CREB: A C^{2+} regulated transcription factor phosphorylated by calmodulin-dependent kinases. *Science*, 252: 1427–1430.

Skene, J.H.P. (1989) Axonal growth-associated proteins. *Annu. Rev. Neurosci.*, 12: 127–156.

Sonnenberg, J.L., Rauscher, F.J., III, Morgan, J.I. and Curran,

T. (1989) Regulation of proenkephalin by Fos and Jun. *Science*, 246: 1622–1625.

Struthers, S., Vale, W.W., Arias, C., Sawchenko, P.E. and Montminy M.R. (1991) Somatotroph hypoplasia and dwarfism in transgenic mice expressing a non- phosphorylatable CREB mutant. *Nature (Lond.)*, 350: 622–624.

Stürmer, C.A.O., Bastmeyer, M., Bähr, M., Strobel, G. and Paschke, K. (1992) Trying to understand axonal regeneration in the CNS of fish. *J. Neurobiol.*, 23: 537–550.

Tetzlaff, W., Alexander, S.W., Miller, F.D. and Bisby, M.A. (1991) Response of facial and rubrospinal neurons to axotomy: changes in mRNA expression for cytoskeletal proteins and GAP-43. *J. Neurosci.*, 11: 2528–2544.

Tölle, T., Herdegen, T., Bravo, R., Zimmermann, M. and Zieglgènsberger, W. (1994) Single application of morphine prior to noxious stimulation differentially modulates expression of FOS, JUN and KROX-24 in rat spinal cord neurons. *Neuroscience*, 58: 305–323.

Treisman, R. (1990) The SRE: a growth factor responsive transcriptional regulator. *Cancer Biol.*, 1: 47–58.

Villegas-Perez, M.-P., Vidal-Sanz, M., Rasminsky, M., Bray, G.M. and Aguayo, A.J. (1993) Rapid and protacted phases of retinal ganglion cell loss follow axotomy in the optic nerve of adult rats. *J. Neurobiol.*, 24: 23–36.

Vogt, P.K. and Bos, T.J. (1990) JUN: oncogene and transcription factor. *Adv. Cancer Res.*, 55: 2–36.

Weiser, M., Baker, H., Wessel, T.C. and Joh, T.H. (1993) Axotomy-induced differential gene induction in neurons of the locus ceruleus and substantia nigra. *Mol. Brain Res.*, 17: 319–327.

Wilkinson, G., Bhatt, S., Ryseck, R. and Bravo, R. (1989) Tissue-specific expression of c-jun and jun B during mouse development. *Development*, 106: 464–473.

Winston, S.M., Hayward, M.D., Nestler, E.J. and Duman, R.S. (1990) Chronic electroconvulsive seizures down-regulate expression of the immediate-early genes *c-fos* and c-jun in rat cerebral cortex. *J. Neurochem.*, 54: 1920–1925.

Wisden, W., Errington, M.L., Williams, S., Dunnett, S.B., Waters, C., Hitchcock, D., Evan, G., Bliss, T.V. and Hunt, S.P. (1990) Differential expression of immediate early genes in the hippocampus and spinal cord. *Neuron*, 4: 603–614.

SECTION IV

Models of Spinal Cord Regeneration

F.J. Seil (Ed.)
Progress in Brain Research, Vol 103

CHAPTER 16

Models of spinal cord regeneration

George F. Martin, Ganesh T. Ghooray, Xian Ming Wang, Xiao Ming Xu and Xun Chang Zou

Department of Cell Biology, Neurobiology and Anatomy, The Ohio State University, College of Medicine, 333 West Tenth Avenue, Columbus, OH 43210, USA

Introduction

Transection of the spinal cord in man results in paralysis and loss of sensation below the lesion and, unfortunately, little regeneration or recovery of normal function (e.g., Windle, 1955; Clemente, 1964; Pettegrew and Windle, 1976; Puchala and Windle, 1977; Kiernan, 1979; Freed et al., 1985; Collins and West, 1989). Adult mammals are good models for spinal cord injury research because their spinal cords respond to trauma more or less like that of man. Dogs were employed to develop the controlled impact technique of Allen (1911), which has been widely used to simulate spinal cord injury in man, and since that time other adult mammals have also been employed (e.g., rats, hamsters, cats and monkeys). The results of such studies have provided a reasonably clear picture of the spinal cord's response to injury and have suggested therapeutic strategies to minimize central hemorrhagic necrosis and maximize axonal sparing (see reviews by Sandler and Tator, 1976; De La Torre, 1981; Balentine, 1985; Faden, 1985; Young, 1985; Beattie et al., 1988). It appears, however, that the spinal cord of adult mammals has more potential for regeneration than previously thought. For example, under certain conditions axons of the mammalian central nervous system regenerate within peripheral nerve grafts (e.g., David and Aguayo, 1981, 1985), suggesting that regeneration can occur if the environment is conducive for it.

A second approach to spinal cord injury research is to employ developing mammals and nonmammalian species whose spinal cords might be expected to regenerate more completely than that of adult mammals. Using this approach, it may be possible to identify the requirements for plasticity and regeneration, as well as factors which limit it. Since reviews are already available on studies that utilize adult mammals, we will restrict the following one to studies which utilized the second approach. Particular emphasis will be placed on the use of developing mammals.

Developing mammals as models of spinal cord injury research

Placental mammals

Placental mammals have been used to study developmental plasticity of the corticospinal tract, the largest descending spinal pathway in man (see review by Davidoff, 1990). Cortical axons grow into the spinal cord postnatally in mammals, making it possible to lesion them in an immature state without intrauterine surgery. Using an orthograde transport technique, Kalil and Reh (1979, 1982) showed that cortical axons grow around a lesion of the medullary pyramids in neonatal hamsters and, based on several lines of evidence, they argued that such growth results from regeneration of cut axons. Tolbert and Der (1987) documented the same phenomenon in neonatal kittens, but concluded that redirection of 'late' arriving axons was the mechanism for plasticity. In the latter experiments, the long lasting fluorescent marker Fast Blue (FB) was injected into the spinal cord between postnatal day (PD) 2 and 6 to prelabel corticospinal neurons, and 5–8 days later the pyramidal tract was cut on one side to transect their axons. When the animals were killed 29–79 days later, there was little evidence for labeled neurons in the cerebral cortex ipsilateral to the lesion. The authors interpreted the lack of labeling to mean that corticospinal neurons failed to survive axotomy and that corticospinal plasticity after pyramidotomy results primarily from growth of late arriving axons around the lesion, not regeneration of cut axons. Merline and Kalil (1990) revisited this issue in neonatal hamsters using a similar approach, and came to the same conclusion.

Cortical axons have also been shown to grow around a lesion of their spinal pathway in neonatal rats (Bernstein and Stelzner, 1983; Schreyer and Jones, 1983; Bates and Stelzner, 1989, 1993), and regeneration of cut axons, as well as new growth, occurs when the lesion is made at cervical levels (Bates and Stelzner, 1993). In the latter experiments, FB was injected into the cervical cord at PD2, 4 and 10, and 2 days later it was removed. The injection labeled corticospinal neurons whose axons were present at the injection site, and its removal made it inaccessible to late arriving axons. Removal of FB also resulted in a lesion which transected the corticospinal tract. Two months after the lesion, another fluorescent marker, Diamidino Yellow (DY), was injected caudal to the lesion. After a 2 day survival to allow for labeling of corticospinal neurons by DY, the animals were killed and perfused so that the spinal cord and brain could be removed and sectioned for examination with a fluorescence microscope. FB labeled neurons were observed in the motor cortex contralateral to the lesion at all ages, suggesting that at least some corticospinal neurons survived axotomy. In the PD2 and 4 cases, a few such neurons also contained DY. It was concluded not only that the latter neurons survived axotomy, as evidenced by the presence of FB, but that they regenerated an axon or axons around the lesion to at least the level of the DY injection. Many cortical neurons contained DY alone, however. Such neurons had apparently not been axotomized, but supported late arriving axons which grew around the lesion. Comparison of the results obtained after lesioning the cervical cord in newborn rats and after lesioning the medullary pyramids in neonatal hamsters and cats suggests that corticospinal neurons survive lesions of the cervical cord better than lesions of the brainstem. Increased survival after cervical lesions might account for the presence of axonal regeneration.

In the neonatal cat, corticospinal plasticity results in sparing of function. Adult cats never show recovery of tactile placing caudal and ipsilateral to a spinal hemisection, but animals operated as neonates do, and return of tactile placing is dependent upon growth of cortical axons around the lesion (Bregman and Goldberger, 1982, 1983a).

The critical period for corticospinal plasticity can be extended by transplants of fetal spinal cord (Bregman et al., 1989). In such experiments, the spinal cord of rats was overhemisected at different ages and, in some cases, the lesion cavity was filled with the transplant. One to 9 months later, orthograde transport techniques were used to label corticospinal axons and it was shown that they grew into the transplant well after the critical period for corticospinal plasticity in animals without transplants. Innervation of the transplant decreased with age, suggesting decreased growth potential.

Marsupials

Although corticospinal axons grow around a lesion of their pathway in neonatal hamsters, cats and rats, brainstem axons do not (e.g., Prendergast and Stelzner, 1976; Bregman and Goldberger, 1982, 1983b). Brainstem-spinal axons grow into the spinal cord prenatally in the above species (Prendergast and Stelzner, 1976; Bregman and Goldberger, 1982, 1983b; Lakke and Marani, 1991), and by birth they may have lost their potential for plasticity. Based on such reasoning, we hypothesized that brainstem axons, like axons from the cerebral cortex, will grow around a lesion of their pathway if it is made early enough during development. That hypothesis might be difficult to test in placental mammals because the prenatal development of brainstem-spinal connections would make it necessary to employ intrauterine surgery. We thought it would be testable in the North American opossum (*Didelphis virginiana*), however, because most brainstem-spinal development occurs postnatally in that species (Cabana and Martin, 1981, 1984; Martin et al., 1993). Opossums are born in a very immature state, 12–13 days after conception (McCrady, 1938), and they remain in an external pouch for 90 days or more (Fig. 1), during which time most of their central nervous system development takes place. The organization of brainstem-spinal connections in opossums is generally comparable to that of placental mammals (Martin, 1969; Martin and Dom, 1970, 1971; Martin et al., 1975, 1979, 1981; Crutcher et al., 1978).

Our initial studies of brainstem-spinal plasticity focused on the rubrospinal tract because rubral axons reach the spinal cord later than axons from

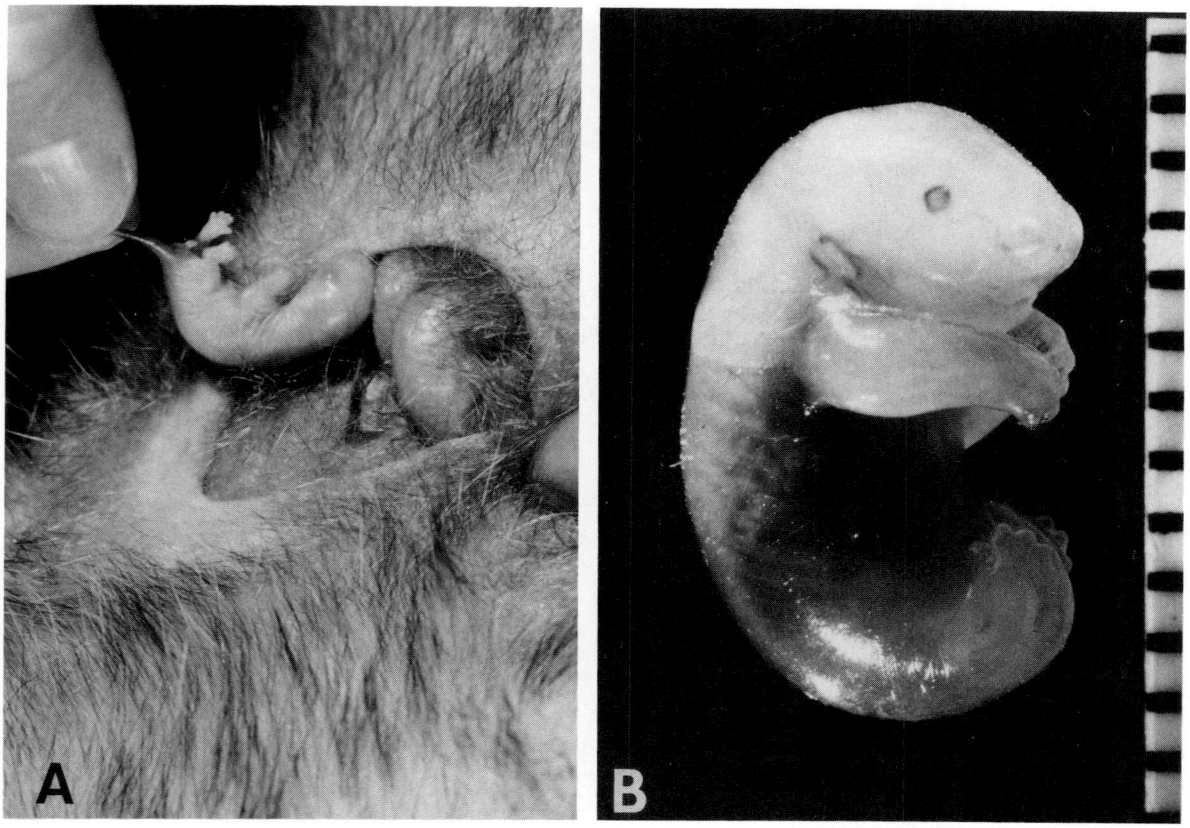

Fig. 1. Photograph of *Didelphis* pups in the pouch (A) and a newborn opossum removed from the pouch (B). A millimeter rule is shown on the right of B.

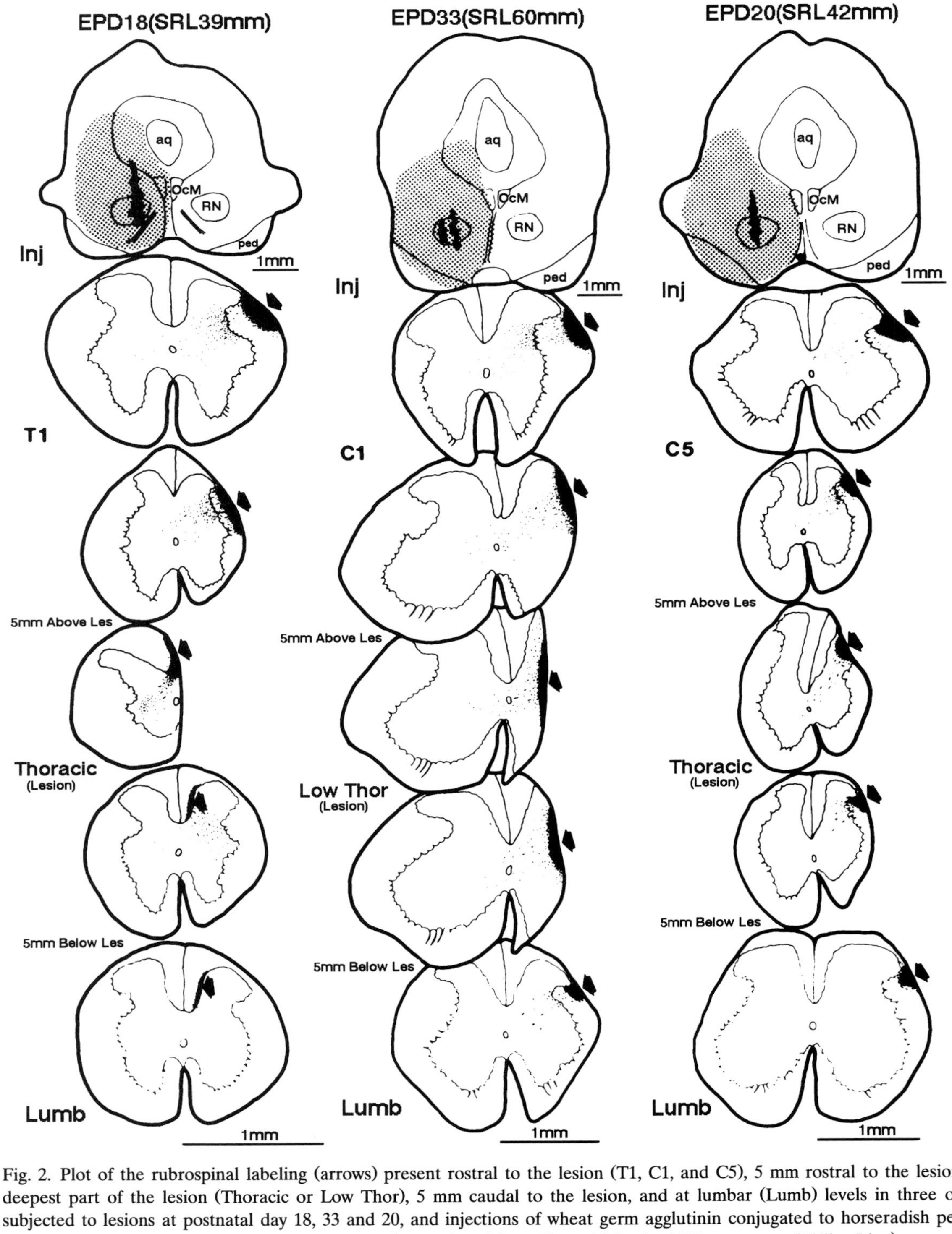

Fig. 2. Plot of the rubrospinal labeling (arrows) present rostral to the lesion (T1, C1, and C5), 5 mm rostral to the lesion, at the deepest part of the lesion (Thoracic or Low Thor), 5 mm caudal to the lesion, and at lumbar (Lumb) levels in three opossums subjected to lesions at postnatal day 18, 33 and 20, and injections of wheat germ agglutinin conjugated to horseradish peroxidase into the red nucleus approximately 30 days later. (Reproduced from Xu and Martin, 1989; courtesy of Wiley-Liss.)

most areas of the brainstem (Cabana and Martin, 1981, 1984; Martin et al., 1992). Since rubrospinal development occurs postnatally in opossums, it was possible to lesion rubral axons at very early stages of development without intrauterine surgery.

In one set of experiments (Martin and Xu, 1988; Xu and Martin, 1989), rubrospinal axons were cut at different stages of development by making unilateral lesions of the lateral funiculus at midthoracic levels of the spinal cord. Approximately 30 days later, the pups were reanesthetized and subjected to injections of one of several retrograde markers several segments caudal to the lesion and ipsilateral to it. After an appropriate survival to allow for retrograde labeling, the animals were reanesthetized, killed, and perfused so that their spinal cords and brains could be removed for sectioning and processing. As expected, there was no evidence for rubrospinal labeling contralateral to the lesion in adult opossums or in older pouch young. In opossums, as in other species, the rubrospinal tract is almost entirely crossed (Xu and Martin, 1991b). In animals younger than PD30, however, rubral neurons were labeled contralateral to the lesion and it was our interpretation that they supported axons which had grown around it to at least the level of the injected marker. That interpretation was supported by the results of orthograde labeling experiments (Martin and Xu, 1988; Xu and Martin, 1989). The location of the rubrospinal tract caudal to the lesion differed from case to case, depending upon the geometry of the lesion; but in most cases rubral axons innervated appropriate areas of the grey matter (Fig. 2).

Assuming that rubral axons grow around a lesion of their spinal pathway during early development, we sought to determine whether such plasticity results from regeneration of cut axons or from new growth. Our initial approach was to determine whether rubrospinal neurons survived axotomy. If not, developmental plasticity could not have resulted from regeneration of cut axons. In experiments designed to address this issue, we labeled rubrospinal neurons at different stages of development by unilateral or bilateral injections of FB into the thoracic cord. After an appropriate survival to allow for retrograde labeling, the rubrospinal tract was cut unilaterally several segments rostral to the injection(s). Thirty days later, the animals were killed so that sections through the red nucleus could be examined for labeled neurons. Rubrospinal neurons were labeled contralateral to the lesion during the critical period for plasticity, but in the cases with bilateral injections, they were not as numerous as those labeled ipsilateral to it. When the number of labeled neurons was compared on the two sides, it was concluded that approximately 75% failed to survive axotomy (Xu and Martin, 1992). In adult animals subjected to the same procedure, only 25% died (Xu and Martin, 1990). The failure of most rubrospinal neurons to survive axotomy during the critical period for plasticity suggested that plasticity did not result primarily from regeneration of cut axons.

In order to address this issue more directly, we performed the experiment shown diagrammatically in Fig. 3. Bilateral injections of FB were made into the rostral lumbar cord during the critical period for rubrospinal plasticity. The intent of the injections was to label rubrospinal neurons that supported axons at the injection site. After approximately 4 days, the rubrospinal tract was lesioned unilaterally 4–5 segments rostral to the injections. Approximately 30 days later, DY was injected between the FB injection and the lesion in order to label rubrospinal neurons that supported axons caudal to the lesion. After a 5-day survival to allow for rubrospinal labeling by DY, sections through the red nucleus were searched for neurons labeled by FB, DY or both markers. Relatively few neurons within the red nucleus contralateral to the lesion were labeled by FB (Fig. 4C), supporting the results of the prelabeling experiments described above. Some of the neurons labeled by FB also contained DY, however (Fig. 4B). It was our interpretation that such neurons had survived axotomy, as evidenced

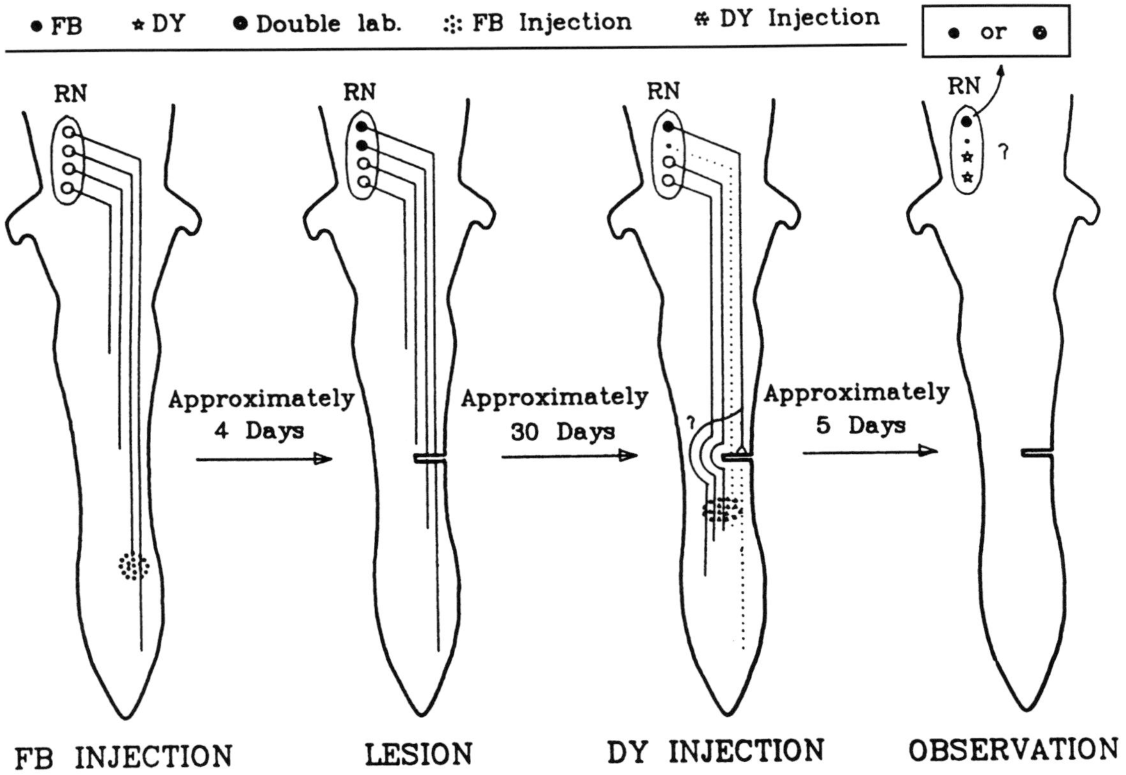

Fig. 3. Schematic drawing of the experimental protocol used for one of the double labeling experiments described in the text. Fast Blue (FB) injections were made into the caudal thoracic or rostral lumbar cord at different ages (FB injection). Approximately 4 days later, after rubrospinal neurons had been labeled by FB, a lesion of their axons was made several segments rostral to the injection (LESION). Approximately 30 days later, a second marker, Diamidino Yellow (DY), was injected into the cord between the FB injection and the lesion (DY INJECTION). Five days later, the animals were killed and the red nucleus (RN) was examined for neurons labeled by one or both markers (OBSERVATION). In some animals, FB was removed by suction at the time of lesioning so that it would not be available to late growing axons during the 30 day survival. (Reproduced from Xu and Martin, 1991; courtesy of Wiley-Liss.)

by the presence of FB, and that they supported an axon or axons which had regenerated around the lesion, as indicated by the presence of DY. Most neurons were labeled by DY alone, however (Fig. 4A). Axons of such neurons were apparently not present at rostral lumbar levels when the FB injections were made, but rather grew around the lesion to incorporate DY during the 30 + day survival. These results suggest that developmental plasticity of the rubrospinal tract, like that of the corticospinal tract (Tolbert and Der, 1987; Merline and Kalil, 1990; Bates and Stelzner, 1993), results primarily from growth of late arriving axons around the lesion. Since late growing axons may have incorporated residual FB as well as DY in the above experiments, we carried out a modified double labeling procedure in which FB was removed by gentle suction at the time of lesioning. Double labeled neurons were still present, however, supporting our interpretation that regeneration of cut axons had occurred.

The relative lack of axonal regeneration in the experiments described above might be related to the failure of most rubrospinal neurons to survive axotomy during the critical period for plasticity (Xu and Martin, 1992). When fetal spinal cord is transplanted into the lesion cavity of spinal cords hemisected at midthoracic levels in neonatal rats, rubrospinal neurons survive axotomy in greater numbers than in lesioned animals without transplants (Bregman and Reier, 1986) and many of the surviving neurons support axons which regenerate into the transplant (Bregman and Bernstein-Goral, 1991; Bernstein-Goral and Bregman, 1993). It is possible that the transplants provided trophic factors which rescued axotomized rubrospinal neurons, making more of them available to support regenerative growth. In that regard, it is interesting that brain-derived neurotrophic factor (BDNF) and neurotrophin-3 (NT-3) rescue rubrospinal neurons from axotomy-induced death in PD3 rats (Diener-Ostfield et al., 1993) and that BDNF rescues rubrospinal neurons from shrinkage after axotomy in adult rats (Tetzlaff et al., 1993).

We have also asked whether reticulospinal and vestibulospinal axons grow around a lesion during development. In these experiments, the caudal thoracic spinal cord was hemisected at different stages of development and, approximately 30 days later, bilateral injections of FB were made several segments caudal to the lesion. After an appropriate survival to allow for FB labeling, the animals were killed and sections through the brainstem were examined for labeled neurons. When the lesion was made relatively late during the critical period for rubrospinal plasticity (PD20), rubral neurons were labeled contralateral to the lesion as expected (Fig. 5A,B), but neurons were not labeled ipsilateral to the lesion in those areas of the pontine reticular formation and lateral vestibular nucleus which project almost exclusively ipsilaterally (the areas within the rectangles, Fig. 5C–E; Martin et al., 1992; Wang et al., 1994). When the same experiment was performed at PD12 or 5, however, neurons were labeled in the latter areas (the areas within the rectangles, Figs. 6C–E) as well as within the contralateral red nucleus (Fig. 6A,B). We have interpreted these results to show that ret iculospinal and vestibulospinal axons, like rubrospinal axons, bypass a lesion of their spinal pathway during early development and that the critical period for reticulospinal and vestibulospinal plasticity ends earlier than that for rubrospinal axons. Since reticular and vestibular axons grow into the spinal cord before axons from the red nucleus (Cabana and Martin, 1981, 1984; Martin et al., 1993), it appears that axons which reach the spinal cord first lose their potential for plasticity before axons which arrive at a later date.

The above results suggest that the end of the critical period for brainstem-spinal plasticity results from loss of growth potential with maturity. It seemed reasonable to ask, therefore, whether the end of the critical period correlates temporally with loss of the ability to synthesize and transport GAP-43, a protein known to be present in regenerating and growing axons (Skene and Willard, 1981; Kalil and Skene, 1986; Meiri et al., 1986; Moya et al., 1989; Skene, 1989). In order to identify GAP-43, we employed a monoclonal antibody (9-lE12) reported to identify all of its known epitopes (Goslin et al., 1988, 1990). As expected, GAP-43 immunostaining was abundant in the lateral funiculus, the location of rubrospinal axons (Martin and Dom, 1970), and in the ventral funiculus, the location of pontine reticulospinal and lateral vestibulospinal axons (Martin et al., 1975, 1979), during the critical periods for rubrospinal, reticulospinal and vestibulospinal plasticity. GAP-43 immunostaining was still present in the lateral and ventral funiculi after the critical period (Fig. 7A) although it decreased with age (compare Figs. 7A and B). One interpretation of these findings is that some of the neurons which support descending spinal axons have the ability to synthesize and transport GAP-43 after the critical period for plasticity and that they retain at least some potential for growth. If so, reduced ability to generate and/or sustain axonal growth is probably not the only factor in loss of developmental plasticity.

Changes in the environment encountered by growing and regenerating axons may also play a

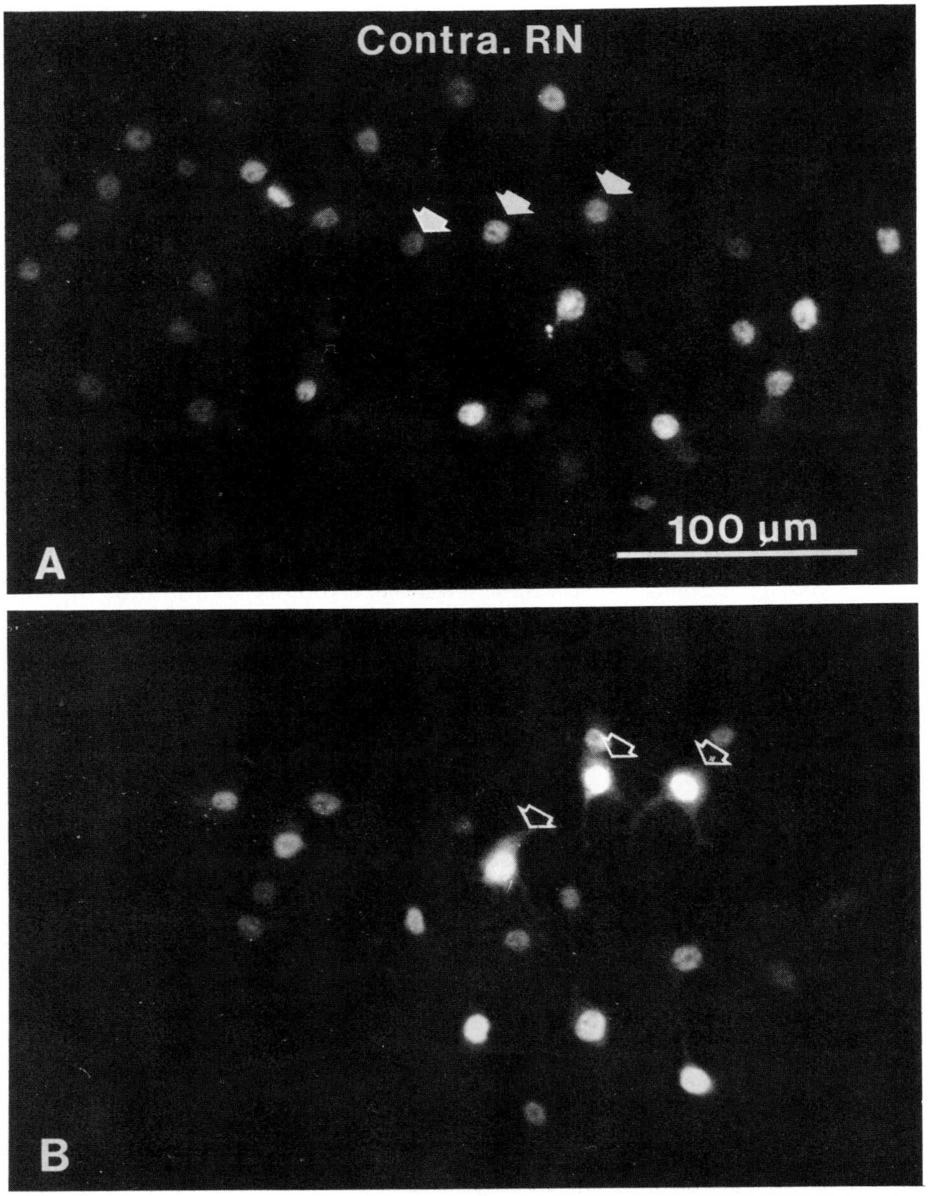

Fig. 4. Fluorescence photomicrographs of neurons labeled by either Fast Blue (FB) or Diamidino Yellow (DY), or by both markers, in the red nucleus contralateral to the lesion (Contra RN) in animals which received bilateral injections of FB and DY and a unilateral lesion of the rubrospinal tract at postnatal day 22. DY single labeled neurons were the most numerous (A, solid arrows),

role in determining the end of the critical period for developmental plasticity. Such changes include the development of myelin, the maturation of glia, and the development of a glial response to lesioning. Schwab and Caroni (1988) have shown that central nervous system myelin is not permissive for axonal growth and that it contains proteins which actually inhibit it (Caroni and Schwab, 1988; Schnell and Schwab, 1990; Kapfhammer et al., 1992). Based on such findings, we asked whether the end of the critical period for brainstem-spinal plasticity correlates temporally with the development of myelin. In order to address this question, we used immunohistochemistry to study the development of myelin basic protein and galactocerebroside-like immunoreactivity in the opossums's spinal cord (Ghooray and Martin, 1993a). The results of such studies showed that myelin basic protein-like immunoreactivity (MBP-LI) is present in the ventral funiculus, the location of pontine reticulospinal and lateral vestibulospinal axons, before it is found in the dorsal part of the lateral funiculus, the location of rubrospinal axons (Fig. 8). The appearance of MBP-LI in each area correlated roughly with the end of the critical period for plasticity of the brainstem-spinal axons contained within it. Such results suggest that the development of myelin may be significant in the end of the critical period for developmental plasticity. Evidence for a cause and effect relationship between myelin formation and loss of developmental plasticity of descending spinal axons has been reported in the chick (Keirstead et al., 1992) and it is discussed in the chapter by Steeves et al. (this volume).

We also studied the development of radial glia and astrocytes immunohistochemically using antibodies against vimentin and glial fibrillary acidic protein (Ghooray and Martin, 1993b). Vimentin is present in radial glia and immature astrocytes

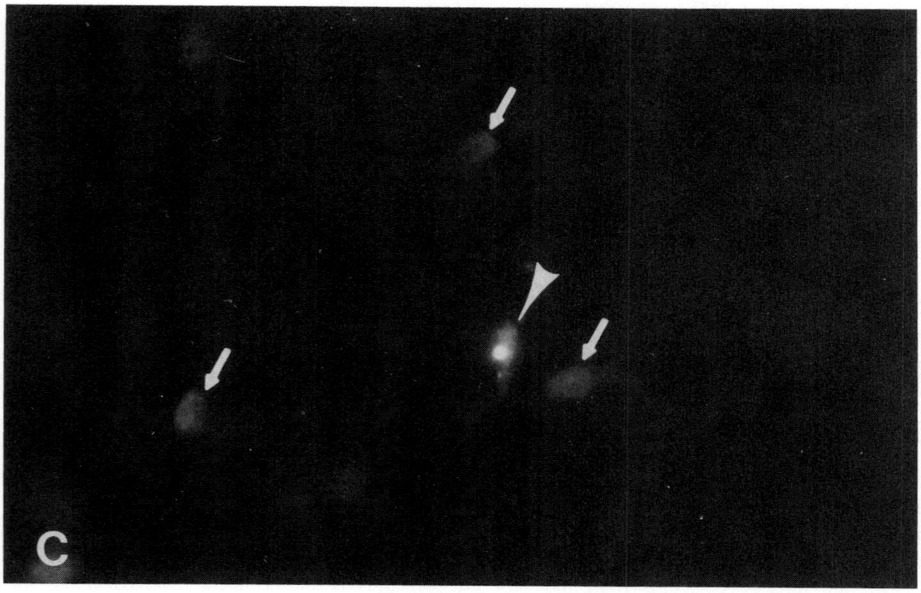

but double labeled neurons were also present (B, open arrows). A few FB single labeled neurons were present (C, long arrows) and small heavily labeled cells could also be identified (C, arrowhead). The bar in A can be used for B and C. (Reproduced from Xu and Martin, 1991; courtesy of Wiley-Liss.)

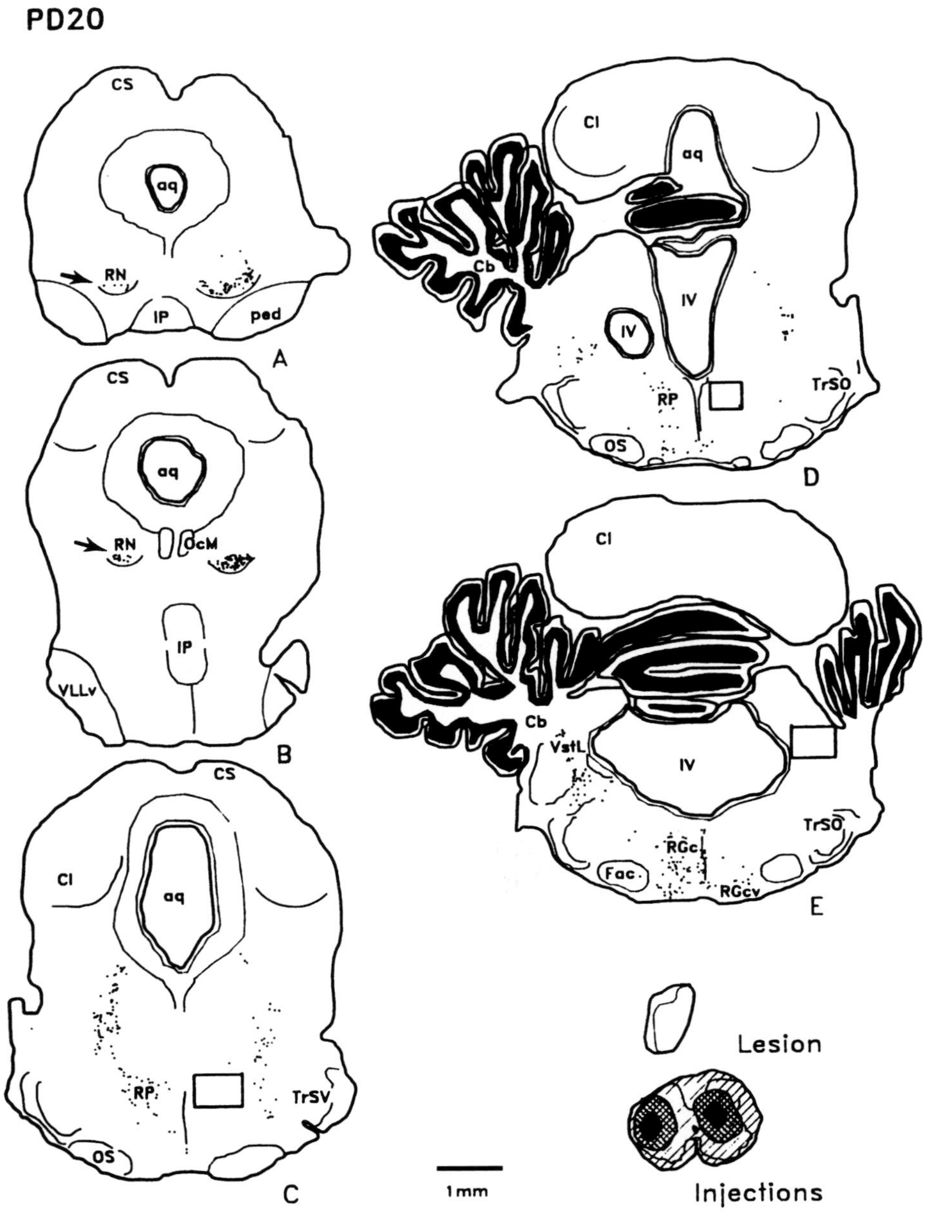

Fig. 5. Plot of labeled neurons (dots) within selected sections of the brainstem of an animal subjected to hemisection of the thoracic cord at postnatal day (PD)20 and bilateral injections of Fast Blue into the lumbar cord 30 days later. Labeled neurons were not present on the side of the lesion in those parts of the pontine reticular and lateral vestibular nuclei which project ipsilaterally (rectangles in sections C–E), but they were present in the contralateral red nucleus (arrows in section A and B). The cerebral aqueduct (aq), the cerebellum (Cb), the inferior colliculus (CI), the superior colliculus (CS), the facial nucleus (Fac), the interpeduncular nucleus (IP), the fourth ventricle (IV), the oculomotor nucleus (OcM), the superior olivary nucleus (OS), the cerebral peduncle (ped), the gigantocellular reticular nucleus (RGc), the ventral gigantocellular reticular nucleus (RGcv), the red nucleus (RN), the pontine reticular nucleus (RP), the oral spinal trigeminal nucleus (TrSo), the ventral sensory trigeminal nucleus (TrsV), and the lateral vestibular nucleus (VstL) are indicated. (Reproduced from Wang et al., 1994; courtesy of Wiley-Liss.).

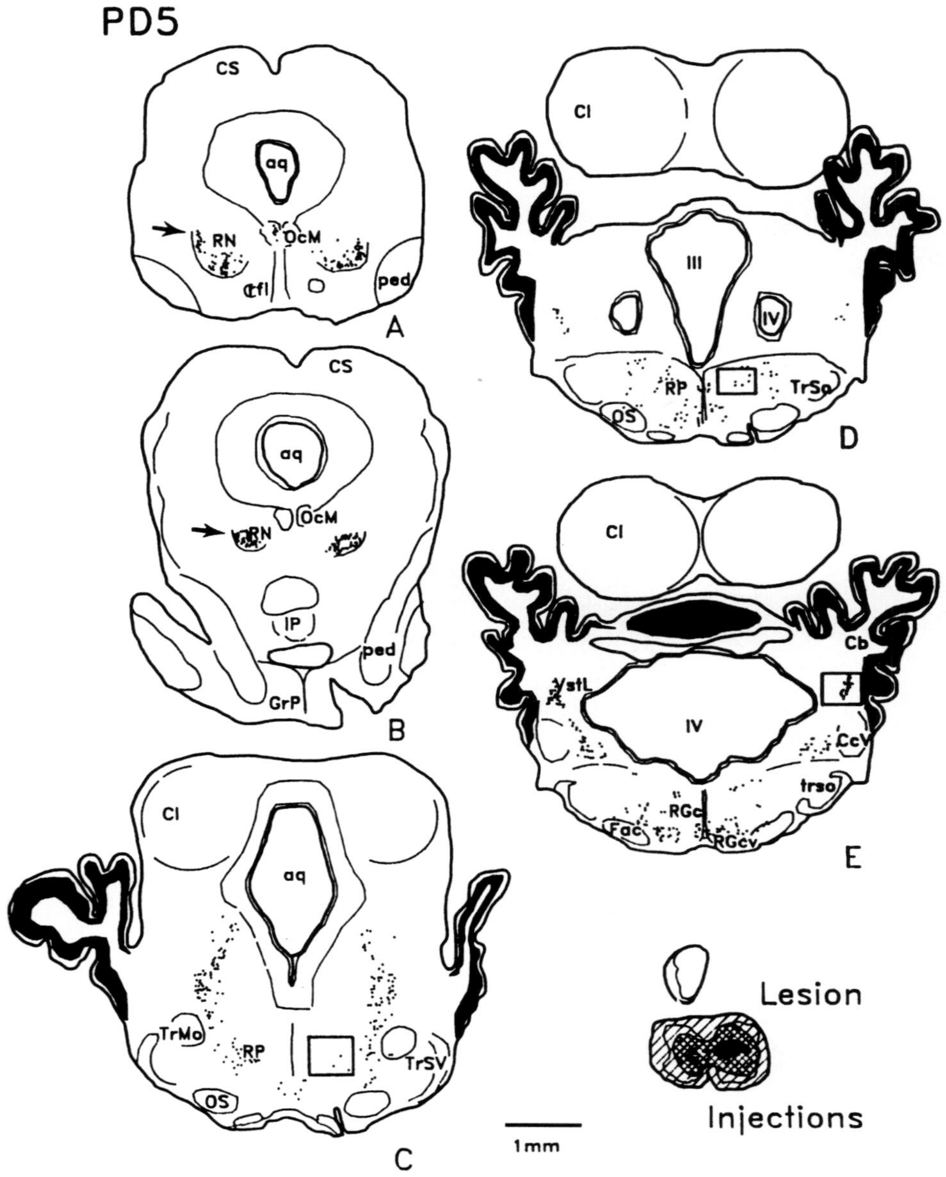

Fig. 6. Plot of labeled neurons (dots) within selected sections of the brainstem from an animal subjected to hemisection of the thoracic cord at postnatal day (PD)5 and bilateral injections of Fast Blue into the lumbar cord approximately 30 days later. Labeled neurons were present ipsilateral to the lesion in those areas of the pontine reticular and lateral vestibular nuclei which project ipsilaterally (rectangles in sections C–E) as well as within the red nucleus contralateral to the lesion (arrows, sections A and B). In addition to the structures referred to in Fig. 5, the pontine nuclei (GrP), the fasciculus retroflexus (rfl) and the motor trigeminal nucleus (TrMo) are indicated. (Reproduced from Wang et al., 1994; courtesy of Wiley-Liss.)

(Pixely and de Vellis, 1984; Voigt, 1989; Yanes et al., 1990; Tohyama et al., 1991), whereas glial fibrillary acidic protein (GFAP) is present within radial glia and mature astrocytes (Eng et al., 1971; Bignami and Dahl, 1976; Levitt and Rakic, 1980). The transition from radial glia to mature-appearing astrocytes occurred earlier in the ventral cord, the location of pontine reticulospinal

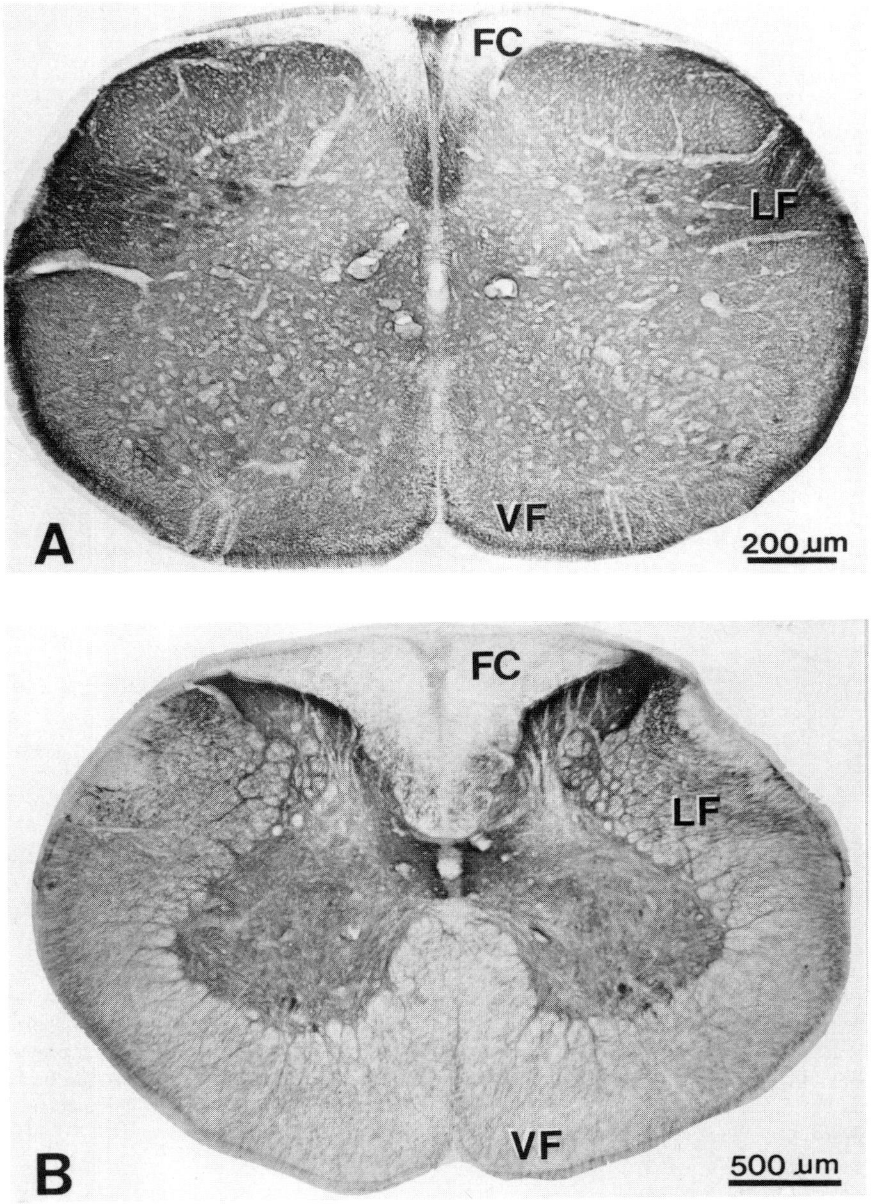

Fig. 7. Photomicrographs of sections through the cervical cord of the opossum (*Didelphis virginiana*) immunostained for GAP-43 at PD47 (A) and PD92 (B). The fasciculus cuneatus (FC), the lateral funiculus (LF) and the ventral funiculus (VF) are indicated.

and lateral vestibulospinal axons, than within the dorsolateral cord, the location of rubrospinal axons (Fig. 9), and in each area it occurred around the end of the critical period for plasticity of the brainstem axons within it. Immature glia may support growing axons (Silver et al., 1982; Silver and Ogawa, 1983; Smith et al., 1986) by mechanical guidance (Singer et al., 1979), the production of extracellular matrix molecules (e.g. Carbonetto et al., 1983, 1987) and the production of trophic and/or tropic factors (e.g. Bregman and Reier, 1986; Repka and Cunningham, 1987; Haun and Cunningham, 1987; Bregman et al., 1989; Bernstein-Goral and Bregman, 1993).

The development of a glial (astrocytic) 'scar' has long been suggested to inhibit axonal regeneration after spinal cord injury in adult mammals and man (see review by Reier et al., 1983). For that reason, we asked whether the development of an astrocytic response to lesioning correlates temporally with the end of the critical period for plasticity (Ghooray and Martin, 1993c). In one set of experiments, the spinal cord of opossum pups was hemisected at midthoracic levels and the animals were allowed to survive 2 weeks before being killed and perfused for GFAP immunohistochemistry. When the spinal cord was hemisected prior to the end of the critical period for rubrospinal plasticity, a relatively mild astrocytic response was observed in the lateral funiculus 2 weeks later. When the hemisection was made near the end of the critical period, hypertrophied astrocytes were present at the junction of the grey matter and lateral funiculus and cystic cavitation was observed.

In a second set of experiments, the pups were allowed to survive 4 weeks after lesioning, the survival time used in the plasticity experiments. Four to 5 days before killing, FB was injected bilaterally 2–3 segments caudal to the lesion to label any rubral neurons whose axons had grown around it. When the lesion was made at later stages during the critical period for rubrospinal plasticity, evidence for a mild astrocytic response was present within the lateral funiculus (Fig. 10B–D) and, as expected, rubral neurons were labeled contralateral to the lesion (Fig. 10E) as well as ipsilateral to it (Fig. 10F). When the lesion was made after the end of the critical period, astrocytic hypertrophy was present at the grey/white interface and cavitation was seen (Fig. 11A–D). In such cases, labeled neurons were not present in the red nucleus contralateral to the lesion (Fig. 11E), but they were present ipsilateral

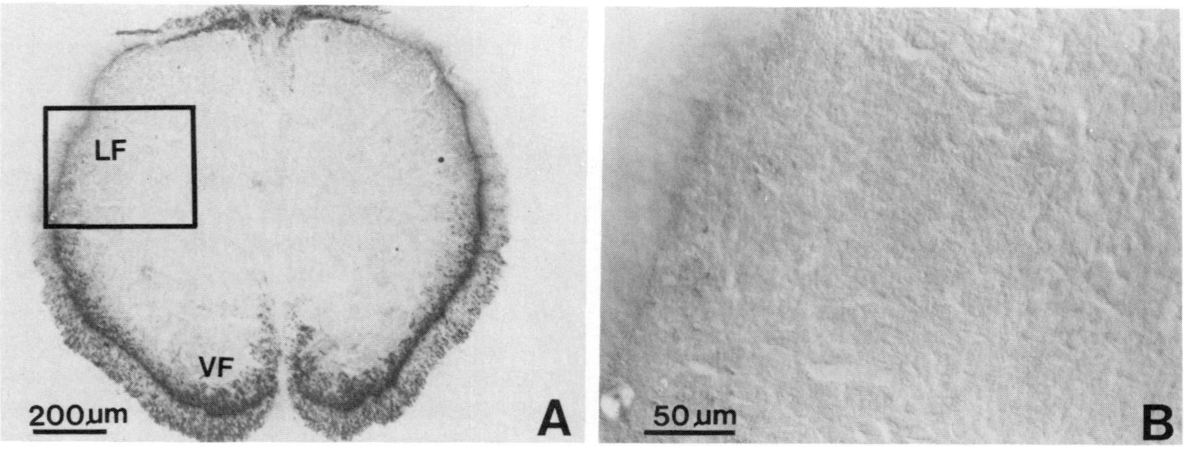

Fig. 8. A photomicrograph of the thoracic cord of the opossum, *Didelphis virginiana*, immunostained for myelin basic protein at PD26 is shown in A. A higher power view of the lateral funiculus is shown in B. The lateral (LF) and ventral (VF) funiculi are indicated in A.

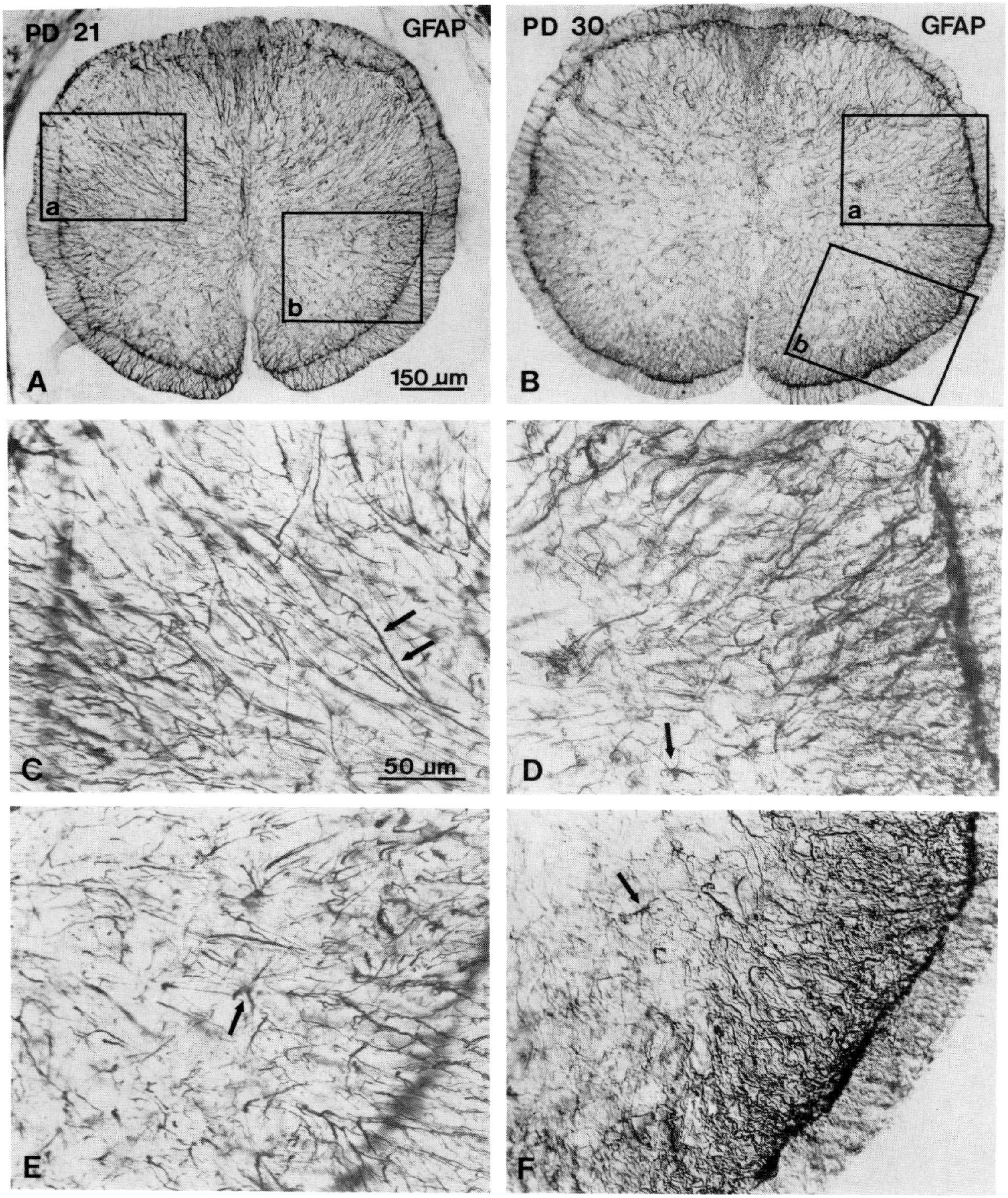

Fig. 9. Photomicrographs from a PD21 opossum showing the distribution of glial fibrillary acid protein (GFAP)-like immunoreactivity in the thoracic cord are presented in A, C and E. The photomicrographs in C and E are higher power views of the areas enclosed by the rectangles labeled 'a' and 'b', respectively, in A. The photomicrographs in B, D and F are from a PD30 opossum showing GFAP-like immunoreactivity in the thoracic cord. Photomicrographs D and F are higher magnifications of the areas enclosed by rectangles labeled 'a' and 'b', respectively, in B. The arrows in C indicate a radial process in the dorsal cord and in D–F they point to mature-appearing astrocytes. (Reproduced from Ghooray and Martin, 1993; courtesy of Wiley-Liss.)

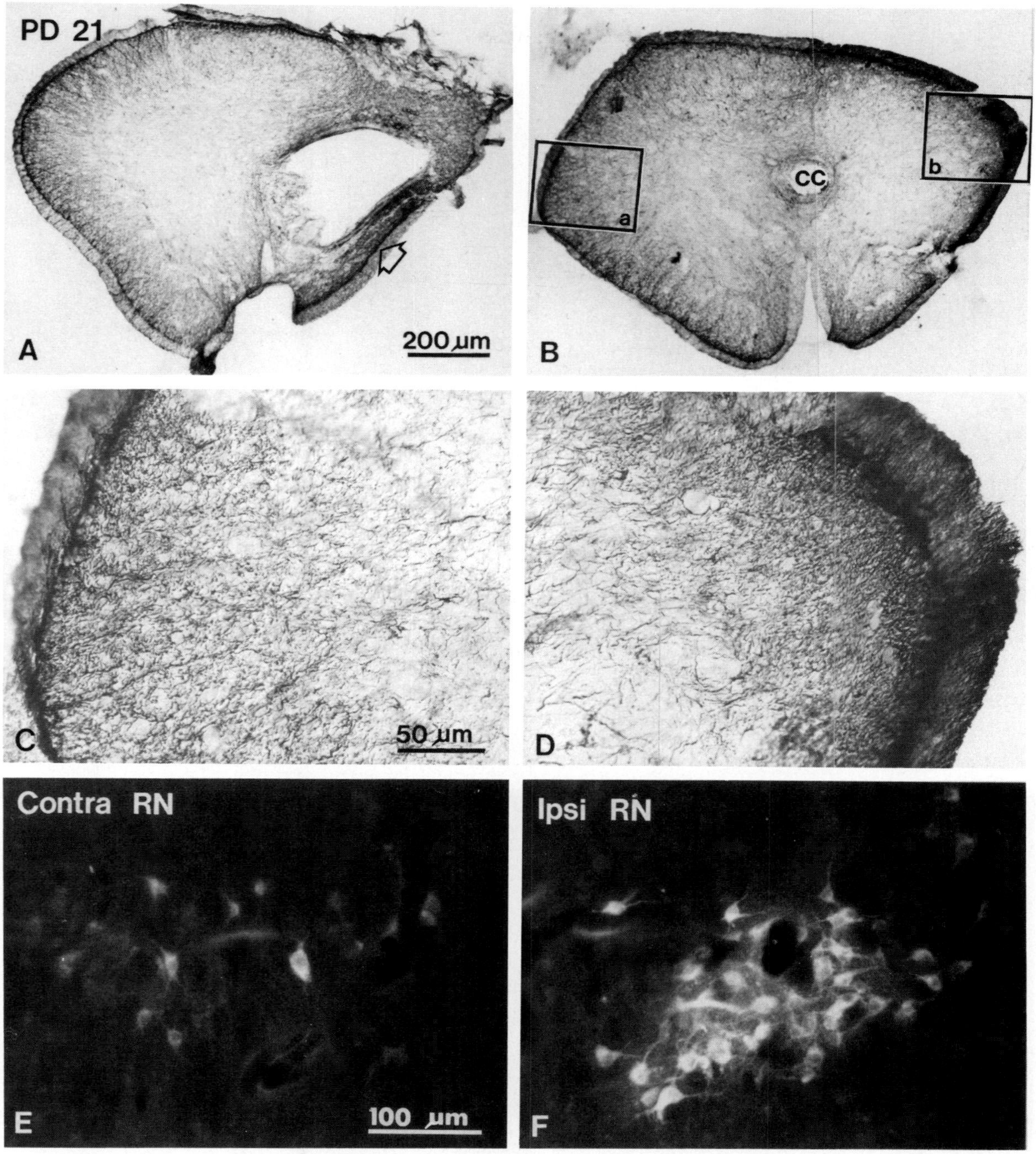

Fig. 10. Photomicrograph A shows the lesion site (GFAP immunostaining) from the spinal cord of an opossum hemisected at PD21 that survived for 4 weeks before death. The section in B is rostral to the lesion site. Higher magnifications of the areas enclosed in rectangles 'a' and 'b' are shown in C and D. A fluorescent photomicrograph showing Fast Blue labeled neurons in the red nucleus contralateral to the lesion (Contra RN) is shown in E and a photomicrograph of labeled neurons in the red nucleus ipsilateral to the lesion (Ipsi RN) is shown in F. The central canal (cc) is indicated in B and the arrow in A indicates the external limiting membrane. (Reproduced from Ghooray and Martin, 1993; courtesy of Wiley-Liss.)

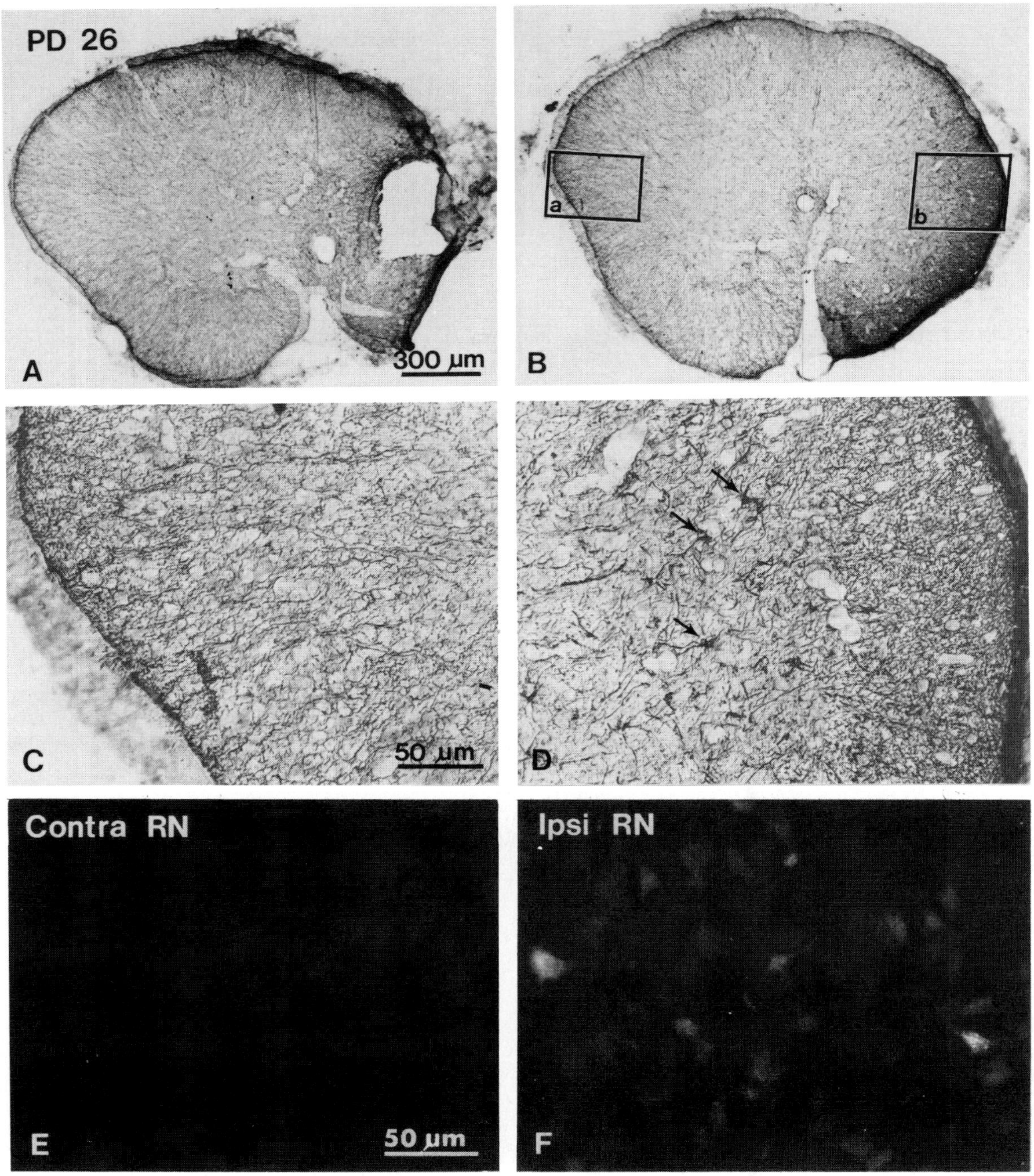

Fig. 11. A photomicrograph of the lesion site (GFAP immunostaining) from the spinal cord of an opossum hemisected at PD26 that survived for 4 weeks is shown in A and a section rostral to the lesion is provided in B. The photomicrographs in C and D are higher magnifications of the areas enclosed in rectangles 'a' and 'b' in panel B. Photomicrographs from the red nucleus contralateral to the lesion (Contra RN) and ipsilateral to it (Ipsi RN) are shown in E and F. Rubral neurons were not labeled contralateral to the lesion, although they were labeled on the ipsilateral side. The arrows in D point to reactive astrocytes. (Reproduced from Ghooray and Martin, 1993; courtesy of Wiley-Liss.)

to it (Fig. 11F). It appears, therefore, that a temporal correlation exists between the end of the critical period for rubrospinal plasticity and the development of hypertrophied astrocytes and cystic cavities at the lesion site. The development of cystic cavities suggests macrophage invasion and phagocytosis of debris, followed by walling off of the resultant cavity.

The Brazilian short-tailed opossum, *Monodelphis domestica*, has also been used for studies of brainstem-spinal plasticity. *Monodelphis* is a pouchless opossum (Fig. 12A) whose young are born in a very immature state, approximately 15 days after conception (Fig. 12B). *Monodelphis* can be bred more easily than *Didelphis*, the species used for the experiments described above, and it is less expensive to maintain. Using *Monodelphis,* we have obtained evidence for brainstem-spinal plasticity similar to that described for *Didelphis*. The thoracic cord was hemisected at PD2, 5, 7, 10 and 15, when brainstem axons are known to be present at that level (Wang et al., 1992), and 2–4 weeks later bilateral injections of FB were made several segments caudal to the lesion. After an appropriate survival for retrograde labeling, the animals were killed so that their spinal cords and brains could be examined with a fluorescence microscope. Rubral neurons were labeled con-

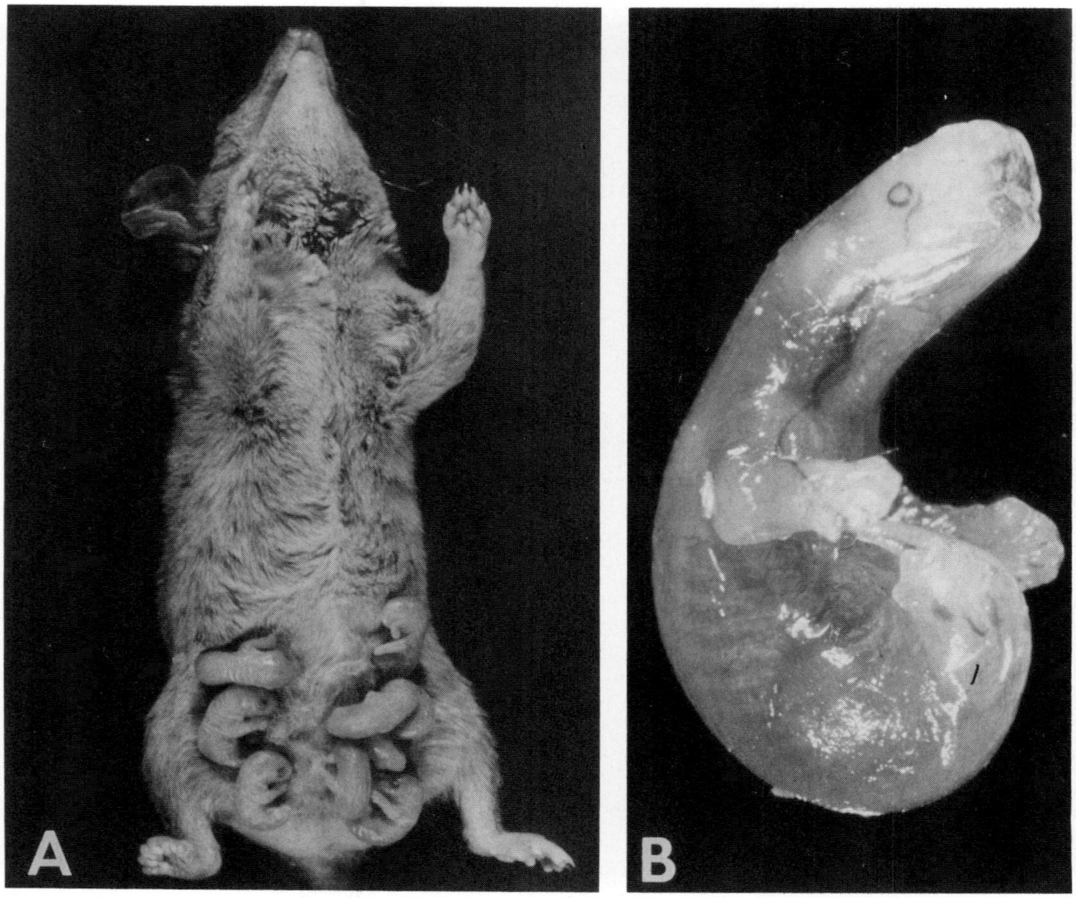

Fig. 12. Photograph of a female *Monodelphis* opossum with young (A) and a newborn *Monodelphis* pup (B). A millimeter rule is provided for B.

tralateral to the lesion, as well as ipsilateral to it, when the injections were made at PD2, 5, 7 (Figs. 13A and B) and 10, but not when it was made at PD15. Neurons were also labeled within the medial pontine reticular formation and the dorsal part of the lateral vestibular nucleus ipsilateral to the lesion, as well as contralateral to it, when the lesion was made at PD2 (Figs. 13C and D). Failure to label reticular and vestibular neurons after PD2 may have been due, in part, to technical problems. In *Monodelphis*, as in *Didelphis*, the red nucleus projects contralaterally and the reticular and vestibular nuclei in question project ipsilaterally (Holst et al., 1991). The earlier loss of rubrospinal plasticity in *Monodelphis* than in *Didelphis* (sometime between PD10 and 15 in *Monodelphis* versus PD26 and 30 in *Didelphis*) is probably a reflection of a more accelerated development in *Monodelphis*.

The developmental history of ascending spinal connections has been reported for *Monodelphis* (Qin et al., 1993), so it may be possible to employ that species to determine whether ascending dorsal root axons, like descending axons from the cerebral cortex and brainstem, are capable of developmental plasticity. In neonatal rats, dorsal root axons do not grow around a lesion of the dorsal columns at cervical levels (Lahr and Stelzner, 1990), although cortical axons do so readily (Bernstein and Stelzner, 1983; Schreyer

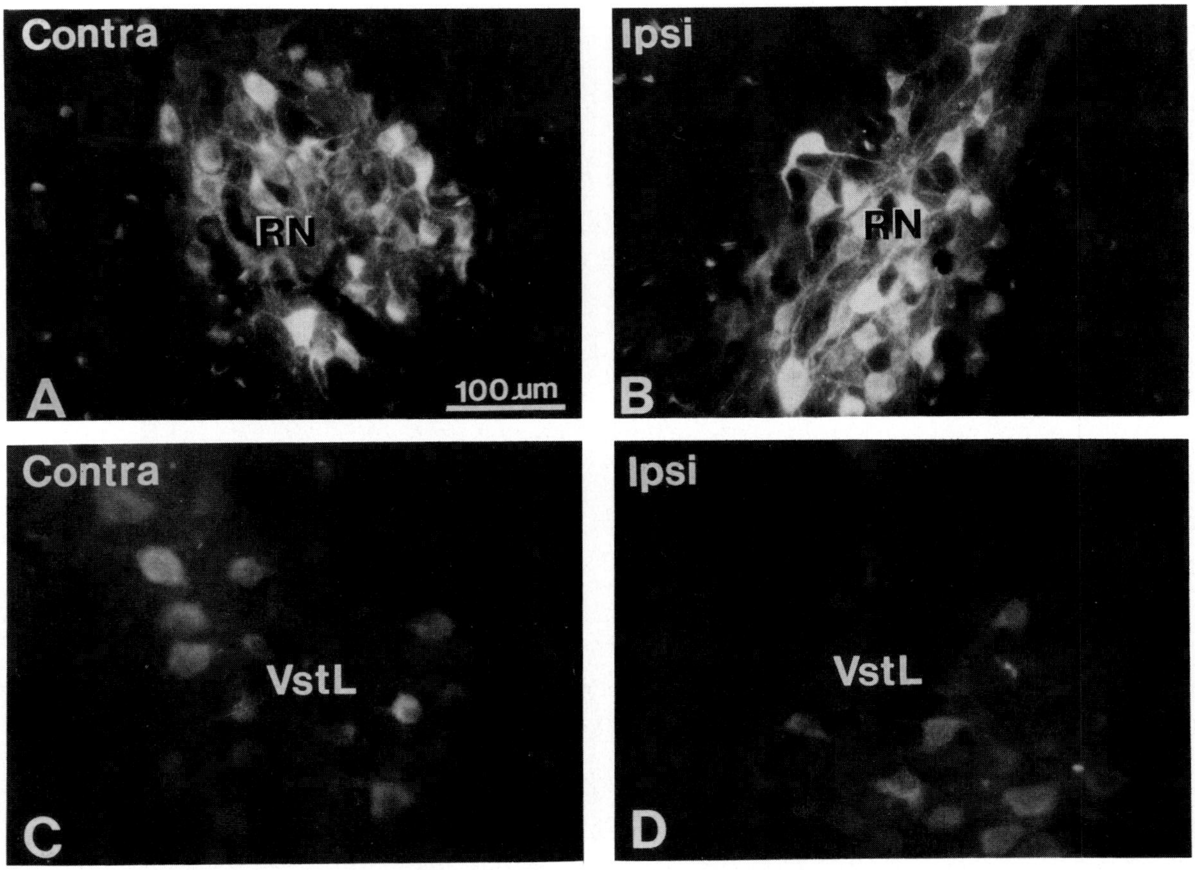

Fig. 13. Photomicrographs A and B document Fast Blue labeling in the red nucleus (RN) contralateral (Contra) and ipsilateral (Ipsi) to a hemisection of the thoracic spinal cord made at PD7 in *Monodelphis*. Labeling in the lateral vestibular nucleus (Vst L) from another animal hemisected at PD2 is shown in C and D.

and Jones, 1983; Bates et al., 1988, 1993). Recent results have shown that dorsal root axons also fail to grow around a lesion of the dorsal columns at thoracic levels in neonates of the same species (Buyan and Stelzner, 1993). Dorsal root axons are relatively mature in newborn rats, since they reach the nucleus gracilis prenatally (Lahr and Stelzner, 1990), and they may have lost their potential for plasticity. In contrast, cortical axons are still growing into the cord at birth (Donatelle, 1977; Schreyer and Jones, 1982) and may retain that capacity. Since the development of the fasciculus gracilis occurs postnatally in *Monodelphis* (Qin et al., 1993), rather than prenatally as in rats and other placental mammals, it may be possible to test that hypothesis.

Monodelphis has also been used for in vitro studies of developmental plasticity. Nicholls and coworkers have shown that the central nervous system of neonates survives in culture medium (Eagle's basal medium) for at least 7 days and that it demonstrates electrical excitability, respiratory activity, reflex responses, cell division and relatively normal ultrastructure (Nicholls et al., 1990; Stewart et al., 1991; Zou et al., 1991; Treherne et al., 1992). Using this model, it has been shown that axons traverse crush lesions of the cervical cord and that conduction across the lesion is reestablished. Axons enter the crush after 3 days and by 5 days they are relatively numerous 2–3 mm distal to it. Growth of axons across the lesion is seen in spinal cords removed prior to PD11, but not in those removed at PD11–14 (Varga et al., 1993), and the critical period for plasticity correlates temporally with the development of myelin-associated inhibitors of neurite growth (Schwab et al., 1993). Use of *Monodelphis* for in vitro studies of spinal cord regeneration is described more completely in the chapter by Nicholls et al. (this volume).

Nonmammalian species as models for spinal cord injury research

Developing birds

The spinal cord of adult birds, like that of adult mammals, does not normally regenerate after transection, but it does during development. When the thoracic cord of chicks is transected prior to embryonic day 13 (E13), anatomical continuity is reestablished and use of retrograde tracing techniques shows that propriospinal and supraspinal axons have grown across the lesion (Shimizu et al., 1990; Hansan et al., 1993). It is of interest that regeneration results in functional recovery. Chicks hatch and locomote normally after transection of the thoracic cord at E2 and E5, when regeneration is robust; but not when the lesion is made at E15, when regeneration no longer occurs. Evidence for functional recovery has also been provided by physiological studies (Valenzuela et al., 1990; Hasan et al., 1991) which indicate that locomotor signals from the brainstem are reestablished during the permissive period for plasticity. It appears from double labeling studies, similar to those described earlier, that regeneration of previously cut axons is a major contributor to the plasticity described above, although growth of late arriving axons also occurs (Hasan et al., 1993). The end of the permissive period for developmental plasticity in chicks correlates temporally with myelin formation, and a cause and effect relationship between those two events has been established experimentally (Keirstead et al., 1992). Use of the embryonic chick as a model for spinal cord regeneration is described in more detail in the chapter by Steeves et al. (this volume).

Lizards

Although regeneration and restitution of function do not occur after transection of the spinal cord in mature mammals and birds, they have been documented after transection of the caudal spinal cord in adult lizards. Most lizards regenerate an amputated tail with at least some regeneration of the caudal spinal cord (Kamrin and Singer, 1955; Simpson, 1968, 1970; Egar et al., 1970). Although the regenerated cord is incomplete, it contains supraspinal and propriospinal axons, some of which have regenerated across the lesion (Duffy et al., 1990, 1992). Most of the axons in the regenerated cord originate immediately rostral to the lesion, however, rather than within the brainstem. In fact, the number of short propriospinal neurons which innervate the caudal cord is greater after tail amputation than in the normal animal (Duffy et al., 1990). Duffy et al. (1992) have suggested that supraspinal axons do not cross the lesion in large numbers because they form synapses immediately rostral to it (see also Bernstein and Bernstein, 1969). Since regeneration does not occur after transection of the spinal cord rostral to levels which innervate the tail, lizards can be used to study segments which do not regenerate normally, as well as segments which do. The chapter by Simpson et al. (this volume) provides a more complete account of lizards as models for spinal cord regeneration.

Salamanders and frogs

Regeneration and restoration of function occur after transection of the spinal cord at all levels in adult salamanders, although it is most robust when the lesion is made at caudal levels (Steffaneli and Capriata, 1943; Steffaneli, 1944, 1950a,b; Steffaneli and Cervi, 1946; Themes, 1950; Santa, 1951; Drummond, 1954; Piatt, 1955a,b; Butler and Ward, 1967; Nordlander and Singer, 1978; Stensaas, 1983; Davis et al., 1989, 1990). After tail amputation in salamanders, the regenerated spinal cord is more complete than after the same manipulation in lizards and it contains motor neurons, interneurons, axonal tracts and dorsal root ganglia (Piatt, 1955a,b). When the spinal cord is transected at thoracic levels, recovery of swimming occurs within 8 weeks, although it is quantitatively different from that in normal animals (Davis et al., 1990). Retrograde tracing studies have shown that recovery of function correlates with growth of propriospinal and supraspinal axons across the lesion (Davis et al., 1989, 1990).

Although regeneration of the transected spinal cord has been documented in adult salamanders, it does not normally occur in adult or juvenile frogs (Piatt and Piatt 1958; Afelt, 1963; Farel, 1971; Beattie et al., 1990). When the thoracic cord is transected in tadpoles, however, and the animals are retained until after metamorphosis, the lumbar cord can be shown to be innervated by most of the supraspinal nuclei which innervate it in the adult animal (Forehand and Farel, 1982; Beattie et al., 1990). It has been suggested that spinal cord regeneration in frogs depends upon hormonal events which occur during metamorphosis (Beattie et al., 1990).

Fish and lampreys

Regeneration of the transected spinal cord and recovery of function are well documented in true fish and lampreys. Of the true fish, the goldfish has been studied most extensively (Windle, 1955; Bernstein, 1964; Bernstein and Bernstein, 1969; Bernstein and Gelder, 1970, 1973; Bernstein et al., 1978; Coggeshall et al., 1982; Bunt and Fill-Moebs, 1984; Bentley and Zottoli, 1993; Sharma et al., 1993). Although regeneration of cut axons occurs after spinal transection in adult goldfish, it may not be complete. Only eleven of the seventeen supraspinal nuclei which normally innervate the spinal cord caudal to the 17th spinal segment do so after transection at the 10th spinal segment (Prasada et al., 1987) and some of the axons which regenerate after transection at the spinomedullary junction enter the first ventral root away from their normal targets (Bentley and Zottoli, 1993). It may be that ventral roots, which are part of the peripheral nervous system, provide a more permissive environment for axonal regeneration than the spinal cord. Such a conclusion would be consistent with the literature in mammals (e.g., David and Aguayo, 1981, 1985). The chapter by Zottoli et al. (this volume) deals with inappropriate pathway choices by regenerating axons in goldfish. It is of interest that axons of Mauthner cells survive separation from their somata for at least 77 days at 14°C in the goldfish (Zottoli et al., 1987) and that neurons which support regenerating axons caudal to the lesion are larger than normal (Sharma et al., 1993).

After transection of the rostral spinal cord in lampreys, recovery of locomotor activity occurs within 3–6 weeks (Rovainen, 1976; Selzer, 1977; McClellan, 1992) and axons which originate within the spinal cord and brainstem regenerate across the lesion (Rovainen, 1976; Selzer, 1977; Wood and Cohen, 1979; Yin and Selzer, 1983; Davis and

McClellan, 1993, 1994a,b). At least some of the axons which traverse the lesion make correct connections (Mackler and Selzer, 1987). Recovery of locomotor activity has been correlated with regeneration of reticulospinal axons known to activate central pattern generators (McClellan, 1990a, 1992; Davis and McClellan, 1993), but mechanoreceptor stimulation also plays a role (McClellan and Sigvardt, 1988; McClellan, 1990b). It is interesting that regeneration of supraspinal axons in the lamprey occurs more slowly than recovery of locomotor function, suggesting that recovery does not necessitate complete restoration of original connections. This issue is discussed by McClellan in this volume.

It is appropriate to ask why regeneration of the spinal cord is so robust in true fish and lampreys. In light of the possible role played by myelin formation in loss of developmental plasticity in opossums and birds (Keirstead et al., 1992; Ghooray and Martin, 1993a; Schwab et al., 1993), it is worth noting that in fish, central nervous system myelin does not inhibit axonal growth (Bastmeyer et al., 1991), and in lampreys, myelin is not present in the spinal cord (Rovainen, 1979). This issue, as well as others related to the presence of spinal cord regeneration in nonmammalian vertebrates, is also discussed in the chapter by McClellan (this volume).

Concluding comments

From the literature reviewed herein it appears that the spinal cord of mammals is capable of greater plasticity during development than at maturity. Cortical and brainstem axons grow around a lesion of their spinal pathway during development and they innervate areas caudal to the lesion which are appropriate to them. It also appears that axons will grow through a complete transection of the cord in vitro. Developmental plasticity of descending spinal axons, at least that reported to date, results primarily from redirection of late growing axons which were not injured by the lesion, rather than regeneration of cut axons. Regeneration of cut axons has been documented, however, and its presence or absence may depend upon the age of the animal at the time of lesioning and/or the distance between the lesion and the axotomized cell body. Distance between the lesion and cell body is particularly interesting. In adult rats, regeneration-related genes are turned on best when axotomy is close to the cell body (see Tetzlaff et al., 1993 and this volume). Unfortunately, such lesions also result in extensive cell death and shrinkage.

Loss of developmental plasticity in mammals may result from decreased ability to initiate and/or sustain axonal elongation with age, but changes in the environment encountered by late growing and regenerating axons probably play a part. Changes in the environment include myelin formation, the transition from radial glia to mature astrocytes, and the development of an astrocytic response to lesioning. Future work should be directed toward identifying the permissive and restrictive factors associated with such changes.

Supraspinal neurons die in large numbers after axotomy in immature mammals, and one explanation for this phenomenon is that they are particularly susceptible to loss of trophic factors. If trophic factors rescue axotomized neurons, as suggested for the neonatal and adult rat, it may be possible to increase the number of neurons available to support regenerating axons. The ability of neurotrophic factors to rescue rubrospinal and corticospinal neurons after axotomy is discussed by Tetzlaff in this volume.

Embryonic chicks as well as adult reptiles, amphibians, fish and lampreys have proven useful for spinal cord injury research because their spinal cords regenerate, at least to some degree, after transection, and regeneration can be correlated with return of function. Using such models, it may be possible to establish the requirements for spinal cord regeneration and functional recovery as well as the mechanisms which underlie them.

Acknowledgements

The authors would like to thank Ms. Mary Ann Jarrell for surgical assistance, tissue processing and plotting related to the experiments from our laboratory described herein, and Mr. Karl Rubin for photographic help. Our studies were supported by USPHS grants NS-25095 and NS-10165 to G.F.M.

References

Afelt, Z. (1963) Variability of reflexes in chronic spinal frogs. In: E. Gutmann and P. Hnik (Eds.), *Central and Peripheral Mechanisms of Motor Function*, Czechoslovak Academy of Science, Prague, pp. 37–41.

Allen, A.R. (1911) Surgery of experimental lesion of spinal cord equivalent to crush injury or fracture dislocation of spinal column. A preliminary report. *J. Am. Med. Assoc.*, 57: 870–880.

Ballentine, J.D. (1985) Hypotheses in spinal cord trauma research. In: D.P. Becker and J.T. Povlishock (Eds.), *Central Nervous System Trauma Status Report*, NIH- NINCDS, Washington, pp. 455–461.

Bastmeyer, M., Beckmann, M., Schwab, M.E. and Stuermer, C.A.O. (1991) Growth of regenerating goldfish axons is inhibited by rat oligodendrocytes and CNS myelin but not by goldfish optic nerve tract oligodendrocytelike cells and fish CNS myelin. *J. Neurosci.*, 11: 626–640.

Bates, C.A. and Stelzner, D.J. (1989) Regrowth of corticospinal axons after spinal injury in the neonatal rat. *Soc. Neurosci. Abstr.*, 15: 321.

Bates, C.A. and Stelzner, D.J. (1993) Extension and regeneration of corticospinal axons after early spinal injury and the maintenance of corticospinal topography. *Exp. Neurol.*, 123: 106–117.

Beattie, M.S., Stokes, B.T. and Bresnahan, J.C. (1988) Experimental spinal cord injury. Strategies for acute and chronic intervention based on anatomic, physiological, and behavioral studies. In: D.G. Stein and B.A. Sabel (Eds.), *Pharmacological Approaches to the Treatment of Brain and Spinal Cord Injury*, Plenum, New York, pp. 43–74.

Beattie, M.S., Bresnahan, J.C. and Lopate, G. (1990) Metamorphosis alters the response to spinal cord transection in *Xenopus laevis* frogs. *J. Neurobiol.*, 21: 1108–1122.

Bentley, A.P. and Zottoli, S.J. (1993) Central nervous system lesion triggers inappropriate pathway choice in adult vertebrate system. *Brain Res.*, 630: 333–336.

Bernstein, D.R. and Stelzner, D.J. (1983) Plasticity of the corticospinal tract following midthoracic spinal injury in the neonatal rat. *J. Comp. Neurol.*, 221: 382–400.

Bernstein, J.J. (1964) Relation of spinal cord regeneration to age in adult goldfish. *Exp. Neurol.*, 9: 161–174.

Bernstein, J.J. and Bernstein, M.E. (1969) Ultrastructure of normal regeneration and loss of regenerative capacity following teflon blockage in goldfish spinal cord. *Exp. Neurol.*, 24: 538–557.

Bernstein, J.J. and Gelder, J.B. (1970) Regeneration of the long spinal tracts in the goldfish. *Brain Res.*, 20: 33–38.

Bernstein, J.J. and Gelder, J.B. (1973) Synaptic reorganization following regeneration of goldfish spinal cord. *Exp. Neurol.*, 41: 402–410.

Bernstein, J.J., Wells, M.R. and Bernstein, M.E. (1978) Spinal cord regeneration. In: C.W. Cotman (Ed.), *Neuronal Plasticity*, Raven Press, New York, pp. 50–71.

Bernstein-Goral, H. and Bregman, B.S. (1993) Spinal cord transplants support the regeneration of axotomized neurons after spinal cord lesions at birth: a quantitative double-labeling study. *Exp. Neurol.*, 123: 118–132.

Bignami, A. and Dahl, D. (1976) Astroglial response to stabbing. Immunofluorescence studies with antibodies to an astrocyte specific protein (GFA) in mammalian and submammalian vertebrates. *Neuropathol. Appl. Neurobiol.*, 2: 99–110.

Bregman, B.S. and Bernstein-Goral, H. (1991) Both regenerating and late-developing pathways contribute to transplant-induced anatomical plasticity after spinal cord lesions at birth. *Exp. Neurol.*, 112: 49–63.

Bregman, B.S. and Goldberger, M.E. (1982) Anatomical plasticity and sparing of function after spinal cord damage in neonatal cats. *Science*, 217: 553–555.

Bregman, B.S. and Goldberger, M.E. (1983a) Infant lesion effect: I. Development of motor behavior following neonatal spinal cord injury in cats. *Dev. Brain Res.*, 9: 103–117.

Bregman, B.S. and Goldberger, M.E. (1983b) Infant lesion effect. III. Anatomical correlates of sparing and recovery of function after spinal cord damage in newborn and adult cats. Dev. *Brain Res.*, 9: 137–154.

Bregman, B.S. and Reier, P.J. (1986) Neural tissue transplants rescue axotomized rubrospinal cells from retrograde death. *J. Comp. Neurol.*, 244: 86–95.

Bregman, B.S., Kunkel-Bagden, E., McAtee, M. and O'Neill, A. (1989) Extension of the critical period for developmental plasticity of the corticospinal pathway. *J. Comp. Neurol.*, 282: 355–370.

Bunt, S.M. and Fill-Moebs, P. (1984) Selection of pathways by regenerating spinal cord fiber tracts. *Dev. Brain Res.*, 16: 307–311.

Butler, E.G. and Ward, M.B. (1967) Reconstitution of the spinal cord after ablation in adult *Triturus*. *Dev. Biol.*, 15: 464–486.

Buyan, L.J. and Stelzner, D.J. (1993) Comparison of the regenerative response of dorsal column axons after neonatal cervical or lumbar lesion. *Soc. Neurosci. Abstr.*, 19: 681.

Cabana, T. and Martin, G.F. (1981) The origin of brainstem-spinal projections at different stages of development in the North American opossum. *Dev. Brain Res.*, 2: 163–168.

Cabana, T. and Martin, G.F. (1984) Developmental sequences in the origin of descending spinal pathways. Studies using retrograde transport techniques in the North American opossum (*Didelphis virginiana*). *Dev. Brain Res.*, 15: 247–263.

Carbonetto, S., Gruver, M.M. and Turner, D.C. (1983) Nerve fiber growth in culture on fibronectin, collagen, and glycosaminoglycan substrates. *J. Neurosci.*, 3: 2324- 2335.

Carbonetto, S., Evans, D. and Cochard, P. (1987) Nerve fiber growth in culture on tissue substrata from central and peripheral nervous systems. *J. Neurosci.*, 7: 610–620.

Caroni, P. and Schwab, M. (1988) Two membrane protein fractions from rat central myelin with inhibitory properties for neurite growth and fibroblast spreading. *J. Cell Biol.*, 106: 1281–1288.

Clemente, C.D. (1964) Regeneration in the vertebrate central nervous system. *Int. Rev. Neurobiol.*, 6: 257–301.

Coggeshall, R.E., Birse, S.G. and Youngblood, C.S. (1982) Recovery from spinal transection in fish. *Neurosci. Lett.*, 32: 259–264.

Collins, G. and West, N. (1989) Prospects for axonal regrowth in spinal cord injury. *Brain Res. Bull.*, 22: 89–92.

Crutcher, K.A., Humbertson, A.0. and Martin, G.F. (1978) The origin of brainstem-spinal pathways in the North American opossum (*Didelphis virginiana*). Studies using the horseradish peroxidase method. *J. Comp. Neurol.*, 179: 169–194.

David, S. and Aguayo, A.J. (1981) Axonal elongation into peripheral nervous system 'bridges' after central nervous system injury in adult rats. *Science*, 214: 931–933.

David, S. and Aguayo, A.J. (1985) Axonal regeneration after crush injury of rat central nervous system fibres innervating peripheral nerve grafts. *J. Neurocytol.*, 14: 1–12.

Davidoff, R.A. (1990) The pyramidal tract. *Neurology*, 40: 332–339.

Davis, B.M., Duffy, M.T. and Simpson, S.B., Jr. (1989) Bulbospinal and intraspinal connections in normal and regenerated salamander spinal cord. *Exp. Neurol.*, 103: 41–51.

Davis, B.M., Ayers, J.L., Koran, L., Carlson, J., Anderson, M.C. and Simpson, S.B., Jr. (1990) Time course of salamander spinal cord regeneration and recovery of swimming: HRP retrograde pathway tracing and kinematic analysis. *Exp. Neurol.*, 108: 198–213.

Davis, G.R. and McClellan, A.D. (1993) Time course of anatomical regeneration of descending brainstem neurons and behavioral recovery in spinal-transected lamprey. *Brain Res.*, 602: 131–137.

Davis, G.R. and McClellan, A.D. (1994a) Extent and time course of restoration of brainstem projections in spinal-transected lamprey. *J. Comp. Neurol.*, 344: 65–82.

Davis, G.R. and McClellan, A.D. (1994b) Long distance axonal regeneration of identified lamprey reticulospinal neurons. *Exp. Neurol.*, 127: 94–105.

De La Torre, J.C. (1981) Spinal cord injury. Review of basic and applied research. *Spine*, 6: 315–335.

Diener-Ostfield, P., DiStefano, P.S., McAtee, M.M. and Bregman, B.S. (1993) Trophic and tropic influence of exogenous NT-3 and BDNF after neonatal spinal cord lesions. *Soc. Neurosci. Abstr.*, 19: 1105.

Donatelle, J.M. (1977) Growth of the corticospinal tract and the development of placing reactions in the postnatal rat. *J. Comp. Neurol.*, 175: 207–232.

Drummond, C.D. (1954) The influence of piromen on the regeneration of the spinal cord in adult *Triturus viridescens*. Undergraduate honors thesis, Brown University, Providence, Rhode Island.

Duffy, M.T., Simpson, S.B., Jr., Liebich, D.R. and Davis, B.M. (1990) Origin of spinal cord axons in the lizard regenerated tail: supernormal projections from local spinal neurons. *J. Comp. Neurol.*, 293: 208–222.

Duffy, M.T., Liebich, D.R., Garner, L.K., Hawrych, A., Simpson, S.B., Jr. and Davis, B.M. (1992) Axonal sprouting and frank regeneration in the lizard tail spinal cord: Correlation between changes in synaptic circuitry and axonal growth. *J. Comp. Neurol.*, 316: 363–374.

Egar, M., Simpson, S.B., Jr. and Singer, M. (1970) The growth and differentiation of the regenerating spinal cord of the lizard, *Anolis carolinensis*. *J. Morphol.*, 131: 131–152.

Eng, L.F., Vanderhaeghen, J.J., Bignami, A. and Gerstl, B. (1971) An acidic protein isolated from fibrous astrocytes. *Brain Res.*, 28: 351–354.

Faden, A.I. (1985) Pharmacological therapy in acute spinal cord injury. In: D.P. Becker and J.T. Povlishock (Eds.), *Central Nervous System Trauma Status Report*, NIH-NINCDS, Washington, pp. 481–487.

Farel, P.B. (1971) Long-lasting habituation in spinal frogs. *Brain Res.*, 33: 405–417.

Forehand, C.J. and Farel, P.B. (1982) Anatomical and behavioral recovery from the effects of spinal cord transection: dependence on metamorphosis in anuran larvae. *J. Neurosci.*, 2: 654–662.

Freed, W., De Medinaceli, L. and Wyatt, R. (1985) Promoting functional plasticity in the damaged nervous system. *Science*, 227: 1544–1552.

Ghooray, G.T. and Martin, G.F. (1993a) The development of myelin in the spinal cord of the North American opossum and its possible role in loss of rubrospinal plasticity. A study using myelin basic protein and galactocerebroside immunohistochemistry. *Dev. Brain Res.*, 72: 67–74.

Ghooray, G.T. and Martin, G.F. (1993b) Development of radial glia and astrocytes in the spinal cord of the North American opossum (*Didelphis virginiana*): an immunohistochemical study using anti-vimentin and anti-glial fibrillary acidic protein. *Glia*, 9: 1–9.

Ghooray, G.T. and Martin, G.F. (1993c) Development of an astrocytic response to lesions of the spinal cord in the North American opossum: an immunohistochemical study using anti-glial fibrillary acidic protein. *Glia*, 9: 10–17.

Goslin, K., Schreyer, D.J., Skene, J.H.P. and Banker, G. (1988) Development of neuronal polarity: GAP-43 distinguishes axonal from dendritic growth cones. *Nature (Lond.)*, 336: 672–674.

Goslin, K., Schreyer, D.J., Skene, J.H.P. and Banker, G. (1990) Changes in the distribution of GAP-43 during the development of neuronal polarity. *J. Neurosci.*, 10: 588–602.

Hasan, S.J., Nelson, B.H. Valenzuela, J.I., Keirstead, H.S., Shull, S.E., Ethell, D.W. and Steeves, J.D. (1991) Functional repair of transected spinal cord in embryonic chick. *Restor. Neurol. Neurosci.*, 2: 137–154.

Hasan, S.J., Keirstead, H.S., Muir, G.D. and Steeves, J.D. (1993) Axonal regeneration contributes to repair of injured brainstem-spinal neurons in embryonic chick. *J. Neurosci.*, 13: 492–507.

Haun, F. and Cunningham, T.J. (1987) Specific neurotrophic interactions between cortical and subcortical visual structures in developing rat: in vivo studies. *J. Comp. Neurol.*, 256: 561–569.

Holst, M-C., Ho, R.H. and Martin G.F. (1991) The origins of supraspinal projections to lumbosacral and cervical levels of the spinal cord in the gray short-tailed Brazilian opossum, *Monodelphis* domestica. *Brain Behav. Evol.*, 38: 273–289.

Kalil, K. and Reh, T. (1979) Regrowth of severed axons in the neonatal central nervous system: establishment of normal connections. *Science*, 205: 1158- 1161.

Kalil, K. and Reh, T. (1982) A light and electron microscopic study of regrowing pyramidal tract fibers. *J. Comp. Neurol.*, 211: 265–275.

Kalil, K. and Skene, J.H.P. (1986) Elevated synthesis of an axonally transported protein correlates with axon outgrowth in normal and injured pyramidal tracts. *J. Neurosci.*, 6: 2563–2570.

Kamrin, R.P. and Singer, M. (1955) The influence of the spinal cord in regeneration of the tail of the lizard, *Anolis carolinensis*. *J. Exp. Zool.*, 128: 611–627.

Kapfhammer, J.P., Schwab, M.E. and Schneider, G.E. (1992) Antibody neutralization of neurite growth inhibitors from oligodendrocytes results in expanded pattern of postnatally sprouting retinocollicular axons. *J. Neurosci.*, 12: 2112–2119.

Keirstead, H.S., Hasan, S.J., Muir, G.D. and Steeves, J.D. (1992) Suppression of the onset of myelination extends the permissive period for the functional repair of embryonic spinal cord. *Proc. Natl. Acad. Sci. USA*, 89: 1164–1168.

Kiernan, J.A. (1979) Hypotheses concerned with axonal regeneration in the mammalian nervous system. *Biol. Rev.*, 54: 155–197.

Lahr, S.P. and Stelzner, D.J. (1990) Anatomical studies of dorsal column axons and dorsal root ganglion cells after spinal cord injury in the newborn rat. *J. Comp. Neurol.*, 293: 377–398.

Lakke, E.A.J.F. and Marani, E. (1991) Prenatal descent of rubrospinal fibers through the spinal cord of the rat. *J. Comp. Neurol.*, 314: 67–78.

Levitt, P. and Rakic, P. (1980) Immunoperoxidase localization of glial fibrillary acidic protein in radial glial cells and astrocytes of the developing Rhesus monkey brain. *J. Comp. Neurol.*, 193 815–840.

Mackler, S.A. and Selzer, M.E. (1987) Specificity of synaptic regeneration in the spinal cord of the larval sea lamprey. *J. Physiol.*, 388: 183–198.

Martin, G.F. (1969) Efferent tectal pathways of the opossum (*Didelphis virginiana*). *J. Comp. Neurol.*, 135: 209–224.

Martin, G.F. and Dom, R. (1970) The rubrospinal tract of the opossum, *Didelphis virginiana*. *J. Comp. Neurol.*, 138: 19–30.

Martin, G.F. and Dom, R. (1971) Reticulospinal fibers of the opossum, *Didelphis virginiana*. II. Course, caudal extent and distribution. *J. Comp. Neurol.*, 141: 467–484.

Martin, G.F., and Xu, X.M. (1988) Evidence for developmental plasticity of the rubrospinal tract. Studies using the North American opossum. *Dev. Brain Res.*, 39: 303–308.

Martin, G.F., Beattie, M.S., Bresnahan, J.C., Henkel, C.K. and Hughes, H.C. (1975) Cortical and brain stem projections to the spinal cord of the American opossum, *Didelphis marsupialis virginiana*. *Brain Behav. Evol.*, 12: 270–310.

Martin, G.F., Humbertson, A.0., Laxson, L.C., Panneton, W.M. and Tschismadia, I. (1979) Spinal projections from the mesencephalic and pontine reticular formation in the North American opossum: a study using axonal transport techniques. *J. Comp. Neurol.*, 187: 373–400.

Martin, G.F., Cabana, T., Humbertson, A.O., Laxson, L.C., and Panneton, W.M. (1981) Spinal projections from the medullary reticular formation of the North American opossum: evidence for connectional heterogeneity. *J. Comp. Neurol.*, 196: 663–682.

Martin, G.F., Wang, X.M. and Xu, X.M. (1992) Developmental plasticity of selected brainstem-spinal pathways. *Soc. Neurosci. Abstr.*, 18: 1321.

Martin, G.F., Pindzola, R.R. and Xu, X.M. (1993) The origins of descending projections to the lumbar spinal cord at different stages of development in the North American opossum. *Brain Res. Bull.*, 30: 303–317.

McClellan, A.D. (1990a) Locomotor recovery in spinal-transected lamprey: role of functional regeneration of descending axons from the brainstem locomotor command neurons. *Neuroscience*, 37: 781–798.

McClellan, A.D. (1990b) Locomotor recovery in spinal-transected lamprey: regenerated spinal coordinating neurons and mechanosensory inputs couple locomotor activity across a spinal lesion. *Neuroscience*, 35: 675–685.

McClellan, A.D. (1992) Functional regeneration and recovery of locomotor activity in spinally transected lamprey. *J. Exp. Zool.*, 261: 274–287.

McClellan, A.D. and Sigvardt, K.A. (1988) Features of entrainment of spinal pattern generators for locomotor activity in the lamprey spinal cord. *J. Neurosci.*, 8: 133–145.

McCrady, E. (1938) The embryology of the opossum. *Amer. Anat. Memoirs*, No. 16, The Wistar Institute of Anatomy and Biology, Philadelphia.

Meiri, K.F., Pfenninger, K.H. and Willard, M.B. (1986) Growth associated protein, GAP-43, a polypeptide that is induced when neurons extend axons, is a component of growth cones and corresponds to pp 46, a major polypeptide of a subcellular fraction enriched in growth cones. *Proc. Natl. Acad. Sci. USA*, 83: 3537–3541.

Merline, M. and Kalil, K. (1990) Cell death of corticospinal neurons is induced by axotomy before but not after innervation of spinal targets. *J. Comp. Neurol.*, 296: 506–516.

Moya, K.L., Jhaveri, S., Schneider, G.E. and Benowitz, L.I. (1989) Immunohistochemical localization of GAP-43 in the developing hamster retinofugal pathway. *J. Comp. Neurol.*, 288: 51–58.

Nicholls, J.G., Stewart, R.R., Erulkar, S.D. and Saunders, N.R. (1990) Reflexes, fictive respiration and cell division in the brain and spinal cord of the newborn opossum, *Monodelphis domestica*, isolated and maintained in vitro. *J. Exp. Biol.*, 152: 1–15.

Nordlander, R.H. and Singer, M. (1978) The role of ependyma in regeneration of the spinal cord in the urodele amphibian tail. *J. Comp. Neurol.*, 180: 349- 374.

Pettegrew, R.K. and Windle, W.F. (1976) Factors in recovery from spinal cord injury. *Exp. Neurol.*, 53: 815–829.

Piatt, J. (1955a) Regeneration of the spinal cord in the salamander. *J. Exp. Zool.*, 29: 177–208.

Piatt, J. (1955b) Regeneration in the central nervous system of amphibia. In: W.F. Windle and L. Chas (Eds.), *Regeneration in the Central Nervous System*, Thomas, Springfield, IL, pp. 20–46.

Piatt, J. and Piatt, M. (1958) Transection of the spinal cord in the adult frog. *Anat. Rec.*, 131: 81–95.

Pixley, S.K.R. and deVellis, J. (1984) Transition between immature radial glia and mature astrocytes studied with a monoclonal antibody to vimentin. *Dev. Brain Res.*, 15: 201–209.

Prasada Rao, P.D., Jadhao, A.G. and Sharma, S.C. (1987) Descending projection neurons to the spinal cord of the goldfish, *Carassius auratus*. *J. Comp. Neurol.*, 265: 96–108.

Prendergast, L.J. and Stelzner, D. (1976) Changes in the magnocellular portion of the red nucleus following thoracic hemisection in the neonatal and adult rat. *J. Comp. Neurol.*, 166: 163–172.

Puchala, E. and Windle, W.F. (1977) The possibility of structural and functional restitution after spinal cord injury. A review. *Exp. Neurol.*, 55: 1–42.

Qin, Y.Q., Wang, X.M. and Martin, G.F. (1993) The early development of major projections from caudal levels of the spinal cord to the brainstem and cerebellum in the gray short-tailed Brazilian opossum *Monodelphis domestica*. *Dev. Brain Res.*, 75: 75–90.

Reier, P.J., Stensaas, L.J. and Guth, L. (1983) The astrocytic scar as an impediment to regeneration in the central nervous system. In: C.C. Kao, R.P. Bunge and P.J. Reier (Eds.), *Spinal Cord Reconstruction*, Raven Press, New York, pp. 163–195.

Repka, A. and Cunningham, T.J. (1987) Specific neurotrophic interactions between cortical and subcortical visual structures in developing rat: in vitro studies. *J. Comp. Neurol.*, 256: 552–560.

Richardson, P.M., Issa, V.M.K. and Aguayo, A.J. (1984) Regeneration of long spinal axons in the rat. *Neurocytology*, 13: 165–182.

Rovainen, C.M. (1976) Regeneration of Muller and Mauthner axons after spinal transection in larval lampreys. *J. Comp. Neurol.*, 168: 545–554.

Rovainen, C.M. (1979) Neurobiology of lampreys. *Physiol. Rev.*, 59: 1007–1077.

Sandler, A.N. and Tator, C.H. (1976) Review of the effect of spinal cord trauma on the vessels and blood flow in the spinal cord. *J. Neurosurg.*, 45: 638–646.

Santa, B. (1951) Il fenomeno delliperrigenerazione in umo studio sperimentale sulla coda di larve di Hyla arborea. *Arch. Zool. Ital.*, 36: 105–132.

Schnell, L. and Schwab, M.E. (1990) Axonal regeneration in the rat spinal cord produced by an antibody against myelin-associated neurite growth inhibitors. *Nature (Lond.)*, 343: 269–272.

Schreyer, D.J. and Jones, E.G. (1982) Growth and target finding by axons of the corticospinal tract in prenatal and postnatal rats. *Neuroscience*, 7: 1837- 1853.

Schreyer, D.J. and Jones, E.G. (1983) Growing corticospinal axons by-pass lesions of neonatal rat spinal cord. *Neuroscience*, 9: 31–40.

Schwab, M. and Caroni, P. (1988) Oligodendrocytes and CNS myelin are nonpermissive substrates for neurite growth and fibroblast spreading in vitro. *J. Neurosci.*, 8: 2381–2393.

Schwab, M.E., Bandtlow, C.E., Varga, Z. and Nicholls, J. (1993) Developmental expression of myelin-associated neurite growth inhibitors correlates with the loss of regeneration after spinal cord lesions in the opossum. *Soc. Neurosci. Abstr.*, 19: 682.

Selzer, M. (1977) Mechanisms of functional recovery and regeneration after spinal cord transection in larval sea lampreys. *J. Physiol.*, 277: 395–408.

Sharma, S.C., Jadhao, A.G. and Prasada Rao, P.D. (1993) Regeneration of supraspinal projection neurons in the adult goldfish. *Brain Res.*, 620: 221- 228.

Shimizu, I., Oppenheim, R.W., O'Brien, M. and Shneiderman, A. (1990) Anatomical and functional recovery following spinal cord transection in the chick embryo. *J. Neurobiol.*, 21: 918–937.

Silver, J. and Ogawa, M.Y. (1983) Postnatally induced formation of the corpus callosum in acallosal mice on glial-coated cellulose bridges. *Science*, 220: 1067–1069.

Silver, J., Lorenz, S.E., Wahlstein, D. and Coughlin, J. (1982) Axonal guidance during development of the great cerebral commissures: descriptive and experimental studies, in vivo, on the role of preformed glial pathways. *J. Comp. Neurol.*, 210: 10–29.

Simpson, S.B., Jr. (1968) Morphology of the regenerated spinal cord in the lizard, *Anolis carolinensis*. *J. Comp. Neurol.*, 134: 193–210.

Simpson, S.B., Jr. (1970) Studies on regeneration of the lizard tail. *Am. Zool.*, 10: 157–165.

Singer, M., Nordlander, R.H. and Egar, M. (1979) Axonal guidance during embryogenesis and regeneration in the spinal cord of the newt: the blueprint hypothesis of neuronal pathway patterning. *J. Comp. Neurol.*, 185: 1–22.

Skene, J.H.P. (1989) Axonal growth-associated proteins. *Annu. Rev. Neurosci.*, 12: 127–156.

Skene, J.H.P. and Willard, M. (1981) Axonally transported proteins associated with axon growth in rabbit central and peripheral nervous system. *J. Cell Biol.*, 89: 96–103.

Smith, G.F., Miller, R.H. and Silver, J. (1986) Changing role of forebrain astrocytes during development, regenerative failure, and induced regeneration upon transplantation. *J. Comp. Neurol.*, 251: 23–43.

Steffaneli, A. (1944) Ossevazioni sullistogenesi del midollo spinale della rigenerata de tritoni. *Boll. Soc. Ital. Biol. Sper.*, 19: 252–253.

Steffaneli, A. (1950a) Some comments on regeneration in the central nervous systems. In: P. Weiss (Ed), *Genetics Neurology*, University of Chicago Press, Chicago, IL, pp 210–211.

Steffaneli, A. (1950b) I processi della rigenerazione del midollo spinale delle larva de Anfibi anuri nella sua relazione con la corda dorsale. Att: Acad. Naz. Lince: Rend Cl. Sci. Fis. Mat. Nat. Ser. VIII 8: 498–504.

Steffaneli, A. and Capriata, A. (1943) La rigenerazione del midollo spinale della coda rigenerata dei tritoni. *Ric. Morfol.*, 20–21: 607–633.

Steffaneli, A. and Cervi, M. (1946) La modalita del riallacciamento dei monconi di midollo spinale di tritoni adulti, separati asportando un segmente di midollo nella regione basale della corda. *Boll. Soc. Ital. Biol. Sper.*, 22: 756–757.

Stensaas, L.J. (1983) Regeneration in the spinal cord of the newt *Notophthalmus (triturus) pyrrhogaster*. In: C.C. Kao, R.B. Bunge and P.J. Reier (Eds.), *Spinal Cord Reconstruction*, Raven Press, New York, pp. 121–149.

Stewart, R.R., Zou, D.-J., Treherne, J.M., Mølgird, K., Saunders, N.R. and Nicholls, J.G. (1991) The intact central nervous system of the newborn opossum in long-term culture: fine structure and GABA-mediated inhibition of electrical activity. *J. Exp. Biol.*, 161: 25–41.

Tetzlaff, W., Kobayashi, N.R. and Bedard, A.M. (1993) BDNF prevents atrophy of rubrospinal neurons after axotomy. *Soc. Neurosci. Abstr.*, 19: 1104.

Themes, G. (1950) Comportamento del midollo spinale caudale delle larve d. Hyla dopo riallacciamento ritardato con il restante neurasse. *Rend. Semin. Sc. Cagliari*, 20: 1–5.

Tohyama, T., Lee, V.M.-Y., Rorke, L.B. and Trojanowski, J.Q. (1991) Molecular milestones that signal axonal maturation and the commitment of human spinal cord precursor cells to the neuronal or glial phenotype in development. *J. Comp. Neurol.*, 310: 285–299.

Tolbert, D.L. and Der, T. (1987) Redirected growth of pyramidal tract axons following neonatal pyramidotomy in cats. *J. Comp. Neurol.*, 260: 299–311.

Treherne, J.M., Woodward, S.K.A., Varga, Z.M., Ritchie, J.M. and Nicholls, J.G. (1992) Restoration of conduction and growth of axons through injured spinal cord of neonatal opossum in culture. *Proc. Natl. Acad. Sci. USA*, 89: 431–434.

Valenzuela, J.I., Hasan, S.J. and Steeves, J.D. (1990) Stimulation of the brainstem reticular formation evokes locomotor activity in embryonic chicken, in ovo. *Dev. Brain Res.*, 56: 13–18.

Varga, Z., Erulkar, S. and Nicholls, J. (1993) A critical time period for growth of neurites across a lesion in neonatal opossum spinal cord in culture. *Soc. Neurosci. Abstr.*, 19: 422.

Voigt, T. (1989) Development of glial cells in the cerebral wall of ferrets: direct tracing of their transformation from radial glia into astrocytes. *J. Comp. Neurol.*, 289: 74–88.

Wang, X.M., Xu, X.M., Qin, Y.Q. and Martin, G.F. (1992) The origins of supraspinal projections to the cervical and lumbar spinal cord at different stages of development in the gray short-tailed Brazilian opossum, *Monodelphis domestica*. *Dev. Brain Res.*, 68: 203–216.

Wang, X.M., Qin, Y.Q., Xu, X.M. and Martin, G.J. (1994) Developmental plasticity of reticulospinal and vestibulospinal axons in the North American opossum, *Didelphis virginiana*. *J. Comp. Neurol.*, in press.

Windle, W.F. (1955) *Regeneration in The Central Nervous System*. Charles C. Thomas, Springfield, IL.

Wood, M.R. and Cohen, M.J. (1979) Synaptic regeneration in identified neurons of the lamprey spinal cord. *Science*, 206: 344–347.

Xu, X.M. and Martin, G.F. (1989) Developmental plasticity of the rubrospinal tract. Studies using the North American opossum. *J. Comp. Neurol.*, 279: 368–387.

Xu, X.M. and Martin, G.F. (1990) The response of rubrospinal neurons to axotomy in the adult opossum, *Didelphis virginiana*. *Exp. Neurol.*, 108: 46–54.

Xu, X.M. and Martin, G.F. (1991a) Evidence for new growth and regeneration of cut axons in developmental plasticity of the rubrospinal tract in the North American opossum. *J. Comp. Neurol.*, 313: 103–112.

Xu, X.M. and Martin, G.F. (1991b) Ipsilaterally projecting rubrospinal neurons in adult and developing opossums. *Anat. Rec.*, 231: 538–547.

Xu, X.M. and Martin, G.F. (1992) The response of rubrospinal neurons to axotomy at different stages of development in the North American opossum. *J. Neurotrauma*, 9: 93–105.

Yanes, C., Monzon-Mayor, M., Ghandour, M.S., deBarry, J. and Gombos, G. (1990) Radial glia and astrocytes in developing and adult telencephalon of the lizard *Gallotia galloti* as revealed by immunohistochemistry with anti-GFAP and anti-vimentin antibodies. *J. Comp. Neurol.*, 295: 559–568.

Yin, H.S. and Selzer, M.E. (1983) Axonal regeneration in lamprey spinal cord. *J. Neurosci.*, 3: 1135–1144.

Young, W. (1985) Blood flow, metabolic and neurophysiological mechanisms in spinal cord injury. In: D.P. Becker and J. T. Povlishock (Eds.), *Central Nervous System Trauma Status Report*, NIH-NINCDS, Washington, pp. 463–473.

Zottoli, S.J., Marek, L.E., Agostini, M.A. and Strittmatter, S.L. (1987) Morphological and physiological survival of goldfish Mauthner axons isolated from their somata by spinal cord crush. *J. Comp. Neurol.*, 255: 272–282.

Zou, D.-J., Treherne, J.M., Stewart, R.R., Saunders, N.R. and Nicholls, J.G. (1991) Regulation of $GABA_B$ receptors by histamine and neuronal activity in the isolated spinal cord of neonatal opossum in culture. *Proc. R. Soc. Lond. B*, 246: 77–82.

F.J. Seil (Ed.)
Progress in Brain Research, Vol 103

CHAPTER 17

Functional regeneration and restoration of locomotor activity following spinal cord transection in the lamprey

Andrew D. McClellan

Division of Biological Science, 105 Lefevre Hall, University of Missouri, Columbia, MO 65211, USA

Introduction

Specific neural networks in the nervous system control rhythmic motor acts such as walking, running, swimming, flying and eating. In particular, locomotor movements are used by many animals during a variety of behaviors and are critical for survival. The neural networks that control locomotor function are usually divided into four components (reviewed in Stein, 1978; Grillner, 1981; McClellan, 1989): (1) central pattern generators (CPGs) in the spinal cord produce the basic pattern of rhythmic motor activity; (2) coordinating systems couple CPG oscillators distributed along the spinal cord; (3) sensory inputs modulate the activity produced by spinal CPG networks; and (4) brainstem command or initiation systems activate the CPGs and initiate locomotor activity (Fig. 1A). The output elements of the command system are thought to be reticulospinal (RS) neurons that activate the spinal CPG networks.

Severe spinal cord injury, such as a complete transection, can disrupt descending command axons, and this leads to paralysis below the lesion. The degree of behavioral recovery following spinal cord injury depends on the phylogeny and developmental stage of the animal (reviewed in McClellan, 1990a, 1992). Most postembryonic 'higher' vertebrates, such as birds and mammals, display very limited recovery following severe spinal cord injury because of restricted regeneration in the central nervous system (CNS) (Kiernan, 1979; Eidelberg, 1981). In reptiles, regeneration does occur in the tail region but not in the spinal cord proper (see Simpson and Duffy, this volume). In 'lower' vertebrates, such as lamprey, jawed fish and some amphibians, as well as in some developing higher vertebrates, behavioral recovery does occur following spinal cord injury because transected axons regenerate across the lesion and make synaptic connections within the CNS.

Spinal cord injury and recovery of locomotor function in the lamprey

The lamprey, a 'lower' vertebrate, has a number of unique and powerful technical advantages that make it ideally suited for studying locomotor function and spinal cord regeneration (reviewed in McClellan, 1989, 1992): (1) the lamprey CNS can repair itself after spinal cord injury and this results in almost complete behavioral recovery; (2) the lamprey CNS has many features in common with the nervous systems in higher vertebrates, yet is comparatively simple; (3) the CNS contains several classes of large, individually identifiable neurons; (4) locomotor movements and

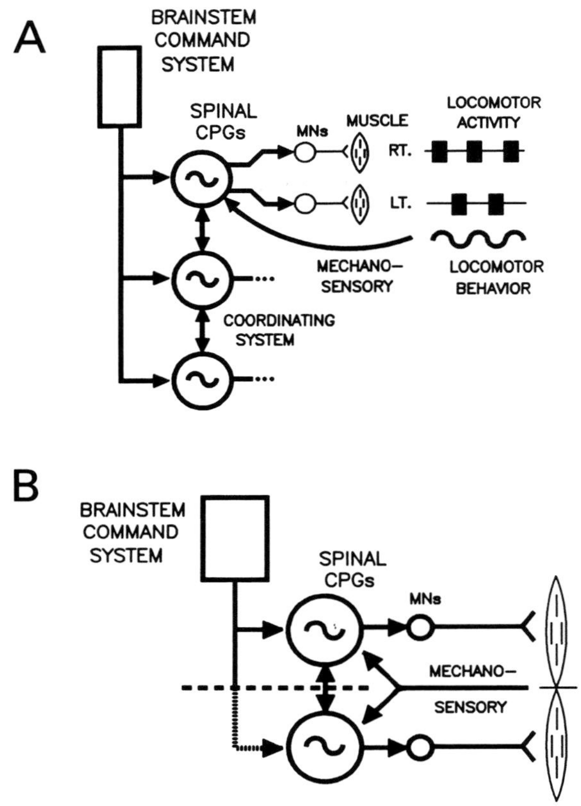

Fig. 1. A. Summary of locomotor system. Neurons in brainstem command systems activate spinal central pattern generators (CPGs), which in turn activate motoneurons to initiate locomotor behavior. B. Summary of previous results from the lamprey (McClellan, 1988a, 1990a,b) following a spinal cord transection (horizontal dashed line). Restoration of locomotor initiation below the transection is mediated by functional regeneration of descending axons (dotted line) from brainstem command systems that can directly activate spinal CPGs. Recovery of locomotor coupling across the lesion is dependent on restoration of spinal coordinating pathways, as well as contributions from mechanosensory inputs.

activity are easy to quantitate, which allows assessment of locomotor function at various recovery times following spinal cord injury; (5) the relatively thin CNS (~ 100–400 μm) in larval animals often permits histological processing in whole-mount preparations; and (6) locomotor activity can be elicited in in vitro nervous system preparations which allow control of the ionic or pharmacological make up of the bath, elimination of mechanosensory inputs, and stable conditions for intracellular recording. Recovery of locomotor behavior following spinal cord transection depends on restoration of at least two functions: recovery of locomotor initiation *below* the transection, and recovery of locomotor coordination *across* the lesion. These two functions were examined in spinal cord-transected larval lamprey (*Petromyzon marinus*) at relatively long recovery times after the restoration of locomotor function.

Restoration of locomotor initiation below the transection

In principle, the locomotor networks below a spinal cord transection could receive inputs from several sources (Fig. 1B): (a) restored descending projections from brainstem command systems; (b) inputs from spinal neurons, such as descending propriospinal neurons (Rovainen, 1985; Dale, 1986) located above or below the lesion; and (c) mechanosensory inputs. In behaviorally recovered spinal cord-transected lamprey, locomotor patterns in whole animal and in in vitro preparations were similar to those in normal animals (McClellan, 1988a, 1990a). These and additional experiments suggest that descending propriospinal relay neurons located above the transection and mechanosensory inputs do not contribute significantly to the activation of spinal locomotor networks below a spinal transection site. Rather, the results strongly suggest that descending command axons can regenerate through the transection site and make functional synaptic connections to activate directly the spinal locomotor networks below the lesion (Fig. 1B). The distance that these axons grow beyond the transection site will be discussed below. These studies were the first convincing demonstration in a vertebrate of functional regeneration of descending command systems following spinal cord transection.

Recovery of locomotor coordination across a spinal cord transection

At least two mechanisms contribute to the recovery of locomotor coordination across a spinal cord transection (Fig. 1B): restoration of spinal coordinating pathways and mechanosensory inputs (McClellan, 1990b; see also Cohen, 1988). Since the coupling produced by either of these mechanisms alone is more variable than observed in recovered spinal cord-transected whole animals, both of these mechanisms contribute to the restoration of locomotor coupling across a spinal cord lesion site.

Time course of recovery following spinal cord transection in lamprey

Our earlier work suggested that recovery of locomotor initiation in spinal cord-transected lamprey was due, in part, to regeneration of descending axons from brainstem neurons. In order to clarify further the mechanisms responsible for recovery of locomotor initiation, we used a multifaceted approach to examine the time course of restoration of locomotor function following complete transections of the rostral spinal cord at 10% body length (BL) (McClellan 1992; Davis and McClellan 1993a, b): (a) kinematic analysis (Davis et al., 1993), (b) muscle recordings (Davis et al. 1993), (c) recordings of in vitro locomotor activity (McClellan, 1994), and (d) anatomical analysis of descending brainstem projections (Davis and McClellan 1994a, b). These approaches provide unique insights into the factors responsible for recovery of locomotor function following spinal cord transection.

Kinematic analysis and muscle activity in whole animals

Locomotor movements and muscle activity were analysed in normal whole animals and compared with those in spinal cord-transected lamprey at fixed recovery times between 2 and 32 weeks post-transection (PT) (Davis et al., 1993). These results were used to determine the time course and completeness of recovery of locomotor function following spinal cord transection (Figs. 2 and 3).

In normal lamprey, locomotor movements consisted of two features: left–right bending at a given level of the body and undulations that traveled toward the tail with increasing amplitude (Fig. 2A, B). These features of locomotor movements were produced by two components of locomotor activity (Fig. 3A, B): left–right alternation (1-2) of muscle activity at a given segmental level and a rostrocaudal phase lag (2, 3 and 3, 4) of motor activity along the same side of the body. In

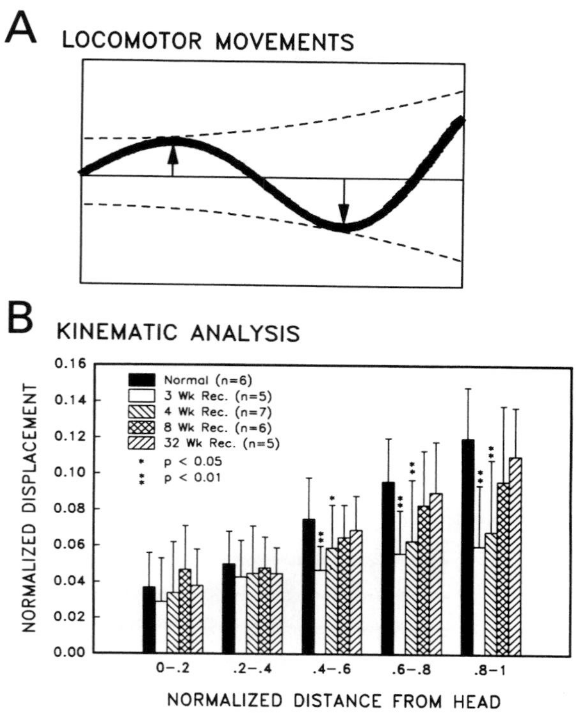

Fig. 2. Summary of kinematic analysis in normal lamprey and animals recovering from spinal cord transection at 10% body length (BL). A. Simulated posture during locomotor movements. Body undulations propagate backwards (not shown) so that the amplitude of locomotor movements (dashed lines) increases toward the tail. Arrows indicate points along the body at which the amplitudes of lateral displacement are maximum. B. Graph of normalized amplitudes of locomotor movements (ordinate) versus normalized distance along the body (abscissa) in normal and spinal cord-transected lamprey. At 3 and 4 weeks post transection (PT), the amplitudes of locomotor movements were attenuated relative to normal, particularly in the caudal half of the body (*$P < 0.05$; **$P < 0.01$). At 8 weeks PT or longer, locomotor movements were not significantly different from normal. (Modified from Davis et al., 1993.)

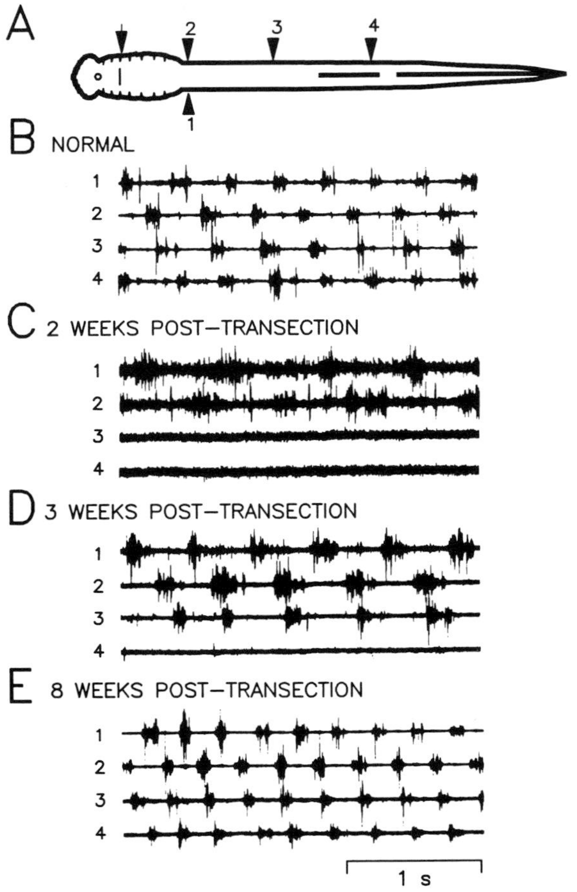

Fig. 3. Summary of muscle activity along the body in normal and spinal cord-transected whole animals. A. Diagram of whole animal showing transection site at 10% BL (arrow, C–E only) and muscle recording sites at approximately 20% (1, 2), 40% (3) and 60% (4) BL. B. In normal animals locomotor activity consisted of a left-right alternation (1, 2) and activity along the body (2–4). C–E. Following spinal cord transection, locomotor activity could be recorded at progressively greater distances below the transection with increasing recovery times. (Modified from Davis et al., 1993.)

particular, muscle activity occurred along the body at least as far as 60% BL, and probably for the entire length of the animal.

Immediately following transection of the rostral spinal cord, the animals were paralysed below the lesion. At about 2 weeks PT, locomotor movements began to appear, but the amplitudes of the movements were reduced, particularly in the caudal body. Presumably, attenuated locomotor movements occurred because muscle activity was limited to the rostral body just below the lesion (1, 2, Fig. 3C). Thus, active muscle contractions in the rostral body produced undulatory movements that were then passively propogated to the caudal body. By 3 weeks PT, locomotor muscle activity could be recorded from the rostral and middle body (1, 2 and 3, Fig. 3D), but locomotor movements were still attenuated, particularly in the caudal half of the body (Fig. 2B). The ranges for parameters of locomotor activity (cycle time, burst proportions and phase lag) were only slightly different than those in normal animals. At this recovery time, descending projections were restored only to the rostral spinal cord (see below). Thus, locomotor activity in the middle body is not mediated directly by restored descending projections from the brain but must have been produced by other mechanisms, such as descending propriospinal relay neurons and/or mechanosensory inputs.

By 8 weeks PT and later, locomotor movements and muscle activity were not significantly different from normal animals (Figs. 2B and 3E). In addition, the parameters for locomotor activity overlapped those in normal animals. By 8 weeks PT, descending brainstem–spinal cord projections were restored only as far as the middle spinal cord (see below), yet locomotor function along the body was normal. Thus, locomotor activity in the caudal body was not mediated directly by restored descending projections from the brain but must have been produced by other mechanisms, as mentioned above. In summary, following spinal cord transection there was a gradual recovery of locomotor movements during which locomotor activity appeared at progressively greater distances below the healed transection site.

In vitro brain / spinal cord preparations

In order to examine the mechanisms that contribute to the time course of behavioral recovery in whole animals, locomotor activity was ex-

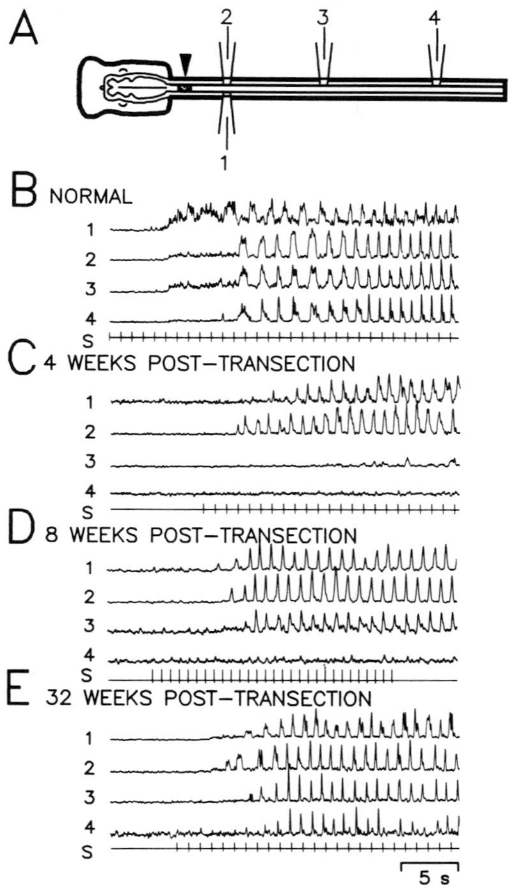

Fig. 4. Summary of locomotor activity along the spinal cord in in vitro brain/spinal cord preparations from normal and spinal cord-transected lamprey. A. Diagram of an in vitro brain/spinal cord preparation showing the transection site at ~10% BL (arrowhead, C–E only) and ventral root recording electrodes at approximately 20% (1, 2), 40% (3) and 60% (4) BL. B. In normal animals, chemical microstimulation in brainstem locomotor regions (S) elicited in vitro locomotor activity which consisted of a left-right alternation (1, 2) and activity along the spinal cord (2–4). C–E. In spinal cord-transected lamprey, in vitro locomotor activity could be recorded at progressively greater distances below the transection with increasing recovery times. (Modified from McClellan, 1994.)

amined in in vitro brain/spinal cord preparations (Fig. 4A) from normal and spinal cord-transected lamprey (McClellan, 1994). Under in vitro conditions, mechanosensory inputs and descending propriospinal relay pathways could be eliminated so that contributions from restored descending brainstem projections could be examined. Locomotor activity was elicited by chemical microstimulation in brainstem locomotor regions (McClellan, 1986), a technique that is thought to activate neurons in the command system. Brainstem-evoked locomotor activity was recorded from spinal ventral roots. The in vitro preparations could be partitioned into a brain pool and several spinal pools (not shown in Fig. 4A) so that the contents of each pool could be manipulated independently.

In in vitro preparations from normal lamprey, brainstem-evoked locomotor activity consisted of two features (Fig. 4B): left–right alternation (1, 2) at the same segmental level and a rostrocaudal phase lag (2, 3 and 3, 4) of ipsilateral activity. Locomotor activity occurred along the spinal cord at least to 60% BL, and probably for the entire length of the spinal cord. In addition, experiments in which conduction through descending polysynaptic relay pathways was blocked indicated that brainstem neurons can directly activate the locomotor networks at each level of the spinal cord in normal animals.

In in vitro preparations from spinal cord-transected lamprey, locomotor activity could be recorded at progressively greater distances below the transection with increasing recovery time (Fig. 4C–E). However, at most recovery times the distances that in vitro locomotor activity could be recorded below the transection (Fig. 4C–E) was less than those for muscle activity in spinal cord-transected whole animals (Fig. 3C–E). Specifically, in vitro locomotor activity was present at rostral spinal levels at 4 weeks PT and could be recorded as far as middle and caudal spinal levels by 8 weeks and 16–32 weeks PT, respectively (Fig. 4C–E). At most recovery times, the parameters of locomotor activity overlapped those in normal animals. Furthermore, experiments in which conduction through descending propriospinal relay systems was blocked indicated that regenerated descending axons usually could activate directly the spinal locomotor networks at the greatest distances below the transection site at which locomotor activity could be recorded.

Restoration of descending brainstem projections

In order to determine the projection patterns of descending brainstem neurons (Fig. 5A) in normal and recovering spinal cord-transected animals, horseradish peroxidase (HRP) was applied to the rostral (~ 20% BL), middle (~ 40% BL) or caudal (~ 60% BL) spinal cord (Davis and McClellan, 1993a, 1994a,b). In normal lamprey, relatively large numbers of brainstem neurons project to the rostral (n = 1250), middle (n = 900), and caudal (n = 825) spinal cord (Fig. 5B). Many of these cells are RS neurons located in four reticular nuclei: mesencephalic reticular nucleus (MRN), and the anterior (ARRN), middle (MRRN), and posterior (PRRN) rhombencephalic reticular nuclei (Fig. 5A). Partial lesions of the rostral spinal cord combined with HRP labeling indicated that many of the RS neurons in the ARRN, MRRN, and PRRN project their axons into the lateral spinal tracts, which are important for the initiation of locomotion (McClellan, 1988b; McClellan and Davis, 1992). In other vertebrates, RS neurons in similar areas of the brain have been implicated in initiating locomotion (reviewed in McClellan, 1986).

By 3 weeks PT, axons of a few brainstem neurons had grown through the lesion site and into the rostral spinal cord (20% BL) just below the transection (Fig. 5B). With increasing recovery time, greater numbers of brainstem neurons projected their axons to the rostral spinal cord, until by 32 weeks PT the number was not significantly different from normal. By about 8 weeks PT, brainstem neurons began to project their axons to middle levels of the spinal cord (40% BL), and by 32 weeks PT, about one-half the normal number of brainstem neurons projected their axons to this level of the spinal cord. By 32 weeks PT, only about 6% of the normal number of descending brain neurons projected their axons to caudal levels of the spinal cord (60% BL), typically more than 50 mm below the transection. Thus, with increasing recovery times, axons from brainstem neurons regenerated to progressively more caudal levels of the spinal cord below the transection site. The ARRN and MRRN had the largest percentages of neurons with restored descending projections, while the PRRN had the largest number of neurons with restored descending projections (Davis and McClellan, 1994a).

Summary of time course of locomotor recovery following spinal cord transection

With increasing recovery times following transection of the rostral spinal cord (10% BL), locomotor activity could be recorded at progressively greater distances below the transection in both whole animals and in vitro preparations, but with different time courses (Figs. 3, 4 and 6). Furthermore, at a given recovery time, the distance that in vitro locomotor activity could be recorded below the transection was similar to the extent of anatomical regeneration of descending axons from brainstem neurons, as demonstrated by retrograde tracer experiments (Figs. 4–6) (McClellan, 1994; Davis and McClellan 1994a). These results indicate that regenerated descending axons from brainstem command neurons could activate directly the spinal locomotor networks in the rostral, middle and caudal spinal cord by about 2, 8 and 32 weeks PT. Thus, at most recovery times, locomotor activity in whole animals occurred at greater distances below the spinal cord transection than the extent of regeneration of descending axons from brainstem command neurons. Any locomotor activity that occurred beyond the extent of regeneration of descending axons could not have been activated directly from the brain but must have been due to other mechanisms, such as descending propriospinal relay neurons (Rovainen, 1985; Dale, 1986) and mechanosensory systems (McClellan and Jang, 1993). Presumably, descending propriospinal relay neurons were activated directly or indirectly by brainstem command neurons. At long recovery times, regenerated descending axons could directly activate the locomotor networks in the caudal spinal cord, typically more than 50 mm below the healed spinal cord transection (Fig. 6).

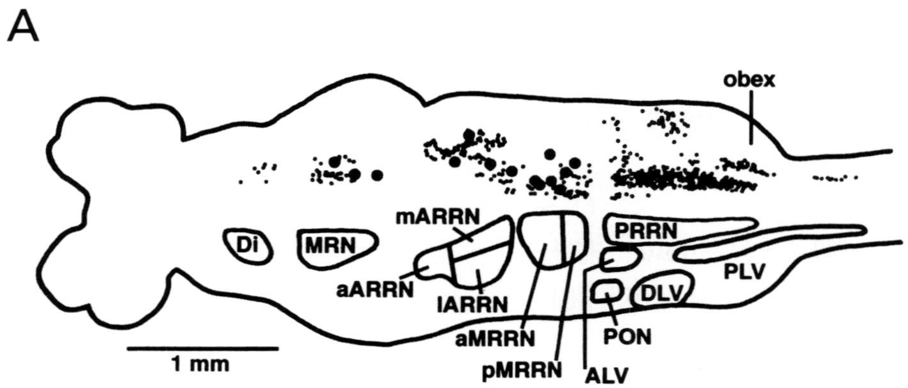

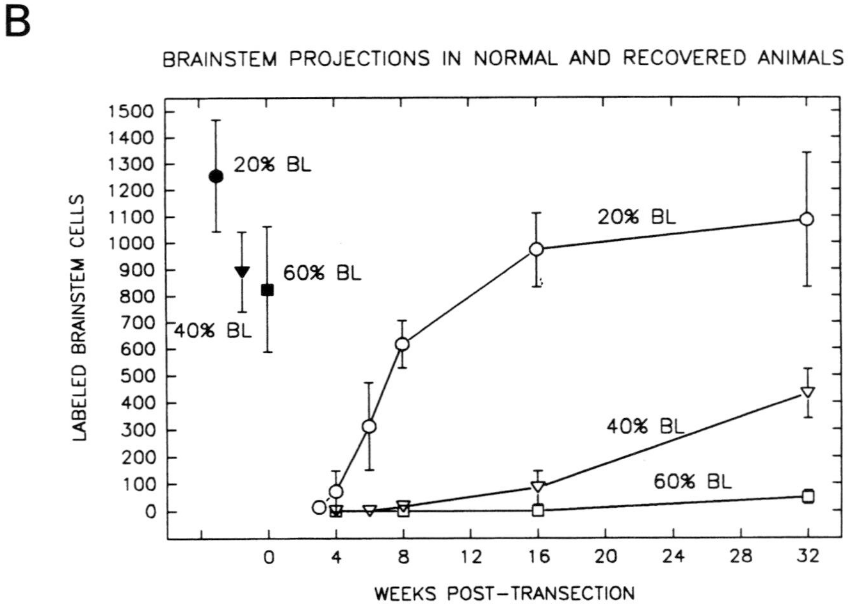

Fig. 5. Summary of descending brain-spinal cord projections in normal and spinal cord-transected lamprey. A. Dorsal view of whole-mount of lamprey brain (spinal cord on far right) from a normal animal. The upper part of the diagram, representing the right side of the animal, shows the pattern of labeling of brain neurons (dots) after application of HRP to the spinal cord at 20% BL. The lower part of the diagram contains outlines of various brain cell groups or subdivisions. B. Total numbers of labeled descending brainstem neurons following application of HRP at 20%, 40%, or 60% BL in normal lamprey (filled symbols) and at various recovery times in spinal cord-transected animals (open symbols). See text for further details. ALV, anterolateral vagal region; ARRN, anterior rhombencephalic reticular nucleus; aARRN, anterior division of ARRN; aMRRN, anterior division of MRRN; Di, diencephalon; DLV, dorsolateral vagal region; lARRN, lateral division of ARRN; mARRN, medial division of ARRN; MRN, mesencephalic reticular nucleus; MRRN, middle rhombencephalic reticular nucleus; PLV, posterolateral vagal region; pMRRN, posterior division of MRRN; PON, posterior octavomotor nucleus; PRRN, posterior rhombencephalic reticular nucleus. (Modified from Davis and McClellan, 1994a.)

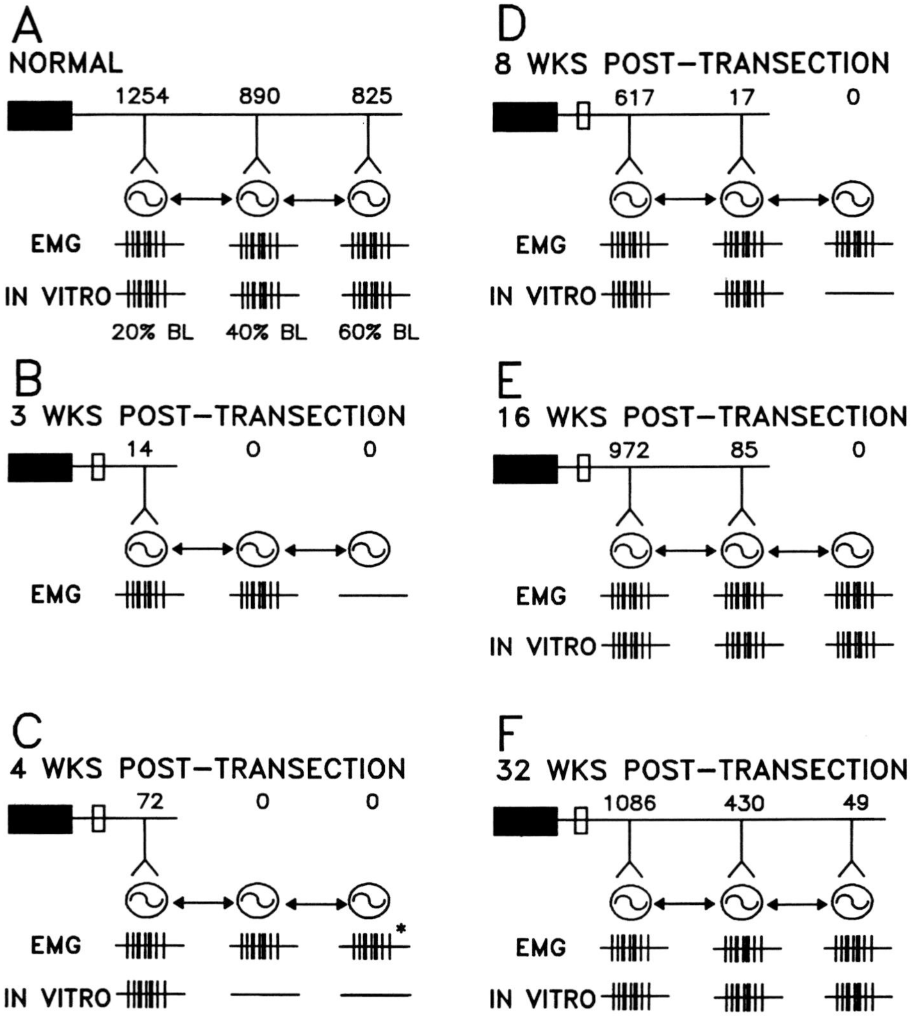

Fig. 6. Overview of locomotor systems in normal lamprey and during recovery of locomotor function in spinal cord-transected animals. Brainstem command system (filled rectangles) send descending axons (horizontal lines) into the spinal cord to activate spinal locomotor networks (circles with oscillator symbols) which are coupled by spinal coordinating systems (lines with double arrows). Numbers above horizontal lines indicate numbers of descending projections to 20%, 40% and 60% BL (see Fig. 5). EMG = muscle activity in whole animals (Fig. 3). IN VITRO = in vitro locomotor activity (see Fig. 4). Spinal cord transection at 10% BL indicated by open rectangles. Labile activity indicated by *. A. In normal animals, descending axons from neurons in brainstem command systems can directly activate the spinal locomotor networks at 20%, 40% and 60% BL and probably along the entire spinal cord. B–F. Between 3 and 32 weeks PT, descending axons from brainstem neurons project to progressively more caudal levels of the spinal cord below the transection and can directly activate the spinal locomotor networks. Locomotor activity can be recorded at progressively greater distances below the transection in whole animals and in in vitro preparations, but with different time courses. See text for further details. (Modified from Davis et al., 1993; Davis and McClellan, 1993a, 1994a; McClellan, 1994.)

Neurons which mediate behavioral recovery

Large reticulospinal Müller cells, which have medial descending axons (Rovainen, 1979), do not appear to contribute significantly to behavioral recovery, since the lateral spinal tracts are important for initiation of locomotor activity in normal and spinal cord-transected animals (McClellan, 1988b, 1990a). Thus, smaller RS neurons in the ARRN, MRRN and PRRN, which project into the lateral tracts of the spinal cord, are likely to be important for behavioral recovery (McClellan, 1990a; Davis and McClellan, 1992).

As discussed above, descending propriospinal systems also contributed to the activation of locomotor networks below the transection, particularly at early recovery times. In preliminary experiments, descending propriospinal neurons were retrogradely labeled in normal and spinal cord-transected lamprey by applying HRP at 40% and 60% BL. Propriospinal neurons, which had short and relatively long descending axons, were distributed along the spinal cord (McClellan et al., unpublished data).

Restored descending projections: regeneration versus development

True axonal regeneration of large identifiable RS neurons

Müller and Mauthner cells are a population of at least 28 large, individually identifiable RS neurons in the lamprey brain (Fig. 7) that are thought to project for the entire length of the spinal cord (Rovainen, 1979). These large RS neurons are not

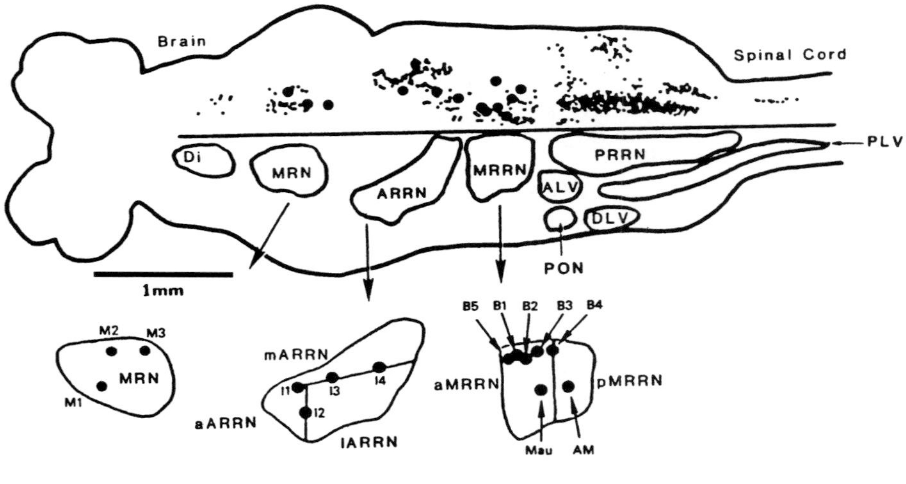

CATEGORY I: M1, I2, AM (P_{rgn} ≥ 60% to middle cord)

CATEGORY II: I3, I4, B3, B4, B5 (P_{rgn} = 20–50% to middle cord)

CATEGORY III: M2, I1, B1, B2, Mau, (P_{rgn} = 20–60% to rostral cord)

CATEGORY IV: M3 (P_{rgn} = 11% to rostral cord)

Fig. 7. True axonal regeneration of large, individually identifiable Müller and Mauthner cells. (Top) Diagram of dorsal view of brain showing positions of Müller cells in the mesencephalic (M1–M3), isthmic (I1–I4), and bulbar (B1–B5) groups, as well as the Mauthner (Mau) and axillary Mauthner (AM) cells. (Bottom) Classification of Müller and Mauthner cells according to their probabilities of regeneration (Prgn) to various levels of the spinal cord. Abbreviations as in legend for Fig. 5. (From Davis and McClellan, 1994b.)

critical for initiation of locomotor activity in normal and spinal cord-transected lamprey (McClellan, 1988b, 1990a). Retrograde labeling experiments indicated that with increasing recovery times following transection of the rostral spinal cord, descending axons of Müller and Mauthner neurons had grown to progressively more caudal levels in the spinal cord below the transection site (Davis and McClellan, 1994b). Since Müller and Mauthner neurons are individually identifiable and do not increase in number during larval stages, these results demonstrated that these neurons are capable of true axonal regeneration. In addition, the results indicated that the axons of some of these neurons had grown at least 57 mm below a rostral spinal cord transection (Davis and McClellan, 1994b). This maximum distance of regeneration is about an order of magnitude greater than previously reported (reviewed in Rovainen, 1979). Furthermore, Müller and Mauthner neurons had different regenerative responses, even though their cell bodies and descending axons were located in similar areas of the nervous system (Fig. 7). These results suggest that differences in regenerative responses may be controlled by intrinsic cell programming.

True axonal regeneration of non-identifiable RS neurons

Restoration of descending brain-spinal cord projections from small or moderate size, non-identifiable RS neurons could be due to true axonal regeneration of pre-existing brain neurons or development of late arriving descending axons (Fig. 8A). In the lamprey, double labeling experiments were used to investigate whether non-identifiable RS neurons are capable of true axonal regeneration (McClellan et al., unpublished data). In control animals, simultaneous application of rhodamine dextran amine (RDA) and fluorescein dextran amine (FDA) to the spinal cord at 20% or 25% BL resulted in substantial double labeling of descending brainstem neurons. In experimental animals (Fig. 8A), RDA was applied to 25% BL, and after allowing for retrograde transport, the spinal cord was completely transected at 10% BL. Eight weeks after the spinal cord transection, FDA was applied to the spinal cord at 20% BL. These experiments resulted in double labeling of many descending brain neurons (Fig. 8B), including RS neurons, indicating that these neurons are capable of true axonal regeneration. Thus, both large identified Müller and Mauthner cells, as well as smaller, non-identifiable RS neurons, are capable of true axonal regeneration, suggesting that this is a common property of RS neurons in the lamprey (also see results in chick: Hasan et al., 1993; Steeves et al., this volume).

Implications for functional regeneration in vertebrates

Conditions required for recovery of locomotor function in the lamprey

In spinal cord-transected lamprey, restoration of the original descending projections and patterns of synaptic connections below the transection were not necessary for recovery of locomotor function. Substantial recovery of locomotor activ-

Fig. 8. True axonal regeneration of non-identifiable reticulospinal (RS) neurons demonstrated by double labeling with retrograde tracers. A. Paradigm for double labeling experiment (brain, left; spinal cord, right). Brain neuron 'a' is retrogradely labeled by application of tracers 1 and 2, indicating that this neuron is capable of true axonal regeneration following spinal cord transection. Neuron 'b' is labeled with tracer 1, indicating that its transected axon did not regenerate or at least did not extend far enough to pick up tracer 2. Neuron 'c' is labeled with tracer 2, indicating that it sent a late arriving axon into the spinal cord after spinal transection. B. Results from double labeling experiment outlined in A in which rhodamine dextran amine (RDA, Tracer 1) was applied to the spinal cord at 25% BL. Two weeks later the spinal cord was transected at 10% BL, and 10 weeks later fluorescein dextran amine (FDA, Tracer 2) was applied to the spinal cord at 20% BL. Neurons in the anterior rhombencephalic reticular nucleus (ARRN) (see Fig. 5A) double labeled with RDA (left) and FDA (right), demonstrating that non-identifiable RS neurons are capable of true axonal regeneration. Calibration bar = 50 μm. See text for further details.

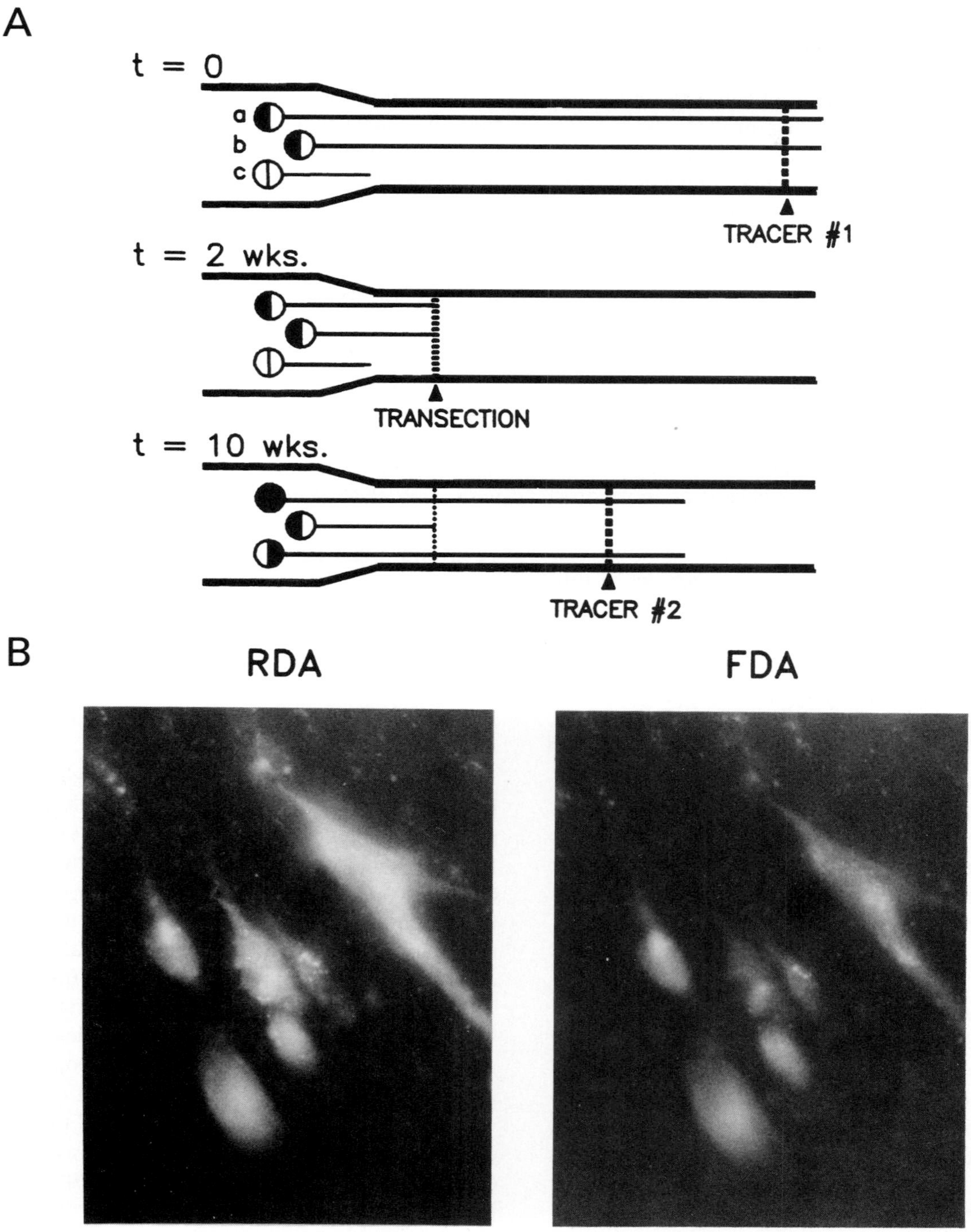
A
t = 0
a
b
c
TRACER #1
t = 2 wks.
TRANSECTION
t = 10 wks.
TRACER #2
B
RDA
FDA

ity could occur at a particular level of the spinal cord even if the descending projections to that level were reduced or absent (Figs. 5B, 6). At least three mechanisms could compensate for reduced or absent descending projections: (1) regenerated descending axons might make unusually strong or numerous synaptic connections with spinal targets; (2) descending propriospinal neurons might substitute for and/or enhance the effects of direct descending activation via brainstem command systems; and (3) mechanosensory inputs, although unable to initiate locomotor activity alone (McClellan, 1990a), might raise the excitability of spinal locomotor networks and facilitate descending activation via brainstem command systems.

If restoration of the original descending projections is not required for recovery of locomotor function, what conditions are necessary? First, at least some neural processes must grow across the transection and result in direct or indirect reconnection between brainstem command neurons and spinal locomotor networks. In addition, these synaptic connections must be strong enough to result in functional activation of spinal locomotor networks below the spinal lesion. Second, depending on the level of the spinal cord injury, restoration of spinal coordinating systems as well as contributions from mechanosensory inputs may be needed to couple locomotor activity across a spinal lesion. Presumably, mechanisms associated with axonal elongation, tract selection and synapse formation are required in both of the above situations.

Spinal cord injury in higher vertebrates

The CNS of adult higher vertebrates is a restrictive environment for axonal regeneration because two myelin proteins (NI-35 and NI-250), which appear after myelination, inhibit axonal regeneration following injury (Schwab, 1990). Thus, in adult higher vertebrates it is not yet possible to study the full complement of mechanisms that may be necessary for regeneration and restoration of function because of very limited axonal regeneration in the CNS. In addition, promotion of axonal regeneration may not be sufficient alone to produce restoration of function. For example, if induction of substantial regeneration were possible in adult higher vertebrates, are there mechanisms in place to control axonal guidance and formation of functionally appropriate synaptic connections?

Under restricted conditions, neurons can regenerate within the CNS of higher vertebrates. For example, substantial axonal regeneration and recovery of function can occur if spinal cord transections are performed before the period of myelination (Hasan et al., 1991, 1993; Keirstead et al., 1992; Varga et al., 1993; Steeves et al., this volume). Limited regeneration results when myelination is temporarily delayed (Salvio and Schwab, 1990) or myelin proteins are blocked with antibodies (Schnell and Schwab, 1990). However, temporary removal of the inhibitory effects of myelin might be detrimental, since both transected axons and undamaged axons may grow into inapproriate areas of the CNS (Schwab and Schnell, 1991).

Requirements for functional regeneration in higher vertebrates

Since axonal regeneration in adult higher vertebrates is severely limited, it is difficult to determine how much regeneration is necessary for recovery of locomotor function following spinal cord injury. Our results from the lamprey indicate that following spinal cord transection, it is not necessary to restore the original organization of descending projections for recovery of function. These data suggest that in higher vertebrates, induction of a minimal or moderate degree of regeneration of descending brainstem projections may be sufficient to produce restoration of locomotor function below a lesion, provided that additional compensatory mechanisms are available (see above). Perhaps more important than the total number of restored descending projections is which systems are restored. Acute lesion studies in mammals indicate that sparing relatively small areas of the spinal cord which include specific tracts can support substantial locomotor function (Windle et al., 1958).

Functional regeneration in lower vertebrates

The lamprey, as well as several other lower vertebrates, can recover locomotor function following spinal cord transection. For example, long distance axonal regeneration can occur in a number of lower vertebrates (reviewed in Davis and McClellan, 1994a). In addition, following spinal cord injury in lower vertebrates, axons of CNS neurons are able to grow in the appropriate direction and sometimes in the appropriate tract (Mackler et al., 1986; Selzer et al., 1988; Lurie and Selzer, 1991; Davis and McClellan, 1992). Furthermore, mechanisms exist for formation of synaptic connections with a high degree of specificity after spinal cord injury (Lee, 1982; Mackler and Selzer, 1987). Therefore, the lamprey and other lower vertebrates offer the opportunity to examine the full complement of mechanisms that lead to recovery of locomotor function following spinal cord transection.

What are some of the reasons that functional regeneration is possible in lower vertebrates (see McClellan, 1992)? First, in several lower vertebrates new neurons appear to be added to the CNS after birth (Holder and Clarke, 1988). Thus, a permissive environment for axonal elongation and synapse formation by newly added neurons may also support axonal regeneration and synaptic reconnection following injury (see Holder and Clarke, 1988). However, in the lamprey and some other lower vertebrates, addition of new neurons to the CNS does not appear to contribute substantially to restoration of locomotor function following spinal cord transection (see Fig. 8). Second, in lower vertebrates, inhibitory mechanisms for axonal regeneration involving myelin appear to be absent or ineffective. The lamprey CNS lacks myelin (Rovainen, 1979), and in fish the CNS myelin appears to lack the inhibitory proteins (Bastmeyer et al., 1991). Interestingly, growing axons from CNS neurons in fish (e.g., retinal ganglion cells) can recognize and are inhibited by CNS myelin from mammals (Bastmeyer et al., 1991). The CNS of adult amphibians (*Xenopus*), but not larvae, appears to contain the myelin inhibitory proteins (Lang et al., 1993), and these differences parallel the capacity for CNS regeneration in these two life stages.

Conclusions

Our studies with spinal cord-transected lamprey have provided a convincing demonstration of functional regeneration of descending command axons following spinal cord transection. Furthermore, correlations of locomotor movements, muscle activity, locomotor activity from in vitro preparations, and projection patterns of descending brainstem neurons have provided unique insights into the mechanisms that contribute to the time course of behavioral recovery following spinal cord transection. With increasing recovery times following transection of the rostral spinal cord, there is a gradual restoration of locomotor activity at progressively greater distances below the transection. During recovery, axons from descending brain neurons regenerate to progressively more caudal areas of the spinal cord below the transection, but with a slower time course than for the rate of behavioral recovery in whole animals. Thus, recovery of locomotor function does not require restoration of the original organization of descending projections to the spinal cord.

There are several important unanswered questions. Do regenerating descending axons make ‘decisions’ to grow into certain areas of the spinal cord, and if so, which guidance cues are involved? Are certain tracts permissive or restrictive substrates for axonal growth? Is synaptic specificity necessary for behavioral recovery in spinal cord-transected lamprey, and if so, what are the controlling mechanisms? Answers to these and other important questions will clarify the cellular and molecular mechanisms that produce the remarkable behavioral recovery following spinal cord transection in the lamprey.

Summary

Lampreys begin to recover locomotor function about 2 weeks following complete transections of the rostral spinal cord at 10% BL. Initially, locomotor movements are attenuated, particularly in the caudal half of the body, and muscle activity is limited to a few millimeters below the transection. Between 2 and 8 weeks PT, locomotor movements and locomotor activity are gradually restored to normal along the body. Locomotor activity from in vitro brain/spinal cord preparations occurs at progressively greater distances below the transection with increasing recovery times, but with a slower time course than in whole animals. Anatomical experiments using retrograde tracers indicate that descending axons from brainstem neurons first project to 20% BL by about 3 weeks PT and are restored to normal by 32 weeks PT. Descending axons first project to 40% BL by 8 weeks PT, and by 32 weeks PT about one-half of the normal numbers of descending projections are restored to this level of the spinal cord. By 32 weeks PT, approximately 6% of the normal numbers of descending projections are restored to 60% BL or more than 50 mm below the transection. Double labeling experiments indicate that most descending brain neurons, including RS neurons, are capable of true axonal regeneration. Taken together, the results indicate that several mechanisms contribute to recovery of locomotor function in spinal cord-transected lamprey: regeneration of descending axons from brainstem command neurons; descending propriospinal relay neurons; and mechanosensory inputs. Results from functional regeneration studies in the lamprey provide information concerning the conditions that may be necessary for locomotor recovery following spinal cord injury in higher vertebrates. In the lamprey, recovery of locomotor function does not require restoration of the original organization of descending projections to the spinal cord. Therefore, our results suggest that in higher vertebrates, induction of a minimal or moderate degree of regeneration of descending brainstem projections may be sufficient to produce restoration of locomotor function below a lesion, provided that additional compensatory mechanisms are available.

Acknowledgements

The comments of Dr G.R. Davis and Andre Hagevik are gratefully acknowledged. Supported by NIH grant NS29043 and American Paralysis Association grant MBl-9108.

References

Bastmeyer, M., Beckmann, M., Schwab, M.E., and Stuermer, C.A.O. (1991) Growth of regenerating goldfish axons is inhibited by rat oligodendrocytes and CNS myelin but not by goldfish optic nerve tract oligodendrocytelike cells and fish CNS myelin. *J. Neurosci.*, 11: 626–640.

Cohen, A.H. (1988) Regenerated fibers of the lamprey spinal cord can coordinate fictive swimming in the presence of curare. *J. Neurobiol.*, 19: 193–198.

Dale, N. (1986) Excitatory synaptic drive for swimming mediated by amino acid receptors in the lamprey. *J. Neurosci.*, 9: 2662–2675.

Davis, G.R. and McClellan, A.D. (1992) Axonal regeneration and pathway selection by brainstem neurons and behavioral recovery in spinal-transected lamprey larvae. *Soc. Neurosci. Abstr.*, 18: 1321.

Davis, G.R. and McClellan, A.D. (1993a) Time course of anatomical regeneration of descending brainstem neurons and behavioral recovery in spinal-transected lampreys. *Brain Res.*, 602: 131–137.

Davis, G.R. and McClellan, A.D. (1993b) Recovery of locomotor function and restoration of descending brainstem projections in spinal cord-transected lamprey. *Soc. Neurosci. Abstr.*, 19: 1316.

Davis, G.R. and McClellan, A.D. (1994a) Extent and time course of restoration of descending brainstem projections in spinal-transected lamprey. *J Comp. Neurol.*, 344: 65–82.

Davis, G.R. and McClellan, A.D. (1994b) Long distance axonal regeneration of identified lamprey reticulospinal neurons. *Exp. Neurol.*, 127: 94–105.

Davis, G.R., Troxel, M.T., Kohler, V.J., Grossmann, E.R. and McClellan, A.D. (1993) Time course of locomotor recovery and functional regeneration in spinal- transected lampreys: kinematics and electromyography. *Exp. Brain Res.*, 97: 83–95.

Eidelberg, E. (1981) Consequences of spinal cord lesions upon motor function, with special reference to locomotor activity. *Prog. Neurobiol.*, 17: 185–202.

Grillner, S. (1981) Control of locomotion in bipeds, tetrapods and fish, In: V. Brooks (Ed.), *Handbook of Physiology,*

Motor Control, American Physiological Society, Washington DC, pp. 1179–1236.

Hasan, S.J., Nelson, B.H., Valenzuela, J.I., Keirstead, H.S., Shull, S.E., Ethell, D.W. and Steeves, J.D. (1991) Functional repair of transected spinal cord in embryonic chick. *Rest. Neurol. Neurosci.*, 2: 137–154.

Hasan, S.J., Keirstead, G.D., Muir, G.D. and Steeves, J.D. (1993) Axonal regeneration contributes to repair of brainstem-spinal neurons in embryonic chick. *J. Neurosci.*, 13: 492–507.

Holder, N. and Clarke, J.D.W. (1988) Is there a correlation between continuous neurogenesis and directed axon regeneration in the vertebrate nervous system? *Trends Neurosci.*, 11: 94–99.

Keirstead, H.S., Hasan, S.J., Muir, G.D. and Steeves, J.D. (1992) Suppression of the onset of myelination extends the permissive period for the functional repair of embryonic spinal cord. *Proc. Natl. Acad. Sci. USA*, 89: 11664–11668.

Kiernan, J.A. (1979) Hypotheses concerned with axonal regeneration in the mammalian nervous system. *Biol. Rev.*, 54: 155–197.

Lang, D., Rubin, B., Schwab, M.E. and Stuermer, C.A.O. (1993) Neurite growth inhibitors (NI) of mammalian CNS myelin are present in *Xenopus* spinal cord but not in the optic nerve. *Soc. Neurosci. Abstr.*, 19: 1738.

Lee, M.T. (1982) Regeneration and functional reconnection of an identified vertebrate central neuron. *J. Neurosci.*, 2: 1793–1811.

Lurie, D.I. and Selzer, M.E. (1991) Preferential regeneration of spinal axons through the scar in hemisected lamprey spinal cord. *J. Comp. Neurol.*, 313: 669–679.

Mackler, S.A. and Selzer, M.E. (1987) Specificity of synaptic regeneration in the spinal cord of the larval sea lamprey. *J. Physiol. (London)*, 388: 183–198.

Mackler, S.A., Yin, H-S. and Selzer, M.E. (1986) Determinants of directional specificity in the regeneration of lamprey spinal axons. *J. Neurosci.*, 6: 1814–1821.

McClellan, A.D. (1986) Command systems for initiating locomotor responses in fish and amphibians — parallels to initiation of locomotion in mammals. In: S. Grillner, P. Stein, D. Stuart, H. Forssberg and R. Herman (Eds.), *Neurobiology of Vertebrate Locomotion*, Wenner-Gren Symposium Series, Vol. 45, Macmillan, London, pp. 3–20.

McClellan, A.D. (1988a) Functional regeneration of descending command pathways for locomotion in the lamprey demonstrated in the in vitro lamprey CNS. *Brain Res.*, 448: 339–345.

McClellan, A.D. (1988b) Brainstem command systems for locomotion in the lamprey: localization of descending pathways in the spinal cord. *Brain Res.*, 457: 338–349.

McClellan, A.D. (1989) Control of locomotion in a lower vertebrate, the lamprey: brainstem command systems and spinal cord regeneration. *Am. Zool.*, 29: 37–51.

McClellan, A.D. (1990a) Locomotor recovery in spinal-transected lampreys. Regenerated coordinating neurons and mechanosensory inputs couple locomotor activity across a spinal lesion. *Neuroscience*, 35: 675–685.

McClellan, A.D. (1990b) Locomotor recovery in spinal-transected lampreys. Role of functional regeneration of descending axons from brainstem locomotor command neurons. *Neuroscience*, 37: 781–798.

McClellan, A.D. (1992) Functional regeneration and recovery of locomotor activity in spinal-transected lamprey. *J. Exp. Zool.*, 261: 274–287.

McClellan, A.D. (1994) Time course of locomotor recovery and functional regeneration in spinal-transected lamprey: in vitro brain/spinal cord preparations. *J. Neurophysiol.*, in press.

McClellan, A.D. and Davis, G.R. (1992) Reticulospinal neurons and descending initiation pathways for locomotion in the lamprey. *Soc. Neurosci. Abstr.*, 18: 314.

McClellan, A.D. and Jang, W. (1993) Mechanosensory inputs to the central pattern generators for locomotion in the lamprey spinal cord: resetting, entrainment, and computer modeling. *J. Neurophysiol.*, 70: 2442–2454.

Rovainen, C.M. (1979) Neurobiology of lampreys. *Physiol. Rev.*, 59: 1007–1077.

Rovainen, C.M. (1985) Effects of groups of propriospinal interneurons on fictive swimming in the isolated spinal cord of the lamprey. *J. Neurophysiol.*, 54: 299–317.

Salvio, T. and Schwab, M.E. (1990) Lesioned corticospinal tract axons regenerate in myelin-free rat spinal cord. *Proc. Natl. Acad. Sci. USA*, 87: 4130–4133.

Schnell, L. and Schwab, M.E. (1990) Axonal regeneration in the rat spinal cord produced by an antibody against myelin-associated neurite growth inhibitors. *Nature (London)*, 343: 269–272.

Schwab, M.E. (1990) Myelin-associated inhibitors of neurite growth and regeneration in the CNS. *Trends Neurosci.*, 13: 452–456.

Schwab, M.E. and Schnell, L. (1991) Channeling of developing rat corticospinal tract axons by myelin-associated neurite growth inhibitors. *J. Neurosci.*, 11: 709–721.

Selzer, M.E., Lurie, D. and Mackler, S.A. (1988) Pathfinding and synaptic specificity of regenerating spinal axons in the lamprey. In: H. Flohr (Ed.), *Post-Lesion Neural Plasticity*, Springer-Verlag, Berlin, pp. 233–248.

Stein, P.S.G. (1978) Motor systems, with special reference to locomotion. *Annu. Rev. Neurosci.*, 1: 61–81.

Varga, Z., Erulkar, S. and Nicholls, J. (1993) A critical time period for growth of neurites across a lesion in neonatal opossum spinal cord in culture. *Soc. Neurosci. Abstr.*, 19: 422.

Windle, W.F., Smart, J.O. and Beers, J.J. (1958) Residual function after subtotal spinal cord transection in adult cats. *Neurology*, 8: 518–521.

F.J. Seil (Ed.)
Progress in Brain Research, Vol 103

CHAPTER 18

Spinal cord regeneration in adult goldfish: implications for functional recovery in vertebrates

Steven J. Zottoli, Adrienne P. Bentley, Deborah G. Feiner, John R. Hering, Brian J. Prendergast and Heather I. Rieff

Department of Biology and Neuroscience Program, Williams College, Williamstown, MA 01267, USA

Introduction

The spinal cord of adult teleost fish has a high degree of regenerative capacity after injury (see reviews by Windle, 1955, 1956 and Bernstein, 1988). After spinal cord transections at the high thoracic to cervical levels, fish (*Carassius vulgaris*; *Carassius auratus*; *Cyprinus carpio*; *Oryzias latipes*) first lay on their sides and then gradually recovered some motor behaviors from about 15 days to 2 months postoperatively (Koppányi and Weiss, 1922; Tuge and Hanzawa, 1935,1937; Pearcy and Koppányi, 1941; reviewed by Koppányi, 1955). Although many animals appeared 'normal', some adult fish had partial or no behavioral regeneration 2–3 months postoperatively (Tuge and Hanzawa, 1937; Pearcy and Koppányi, 1941). Cases of incomplete behavioral regeneration were most apparent when fish were lesioned at the cervical spinal cord level. Specifically, none of the fish with cervical spinal wounds recovered equilibrium during postoperative intervals of 40–64 days, although swimming became more coordinated (Tuge and Hanzawa, 1935, 1937). Such results indicate that the success of behavioral regeneration in adult teleost fish may be determined, in part, by the level of spinal cord damage. To determine what factors may limit behavioral regeneration at more rostral lesion sites, we have studied the response of central nervous system (CNS) neurons to spinal cord crush at the spinomedullary level (SML, the junction between the spinal cord and medulla oblongata; this level is the equivalent of the cervical spinal cord level of Tuge and Hanzawa [1935] and is just rostral to the first ventral root). Many injured CNS cells, including vestibulospinal and reticulospinal neurons, do not make the same pathway choice as they made during development. Instead they extend axons into the first ventral root, away from their normal target areas in the spinal cord. This shift in direction may limit behavioral recovery.

Behavioral recovery after SML crush

Thirty-one adult goldfish (*Carassius auratus*; 10–12 cm in body length; Hunting Creek Fisheries) were tested for fast startle responses (C-starts) preoperatively (see Eaton et al., 1988 for behavioral techniques). After testing, fish were anesthetized with 0.03% ethyl-*m*-aminobenzoate and then placed in an operation chamber where chilled water with 0.012% anesthetic was recirculated over the gills. Portions of the skull were removed, and the brain and rostral spinal cord were exposed by suctioning away overlying fat. A complete crush wound was made at the SML level using No. 5 Dumont forceps. The tips of the forceps were lowered on either side of the spinal cord until they touched the ventral portion of the chondrocranium, then moved rostrally to the caudal edge of the vagal lobes (i.e., the spino-medullary level, SML). The tips were then closed and pressure was applied for approx. 2 sec. This procedure was then repeated. The cord was not severed by this crush but a distinct line was present where the forceps had been closed. The location of the SML crush (Fig. 1) was just rostral to the exit of the first ventral root and, as a result, motoneuron axons rostral but not caudal to the lesion would be damaged. The brain was covered with a petroleum jelly–paraffin oil mixture to a level just below the skull. A piece of thin plastic, the size of the hole, was placed on the mixture, and the skull was capped as described previously (Zottoli, 1977) except that a different sealing material (Imprint, 3M) was used. After the operation, the recirculating anesthetic solution was replaced with conditioned tap water and the fish recovered in approx. 10–15 min. Fish were kept in individually aerated tanks at about 22°C and fed Hikari Staple food (Kamihata Co., Ltd.) three times a week.

We have focused on equilibrium and C-start behavior, which are profoundly influenced by a wound at the SML level. Fish were observed immediately after an SML crush and 10 days postoperatively. During this initial period they lay on their sides with no movement caudal to the wound. Subsequent behavioral assessment of equilibium was made biweekly. Once equilibrium returned, fish were tested for C-starts. The behavioral status of 31 goldfish is shown in Fig. 2, at 5 months (A) and 12 months (B) postoperatively. A

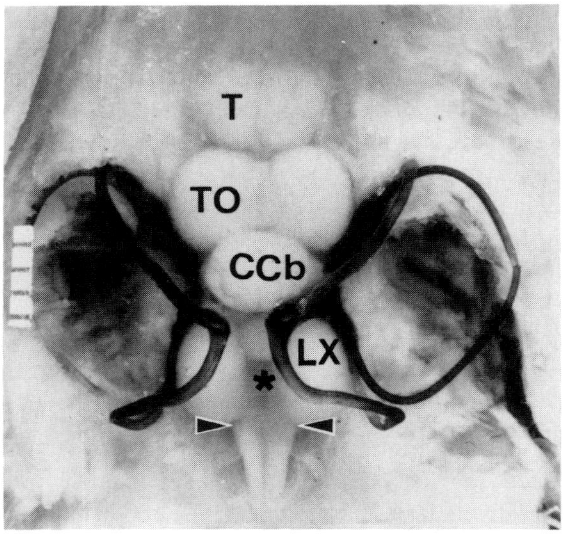

Fig. 1. Dorsal view of the goldfish (*Carassius auratus*) brain and the spino-medullary crush site. The anterior, posterior and horizontal semicircular canals were filled with India ink. The spino-medullary level (SML) crush site is between the arrowheads just caudal to the vagal lobes (LX) at the junction of the spinal cord and medulla oblongata. The medulla oblongata is designated by an asterisk. Abbreviations: T, telencephalon; TO, optic tectum; CCb, corpus cerebellum; LX, vagal lobe. Calibrations in mm. Rostral is at the top and caudal at the bottom. (Modified from Zottoli et al., 1994.)

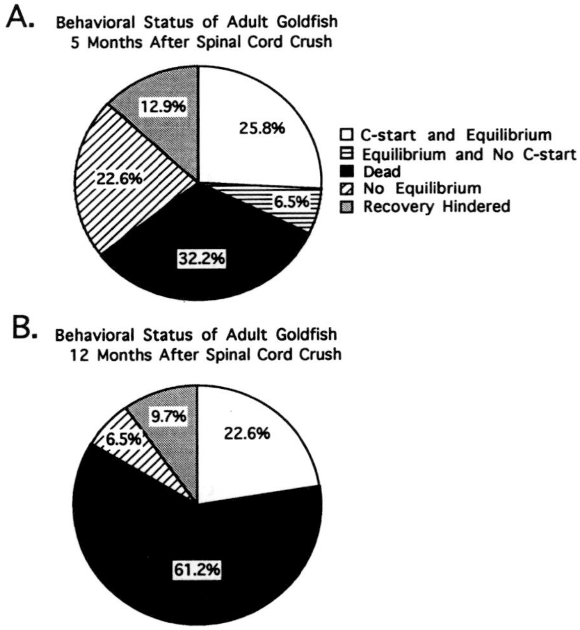

Fig. 2. Behavioral status of goldfish 5 and 12 months after SML crushes. Thirty-one fish were classified based on the recovery of equilibrium and C-starts at two postoperative intervals. A number of fish died during the course of this study and others were hindered as a result of physical abnormalities (e.g., kinks in the tail or arched bodies). The fish that did not regain equilibrium contributed to the increased proportion of dead animals at 12 months postoperatively.

number of fish died during the postoperative interval and others developed physical abnormalities that hindered the recovery of equilibrium (e.g., arched bodies or kinked tails). The behavioral status of those that remained varied. Although about one-quarter of the fish recovered both equilibrium and C-starts, many never recovered equilibrium. The death of some of this latter group contributed to the increased mortality at 12 months.

What factors are responsible for the inability of some fish to recover all behaviors? Although the age of the individual fish (Bernstein, 1964) and wound variability are two possible contributors, we believe that neither of these had a major effect on recovery of behavior, especially at such long postoperative intervals. Rather, recent results indicate that the selection of a peripheral nervous system (PNS) pathway diverts regenerating CNS axons toward totally inappropriate targets. Such a pathway choice could possibly delay, impair, or prevent the return of some behaviors (Bentley and Zottoli, 1993).

Pathway choice of vestibulospinal and reticulospinal neurons after SML crush

Bentley and Zottoli (1993) have shown that the normal pool of motoneuron somata that send axons into PNS by way of the first ventral root (determined by retrograde somata labeling by application of horseradish peroxidase (HRP) on the left root) is entirely ipsilateral to the filled root and extends over a distance of 2.6 ± 0.2 mm (mean ± S.E.M.; n = 5), centered approximately on the SML junction (Fig. 3A1, B1). After an SML crush, the population of somata that project axons into the first ventral root differed from normal pools in two fundamental ways: (1) a new population of somata was labeled on the contralateral side and (2) the extent and composition of labeled cell bodies was different on the ipsilateral side (Fig. 3A2, B2). The new somata found both ipsilateral and contralateral to the labeled ventral root included vestibulospinal and reticulospinal neurons whose axons are normally confined to the CNS (Lee et al., 1993). Examples of regenerating reticulospinal neurons that send axons into the first ventral root are shown in Fig. 4. These neurons are located in the medulla ob-

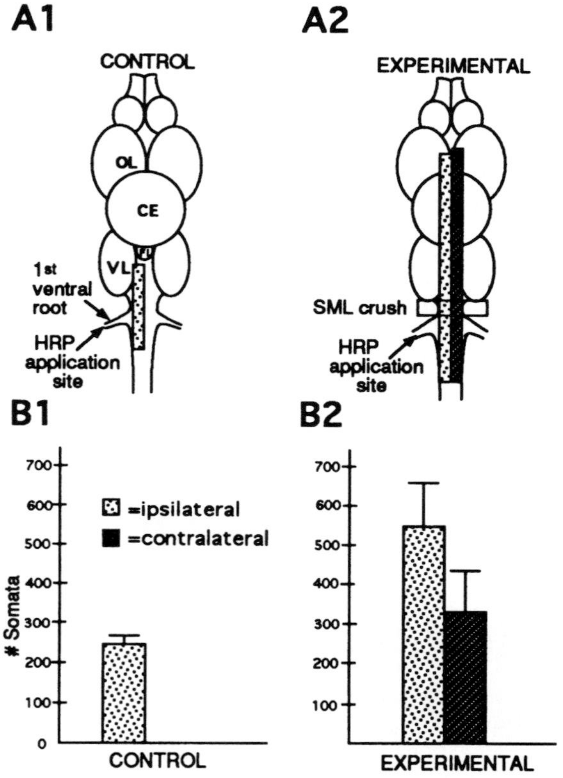

Fig. 3. Distribution and number of neuronal somata labeled after application of horseradish peroxidase (HRP) to the first ventral root. A1, A2. Comparison of the distribution of HRP filled cell bodies in the normal (A1) and experimental (A2) goldfish central nervous system. A1. Crystalline HRP applied to the left first ventral root of normal fish filled motoneuronal somata that were exclusively ipsilateral, and the somata extended 2.6 mm ± 0.2 rostrocaudally (mean ± S.E.M.). A2. In contrast to normal fish, HRP applied to the ventral root in experimental goldfish (70–240 days after SML crush) filled somata both ipsi- and contralaterally over a significantly greater rostrocaudal extent (ipsilateral = 12.7 mm ± 1.0; contralateral = 13.2 mm ± 0.7). B1, B2. Histograms of the numbers of somata filled ipsi- and contralaterally for normal (B1) and experimental (B2) fish. Although the number of ipsilateral experimental somata was not significantly different from controls ($P < 0.06$), the neuronal composition was different. VL, vagal lobe; FL, facial lobe; CE, cerebellum; OL, optic lobe. (From Bentley and Zottoli, 1993.)

longata rostral to the normal motoneuron pool. The left Mauthner axon (M-axon) contains HRP, which indicates that it too has regenerating sprouts in the first root.

The number of regenerated fibers in the ventral root was twice the number counted in the CNS (Bentley and Zottoli, 1993). The higher fiber counts in the PNS may indicate a pathway preference of regenerating CNS axons that is parallel to that in mammalian systems (Richardson et al., 1980). To help determine the pathway preference of individual reticulospinal neurons that are involved in specific behaviors, we have studied the choice made by Mauthner sprouts after they have traversed an SML crush (i.e., PNS vs. CNS) (Zottoli, et al., unpublished observations).

Pathway choice of an identified reticulospinal neuron, the Mauthner cell, after SML crush

The reticulospinal system is one of the most conserved networks in the brain, with organization of nuclei and topographic arrangement of neurons being remarkably similar in various organisms (see Nissanov and Eaton, 1989 and Lee et al., 1993, for references). The Mauthner cell (M-cell) is an identified reticulospinal neuron found in most fish and amphibians (Zottoli, 1978). This cell is involved in the initiation of C-starts, which are thought to be used in escape from predation (Zottoli, 1977; Eaton et al., 1981). To determine the initial pathway choice of this neuron after an

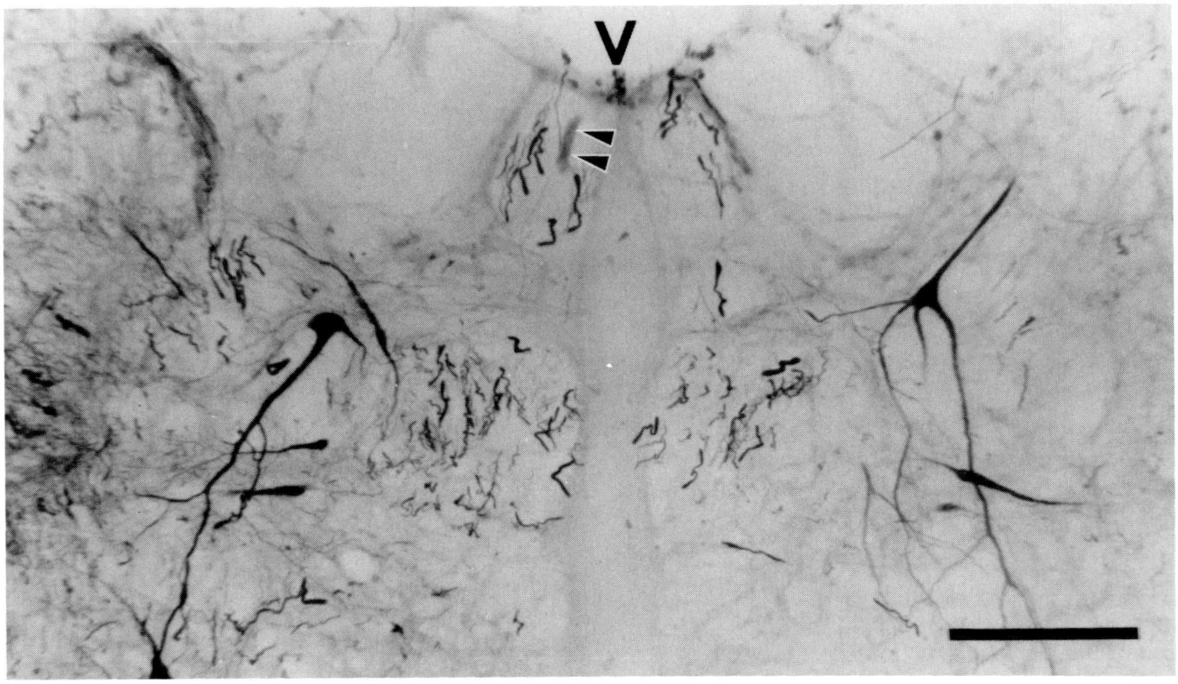

Fig. 4. Photomicrograph of somata and fibers labeled by application of HRP to the left first ventral root of the goldfish 142 days post SML crush. Large reticulospinal somata are labeled with HRP on both sides of the medulla oblongata. These cells are located about 400 μm caudal to the M-cells, a level that is rostral to the normal motoneuron pool of the first ventral root. The left Mauthner axon (double arrowheads) also contains HRP, which indicates that it had sprouts that projected into the root. Many axons within the fasiculus longitudinalis medialis (FLM) contain HRP, which is not the case in control animals. V, ventricle. Dorsal is up and the midline is in the middle of the photograph. Scale bar = 200 μm.

SML crush, we have iontophoretically injected 19 M-axons in 13 goldfish with Lucifer Yellow, 30–42 days post crush (Zottoli et al., unpublished data). Such a procedure is relatively simple since the M-axons are within 100 μm of the surface of the medulla oblongata and are visible with the aid of a dissecting microscope (Fig. 5; Zottoli et al., 1994).

There is a remarkable association between the M-axon sprouts that cross the SML crush wound and the first ventral root. Specifically, 85.7% of regenerating M-axons that traversed the wound and were long enough to be faced with the choice of PNS and/or CNS had sprouts that were either within or in close proximity to the first ventral root. Furthermore, all sprouts of each individual M-axon oriented toward or into the root. There was no instance of an M-axon sending one sprout into the ventral root and another into the spinal cord. The M-axon is capable of regenerating past

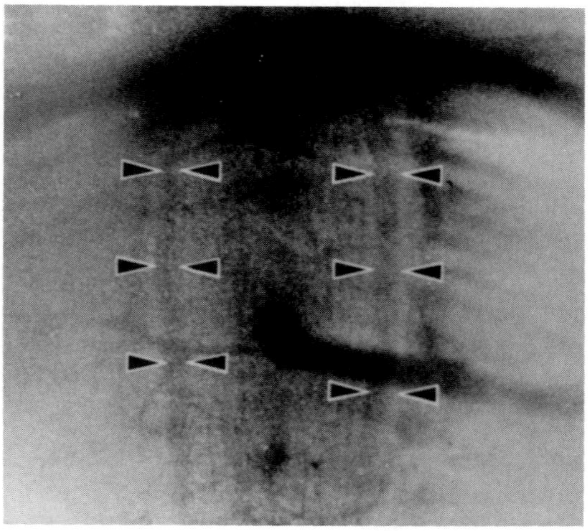

Fig. 5. Visibility of the M-fibers in a living fish. The medulla oblongata can be exposed by tearing the choroid plexus, separating the vagal lobes and wicking away cerebrospinal fluid. The M-fibers lie about 150 μm below the surface of the medulla (designated by asterisk in Fig. 1) and are visible with the aid of a dissecting microscope. The midline of the brain is centered on the picture and the fibers can be seen to either side of the midline (between arrowheads). The fibers are approximately 80–100 μm in diameter. Rostral is at the top and caudal at the bottom. (Modified from Zottoli et al., 1994.)

the ventral root, as indicated in one case where sprouts bypassed the ventral root and continued down the spinal cord. An example of the growth of an M-axon into a ventral root is presented in Fig. 6. These results indicate that at early stages of regeneration the M-axon prefers the first ventral root. Whether this pathway choice is permanent or temporary is not yet known.

Does the Mauthner cell participate in the return of C-start behavior?

The C-start returns after SML crush (Zottoli and Freemer, 1991). This behavioral recovery is lost if the cord is recrushed, confirming the role of axonal regeneration across the wound site. However, significant differences exist between C-starts of experimental fish and sham-operated controls. The differences include lower probability of response, longer latency from stimulus presentation to initiation of the response (Stage 1 latency), smaller turning angles and shorter distances traveled by the center of mass. A comparison of C-starts evoked preoperatively (Fig. 7A1, B1), at the time of behavioral recovery (2.5 months; Fig. 7A2, B2) and 12 months post crush (Fig. 7A3, B3) is presented in Fig. 7. The recovered responses represent some of the most robust ones we have encountered. The most dramatic change is the increase in response latency from 11.6 msec preoperatively to 37.6 msec 2.5 months postoperatively. It is interesting that the response latency then decreased to 27.6 msec at 12 months postoperatively. Such changes in latency may be indicative of plasticity of neuronal wiring or of an increased efficacy of the newly established connections. We have speculated that the longer response latency and the reduced movement in recovered C-starts may compromise the animal's ability to escape predators. Thus, the term 'behavioral regeneration' has been used in preference to 'functional regeneration' (Zottoli and Freemer, 1991).

Our results at about 1 month postoperatively indicate that those Mauthner cells that regenerate into the PNS are unlikely to participate in the

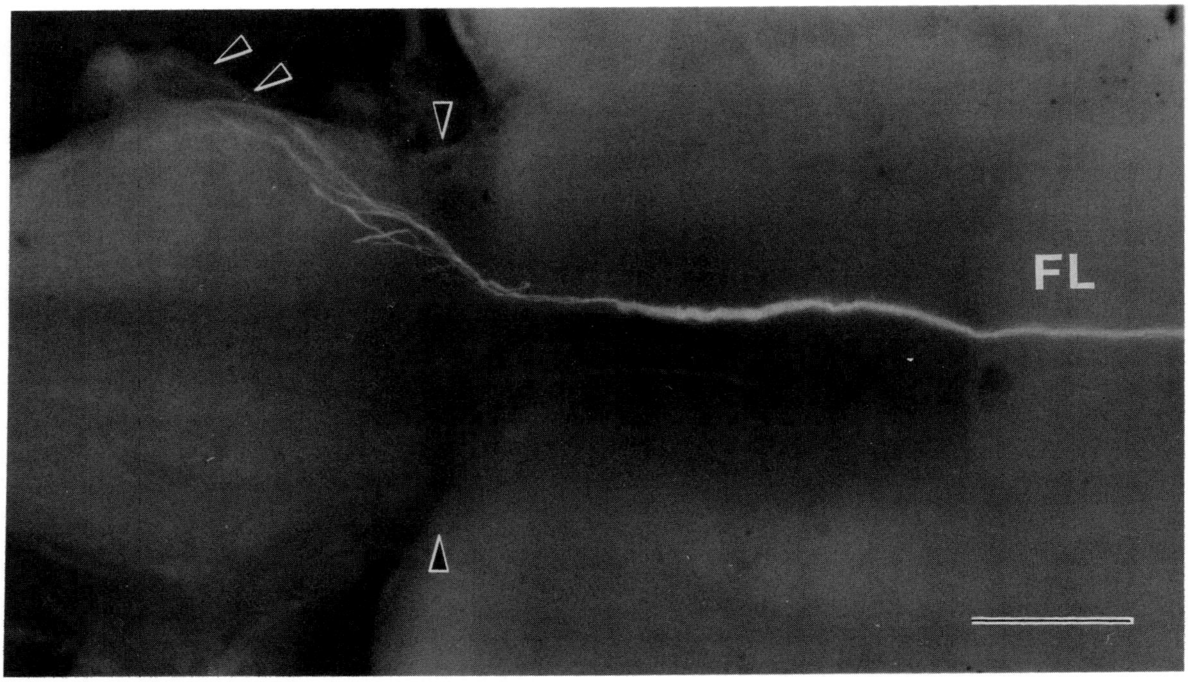

Fig. 6. Regrowth of a right Mauthner axon damaged 32 days previously by whole SML crush. The brain was viewed from its ventral aspect with a fluorescent microscope. The sprouts of this right axon (ventral view of brain) emanate from the parent axon rostral to the wound, cross the wound site (between arrowheads) and project into the first ventral root (double arrowheads). Note that all branches of this axon are either in or oriented toward the root. Rostral is to the right. FL = facial lobe. Scale bar = 500 μm.

initial return of C-start behavior. Although some M-axons with sprouts that remain in the CNS may contribute to C-start recovery, other reticulospinal neurons must be involved in a number of cases. Reticulospinal neurons can elicit C-starts in the absence of the M-cell. Specifically, if both M-cells are lesioned, C-starts have a longer response latency but otherwise appear kinematically identical to those in which the M-cell is present (Eaton et al., 1982). The identity of non-M-cells that participate in this C-start production is not known. Two pairs of candidate neurons have been identified based on the similarities between their dendritic and axonal projections and those of the M-cell. These segmentally homologous neurons (Lee et al., 1993) are shown in Fig. 8. They may be the neurons responsible for behavioral regeneration of C-starts, and therefore it is important to physiologically identify these cells as a first step to ultimately learning how they may participate in the return of C-start behavior.

The long-term fate of regenerating M-cells that choose the PNS in the recovery of C-starts is not clear at this time. Changes in recovered C-start behavior over time, especially a reduction in response latency, indicate a possible plasticity in regenerated neuronal connections that may involve the contribution of additional cells such as M-cells (see above). The one case in which an M-axon bypassed the ventral root and continued down the spinal cord indicates that these cells have the capacity to regenerate in appropriate directions toward motoneuron targets. M-axons can extend up to 3 mm beyond a crush wound by 60 days postoperatively (Zottoli et al., 1988). Furthermore, physiological evidence indicates that

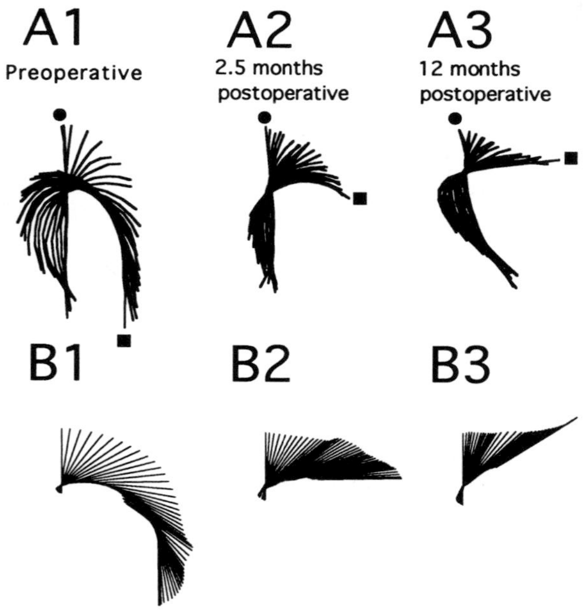

Fig. 7. C-start behavior prior to and 2.5 and 12 months post crush at the SML. A1–A3. Midlines of the fish superimposed to show the actual movement over time. The goldfish midlines are generated every 2 msec starting just before the animal begins a C-start, but only every other one is shown here (i.e., each line represents 4 msec in time). The dot represents the rostral end of the animal just before the animal responds and the square designates the nose at the end of the trial. B1–B3. Linear regression of the rostral 40% of each midline shown in A. Every midline is included in this series (i.e., each line represents 2 msec). A1, B1. Preoperatively C-starts had a short Stage 1 latency (time from stimulus to detectable movement; 11.6 msec). A2, B2. This recovered C-start at 2.5 months post crush has a much longer Stage 1 latency (37.6 msec) and all of the response parameters (e.g., angle and center of mass straight line movement 70 msec after Stage 1 latency, velocity of center of mass movement) are reduced from corresponding preoperative measures. A3, B3. This C-start has a shorter Stage 1 latency (27.6 msec) than that at 2.5 months but is otherwise similar. (For more information on the stimulus and analysis techniques, see Eaton et al., 1988.)

some regenerated M-axons can form functional synapses below the wound since their axonal stimulation can evoke electromyographic responses in trunk musculature (Zottoli et al., 1989). It is possible that sprouts within the ventral root at 33 postoperative days may eventually be retracted in favor of those those that project down the spinal cord. Thus, it is important to determine pathway choice of the M-cell at longer postoperative intervals.

Why do regenerating CNS neurons choose the first ventral root?

Ramón y Cajal (1928) described CNS sprouts that entered anterior (ventral) roots of young cats after spinal cord injury. He stated, "Such strange migrating sprouts are the more abundant the nearer the root is to the wound, provided always that the degenerated roots have been largely replaced by *bands of Bünger*." He suggested that the Schwann cells induce growth and attract these sprouts. Our results confirm the centrifugal growth described by Cajal and his attraction hypothesis provides one explanation of why regenerating CNS axons choose the ventral root. Alternatively, regenerating motoneuron axons might provide a pathway that can be followed by regenerating CNS axons into the PNS. An SML crush severs axons of rostral motoneurons that project into the first ventral root. Presumably these motor axons regenerate toward their normal targets by way of the first root. This hypothesis of pathway guidance does not require Schwann cell attraction but would require interactions between regenerating motoneuron axons and regenerating CNS neurons that come in contact with them. Observations of the second ventral root might help distinguish between the two hypotheses. If this root was not damaged by an SML crush, then there would be no attraction of regenerating sprouts by Schwann cells. Therefore, if regenerating CNS neurons exited this second root, the second hypothesis would be more attractive.

Once CNS axons are within the PNS, they might be expected to continue the entire length of the nerve toward the periphery, as is the case of mammalian CNS neurons exposed to peripheral nerve segments (David and Aguayo, 1981, 1985). Further studies on the growth of regenerating CNS fibers into the PNS will provide interesting information on the long-term viability of misdirected CNS sprouts, their maximal growth and

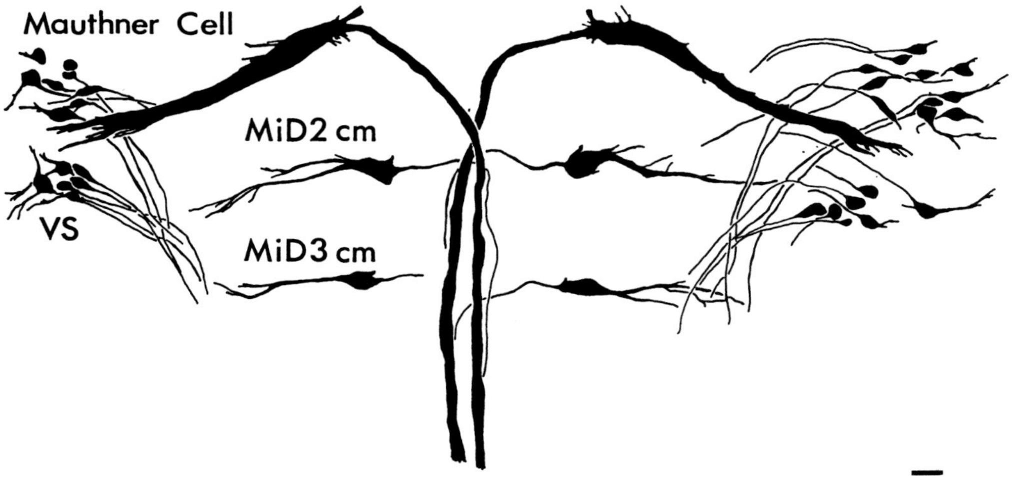

Fig. 8. Horizontal view of three pairs of segmentally homologous neurons, the Mauthner series. The Mauthner cells, MiD2cm and MiD3cm, respectively, are shown. These three pairs of neurons have lateral dendrites and decussating axons that enter the fasciculus longitudinalis medialis. These neurons also have prominent ventral dendrites that are not apparent in the horizontal plane. Scale bar = 50 μm. (Modified from Lee et al., 1993.)

their interaction with Schwann cells (Ramón y Cajal, 1928; Aguayo et al., 1982). Finally, if these sprouts continue to extend in the PNS, their ultimate interaction with peripheral targets (e.g., muscle fibers) can be determined.

Conclusions

Many CNS neurons damaged by SML crush in adult goldfish extend sprouts that choose a PNS pathway. We suggest that this inappropriate choice delays, impairs, or prevents recovery of behaviors, including equilibrium and C-starts. If this pathway choice is responsible for the limited regenerative capacity, it may also explain limited behavioral recovery in nonmammalian (e.g., adult lamprey: Ayers et al., 1982; Cohen and Baker, 1988; Margolin and Ayers, 1988; Cohen, et al., 1989; goldfish: Tuge and Hanzawa, 1937; frogs: Piatt and Piatt, 1958; and salamanders: Davis et al., 1990) and mammalian vertebrates alike.

The goldfish PNS may present a more permissive environment to regenerating fibers than the CNS after SML crush. Such a pathway preference demonstrates a parallel to mammalian systems (Ramón y Cajal, 1928; David and Aguayo, 1981, 1985) and makes the goldfish more valuable as a model system for regeneration.

While advances have been made in techniques that allow mammalian CNS neurons to regenerate over distances longer than 1 mm, such as peripheral nerve implants, conditioned media, and antibodies that neutralize inhibitory substances (Richardson et al., 1980; David and Aguayo, 1981, 1985; Caroni and Schwab, 1988; Aguayo et al., 1990; Lavie et al., 1990; Schnell and Schwab, 1990; Schwab, 1990), there is no guarantee that regenerating sprouts will make appropriate pathway choices (Aguayo et al., 1991), that behavioral recovery will result in the return of function or that neurons normally involved in a behavior will contribute equally to the recovery. The adult goldfish nervous system provides an exciting model to address these issues.

Acknowledgements

We thank Don Faber for reviewing an earlier version of this manuscript. This research was supported in part by NSF grant 8809445 and an Essel Foundation Grant to Williams College.

References

Aguayo, A.J., David, S., Richardson, P.M. and Bray, G.M. (1982) Axonal elongation in peripheral and central nervous system transplants. In: S. Fedoroff and L. Hertz (Eds.), *Advances in Cellular Neurobiology*, Vol. 3, Academic Press, New York, pp. 215–234.

Aguayo, A.J., Bray, G.M., Rasminsky, M., Zwimpfer, T., Carter,D. and Vidal-Sanz, M. (1990) Synaptic connections made by axons regenerating in central nervous system of adult mammals. *J. Exp. Biol.*, 153: 199–224.

Aguayo, A.J., Rasminsky, M., Bray, G.M., Carbonetto, S., McKerracher, L., Villegas-Pérez, N., Vidal-Sanz, M. and Carter, D.A. (1991) Degenerative and regenerative responses of injured neurons in the central nervous system of adult mammals. *Phil. Trans. R. Soc. Lond. B*, 331: 337–343.

Ayers, J., Currie, S., Kinch, J. and Pereira, W. (1982) Adult lampreys can recover from complete spinal cord transection. *Soc. Neurosci. Abstr.*, 8: 868.

Bentley, A.P. and Zottoli, S.J. (1993) Central nervous system lesion triggers inappropriate pathway choice in adult vertebrate system. *Brain Res.*, 630: 333–336.

Bernstein, J.J. (1964) Relation of spinal cord regeneration to age in adult goldfish. *Exp. Neurol.*, 9: 161–174.

Bernstein, J.J. (1988) Successful spinal cord regeneration: known biological strategies. In: P.J. Reier, R.P. Bunge and F.J. Seil (Eds.), *Current Issues in Neural Regeneration Research*, Alan R. Liss, Inc., New York, pp. 331–341.

Caroni, P. and Schwab, M.E. (1988) Antibody against myelin-associated inhibitor of neurite growth neutralizes non-permissive substrate properties of CNS white matter. *Neuron*, 1: 85–96.

Cohen, A.H. and Baker, M.T. (1988) Functional and non-functional regeneration in the spinal cord of adult lampreys. In: P.J.Reier, R.P. Bunge, and F.J. Seil (Eds.), *Current Issues in Neural Regeneration Research*, Alan R. Liss, New York, pp. 387–396.

Cohen, A.H., Baker, M.T. and Dobrov, T.A. (1989) Evidence for functional regeneration in the adult lamprey spinal cord following transection. *Brain Res.*, 496: 368–372.

David, S. and Aguayo, A.J. (1981) Axonal elongation into peripheral nervous system 'bridges' after central nervous system injury in adult rats. *Science*, 214: 931–933.

David, S. and Aguayo, A.J. (1985) Axonal regeneration after crush injury of rat central nervous system fibres innervating peripheral nerve grafts. *J. Neurocytol.*, 14: 1–12.

Davis, B.M., Ayers, J.L., Koran, L., Carlson, J., Anderson, M.C. and Simpson, S.B., Jr. (1990) Time course of salamander spinal cord regeneration and recovery of swimming: HRP retrograde pathway tracing and kinematic analysis. *Exp. Neurol.*, 108: 1–16.

Eaton, R.C., Lavender, W.A. and Wieland, C.M. (1981) Identification of Mauthner initiated response patterns in goldfish: evidence from stimultaneous cinematography and electrophysiology. *J. Comp. Physiol.*, 144: 521–531.

Eaton, R.C., Lavender, W.A. and Wieland, C.M. (1982) Alternative neural pathways initiate fast-start responses following lesions of the Mauthner neuron in goldfish. *J. Comp. Physiol.*, 145: 485–496.

Eaton, R.C., DiDomenico, R. and Nissanov, J. (1988) Flexible body dynamics of the goldfish C-start: implications for reticulospinal command mechanisms. *J. Neurosci.*, 8: 2758–2768.

Koppányi, T. and Weiss, P. (1922) Functionelle Regeneration des Rückenmarks bei Anamniern. *Anz. Akad. Wiss. Wien, math. nature. Kl.*, 59: 206.

Koppányi, T. (1955) Regeneration in the central nervous system of fishes. In: W.F. Windle (Ed.), *Regeneration in the Central Nervous System*, Charles C. Thomas, Springfield, pp. 3–19.

Lavie, V., Murray, M., Solomon, A., Ben-Bassat, S., Belkin, M., Rumelt, S. and Schwartz, M. (1990) Growth of injured rabbit optic neurons within their degenerating optic nerve. *J. Comp. Neurol.*, 298: 293–314.

Lee, R.K.K., Eaton, R.C. and Zottoli, S.J. (1993) Segmental arrangement of hindbrain neurons in the goldfish, *Carassius auratus*. *J. Comp. Neurol.*, 329: 539–556.

Margolin, L. and Ayers, J. (1988) Development and recovery of command function by the pontine locomotor region in the lamprey. *Soc. Neurosci. Abstr.*, 14: 653.

Nissanov, J. and Eaton, R.C. (1989) Reticulospinal control of rapid escape turning maneuvers in fishes. *Amer. Zool.*, 29: 103–121.

Piatt, J. and Piatt, M. (1958) Transection of the spinal cord in the adult frog. *Anat. Rec.*, 131: 81–95.

Pearcy, J.F. and Koppányi, T. (1941) A further note on regeneration of the cut spinal cord in fish. *Proc. Soc. Exp. Biol. Med.*, 22: 17–19.

Ramón y Cajal, S. (1928) In: J. DeFelipe and E.G. Jones, (Eds.), *Cajal's Degeneration & Regeneration of the Nervous System*, translated by Raoul M. May, Oxford University Press, Oxford, 1991, pp. 10, 43–51, 118, 536.

Richardson, P.M., McGuinness, U.M. and Aguayo, A.J. (1980) Axons from CNS neurones regenerate into PNS grafts. *Nature (Lond.)*, 284: 264–265.

Schnell, L. and Schwab, M.E. (1990) Axonal regeneration in the rat spinal cord produced by an antibody against myelin-associated neurite growth inhibitors. *Nature (Lond.)*, 343: 269–272.

Schwab, M.E. (1990) Myelin-associated inhibitors of neurite growth and regeneration in the CNS. *Trends Neurosci.*, 13: 452–456.

Tuge, H. and Hanzawa, S. (1935) Physiology of the spinal fish, with special reference to the postural mechanism. *Sci. Rep.Tohoku Imp. Univ., Biol.*, 10: 589–606.

Tuge, H. and Hanzawa, S. (1937) Physiological and morphological regeneration of the sectioned spinal cord in adult teleosts. *J. Comp. Neurol.*, 67: 343- 365.

Windle, W.F. (Ed.) (1955) *Regeneration in the Central Nervous System*. Charles C. Thomas, Springfield, Ill.

Windle, W.F. (1956) Regeneration of axons in the vertebrate central nervous system. *Physiol. Rev.*, 36: 427–440.

Zottoli, S.J. (1977) Correlation of the startle reflex and Mauthner cell auditory responses in unrestrained goldfish. *J. Exp. Biol.*, 66: 65–81.

Zottoli, S.J. (1978) Comparative morphology of the Mauthner cell in fish and amphibians, In: D. Faber and H. Korn (Eds.), *Neurobiology of the Mauthner Cell*, Raven Press, New York, pp. 13–45.

Zottoli, S.J. and Freemer, M.M. (1991) Behavioral recovery of the goldfish startle response after spinal cord crush. *Soc. Neurosci. Abstr.*, 17: 942.

Zottoli, S.J., Agostini, M.A., Danielson, P.D., Lee, E.J., Laidley, T.L., Markstein, E.A. and Scalise, T.L. (1988) Pathway selection of regenerating Mauthner axons of the adult goldfish. *Soc. Neurosci. Abstr.*, 14: 54.

Zottoli, S.J., Northen, S.C. and Scalise, T.L. (1989) Regeneration of the goldfish Mauthner cell does not underlie behavioral recovery of the startle response. *Soc. Neurosci. Abstr.*, 15: 333.

Zottoli, S.J., Bentley, A.P., Prendergast, B.J. and Rieff, H.I. (1994) Comparative studies on the Mauthner cell of teleost fish in relation to sensory input. *Brain Behav. Evol.*, in press.

F.J. Seil (Ed.)
Progress in Brain Research, Vol 103

CHAPTER 19

The lizard spinal cord: a model system for the study of spinal cord injury and repair

Sidney B. Simpson Jr. and Mark T. Duffy

Department of Biological Sciences, University of Illinois at Chicago, Chicago, IL 60607, USA

Introduction

Our laboratory has been engaged in a detailed analysis of spinal cord regeneration in two inframammalian model systems, the urodele amphibian, *Notophthalmus (Triturus) viridescens*, and the iguanid lizard, *Anolis carolinensis*. In this chapter we will review our studies on the lizard and comment briefly on results from other systems, inframammalian and mammalian, as they relate to our findings in the lizard.

The regenerated tail spinal cord of *Anolis*

Cellular organization

Autotomy of the tail in *Anolis* results in the formation of a regeneration blastema that grows and differentiates, ultimately replacing the lost portion of the tail. Internally, the injured tail spinal cord also regenerates but is quite deficient when compared with the original (Simpson, 1968, 1970; Egar et al., 1970; Alibardi et al., 1992). The regenerated cord consists of an epithelial tube primarily made up of ependymal epithelial cells that grow from the ependymal cell lining of the injured spinal cord. Enclosed within the ependymal tube are some 2,000 to 4,000 descending central axons that have grown from the injured cord. The ependymal cells in the regenerate surround the central canal. They are linked by tight junctions at their luminal ends and extend long processes that abut on the basal lamina at the pial surface. These processes, reminiscent of the embryonic neuroepithelial cells, radiate like spokes of a wagon wheel and define longitudinal channels that contain the descending central axons (Simpson, 1968, 1970). Thus, all but a few stray descending central axons are fasciculated within the channels of the ependymal tube (Fig. 1).

Originally it was believed that the cellular content of the regenerated cord was exclusively the ependymal cells (Simpson, 1970). However, we now know that the regenerated spinal cord contains small numbers of neurons of a type known as cerebrospinal fluid contacting neurons (CSFCNs). This class of neuron has been extensively described in the literature (Vigh and Vigh-Teichmann, 1973; Vigh-Teichmann et al., 1979; Vigh et al., 1980; Fujita et al., 1988). CSFCNs are present in the embryonic and adult spinal cords of every vertebrate that has been examined (Vigh and Vigh-Teichmann, 1973; Scott et al., 1982; Oksche, 1988). The function(s) of these neurons is unknown. Suggested functions range from chemosensory (Vigh and Vigh-Teichmann, 1973) to neurosecretory (Fujita et al., 1988; Oksche, 1988) to mechanosensory (Alibardi et al., 1993a). CSFCNs were first described in the cord regenerates of three Australian lizards (Alibardi and

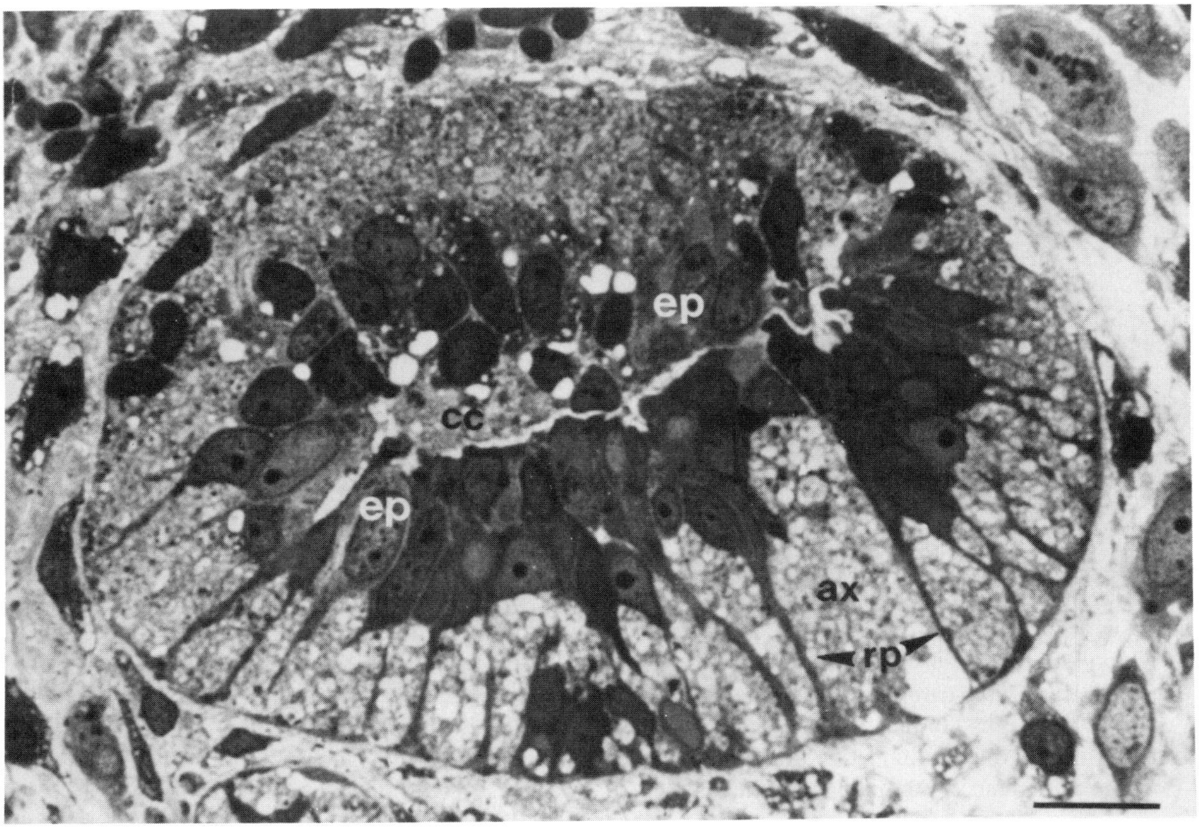

Fig. 1. Light photomicrograph of a 1 μm thick transverse section of the regenerated tail spinal cord stained with methylene blue. The regenerated spinal cord is made up of descending axons (ax) fasciculated by radial processes (rp) of ependymal cells (ep) which line the central canal (cc). No neuronal cell bodies are present in this section. The spinal cord is surrounded by fibroblasts and connective tissue. Calibration bar = 10 μm. (From Duffy et al., 1990.)

Meyer-Rochow, 1988), and later in the lizard, *Anolis*, by Alibardi et al. (1992).

The CSFCNs that differentiate in the regenerated spinal cord are indistinguishable from those found in the normal adult cord. In the regenerated cord these cells appear as rounded or plump spindle-shaped electron-lucent cells (Fig. 2). Their luminal ends are connected to surrounding ependymal cells via tight junctions. Their luminal ends project into the central canal as a cluster of stereociliar tufts (Fig. 3). The stereocilia are shorter and wider than the cilia of the surrounding ependymal cells (Alibardi et al., 1993a). They also have a characteristic flattened tip. The tufts contact Reissner's fiber inside the central canal. The CSFCNs exhibit clusters of rough endoplasmic reticulum, resembling Nissl bodies. Synapses are rarely observed, but have been found on the perikarya of these cells. Each CSFCN has a large axon-like process that projects to the pial surface, joins the fasciculated descending axons, and then ascends rostrally within the regenerated cord. These CSFCNs accumulate ^{3}H-GABA, while surrounding ependymal cells do not (Alibardi et al., 1993b). Previous studies of CS-FCNs in the normal cord of other vertebrates

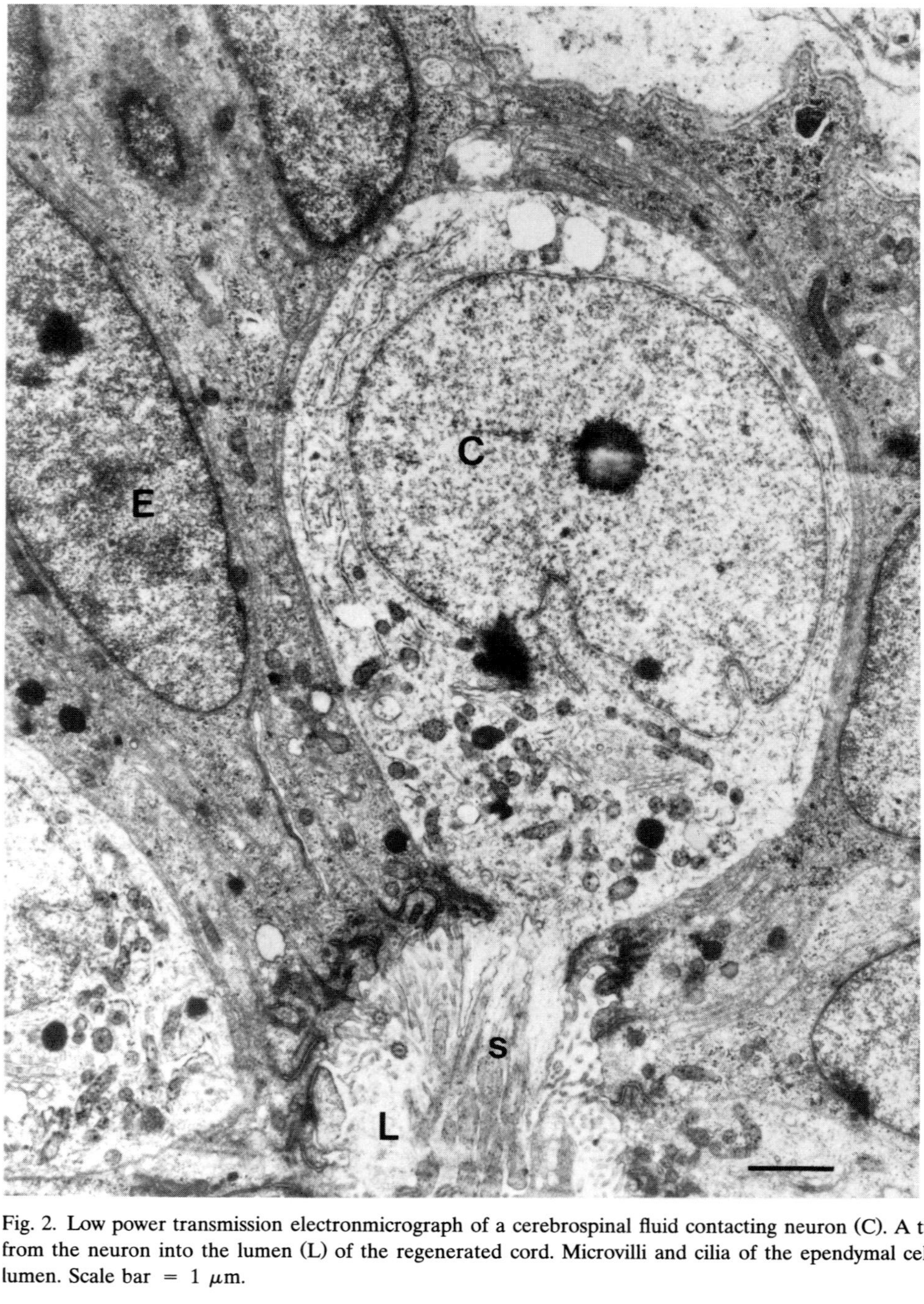

Fig. 2. Low power transmission electronmicrograph of a cerebrospinal fluid contacting neuron (C). A tuft of stereocilia (s) project from the neuron into the lumen (L) of the regenerated cord. Microvilli and cilia of the ependymal cells (E) also project into the lumen. Scale bar = 1 μm.

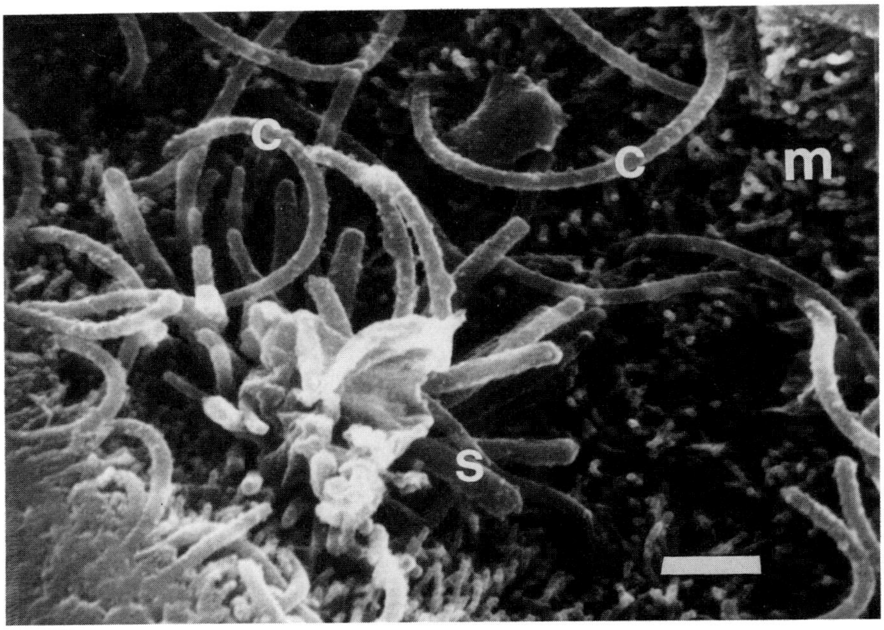

Fig. 3. Scanning electronmicrograph of a tuft of stereocilia (s) from a cerebrospinal fluid contacting neuron projecting up into the lumen of the regenerated spinal cord. Surrounding the stereocilia are cilia (c) and microvilli (m) of the ependymal cells. Scale bar = 1 μm.

demonstrated GABA immunoreactivity in these cells (McLaughlin et al., 1975; Barberm et al., 1982; Dale et al., 1987; Brodin et al., 1990).

In young regenerates, the CSFCNs are rather evenly distributed along the length of the regenerate. Thymidine labeling experiments have shown that young neuroblast-like cells differentiate from the rapidly dividing subterminal ependymal cells and subsequently differentiate into CSFCNs (Alibardi et al., 1992). Among these differentiating cells one encounters images that are reminiscent of degenerating cells.

Mature regenerates (6 months or older) exhibit only mature CSFCNs and their distribution is nonuniform. While two to three small clusters of CSFCNs ranging from 2 to 20 cells per cluster are found along the length of the mature regenerated cord, most of them are localized in the distal-most region of the regenerated cord (Duffy et al., 1993). Here, within a 1.0 mm segment, as many as 60 CSFCNs can be found. Labeling experiments using horseradish peroxidase (HRP) and fluorescent dyes demonstrated that the most distal group of CSFCNs send axons rostrally as far as the transition zone. None appear to project past two vertebral segments rostral to the level of cord injury. Interestingly enough, none of the CSFCNs in more rostral regions of the regenerated cord sends axons into the old cord. Thus those CSFCNs that project rostrally beyond the regenerated cord proper seem to end in either the transition zone (where many of the descending axons also end) or immediately rostral to the transition zone. The latter area is where the majority of the descending axons in the regenerate have their origin. Ascending axons of CSFCNs have also been described in larval *Xenopus* (Chen and Heathcote, 1993); some may even reach the developing hindbrain (Nordlander, 1991, personal communication).

The presence or absence of glial cells, other than the ependymal tanycytes, would seem to depend upon the species of lizard. Astrocyte-like profiles have been described (Egar et al., 1970; Alabardi, 1990) but they are rare. Oligodendroglia are not seen in the regenerated cord of *Anolis* (Simpson, 1968; Egar et al., 1970). However, they have been described in the mature regenerated cord of other lizards, as well as in *Sphenodon* (Alibardi, 1990). In these cases it was unclear whether they differentiated from the outgrowing ependymal cells or migrated into the regenerated cord from the normal cord.

Thus the cellular component of the regenerated cord in *Anolis* consists primarily of ependymal cells. The outgrowing ependymal cells of the young regenerate exhibit a very limited potential for both neurogenesis and gliogenesis. This limited potential is probably due to the absence of appropriate interactions between the outgrowing ependymal-neuroepithelial cells and the surrounding mesenchymal-mesodermal cells in the blastema. Problems in the normal signaling are reflected in both the restricted cellular potential of the regenerated cord and the absence of a segmented vertebral column. The latter is replaced by a continuous elastic-hyaline cartilage tube that surrounds the regenerated cord (Simpson, 1964). The lack of proper ependyma-mesenchyme interactions may likewise explain why in urodeles rather complete cellular replacement (glia and neurons) occurs during tail cord regeneration, yet no new neurons are produced during thoracic cord regeneration (Davis et al., 1990).

Origin of the descending central axons

As mentioned earlier, the regenerated tail cord of *Anolis* contains between 2,000 and 4,000 unmyelinated, descending central axons of various diameters (Simpson, 1968, 1970). The origins of the fiber projections to the normal tail spinal cord and the regenerated tail cord have been mapped using a variety of retrograde markers (Duffy et al., 1990, 1992). Application of HRP to the severed normal tail spinal cord labeled neurons in the nucleus paraventricularis, the interstitial nucleus of the fasciculus longitudinalis, the nucleus ruber, the medullary reticular formation and the vestibular nuclei (Fig 4). When HRP was applied to the regenerated tail spinal cord, only 4% of the neurons labeled in the normal tail cord were labeled in the regenerate. The majority of the supraspinal neurons labeled from the regenerated cord were confined to the rhombencephalic nuclei (Fig. 5a). The absence of labeling in the more rostral nuclei was not due to their death or atrophy. HRP applied immediately rostral to the regenerated tail cord (i.e., the transition zone) resulted in the labeling of normal to supernormal numbers of supraspinal neurons in all areas (Fig. 5b). The HRP studies thus suggested that many of the central axons in the regenerate were likely to be of long propriospinal or local spinal origin. This was verified using an assay that was independent of the retrograde tracing method. Actual counts of central axons were made in the regenerated cords, before and after complete spinal transections at various levels. The axon counts were made from electronmicrograph montages. The data demonstrated that the number of central axons in the regenerated cord was significantly reduced only when the cord transection was made within one spinal segment rostral to the regenerated cord proper. This was consistent with our HRP studies and confirmed the local origin of most of the axons in the regenerated cord.

Next, the number of spinal neurons contributing axons to the regenerate proper and to the transition zone immediately rostral to the regenerated cord were assayed with HRP. The results are presented in Fig. 6. When HRP was applied to the regenerate proper, there was a 134% increase in the labeled spinal neurons when compared with those labeled from a normal cord at the same level. Moreover, application of HRP to the transition zone rostral to the regenerated cord resulted in a spinal neuron labeling increase of 233% over normal. These results demonstrate that the majority of the descending central axons in the regenerate are of local spinal origin. They

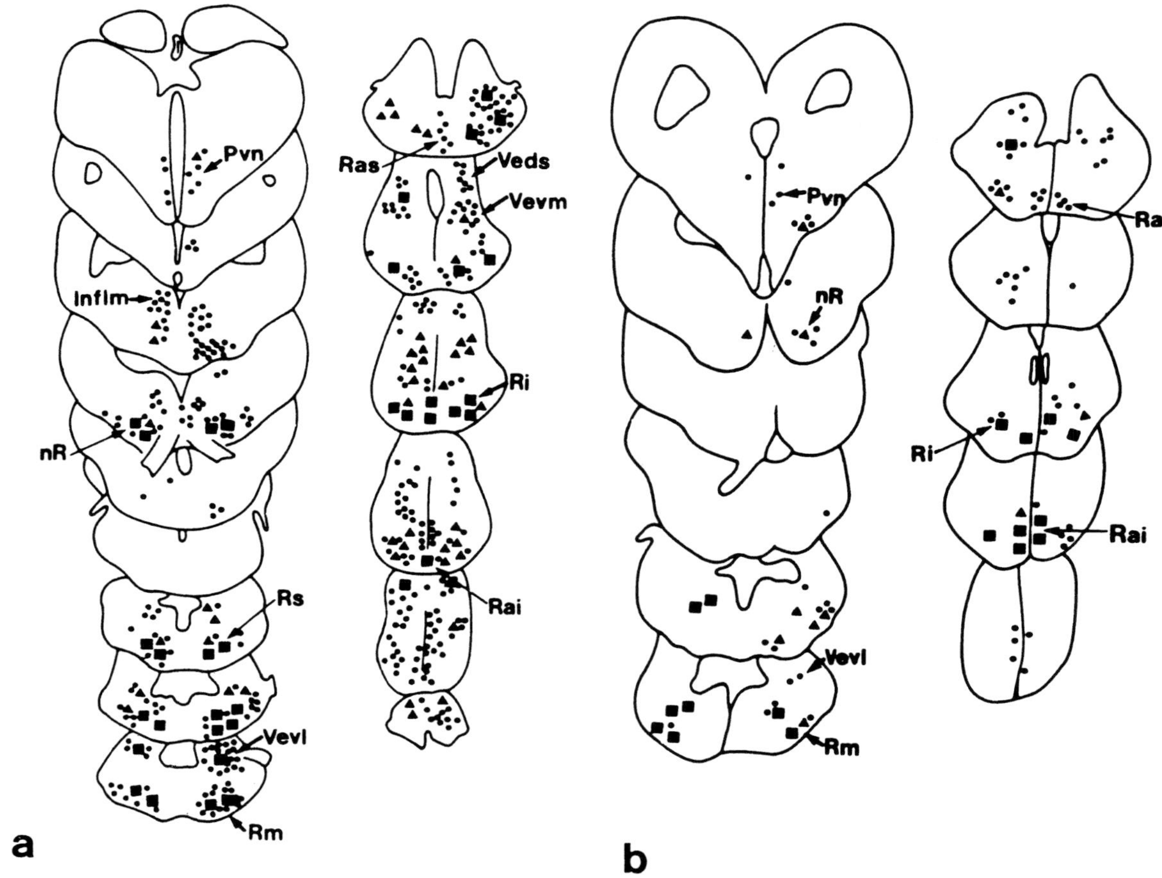

Fig. 4. Distribution of HRP labeled supraspinal neurons following application of HRP to a transection of the lumbar enlargement (a) and the tail spinal cord (b). For these schematics, tracings from five adjacent 50 μm tissue sections were collapsed so that each panel in a and b represents 250 μm of tissue. All HRP labeled cells are shown. The supraspinal projections to the two levels of the spinal cord are similar and differ primarily in the number of neurons arising from the different nuclei. ●, single HRP labeled neurons; ▲, five HRP labeled neurons; ■, ten HRP labeled neurons. Inflm, interstitial nucleus of the fasciculus longitudinalis medialis; Pvn, nucleus paraventricularis; Rai, nucleus raphe inferioris; Ras, nucleus raphe superioris; Ri, nucleus reticularis inferioris,; Rm, nucleus reticularis medius; Rs, nucleus reticularis superioris; nR, nucleus ruber; Veds, nucleus vestibulares descendens; Vevl, nucleus vestibulares ventrolateralis; Vevm, nucleus vestibulares ventromedialis. (From Duffy et al., 1990.)

also suggest that many of the axons both rostral to and within the regenerate are the products of sprouting of uninjured axons.

To gain some estimate of the proportion of directly regenerating axons to sprouting axons, we performed double labeling experiments where fluorescein-conjugated latex beads were applied to the injured spinal cord at the time of autotomy and HRP was applied to the transition zone of the subsequent mature regenerate. With this protocol, double labeled neurons should represent neurons whose axons were injured during transection and subsequently regenerated. In this study (Duffy et al., 1992) 28% of the local spinal neurons were double labeled, while 7% of the supraspinal neurons were double labeled.

The potential contribution of new neurons to the number of axons in the regenerated cord was

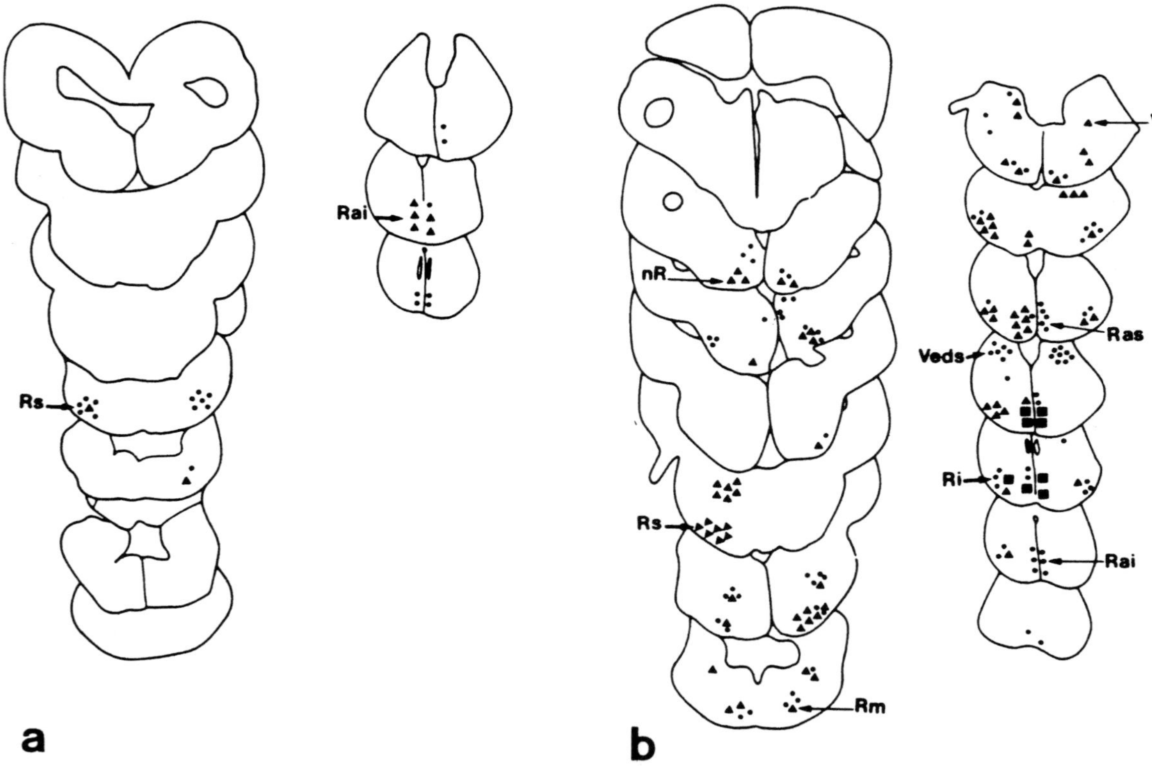

Fig. 5. Distribution of HRP labeled supraspinal neurons following application of HRP directly to the regenerated tail spinal cord (a) and following application of HRP to the transition zone immediately rostral to a regenerated tail (b). Each panel represents 250 μm. All HRP labeled cells are shown. (a) HRP labeled cells are seen in mesencephalic and medullary reticular formation (Rs and Rai, respectively). In other cases, HRP labeled cells are seen in other mesencephalic and medullary reticular nuclei, but in no cases are cells seen in the nucleus ruber or in nuclei rostral to the mesencephalon. (b) In this particular case, the nucleus paraventricularis and the interstitial nucleus of the fasciculus longitudinalis medialis are not labeled, although in other cases using the same protocol, labeled cells were seen in these nuclei. ●, single HRP labeled neurons; ▲, five HRP labeled neurons; ■, ten HRP labeled neurons. Rai, nucleus raphe inferioris; Ras, nucleus raphe superioris; Ri, nucleus reticularis inferioris; Rm, nucleus reticularis medius; Rs, nucleus reticularis superioris; nR, nucleus ruber; Veds, nucleus vestibulares descendens; Vevl, nucleus vestibulares ventrolateralis. (From Duffy et al., 1990.)

assessed by using repeated ^{3}H-thymidine labeling. Since the majority of the axons in the regenerate come from the 7.0 mm of normal cord rostral to the regenerate, we focused on this area. In injection protocols where control tissues (duodenal epithelium and blastema cells) were labeled to 84% and 90% respectively, no positively labeled neurons were seen (Duffy et al., 1992). The telencephalons of the same lizards were used as a control to establish that new neurons could be born, migrate and differentiate within the time frame of the experiments. The telencephalon is a superb internal control since it continuously produces new neurons in the adult lizard (Garcia-Verdugo et al., 1984; Davila et al., 1986).

Thus the descending central axons in the regenerated cord of *Anolis* comprise a sampling of most of the axons that normally project to the tail cord. However, with regard to number, few supraspinal axons extend into the regenerate proper. The remainder reside in the transition zone rostral to the regenerate proper. Clearly the majority of the axons in the regenerate are of local spinal origin and many of these are the result of sprouting. Some of these sprouted axons had to have traversed several millimeters of the normal spinal cord to end up in either the transition zone or the regenerate cord. It is worth noting that the proliferative response of the ependymal epithelium also extended several mil-

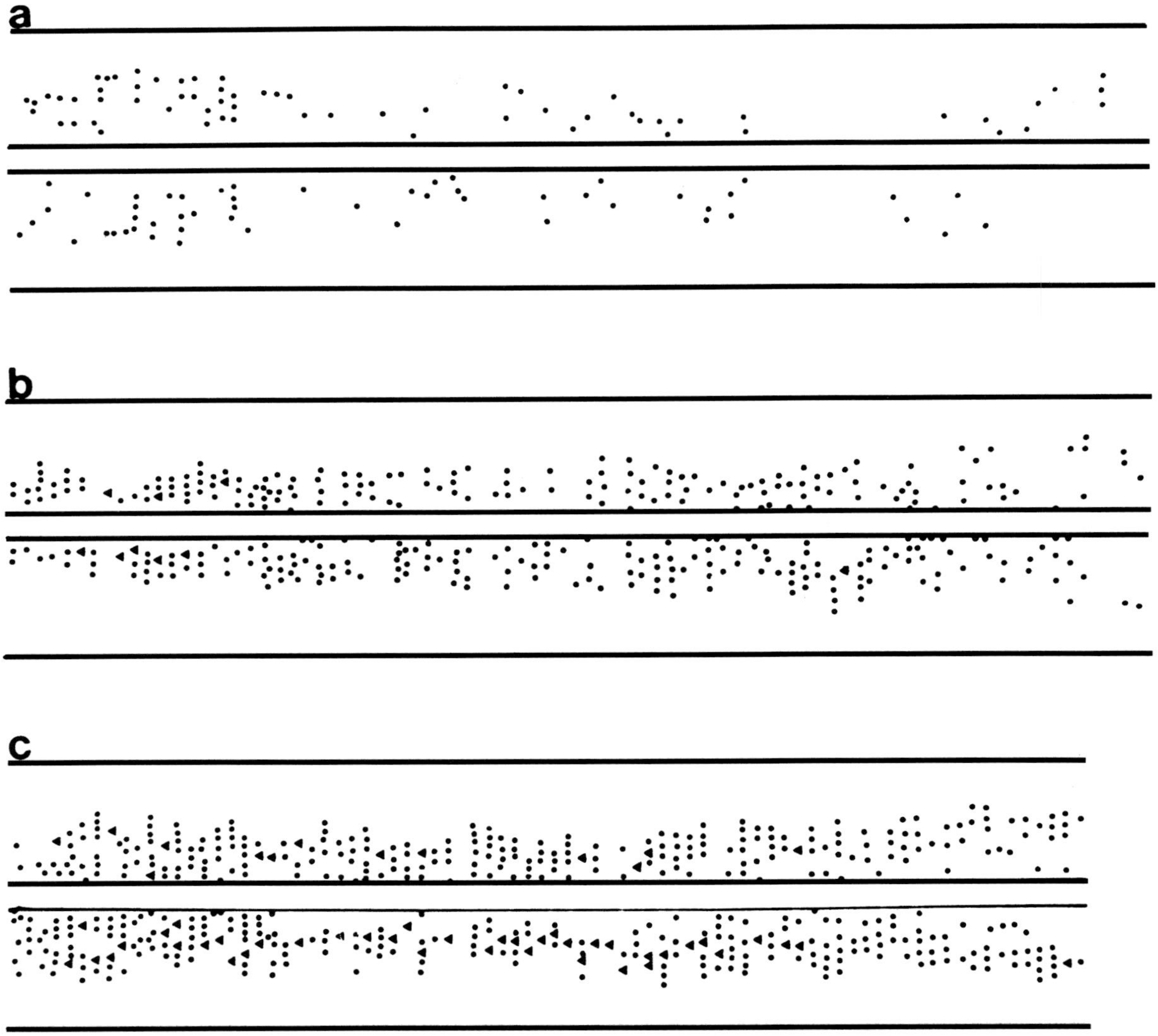

Fig. 6. Distribution of HRP labeled spinal cord neurons following application of HRP to normal tail (a), directly to the regenerated tail spinal cord (b), and to the transition zone immediately rostral to a regenerated tail (c). The portions of the tail spinal cord in (a) and (c) are from the site of HRP application (left side of schematic) to the caudal end of the lumbar enlargement (right side). In (b), the orientation is the same but the left side represents the junction of regenerated and normal spinal cord. All HRP labeled cells are shown. ●, single HRP labeled neurons; ▲, five HRP labeled neurons. The greatest number of labeled neurons is seen following application of HRP to the transition zone between the normal and regenerated portions of the spinal cord (c). The least HRP labeled neurons are seen following application of HRP to normal spinal cord in nonregenerate lizards (a). (From Duffy et al., 1990.)

limeters rostral to the transition zone (Duffy et al., 1992).

These studies also point to the transition zone as being key to axon access to the regenerated cord. While the transition zone appears to act as a 'filter', it is not a selective filter, at least with regard to axon type. Some axons of all origins grow through this zone but the majority do not. Axon trapping in this zone appears to be sufficient to maintain the cell body of origin.

The transition zone: gate-keeper to the regenerated cord

Previous studies with the goldfish (Bernstein and Bernstein, 1969) and the rat (Bernstein et al., 1978) suggested that blockage of axon regeneration could be due to synaptic capture by denervated neurons in the injured cord. We recently investigated this possibility in the lizard by looking at cellular and synaptic changes in the transition zone (Duffy et al., 1992). First, a combination of repeated ^{3}H-thymidine injections during regeneration followed by HRP labeling of the mature regenerate failed to reveal any double labeled neurons. This confirmed our earlier thymidine labeling studies and suggested that there is no significant contribution of axons from newly formed neurons. Second, morphometric studies based on electronmicrographs of the transition zone revealed a number of important changes. Ventral horn neurons in the transition zone rostral to the regenerated cord exhibited a significant ($P < 0.001$) increase (112%) in size over those in the normal tail cord. This increase in size is probably due to the fact that motor as well as sensory innervation to the entire regenerated portion of the tail comes from the three spinal segments rostral to the regenerated tail. The alterations in spinal circuitry, however, extend well beyond these three rostral segments. Acute transection of the spinal cord in the lumbar region did not alter neuron size in either the normal or regenerate.

The number of synaptic contacts on the ventral horn neuronal somata in the transition zone were counted and compared with those from a comparable level of normal cord. Synapses on the ventral horn neurons in the transition zone were more than twice the number seen on neurons in the normal cord (Fig. 7). This increased number of synapses returned to normal when animals with regenerated cords had their spinal cords transected at the lumbar level. This suggests that the increase in synaptic contacts seen in the transition zone are due to axons arising from supraspinal and/or long propriospinal axons. The density of synaptic contacts also followed the same trend. However the density of synaptic contacts did not increase proportional to the increase in number of contacts because the size of the neurons was also greatly increased.

These results suggest that increased synaptogenic activity in the transition zone could be an important mechanism for inhibiting central nervous system (CNS) axonal regeneration. Our results, however, fail to explain why some axons are trapped and some are not.

Response of non-tail spinal cord to transection

As we have seen, the tail cord regenerates. Paradoxically, transection of the lizard spinal cord rostral to the tail region leads to connective tissue and glial scarring as well as the formation of ependymal cysts. Histologically the wounded cord looks very much like what one would see in a transected mammalian cord.

We know that the lizard thoracic spinal cord is capable of regeneration. One can transplant a segment of thoracic cord to the tail, in place of the tail cord. Once such a homograft has healed, one can transect the tail through the graft. A blastema forms, and the grafted thoracic cord regenerates just like the tail cord (Simpson and Pollack, 1985). This suggests that the failure of the thoracic cord to regenerate is due to the absence of an appropriate mesodermal wound tissue, rather than some inability of the cord, per se, to respond and regenerate. This interpretation is supported by another experiment that can be

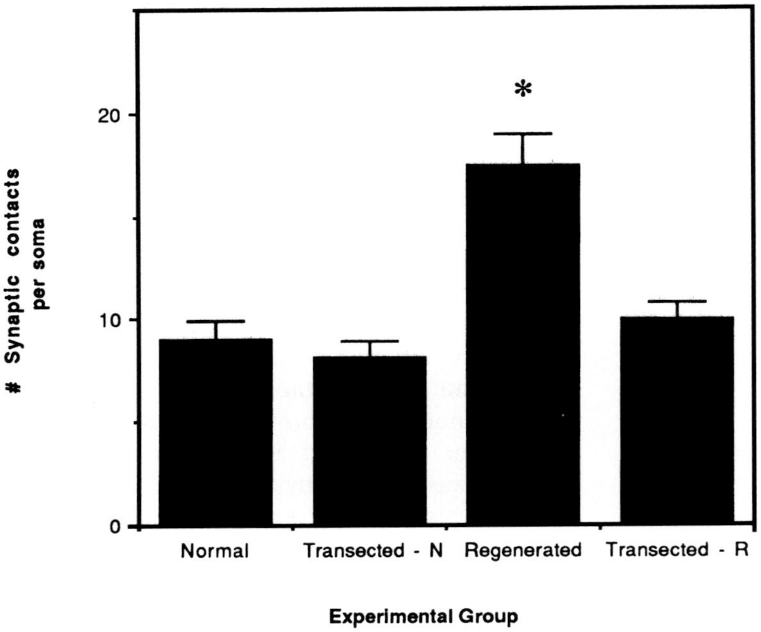

Fig. 7. Comparison of mean number of axosomatic contacts on ventral horn neurons. Neurons were selected from the 5th to 7th tail spinal cord segment in unoperated lizards (Normal), acutely transected lizards with normal tails (Transected-N), from lizards with regenerated tails (Regenerated) and regenerated lizards with 21-day-old lumbar transections (Transected-R). Ventral horn neurons rostral to regenerated spinal cord averaged significantly more synapses per soma (*) than all other groups ($P < 0.001$). Error bars = SEM. (From Duffy et al., 1992.)

performed on the mature regenerated tail. A regenerated tail can be amputated and it will regenerate again. The regenerated spinal cord also regenerates a second time. However, if one makes a small dorsal incision in the regenerated tail, transects the regenerated spinal cord, and then tightly sutures the dorsal incision (i.e., to block blastema formation), the transected regenerated cord does not regenerate. Again, the ependyma apparently needs a specific set of signals, provided normally by the blastema cells, for its proper proliferation and morphogenesis.

We have tried the obvious experiment of grafting early blastema cells from a regenerating tail to a transection site in the thoracic cord. Unfortunately, these cells are on their own time course with respect to differentiation. They begin almost immediately to differentiate into cartilage and muscle. They do not maintain their blastemal characteristics long enough to support a sustained outgrowth of the ependyma. This interdependence between the ependymal epithelium and the mesodermal blastema was previously described as the ‘ependyma-mesenchyme hypothesis’ of spinal cord regeneration (Simpson, 1983). Functional recovery following transection of the mammalian spinal cord will, we posit, require replication of the mesodermal signals needed to stimulate and direct the ependyma to fasciculate and guide regenerating CNS axons from one stump to the other.

Generalizations

The lizard model that we have just reviewed is one of several inframammalian models (also see McClellan, this volume; Zottoli et al., this volume) that continue to contribute to our understanding of spinal cord injury and repair. While our understanding of spinal cord regeneration in nonmammalian species is far from complete, there are some important provisional generalizations that emerge from the literature.

The first generalization that can be made is that in transection injuries, glial cells, often ependymal cells, are the first to bridge the injury gap and they are responsible for guiding regenerating CNS axons across the gap. This role of the glia, especially the ependymal epithelium, was first proposed based on studies of lizard cord regeneration (Simpson, 1968, 1970; Egar et al., 1970). Subsequently the ependymal cells have been shown to guide regenerating CNS axons in larval anurans (Michel and Reier, 1979) and in larval and adult urodeles (Egar and Singer, 1972; Nordlander and Singer, 1978; Singer et al., 1979) during tail regeneration and during regeneration at thoracic levels in adult urodeles (Simpson, 1983). The same role for the ependyma has also been demonstrated during tail regeneration in the fish, *Sternarchus* (Anderson et al., 1983), and, although not explicitly stated, is suggested by descriptions of thoracic cord regeneration in the goldfish (Bernstein and Bernstein, 1969). In lizards and urodele amphibians, the ependymal cells fasciculate the outgrowing CNS axons into preformed longitudinal channels, while in larval anurans and the fish, *Sternarchus*, the ependymal cells form guidance channels in the form of grooves and gutters. A recent study in the larval sea lamprey also points to glial processes, as yet unidentified, that bridge a transection gap and guide regenerating CNS axons (Pijak et al., 1993). In studies that have related cord regeneration to functional recovery in urodele amphibians, it has been noted that functional recovery from a transection is correlated with the uniting of the regenerating ependymal tubes (Butler and Ward, 1967; Davis et al., 1990).

A second generalization is that among tailed vertebrates that regenerate their spinal cords, cord regeneration from a thoracic level transection is quite different from cord regeneration as it occurs during tail regeneration. That the rules for cord regeneration might be different in the two situations was first suggested by Goss (1969). Certainly, during tail regeneration in adult urodeles where the outgrowing ependyma contacts a mesenchymal blastema, the fidelity of cellular replacement, both neurons and glia, is impressive (Nordlander and Singer, 1978), while at thoracic levels, where no blastema forms, no new neurons appear and less than 10% of the descending CNS axons actually grow across the injury gap (Davis et al., 1990). In the lizard the difference is even more dramatic. Limited cord regeneration occurs during tail regeneration, while no cord regeneration occurs at thoracic levels (Simpson, 1970). These examples suggest that important interactions occur between the generative ependymal epithelium and the surrounding mesodermally derived wound tissues (Simpson, 1983).

A third generalization suggests that the rules that govern spinal cord regeneration from a crush injury are different from those governing cord regeneration from a transection. The crucial difference may well be the integrity of the pial membrane. This generalization is weaker than those discussed above. This is due primarily to lack of good data on crush injured cords in nonmammalian species. We draw our support for this generalization from comparison of thoracic cord regeneration in urodeles. Studies of thoracic cord regeneration following suction ablation of the spinal cord, keeping the meninges intact, in the salamander, *Notophthalmus pyrrhogaster* (Stensaas, 1983), gave results that were very different from those reported for complete transection of the cord in *Notophthalmus viridescens* (Simpson, 1983; Davis et al., 1990). When the pial basement membrane remained intact, regenerating CNS axons followed the basement membrane rather than being fasciculated and guided by the ependyma (Stensaas, 1983). Additionally, outgrowth of the ependyma was aberrant and retarded when compared with a complete transection injury in *N. viridescens* (Simpson, 1983). One interpretation of this difference is that the intact meninges prevented proliferating mesodermal cells from interacting with the ependyma, thus interfering with ependymal growth and morphogenesis. Whether or not axonal guidance via the pial basement membrane is as efficient as ependymal guidance in terms of functional recovery remains to be seen.

A fourth generalization is that collateral sprouting (Seil, 1989) of uninjured and injured CNS axons is a characteristic response to cord injury in inframammalian species, as it is in mammalian species. Studies of spinal cord injury in the larval sea lamprey have shown that regenerating spinal axons branch profusely, often leading to synapses in inappropriate sites (Wood and Cohen, 1981). Sprouting is also seen in injured goldfish cords (see Zottoli et al., this volume). Sprouting in urodele amphibians has not been systematically studied. In lizards, sprouting of supra- and infraspinal axons is profuse (Duffy, 1990).

A fifth, and last generalization is that the regeneration of very few descending spinal axons can lead to an impressive return of function. At the same time, 100% return of function is rarely if ever achieved. Excellent regenerators such as the larval sea lamprey (Frank, 1982; McClellan, 1990) and the urodele amphibians (Davis et al., 1990) are anatomically and physiologically incomplete. In the case of the newt, *Notophthalmus viridescens*, only 10% of the normal component of descending spinal axons regenerate across a thoracic transection. Yet functionally, coordinated swimming returns to within 95% of normal. Studies on cord regeneration in goldfish also suggest that return of function, while impressive, is never 100% (Zottoli and Freemer, 1991; Zottoli et al., this volume). These generalizations are provisional. We hope they will stimulate discussion and experimentation. Until we can explain cord regeneration in the inframammalian species, it is unlikely that we will bring about functional regeneration in mammals.

References

Alibardi, L. (1990) Cerebrospinal fluid contacting neurons inside the regenerating spinal cord of *Xenopus* tadpoles. *Boll. Zool.*, 57: 309–315.

Alibardi, L. and Meyer-Rochou, V.B. (1988) Ultrastructure of the neural component of the regenerating spinal cord in the tail of three species of New Zealand lizards (*Leiolopisma nigri plantare maccanni*, *Lampropholis delicate* and *Hoplodactylus maculaturm*). *N.Z. J. Zool.*, 15: 535–550.

Alibardi, L., Gibbons, J. and Simpson, S.B., Jr. (1992) Fine structure of cells in the young regenerating spinal cord of the lizard, *Anolis carolinensis*, after H^3-thymidine administration. *Biol. Struct. Morphog.*, 4: 45–52.

Alibardi, L., Wibel, R. and Simpson, S.B., Jr. (1993a) Scanning and transmission electron microscopic observations on the central canal of the regenerating tail spinal cord in the lizard, *Anolis carolinensis*. *Boll. Zool.*, 60: 245–252.

Alibardi, L., Gibbons, J. and Simpson, S.B., Jr. (1993b) ^3H-GABA administration during tail regeneration of lizards and autoradiographic localization. *J. Hirnforsch.*, 34: 67–77.

Anderson, M.J., Waxman, S.G. and Laufer, M. (1983) Fine structure of regenerated ependyma and spinal cord in *Sternarchus albifrons*. *Anat. Rec.*, 205: 73–83.

Barber, R.P., Vaughn, J.E.,and Roberts, E. (1982) The cytoarchitecture of GABAergic neurons in rat spinal cord. *Brain Res.*, 238: 305–328.

Bernstein, J.J. and Bernstein, M.E. (1969) Ultrastructure of normal regeneration and loss of regenerative capacity following Teflon blockage in goldfish spinal cord. *Exp. Neurol.*, 24: 538–657.

Bernstein, J.J., Bernstein, M.E. and Wells, M.R. (1978) Spinal cord regeneration and axonal sprouting in mammals. In: S.G. Waxman (Ed.), *Physiology and Pathobiology of Axons*, Raven Press, New York, pp. 407–420.

Brodin, L., Dale, N., Christenson, J., Storm-Mathisen, J., Hökfelt, T. and Grillner, S. (1990) Three types of GABA-immunoreactive cells in the lamprey spinal cord. *Brain Res.*, 508: 172–175.

Butler, E.G. and Ward, M.B. (1967) Reconstruction of the spinal cord after ablation in the adult *Triturus*. *Dev. Biol.*, 15: 464–486.

Chen, A. and Heathcote, R. D. (1993) The influence of the notochord on a specific population of spinal cord cells. *Soc. Neurosci. Abstr.*, 19: 1712.

Dale, N., Roberts, A., Ottersen, O.P. and Storm-Mathisen, J. (1987) The morphology and distribution of 'Kolmer-Agdur cells', a class of cerebrospinal fluid contacting neurons revealed in the frog embryo spinal cord by GABA immunocytochemistry. *Proc. R. Soc. Lond. B*, 232: 193–203.

Davis, B.M., Ayers, J.L., Koran, L., Carlson, J., Anderson, M.C. and Simpson, S.B., Jr. (1990) Time course of salamander spinal cord regeneration and recovery of swimming: HRP retrograde pathway tracing and kinematic analysis. *Exp. Neurol.*, 108: 198–213.

Duffy, M.T., Simpson, S.B., Jr., Liebich, D.R. and Davis, B.M. (1990) Origin of spinal cord axons in the lizard regenerated tail: supernormal projections from local spinal neurons. *J. Comp. Neurol.*, 293: 208–222.

Duffy, M.T., Liebich, D.R., Garner, L.K., Hawrych, A., Simpson, S.B., Jr. and Davis, B.M. (1992) Axonal sprouting and frank regeneration in the lizard tail spinal cord: correlation between changes in synaptic circuiting and axonal growth. *J. Comp. Neurol.*, 316: 363–374.

Duffy, M.T., Hawrych, A., Liebich, D. and Simpson, S.B., Jr. (1993) Regeneration of cerebrospinal fluid contacting neurons (CSFCN's) in the regenerated tail spinal cord of the lizard, *Anolis carolinensis*. *Soc. Neurosci. Abstr.*, 19: 1716.

Egar, M., Simpson, S.B., Jr. and Singer, M. (1970) The growth and differentiation of the regenerating spinal cord of the lizard, *Anolis carolinensis*. *J. Morphol.*, 131: 131–152.

Egar, M. and Singer, M. (1972) The role of the ependyma in spinal cord regeneration in the urodele *Triturus*. *Exp. Neurol.*, 37: 422–430.

Frank, E. (1982) Adaptive and maladaptive regeneration in the spinal cord. In: J.G. Nicholls (Ed.), *Repair and Regeneration of the Nervous System*, Springer Verlag, Berlin/Heidelberg, pp. 243–254.

Fujita, T., Kanno, T. and Kobayashi, S. (1988) *The Paraneuron*, Springer Verlag, Berlin, pp. 273–277.

Goss, R. (1969) *Principles of Regeneration*, Academic Press, New York, p. 209.

McClellan, A. D. (1990) Locomotor recovery in spinal-transected lamprey: role of functional regeneration of descending axons from brainstem locomotor command neurons. *Neuroscience*, 37: 781–798.

McLaughlin, B.J., Barber, R., Saito, K., Roberts, E. and Wu, J.T. (1975) Immunocytochemical localization of glutamate decarboxylase in rat spinal cord. *J. Comp. Neurol.*, 164: 305–322.

Michel, M.E. and Reier, P.J. (1979) Axonal-ependymal associations during early regeneration of the transected spinal cord in Xenopus laevis tadpoles. *J. Neurocytol.*, 8: 529–548.

Nordlander, R. and Singer, M. (1978) The role of ependyma in regeneration of the spinal cord in the urodele amphibian tail. *J. Comp. Neurol.*, 180: 349–374.

Oksche, A. (1988) Sensory and secretory potencies and differentiation of the central nervous system. *Acta Anat.*, 132: 216–224.

Pijak, D.S., Lurie, D.J. and Selzer, M.E. (1993) Longitudinal glial fibers precede regenerating axons into a spinal transection in the larval sea lamprey. *Soc. Neurosci. Abstr.*, 19: 682.

Scott, D.E., Gash, D.M., Sladek, J.R., Clayton, C., Mitchell, J.A., Calderon, S. and Paull, W.K. (1982) Organization of the mammalian cerebral ventricular system: ultrastructural correlates of CSF-neuropeptide secretion. In: E.M. Rodriquez and T.B. van Wiersma (Eds.), *Cerebrospinal fluid and peptide hormones. Frontiers of Hormone Research*, Vol. 9, S. Karger, Basel, pp. 15–35.

Seil, F. J. (1989) Axonal sprouting in response to injury. In F.J. Seil (Ed.), *Neural Regeneration and Transplantation, Frontiers of Clinical Neuroscience*, Vol. 6, Alan R. Liss, New York, pp. 123–135.

Simpson, S.B., Jr. (1964) Analysis of tail regeneration in the lizard *Lygosoma laterale*. I. Initiation of regeneration and cartilage differentiation. The role of the ependyma. *J. Morphol.*, 114: 425–435.

Simpson, S.B., Jr. (1968) Morphology of the regenerated spinal cord in the lizard, *Anolis carolinensis*. *J. Comp. Neurol.*, 134: 193–210.

Simpson, S.B., Jr. (1970) Studies on regeneration of the lizard's tail. *Am. Zool.*, 10: 157–165.

Simpson, S.B., Jr. (1983) Fasciculation and guidance of regenerating central axons by the ependyma. In: C.C. Kao, R.P. Bunge and P.J. Reier (Eds.), *Spinal Cord Reconstruction*, Raven Press, New York, pp. 151–162.

Simpson, S.B., Jr. and Pollack, K. (1985) Ependyma-mesenchyme interactions during spinal cord regeneration. *Soc. Neurosci. Abstr.*, 10: 1027.

Singer, M., Nordlander, R. and Egar, M. (1979) Axonal guidance during embryogenesis and regeneration in the spinal cord of the newt: the blueprint hypothesis of neuronal pathway patterning. *J. Comp. Neurol.*, 185: 1–22.

Stensaas, L.J. (1983) Regeneration in the spinal cord of the newt *Notopthalmus (Triturus) pyrrhogaster*. In: C.C. Kao, R.P. Bunge and P.J. Reier (Eds.), *Spinal Cord Reconstruction*, Raven Press, New York, pp. 121–149.

Vigh, B. and Vigh-Teichmann, I. (1973) Comparative ultrastructure of the cerebrospinal fluid contacting neurons. *Int. Rev. Cytol.*, 35: 189–251.

Vigh, B., Vigh-Teichmann, I., Sikora, K. and Jennes, L. (1980) Scanning electron microscopy of the cerebrospinal fluid contacting neurons of the central canal in various vertebrates. *Verb. Anat. Ges.*, 74: 707–714.

Vigh-Teichmann, I., Vigh. B. and Aros, B. (1979) Ciliated neurons and different types of synapses in anterior hypothalamic nuclei of reptiles. *Cell Tissue Res.*, 174: 139–160.

Wood, M. R. and Cohen, M. J. (1981) Synaptic regeneration and glial reactions in the transected spinal cord of the lamprey. *J. Neurocytol.*, 10: 57–79.

Zottoli, S. J. and Freemer, M.M. (1991) Behavioral recovery of the goldfish startle response after spinal cord crush. *Soc. Neurosci. Abstr.*, 17: 942.

F.J. Seil (Ed.)
Progress in Brain Research, Vol 103

CHAPTER 20

Permissive and restrictive periods for brainstem-spinal regeneration in the chick

John D. Steeves[1,2], Hans S. Keirstead[1], Douglas W. Ethell[1], Sohail J. Hasan[1], Gillian D. Muir[1], David M. Pataky[1], Christopher B. McBride[1], Barbara Petrausch[1] and Thomas J. Zwimpfer[1,3]

Departments of [1]Zoology, [2]Anatomy, and [3]Surgery, University of British Columbia, c / o Biological Sciences Building, 6270 University Boulevard, Vancouver, British Columbia, V6T 1Z4, Canada

Introduction and rationale

Damage to adult central nervous system (CNS) axons, as in spinal cord injuries, most often results in aborted attempts at regeneration followed by degeneration (Ramón y Cajal, 1928; Björklund et al., 1971). However, it has been demonstrated that some adult CNS axons will anatomically regenerate if they are allowed to project through a peripheral nervous system environment (Tello, 1911; David and Aguayo, 1981). These observations served to dispel previous suggestions that the lack of CNS axonal regeneration in higher adult vertebrates (i.e., birds and mammals) was wholly due to the irreversible suppression of intrinsic neuronal growth programs. Nevertheless, distinct types of CNS neurons may possess intrinsically different responses with regard to axotomy, cell survival and any subsequent axonal outgrowth (Tetzlaff et al., 1991; Fawcett, 1992).

In short, both intrinsic neuronal growth programs and extraneuronal environmental conditions must be favorable for functional axonal regeneration. Such a situation is evident during embryonic development and is indeed necessary to support the accurate growth of CNS axons. If it is accepted that many of the events underlying adult axonal regeneration are in part a recapitulation of axonal development (Holder and Clarke, 1988; Treherne et al., 1992), then a documentation of the regenerative capacity of the injured embryonic spinal cord should help elucidate some of the developmental events necessary to promote functional regeneration of adult CNS axons.

Because most mammals are viviparous, it is difficult to examine in utero the detailed aspects of spinal cord development and/or axonal repair. Since chickens are oviparous, the embryo is more readily accessible and will often survive experimental manipulations (e.g., surgery) that a mammalian embryo will not endure. A further advantage is the relatively accelerated rate of neurodevelopment in the chicken. Hatchling chicks are precocial and their CNS (especially those brainstem and spinal systems concerned with locomotion) can be considered fully developed and adult-like in function at the time of hatching (Okado and Oppenheim, 1985; Shimizu et al., 1990; Glover and Pettursdottir, 1991; Hasan et al., 1991, 1993; Shiga et al., 1991; Glover, 1993).

The available evidence suggests that spinal cord neurons concerned with vertebrate locomotion are predominantly activated by direct input from the phylogenetically older brainstem-spinal pathways of the extrapyramidal motor system (for reviews see Armstrong, 1986; Jordan, 1986; Grillner and Dubuc, 1988). Even in primates, the pyramidal tract (corticospinal pathway) does not appear to be essential for the direct activation of spinal cord locomotor neurons (Lawrence and Kuypers, 1968a,b), and like all nonmammalian vertebrates, birds do not possess a corticospinal tract (Webster et al., 1990). Therefore, a good proportion of the integrated descending locomotor output is directed to the cord via reticulospinal pathways originating in the pons and medulla (Lawrence and Kuypers, 1968a,b; Steeves and Jordan, 1984; Steeves et al., 1987). Locomotor paralysis, as a result of an adult spinal cord injury, is often the consequence of irreversible damage to these descending supraspinal projections. Furthermore, it is well established that the overall structure and function of the vertebrate brainstem and spinal cord has remained relatively unchanged throughout evolutionary history (Sarnat and Netsky, 1981; McClellan, 1990).

Studies of the development and organization of brainstem and spinal locomotor mechanisms indicate that birds are very similar to all other vertebrates (Bekoff, 1976; Okado and Oppenheim, 1985; Sholomenko and Steeves, 1987; Steeves et al., 1987; Webster and Steeves, 1988; Valenzuela et al., 1990; Hasan et al., 1991; Sholomenko et al., 1991a,b,c; O'Donovan et al., 1992). For example, from previous work in our laboratory we have shown that the anatomical, physiological, and pharmacological organization of avian brainstem-spinal locomotor circuits is analogous to that of all other vertebrates, including mammals (Sholomenko and Steeves, 1987; Steeves et al., 1987; Webster and Steeves, 1988, 1991; Valenzuela et al., 1990; Sholomenko et al., 1991a,b,c). Moreover, after a complete or incomplete spinal cord injury, adult birds suffer the same motor deficits as adult mammals (Sholomenko and Steeves, 1987; Webster and Steeves, 1991).

Anatomical and physiological evidence for regeneration in the developing chick

We have determined the duration of the 21 day development period over which an embryonic chick is capable of axonal repair after a complete transection of the thoracic spinal cord. Details of the experimental methods are available elsewhere (Hasan et al., 1991, 1993; Keirstead et al., 1992; Steeves et al., 1993). In brief, approximately 5–7 days after transection, neuroanatomical repair can be evaluated with a restricted injection into the lumbar cord (caudal to the transection site) of a fluorescent retrograde tracing dye (Hasan et al., 1991). Functional (physiological) repair of descending supraspinal pathways can be evaluated with behavioral observations of locomotor functions by posthatching (P) chicks and can also be directly tested by focal electrical stimulation of brainstem locomotor regions known to have direct projections to the lumbar cord (Valenzuela et al., 1990; Hasan et al., 1991, 1993).

If the thoracic spinal cord of an embryonic chick is transected prior to embryonic day 13 (E13), the animal will subsequently effect complete neuroanatomical and physiological repair resulting in total functional recovery (Shimizu et al., 1990; Hasan et al., 1991, 1993). We have called the developmental period prior to E13 the permissive period for functional spinal cord repair. If the spinal cord is transected on E13 or E14, the repair of descending supraspinal pathways progressively diminishes, resulting in minimal if any functional recovery (Shimizu et al., 1990; Hasan et al., 1991, 1993). By E15, a thoracic transection results in no axonal repair/regeneration or functional recovery and the chick, upon hatching, is as paralyzed as a bird or mammal transected as an adult (Sholomenko and Steeves, 1987; Shimizu et al., 1990; Hasan et al., 1991, 1993; Webster and Steeves, 1991; Keirstead et al., 1992). For these reasons we have called the developmental period after E13 the restrictive period for functional spinal cord repair.

Several neuroanatomical responses could underlie this repair process, including: (1) neurogenesis of new descending brainstem-spinal neurons, (2) subsequent projections from late developing brainstem-spinal neurons, and (3) axonal regeneration of previously axotomized brainstem-spinal projections. Brainstem-spinal projections to the lumbar cord develop over a period extending from approximately E3 to E11 (Okado and Oppenheim, 1985; Shimizu et al., 1990; Glover and Pettursdottir, 1991; Hasan et al., 1991; Shiga et al., 1991; Glover, 1993), with the first functional synaptic connections evident on E6–E7 (Bekoff, 1976; Shiga et al., 1991; Sholomenko and O'Donovan, 1994). By E11 of normal embryonic development, the distribution and number of retrograde labeled brainstem-spinal neurons is equivalent to those labeled in a chick after hatching (Okado and Oppenheim, 1985; Shimizu et al., 1990; Hasan et al., 1991; Shiga et al., 1991). Interestingly, there is no evidence for the overproduction of brainstem-spinal neurons during development or any subsequent neuronal death at later stages of development (Oppenheim, 1991). It is also known that brainstem-spinal neurons become postmitotic very early in development, usually prior to E5 (McConnell and Sechrist, 1980) and well before E12. Therefore, it is unlikely that our findings of complete functional repair of an E7–E12 transected cord is dependent on the neurogenesis of additional brainstem-spinal neurons (Hasan et al., 1991, 1993). If spinal repair was not in part due to 'true' axonal regeneration, but only due to subsequent axonal projections from late developing neurons, a reduced number of brainstem-spinal neurons should be retrogradely labeled after an E11–E12 transection. The similar number and distribution of retrograde labeled brainstem-spinal neurons in both E11-transected embryos and sham-operated control embryos argues in favor of axonal regeneration contributing to the repair process (Hasan et al., 1991). Needless to say, these potential repair mechanisms are not mutually exclusive.

To determine to what extent 'true' axonal regeneration was contributing to this repair process, we used a double retrograde tract tracing protocol (Fig. 1) (Hasan et al., 1993). On E8–E13, the caudal thoraco-lumbar cord was injected with 0.1–0.6 μl of the first fluorescent tracer (e.g., rhodamine labeled dextran amine, RDA). One to 2 days later, the upper thoracic cord was completely transected. After an additional 7 days, a different second fluorescent tracer (e.g., cascade blue labeled dextran amine, CBDA) was injected into the thoraco-lumbar cord at least 0.5 cm caudal to the transection site. Finally, 2 days after the second tracer was injected, the CNS was fixed and sectioned. In comparison to nontransected or

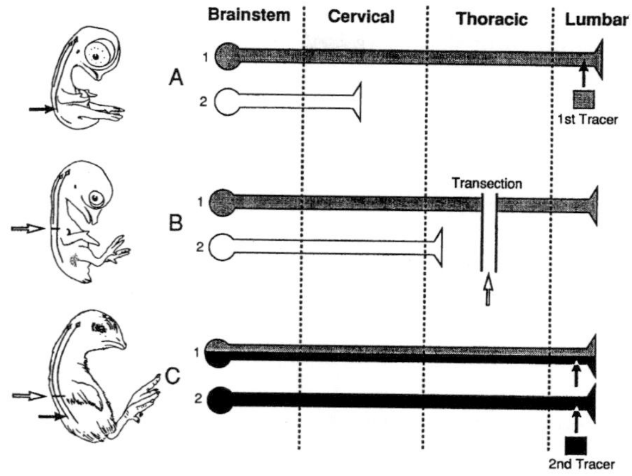

Fig. 1. Schematic representation of experimental procedure for retrograde double labeling of axotomized brainstem-spinal neurons. (A) On E8–E13, the caudal thoraco-lumbar spinal cord was injected with the first fluorescent tracing dye. Note that neuron 1 represents brainstem-spinal neurons that have already projected axons to the level of the lumbar cord at that stage of embryonic development, whereas neuron 2 represents any late developing neurons that have yet to project as far as the caudal thoraco-lumbar injection site. Neuron 1 therefore becomes retrogradely labeled with the first tracing dye, while the late developing neuron 2 remains unlabeled. (B) The upper to mid-thoracic spinal cord was completely transected 1–2 days later. Note that the axon of neuron 1 is severed. However, the late developing neuron 2 has not yet reached the transection site and remained intact. (C) After a further 7–8 days to allow for any repair/regeneration, the second (different colored) fluorescent tracing dye was injected into the thoraco-lumbar cord, approximately 0.5 cm caudal to the transection site. Note that by this late stage of development (E16 or later) all brainstem-spinal projections (i.e., both neuron 1 and 2) will have reached the level of the second injection. Neuron 1 therefore would become retrogradely double labeled with both tracing dyes (or remain labeled by only the first tracing dye should it not have regenerated). Conversely, neuron 2 would be retrogradely labeled by only the second tracing dye. Note that the first retrograde tracing dye does not remain viable for cotransport with the second tracing dye. (From Hasan et al., 1993.)

sham-transected controls, there were relatively normal numbers of double labeled brainstem-spinal neurons following a transection prior to E13 (Fig. 2), whereas the number of double labeled and second labeled brainstem-spinal neurons decreased dramatically after a transection on E13–E14 (Hasan et al., 1993). Thus, damaged embryonic spinal cord is capable of axonal regeneration after an E12 transection, but anatomical and functional repair rapidly diminishes after a transection on E13–E14 and is completely nonexistent after an E15 transection.

Regardless of which currently available anatomical tracing technique is used and no matter how rigorous the methodology, there can be variability in the number or quality of retrograde neuronal labeling (Heimer and Robards, 1981). For optimum uptake of fluorescent dextran amine

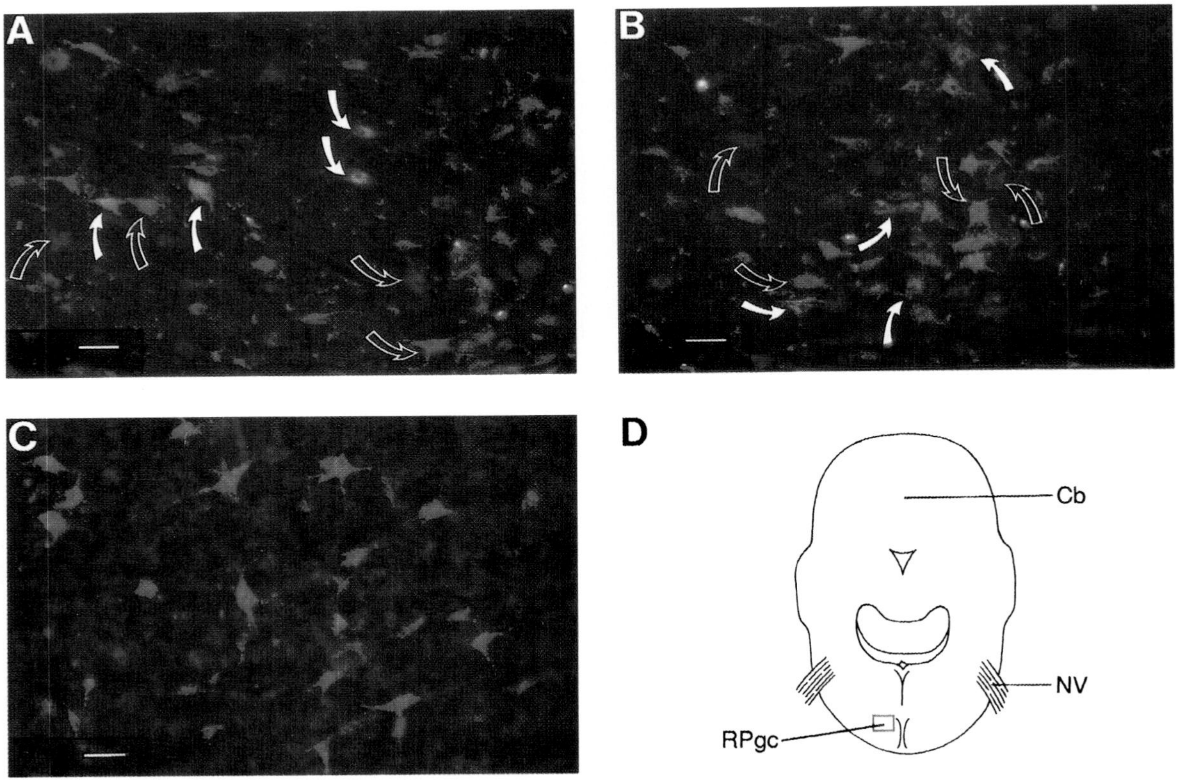

Fig. 2. Photomicrograph of retrogradely labeled gigantocellular reticulospinal neurons within the ventromedial reticular formation of the caudal pons of the chick. Double exposed photomicrograph of P1 hatchling brainstem-spinal projections retrogradely labeled with a lumbar injection of the first tracing dye (0.1 μl of RDA, red) on E10 followed by a lumbar cord injection of the second label (0.3 μl of CBDA, blue) on E20. The embryonic spinal cord was transected on E12, i.e., between the first retrograde tracer injection and the second retrograde tracer injection. After the film has been double exposed, the presence of double labeled (red + blue = pink) reticulospinal neurons indicates regeneration of previously axotomized fibers, whereas the presence of single labeled neurons potentially indicates either no regeneration (red) or repair due to subsequent projections (blue) from late developing reticulospinal neurons. There was a similar number and distribution of retrogradely double labeled neurons in permissive-transected animals and sham-operated control embryos (see Table 1). A few representative single labeled neurons are indicated by open arrows, and a few representative (but not all) double labeled neurons are indicated by solid arrows. Scale bar = 50 μm. (Modified from Hasan et al., 1993.)

tracers, the axons should be damaged by the tracer injection needle (Glover et al., 1986). Since the two different fluorescent dextran amine tracing chemicals are injected at separate times, it is not possible to ensure that the same brainstem-spinal axons will always take up and retrogradely transport both tracers. Consequently, counting retrogradely single labeled or double labeled neurons can lead to mistaken estimates (always underestimates) of the number of projections to an injection site.

By counting the number of retrograde labeled neurons in large numbers of experimental and control animals, an appreciation of the amount of variability inherent to tract tracing techniques is gained. But more importantly, comparisons between experimental and control animals can be made with a higher degree of confidence (see Table 1). By calculating the ratio of double labeled brainstem-spinal neurons (indicating regeneration of previously severed axons) to the number of neurons labeled with only the second fluorescent tracer (potentially indicating repair as a result of subsequent projections from late developing brainstem-spinal neurons), we determined the ratio for 'true' axonal regeneration contributing to the repair of descending pathways after severing the thoracic cord at different stages of development. There was an ever increasing number of double labeled neurons in animals transected between E9 and E12, with a maximum of 30% double labeled neurons within several brainstem-spinal nuclei after an E12 transection. The extent of axonal regeneration after an E13 transection decreased dramatically and no double labeling was ever observed after an E14 (or later) transection (Hasan et al., 1993). For the reasons outlined above, the actual percentage of brainstem-spinal

TABLE 1

Number (mean + SE) of single and double labeled brainstem-spinal neurons after temporally separated injections (shown in parentheses) of two different fluorescent retrograde tracing dyes into the lumbar cord

Tsx	Injection	Rgc (medulla)		VeL (pons)		Nucleus interstitialis (mesencephalon)	
		Experimental	Control	Experimental	Control	Experimental	Control
E10	1st (E8)	27.2 ± 5.2	18.3 ± 3.4	68.6 ± 7.8	52.2 ± 7.2	21.3 ± 4.4	28.1 ± 3.6
	2nd (E18)	33.4 ± 3.3	37.1 ± 6.8	78.9 ± 8.1	81.2 ± 12.5	96.4 ± 8.8	70.0 ± 15.0
	Double	3.6 ± 0.8	4.2 ± 1.2	4.8 ± 0.3	7.8 ± 2.1	5.3 ± 1.6	8.0 ± 2.8
	% Double	10.8	11.3	6.1	9.6	5.5	11.4
E12	1st (E10)	17.7 ± 3.7	14.1 ± 1.1	111.8 ± 22.8	102.0 ± 4.2	88.2 ± 17.8	79.1 ± 9.7
	2nd (E20)	27.7 ± 1.0	22.4 ± 3.2	96.1 ± 27.2	72.8 ± 6.5	80.4 ± 7.7	87.6 ± 2.9
	Double	8.2 ± 1.1	6.5 ± 1.6	20.5 ± 4.5	23.9 ± 7.4	17.8 ± 0.9	22.9 ± 3.1
	% Double	29.6	29.0	21.3	32.8	22.1	26.1
E14	1st (E12)	31.7 ± 6.4	28.9 ± 1.8	85.6 ± 18.1	89.8 ± 9.9	79.5 ± 7.1	68.2 ± 13.4
	2nd (P1)	0.0 ± 0.0	36.3 ± 2.4	0.0 ± 0.0	97.6 ± 6.8	0.0 ± 0.0	72.3 ± 5.6
	Double	0.0 ± 0.0	9.6 ± 1.1	0.0 ± 0.0	21.5 ± 3.9	0.0 ± 0.0	19.5 ± 3.1
	% Double	0.0	26.4	0.0	22.0	0.0	26.9

Data are shown for three representative and spatially separated nuclei. The spinal cord of the experimental animals was transected at the thoracic level; $n = 5$ (E10), 6 (E12), and 5 (E14) for experimentals and $n = 4$ (E10), 5 (E12), and 4 (E14) for controls. Tsx, experimental age of transaction. (From Hasan et al., 1993).

neurons that regenerated during the permissive period for repair was probably greater, although to what degree is unknown.

There are a number of factors that must be considered before accepting the anatomical evidence for axonal regeneration. These factors include: (1) the possibility that the thoracic cord transection was incomplete in the those animals demonstrating axonal regeneration and functional recovery, (2) the possibility that there was direct diffusion of the second retrograde tracing dye across the transection site, resulting in false positive results, (3) the possibility of the first tracing dye remaining viable for prolonged periods after lumbar injection such that any late developing brainstem-spinal projections could retrogradely transport the first and second dyes simultaneously, once again resulting in a false positive result, and (4) the possibility of transsynaptic labeling of brainstem neurons via the initial labeling of intrinsic spinal neurons above the transection site (e.g., propriospinal neurons).

After an animal has functionally recovered from a spinal cord injury, as was the case for chicks transected during the permissive period of development, it is impossible to discern the completeness of the original transection. Histologically, most spinal cords transected during the permissive period appear to be similar to unoperated control animals (Hasan et al., 1991). Therefore, we must rely on examinations of the spinal cord transection site from randomly selected animals, killed immediately after the transection procedure. We have examined dozens of spinal cords, immediately after transection, and only rarely have we observed what appeared to be an incomplete transection. Thus, we are confident that our transection procedure resulted in the complete severing of the spinal cord in the overwhelming majority of cases.

It was also necessary to confirm that the injection of the second retrograde tracing chemical remained confined to the caudal thoraco-lumbar cord. If the tracing dye were to diffuse to (or above) the transection site, then it could falsely label brainstem-spinal neurons that had not regenerated. We have examined the spinal cord injection sites of numerous animals exhibiting double labeled brainstem-spinal neurons and always found the injection sites for the retrograde tracers to be confined to the lumbar spinal cord and always at least 0.5 cm away from the transection site (see Hasan et al., 1991).

Furthermore, it was critical that we discount the possibility that the first injected tracer remained viable for cotransport with the second retrograde tracer. If this were possible, then late developing projections (undamaged by the transection) could retrogradely transport both fluorescent chemicals simultaneously and give false positive evidence for axonal regeneration. We discounted this possibility by injecting the first retrograde tracer into the lumbar spinal cord of numerous chicks on E10 and then immediately transecting the thoracic cord (rostral to the injection site). This protocol prevented the first tracer from being retrogradely transported to the neuronal cell bodies of origin for brainstem-spinal pathways. The same animals were then injected with the second retrograde tracer on E18 or later. Subsequent examination revealed only the second tracer within brainstem-spinal neuronal cell bodies, indicating that repair had occurred over the intervening recovery period, but the first tracer had not remained viable for cotransport. Note that these experiments also confirmed that the spinal cord was completely severed by the transection procedure and that the first tracer never diffused to (or above) the transection site.

False positive results for axonal regeneration as a result of transsynaptic labeling of brainstem-spinal neurons is unlikely due to the short survival times after the injection of the second retrograde tracer (48 h or less). Transsynaptic labeling was also ruled out since the only retrogradely labeled brainstem nuclei were those that have direct projections to the lumbar cord (Okado and Oppenheim, 1985; Webster and Steeves, 1988, 1991; Shimizu et al., 1990; Shiga et al., 1991). Brainstem neurons (e.g., within the medial vestibular nu-

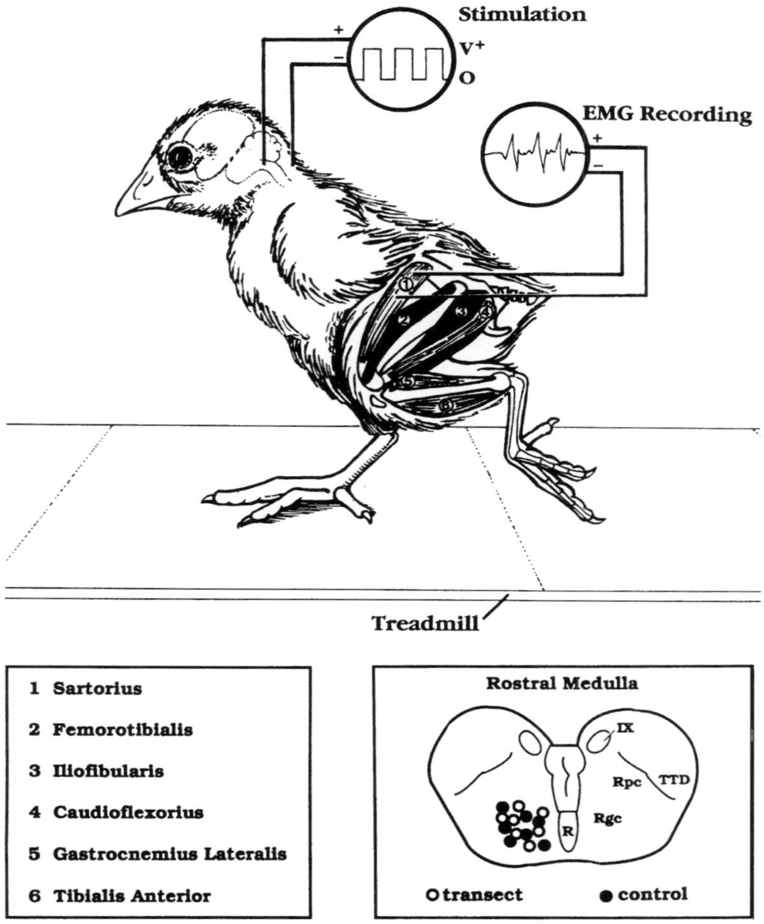

Fig. 3. Schematic representation of experimental procedures used for in vivo focal electrical stimulation (range of effective current strength was 15–50 μA) of brainstem locomotor regions in surgically decerebrate P1–P7 chicks that had previously been transected at different stages of embryonic development (E9–E15). Similar experiments were also undertaken in sham-operated and unoperated P1–P2 hatchling chicks. Video recordings monitored any evoked locomotion and electromyographic (EMG) recordings were used to specifically monitor brainstem-evoked locomotor activity in muscles of the right leg. The positions of the six muscles numbered in the lower left panel are shown on the diagram of the chick and included: (1) the sartorius (hip flexor, knee extensor), (2) the femorotibialis (knee extensor), (3) the iliofibularis (hip extensor, knee flexor), (4) the caudioflexorius (hip extensor, knee flexor), (5) the gastrocnemius lateralis (ankle extensor), and (6) the tibialis anterior (ankle flexor). In addition, either the sartorius, femorotibialis, or gastrocnemius lateralis muscles of the left leg were implanted to record alternating locomotor activity. For examples of EMG recordings during locomotion see Fig. 8. EMG recordings were also made from the pectoralis major (wing depressor) muscle (not shown). Evoked movements of the wings confirmed that the animal was in a healthy state after the surgical decerebration. More importantly, descending locomotor pathways to cervical/brachial cord neurons controlling wing movements would not have been interrupted by the thoracic cord transection procedure; thus every animal served as its own control for functional assessments. Finally, brainstem-evoked wing flapping confirmed that the focal electrical stimulating current activated the brainstem locomotor regions. Lower right panel shows the positions of effective brainstem locomotor stimulation sites within the ventromedial reticular formation of the rostral medulla in hatchling chicks which were either sham-operated (open circles) controls or experimental (previously transected) hatchlings (closed circles). IX, N. nervi glossopharyngei; R, N. raphé; Rgc, N. reticularis gigantocellularis; Rpc, N. reticularis parvocellularis; TTD, N. et tractus descendens nervi trigemini. (From Hasan et al., 1993.)

cleus) which only project as far as the cervical/brachial region were never labeled.

Since it is has been repeatedly documented that many vertebrate animals can spontaneously stand and even make rhythmical stepping movements with their legs after a complete spinal cord transection (for review see Armstrong, 1986), claims of functional recovery must also be interpreted with caution. This is why our assessments of functional recovery also employed focal electrical stimulation of identified brainstem locomotor regions (e.g., the ventromedial pontomedullary reticular formation). Neurons within the vertebrate ventromedial pontomedullary reticular formation have direct axonal projections to the lumbar spinal cord (for birds see Steeves et al., 1987; Webster and Steeves, 1988, 1991), and discrete electrical stimulation or pharmacological activation of these neurons will evoke coordinated locomotion in all decerebrate vertebrates (Fig. 3) examined to date (e.g., Steeves et al., 1987; Noga et al., 1988; McClellan, 1990; Sholomenko et al., 1991a,b,c).

After an embryonic spinal cord transection during the permissive period, brainstem-evoked leg activity can be accepted as a reliable indicator for the functional repair of brainstem-spinal projections if the following criteria are satisfied: (1) the leg activity must commence with the onset of brainstem stimulation and terminate with the offset of stimulation, (2) the leg activity must be evoked in response to a stimulating current that would not activate the spinal cord directly; in other words, the effective stimulating current must be small (< 100 μA) so as not to spread beyond the close confines of the stimulating electrode tip (i.e., an effective radius of less than 100 μm), (3) the pattern of leg muscle activity evoked in a permissive-transected animal should be similar to the pattern of evoked activity in an unoperated or sham operated control animal, (4) the relationship between muscle burst duration and step cycle duration should be similar for corresponding muscles in control and transected animals, and

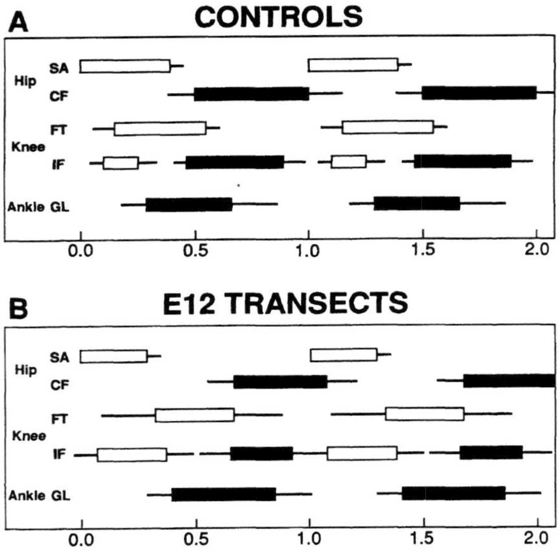

Fig. 4. Summary of temporal relationships for leg muscle activity patterns during brainstem-evoked overground walking (see Fig. 3 for experimental setup). The horizontal axis is time (seconds) normalized for the duration of the step cycle. Two complete step cycles are presented in A and B. Bars represent the proportion of the step cycle during which each muscle is active: solid bars represent stance phase activity and open bars represent swing phase activity. Lines at the end of each bar represent the standard error (SE) for the onset/offset time for each muscle. (A) Mean muscle activity pattern in control hatchlings ($n = 6$). The onset of activity of the sartorius muscle (SA) occurs just prior to the swing phase of the step cycle and was used here to demarcate the beginning of the step cycle. The SA muscle continues to be active throughout most of the swing phase. The femorotibialis (FT) and iliofibularis (IF) muscles are also active during the swing phase. The IF muscle is also normally active during the stance phase (i.e., twice during the step cycle). The caudioflexorius (CF) and gastrocnemius lateralis (GL) muscles alternate with the SA muscle and are therefore primarily active during the stance phase. (B) Mean muscle activity patterns in hatchlings that underwent a thoracic transection at E12 ($n = 6$). There were no significant differences between the muscle activity patterns in E12 transected and sham-operated or unoperated control hatchlings. Chicks transected on E13 through E15 never showed voluntary or evoked locomotor activity; however, sham-operated E14 control animals always displayed normal locomotion. The similarity of the muscle activity patterns and the video-recorded limb movement records (not shown) supports the observation that E12-transected chicks show complete functional recovery due at least in part to 'true' axonal regeneration. (From Hasan et al., 1993.)

(5) the frequency of the brainstem-evoked leg movements should match changes in the strength of the brainstem stimulation current, i.e., an increase in strength should evoke leg movements at a faster frequency. Our findings (Hasan et al., 1991,1993) satisfied all of the above criteria (Figs. 4 and 5).

Cellular factors contributing to functional axonal regeneration

We have approached the search for the cellular factors that underlie the transition between the permissive and restrictive periods for functional regeneration using a number of different tech-

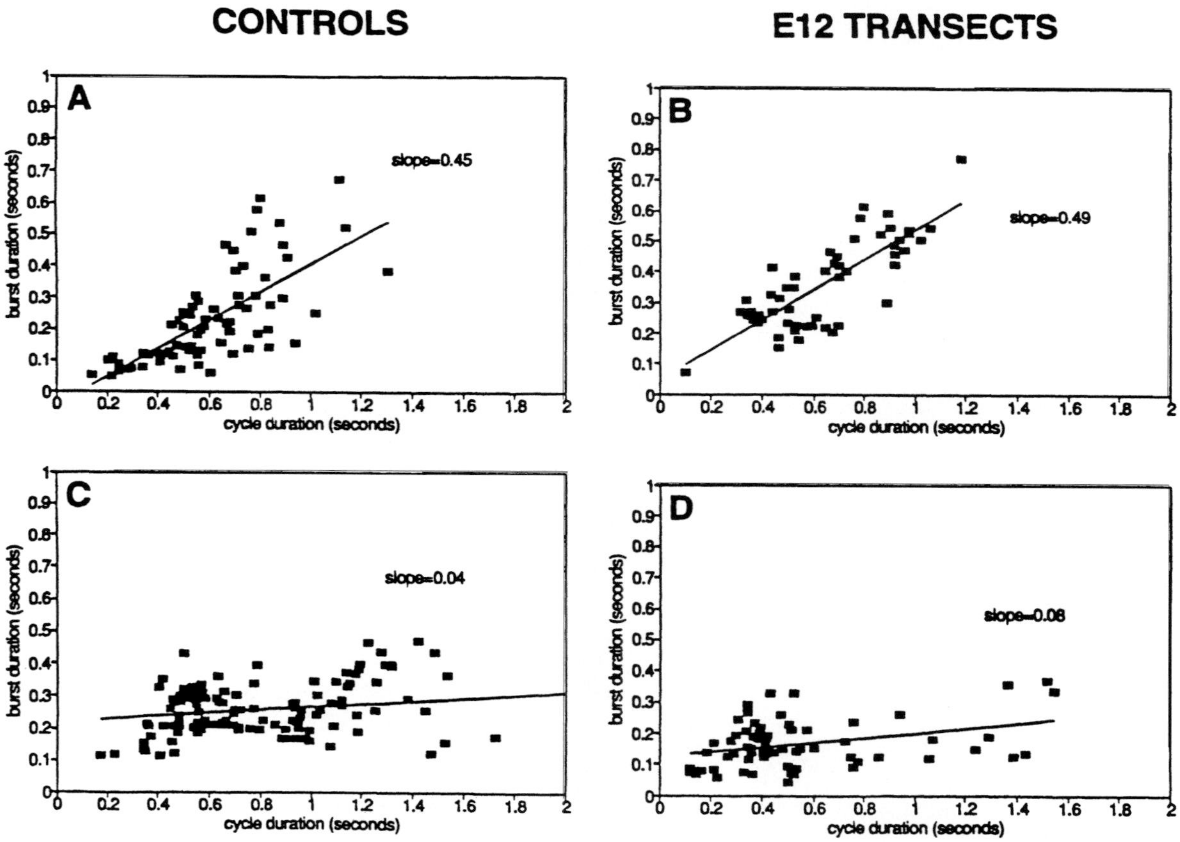

Fig. 5. Linear regression of leg muscle activity (burst) duration versus step cycle duration during brainstem-evoked locomotion in hatchling chicks: A and B are for the gastrocnemius lateralis muscle (GL, active during the stance phase), whereas C and D are for the sartorius muscle (SA, active during the swing phase). Typical of most terrestrial birds and mammals, as the step cycle duration changes, the burst duration of stance phase muscles such as the GL (A and B) changes accordingly. Conversely, the burst duration of swing phase muscles such as the SA (C and D) remains relatively constant during changes in step cycle duration. Thus an increase in velocity (or shorter step cycle duration) is characterized by shorter burst durations within stance phase muscles. Control (sham-operated or unoperated) hatchlings (A and C) show the typical relationships, as do E12-transected hatchlings (B and D). The similarity of the burst duration versus cycle duration relationships in both control and E12-transected animals verifies the complete functional recovery of chicks transected during the permissive period for repair. The coefficients of determination (r^2) = 0.49, 0.06, 0.65 and 0.13 for A, B, C and D, respectively; $n = 6$ for controls and $n = 6$ for E12 spinal-transected animals. (From Hasan et al., 1993.)

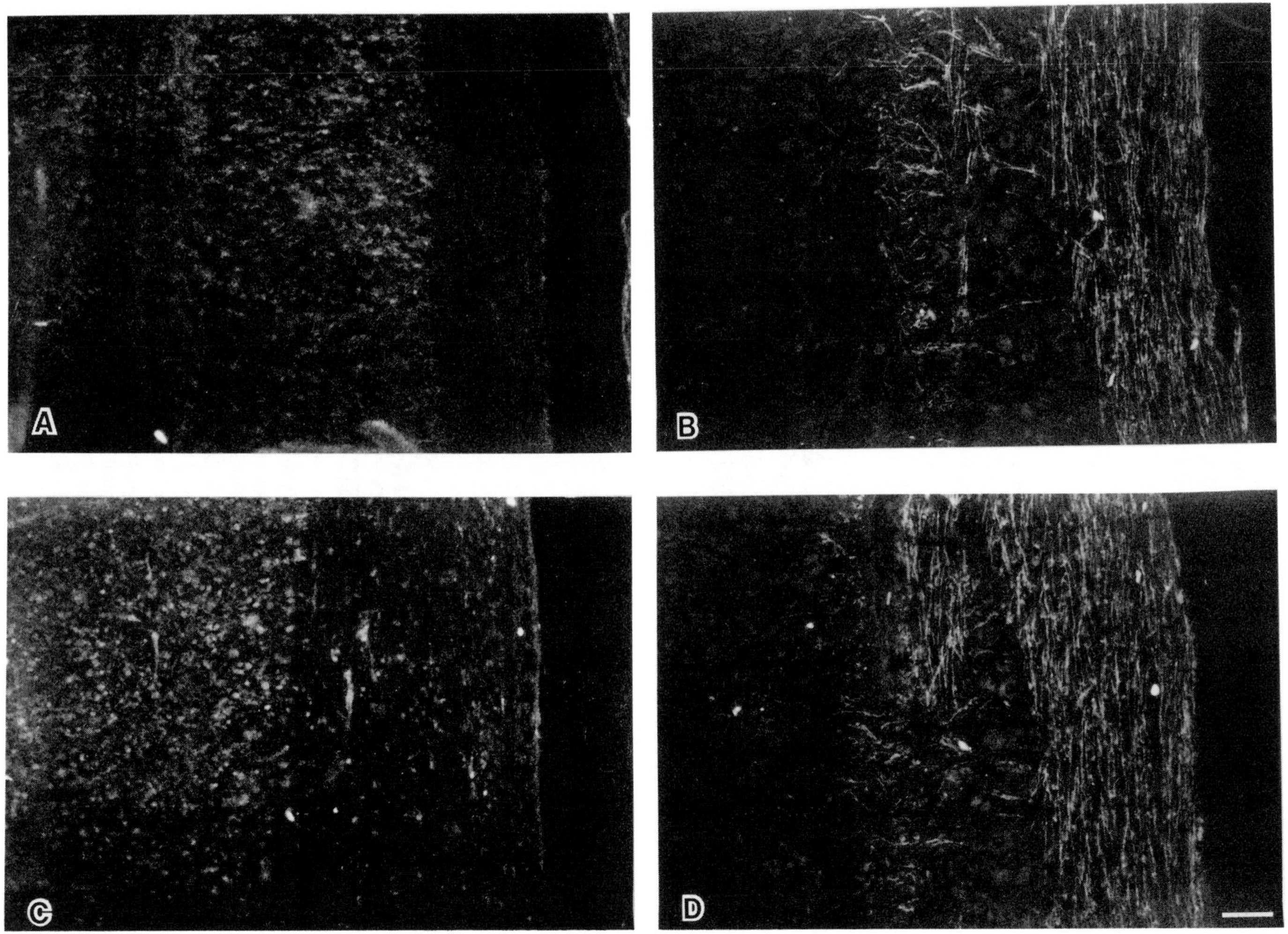

Fig. 6 Myelin basic protein (MBP) immunofluorescence staining of embryonic chicken spinal cord white matter in parasagittal section. (A) Unoperated control E12 thoracic spinal cord, prior to the onset of myelination, showing no MBP staining. (B) Unoperated normally myelinated (control) E15 thoracic spinal cord showing extensive MBP staining within the white matter. MBP immunofluorescence first appears at E13. (C) E15 thoracic spinal cord from a myelination-inhibited animal that received a single 2–3 μl thoracic spinal injection on E9–E12 of homologous or heterologous (guinea pig) serum complement along with an oligodendrocyte-specific antibody that binds complement (e.g., a monoclonal IgG3 antibody to galactocerebroside, GalC; polyclonal O4 antibody). Note the lack of MBP staining, indicating an absence of myelin; similar evidence for the developmental inhibition of myelination was also obtained with CNP or MAG immunostaining (see text). (D) E15 thoracic spinal cord from an immunological control animal that received a single injection of serum complement only on E9–E12; note that MBP staining is comparable to normal (unoperated) E15 spinal tissue, shown in B. Normal myelination was also observed for all other immunological controls. Scale bar = 50 μm for A; 100 μm for B–D. (From Keirstead et al., 1992.)

niques. Initially, we examined whether plasma membrane fractions, isolated from spinal cord tissue at different stages of development, were permissive or restrictive substrates for the in vitro differentiation and outgrowth of processes from immortalized neuronal-glial hybrid cells (NG108-15 cells; Ethell et al., 1993, 1994a). As might be expected from the in vivo results (described

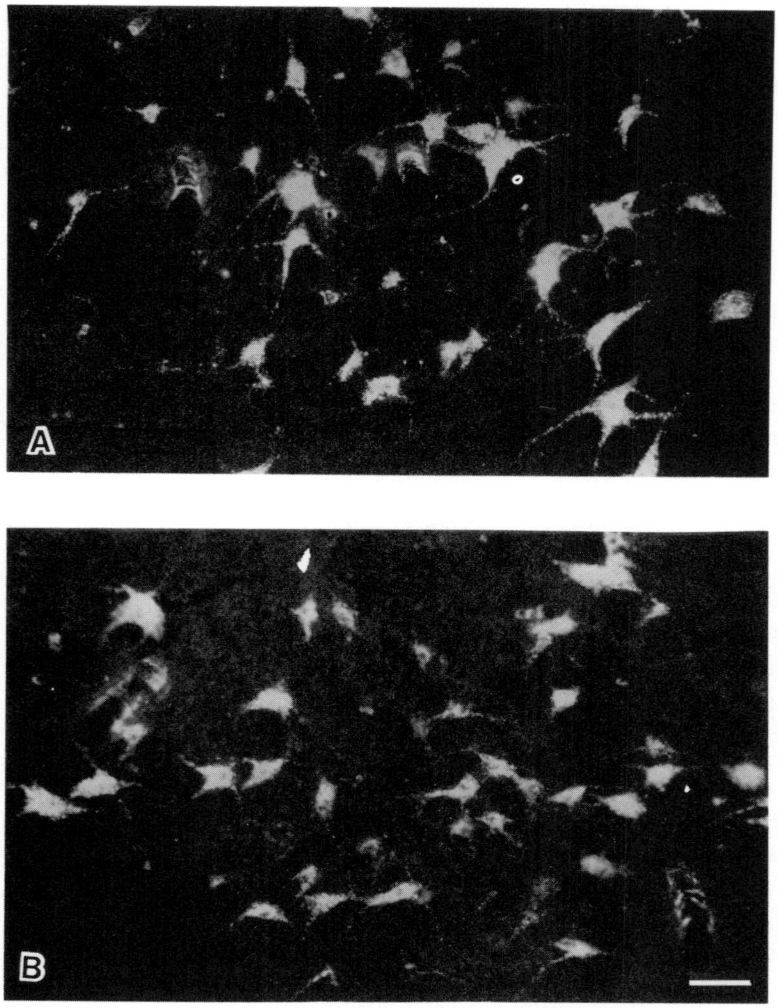

Fig. 7. Photomicrographs of retrogradely labeled gigantocellular reticulospinal neurons within the ventromedial reticular formation of the caudal pons in P4 chicks. Numerous brainstem-spinal neurons were labeled after an injection on P2 of the RDA tracing dye into the caudal thoraco-lumbar spinal cord. (A) Normal myelinated, unoperated (control) hatchling chick brainstem section showing a typical number and distribution of reticulospinal neurons. (B) Experimental hatchling chick that was subjected to immunological inhibtion of the formation of spinal cord myelin on E10, followed by a complete transection of the thoracic cord on E15. Note the similar number and distribution of retrogradely labeled reticulospinal neurons. Comparable anatomical repair/regeneration was evident for several other brainstem-spinal projections in myelination-inhibited chicks. E15-transected chicks where myelination was not immunologically inhibited showed no evidence of neuroanatomical regeneration (not shown). Scale bar = 50 μm. (From Keirstead et al., 1992.)

above), plasma membrane fractions isolated from spinal cord tissue prior to E13 were permissive substrates for the in vitro differentiation of NG108-15 cells, whereas plasma membrane fractions isolated from spinal cord tissue after E13 (including adult) became progressively more restrictive substrates for NG108-15 cells. A subsequent comparison of plasma membrane fractions isolated from rat spinal cord as permissive or restrictive substrates revealed a temporal transition at about the time of birth, presumably befitting of the delayed development of spinal cord pathways in mammals that are not as precocial as chicks (Ethell et al., 1994a).

The exact nature of the inhibitory molecule(s) within these plasma membrane fractions is unknown, but may include any combination of proteins, carbohydrates or lipids. Most structural carbohydrates are either conjugated to proteins as glycoproteins and proteoglycans, or to lipids as glycolipids. For example, previous studies have implicated membrane associated proteins (Caroni and Schwab, 1988) and proteoglycans (Dow et al., 1993) as inhibitors of neurite outgrowth. Recently, we have noted developmental changes in proteoglycan expression that temporally correlate with the transition between the permissive and restrictive period for spinal cord repair in the embryonic chick (Dow et al., 1994). Specifically, the permissive period is characterized by a high ratio of heparan sulphate proteoglycan (HSPG) to chondroitin sulphate proteoglycan (CSPG) expression and this is associated with robust neurite promoting activity within chick dorsal root ganglion (DRG) neurons grown in vitro on E9 proteoglycan fractions immobilized on a laminin substrate. After E13, CSPG synthesis increases and masks the neurite promoting activity of HSPG. Proteoglycan fractions from E17 chick spinal cord are inhibitory to DRG neurite outgrowth. Removal of the influence of CSPGs from E17 proteoglycan extracts enhanced in vitro neurite outgrowth by DRG neurons.

We have also completed an initial examination of lipids as substrates for the differentiation of neurons and immortalized cells in vitro (Ethell et al., 1994b). Lipid fractions were isolated from either the permissive (< E13) or restrictive (> E13) periods of the developing chick spinal cord, as well as from adult bovine spinal cord. All lipid fractions were reformed into vesicles for presentation as a substrate for primary cultures of superior cervical ganglion neurons and two immortalized cell lines, NG108-15 and pheochromocytoma (PC12) cells. No neurite inhibition was detected from any of the purified lipids, indicating that the lipid component of spinal cord plasma membranes is unlikely to inhibit axonal regeneration.

We have also used assays for changes in protein expression at different developmental stages, which have now been supplemented with assays for changes in gene expression. To date we have observed several proteins (Ethell and Steeves, 1993) and gene clones (Rott and Steeves, unpublished observations) that alter their developmental expression over the time of the in vivo transition between permissive and restrictive periods for functional spinal cord regeneration. These cellular and molecular changes are currently being examined further.

It is noteworthy, however, that the onset of myelination in the developing chick spinal cord has been reported to start around E13 (Benstead et al., 1957; Hartman et al., 1979; Macklin and Weill, 1985). Using immunocytochemical protocols for either myelin basic protein (MBP; Keirstead et al., 1992), myelin associated glycoprotein (MAG; Keirstead et al., 1994) or 2′,3′-cyclic nucleotide 3′-phosphodiesterase (CNP; Keirstead et al., 1994), we have independently confirmed these developmental findings, noting that the onset of myelination is coincident with the transition from the permissive to the restrictive period for repair (Keirstead et al., 1992). MBP, MAG and CNP expression are only associated with myelin and, along with proteolipid protein (PLP), constitute the major identifiable proteins expressed during myelination of CNS axons (Hartman et al., 1979; Morell et al., 1989).

Recently, myelin associated proteins have been identified in rat spinal cord that inhibit the anatomical regrowth of axotomized corticospinal fi-

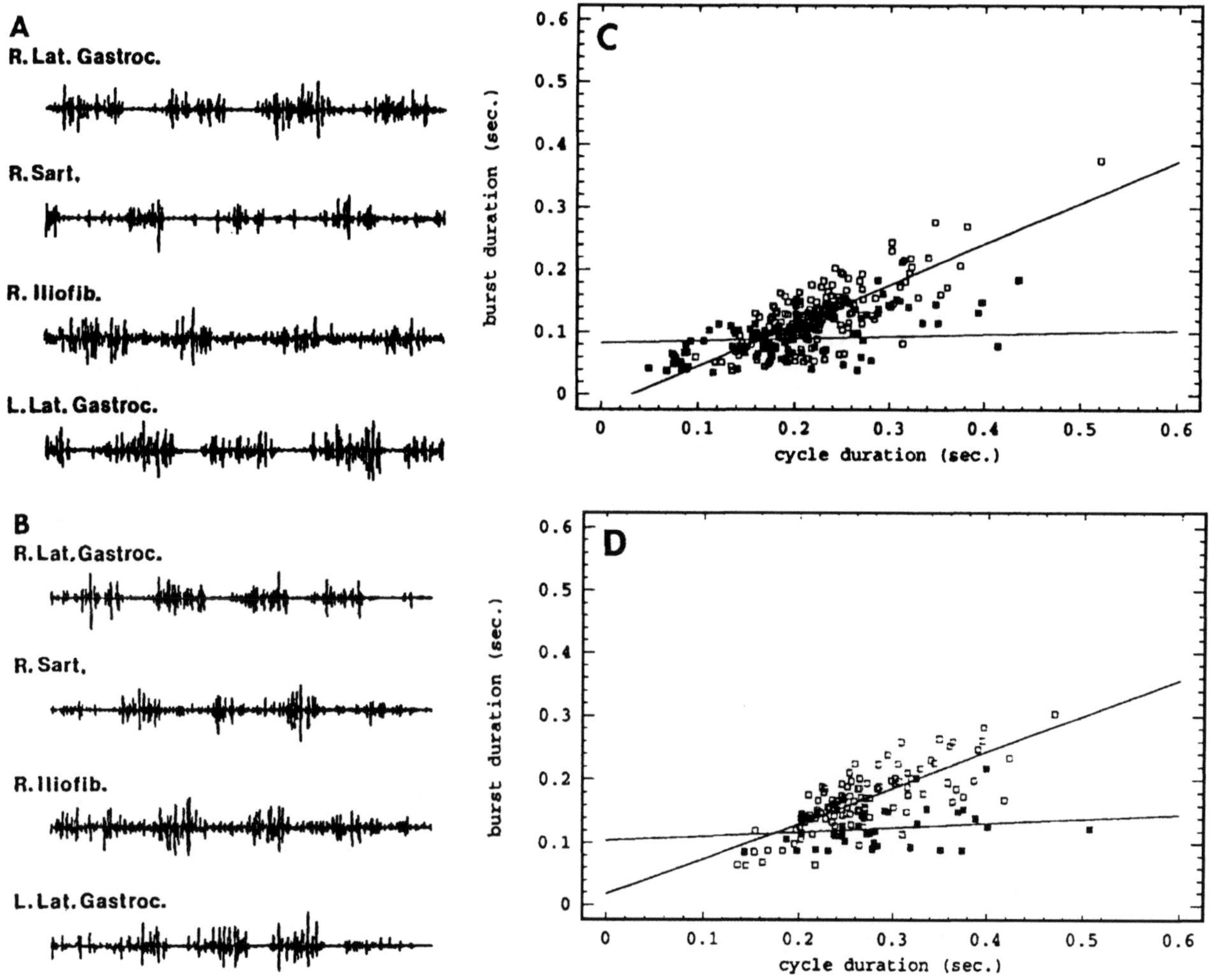

Fig. 8 (A and B) Simultaneous EMG recordings from four leg muscles during voluntary overground walking by a normal myelinated, unoperated (control) chick (A) and a myelination-inhibited, E15-transected chick (B). The control and experimental chicks both exhibit the same locomotor patterns and muscle activity profiles. (C and D) Regression of muscle activity (burst) duration versus step cycle duration for gastrocnemius lateralis (GL) muscle (open squares, active during stance phase) and the sartorius (SA) muscle (filled squares, active during swing phase) during voluntary overground walking in a control (C) and experimental (D) hatchling chick. The slopes of the corresponding regression lines in C and D are not significantly different ($P < 0.05$). The coefficients of determination (r^2) for GL and SA muscles, respectively, are 0.58 and 0.04 in C and 0.59 and 0.08 in D. (From Keirstead et al., 1992.)

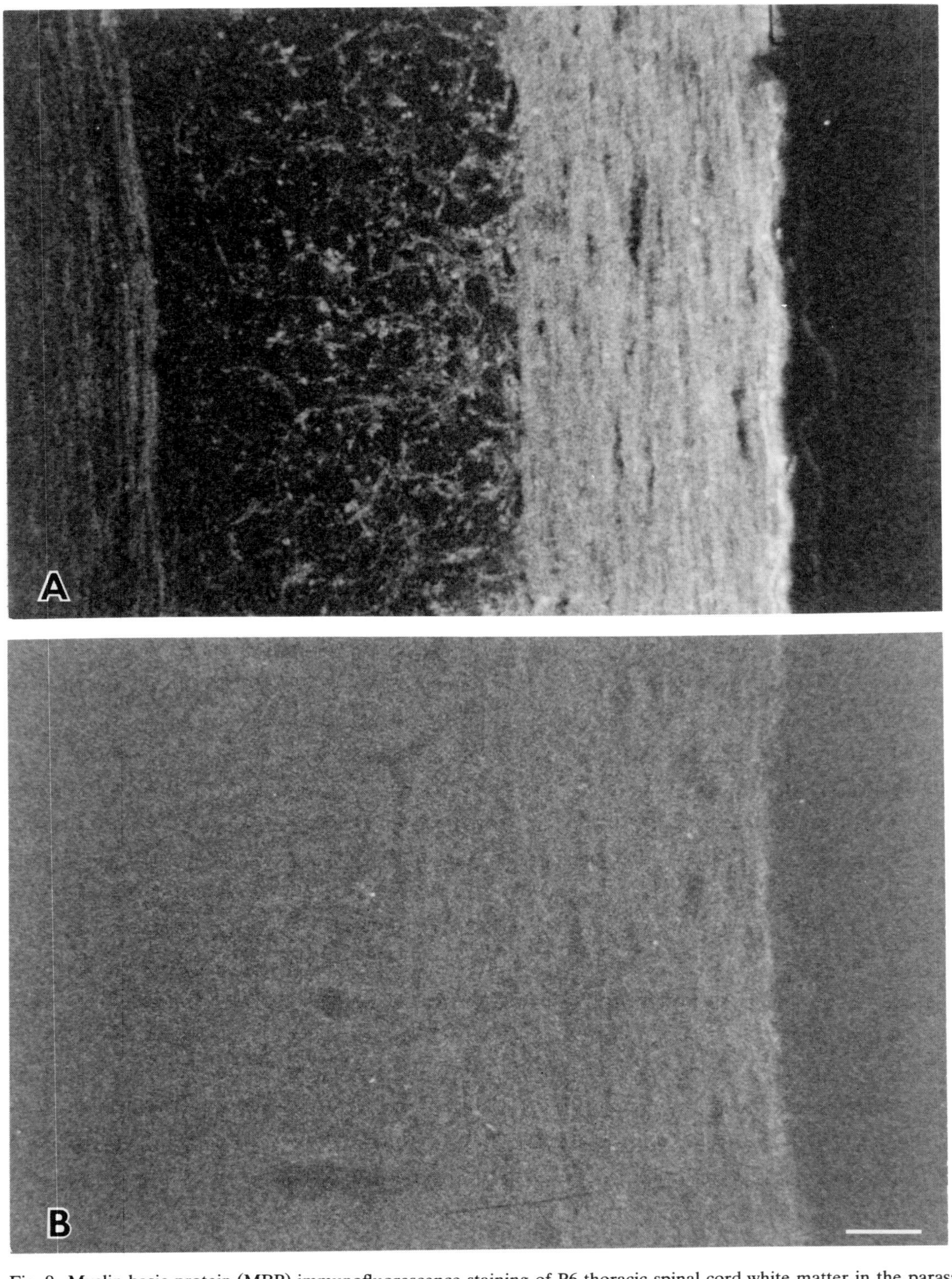

Fig. 9. Myelin basic protein (MBP) immunofluorescence staining of P6 thoracic spinal cord white matter in the parasagittal plane. (A) Control P6 thoracic cord showing robust MBP immunoreactivity characteristic of myelinated CNS fiber tracts. (B) Experimental

bres (Caroni and Schwab, 1988; Schnell and Schwab, 1990). The neutralization of these myelin associated proteins with specific antibodies (e.g., IN-1) facilitated the anatomical regrowth of a small proportion of these transected axons (Schnell and Schwab, 1990). It is not known whether any of the corticospinal regeneration resulted in the formation of functional synapses with spinal neurons. Considering that embryonic chicks displayed both neuroanatomical repair and functional locomotor recovery after cord injury, we decided to use a different approach to assess the potential inhibitory role of myelin in the regeneration of brainstem-spinal projections. We immunologically delayed the developmental onset of myelination until well into the restrictive period for embryonic spinal cord repair. After a subsequent restrictive period transection (e.g., E15) in such an unmyelinated environment, the assessment of spinal cord repair then serves as a direct test of whether myelin inhibits neuroanatomical and functional regeneration.

Antisera against galactocerebroside (GalC) have been shown to inhibit myelination and reversibly demyelinate CNS tissue in vitro (Dubois-Dalcq et al., 1970; Fry et al., 1974; Hruby et al., 1977; Dorfman et al., 1979; Dyer and Benjamins, 1990) and optic nerve (Sergott et al., 1984; Ozawa et al., 1989) and spinal cord (Mastiglia et al., 1989) in vivo. GalC is the major sphingolipid produced by oligodendrocytes and is highly conserved across species (Ranscht et al., 1982). The GalC antibody that we use has been shown to cross-react with chicken and exhibit specificity for oligodendrocytes within the CNS (Ranscht et al., 1982). The proposed mechanism of anti-GalC-induced demyelination in vitro involves microtubule disassembly of oligodendrocyte processes mediated by an influx of extracellular calcium (Dyer and Benjamins, 1990). Although the in vivo mechanism of myelin inhibition has not been characterized, we have found that a single injection of a monoclonal GalC antibody (with homologous complement) into the thoracic spinal cord of an E9–E12 chick embryo (i.e., around the time of oligodendrocyte differentiation) results in a delay in the onset of spinal cord MBP (Fig. 6), CNP and MAG immunoreactivity (i.e., myelination) until E17 (Keirstead et al., 1992, 1994).

We have discounted the possibility of nonspecific binding of the GalC antibody influencing our results by injecting a nonspecific, complement binding antibody (to glial fibrillary acidic protein, GFAP) plus homologous complement into the thoracic spinal cord; this procedure does not alter the development of myelin, nor the response to injury at any developmental stage (Keirstead et al., 1992). Similarly, no effect on CNS myelination is observed if antibody only, serum complement proteins only, vehicle only, or GalC antibody plus heat-inactivated serum are injected into the spinal cord. This indicates that both the GalC antibody and serum complement proteins are necessary to developmentally inhibit myelination. Equally effective inhibition can also be produced by simultaneously injecting (as described above) serum complement along with complement fixing, oligodendrocyte-specific O4 antibody (Sommer and Schachner, 1981).

A thoracic spinal cord transection as late as E15 (i.e., during the normal restrictive period for repair) in an embryo without spinal cord myelin resulted in complete neuroanatomical repair and functional recovery. This is in sharp contrast to (normally myelinated) control embryos transected on E15 which showed no axonal repair/regeneration and, upon hatching, were completely paralyzed. In brief, the number and distribution of retrograde labeled brainstem-spinal neuronal cell bodies in myelination-inhibited E15-transected

P6 thoracic cord that previously received a direct intraspinal injection on P4 of serum complement along with (a complement binding) IgG3 monoclonal antibody to galactocerebroside (GalC). Note the absence of MBP immunoreactivity. States of demyelination can be maintained with prolonged infusion (via an osmotic pump) of complement and an oligodendrocyte-specific antibody that binds complement. The demyelination is transient and remyelination begins within 24–48 h after termination of the immunologically induced demyelination. Scale bar = 50 μm.

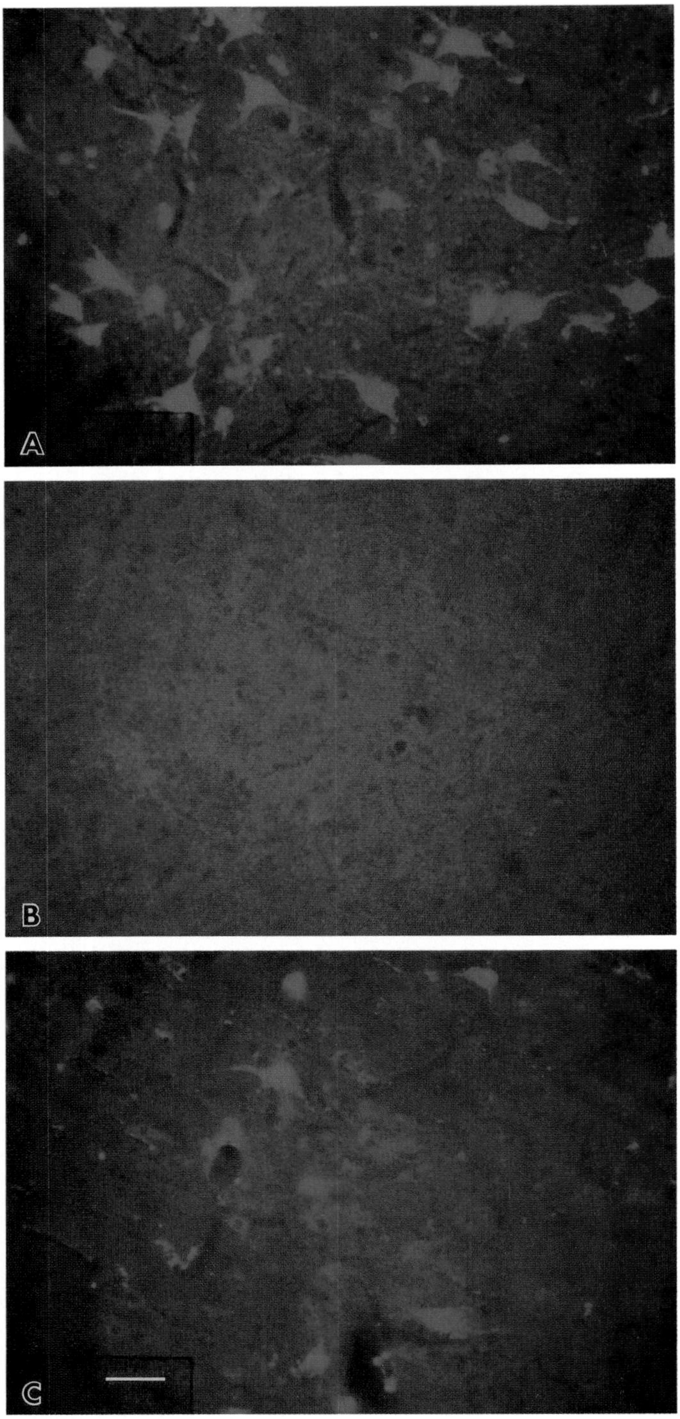

Fig. 10. Photomicrographs of retrogradely labeled gigantocellular reticulospinal neurons within the caudal pons in hatchling chicks in an experiment to determine whether the subsequent transient immunological demyelination of the 'adult' spinal cord can 'rescue'

animals was indistinguishable from nontransected control embryos (Fig. 7) or embryos transected during the permissive period (e.g., E12, when myelin has yet to appear). The locomotor functions of myelination-inhibited E15-transected embryos were similar to untransected control animals or embryos transected during the permissive period (Fig. 8; Keirstead et al., 1992).

These findings demonstrate that, after a spinal transection, the suppression of myelination extends the permissive period for neuroanatomical repair/regeneration, and represent the first observation of functional CNS recovery facilitated by a therapeutic treatment. The results clearly confirm and extend the proposition that the presence of CNS myelin is one factor that contributes to the inhibition of neuronal repair after an adult CNS injury (Keirstead et al., 1992). This suggestion is also supported by the recent evidence for neuronal repair prior to the developmental onset of myelination in neonatal opposums (Treherne et al., 1992), and the functional repair/regeneration in animals (e.g., lamprey) that do not have myelinated CNS fiber tracts (McClellan, 1990).

The more critical goals now requiring answers are: (1) will the immunological therapy outlined above transiently remove myelin from the adult avian and mammalian CNS (i.e., transient demyelination), (2) will demyelination of the CNS after a traumatic injury 'rescue' disrupted pathways, and (3) does demyelination alone facilitate neuroanatomical regeneration to a sufficient degree to promote functional recovery after a CNS injury? Our preliminary evidence suggests yes to the first two questions, but no to the third and ultimately most important goal (Keirstead et al., unpublished observations).

In brief, recent data have shown that direct spinal cord infusion (via an osmotic pump) of serum complement proteins along with an oligodendrocyte-specific antibody (e.g., GalC or O4) that binds to complement will transiently demyelinate several segments of the spinal cord in hatchling chicks or neonatal mice (Fig. 9). Demyelination begins within 12 h after the start of infusion and can be maintained for as long as the complement and antibody are infused. To date, 14 days has been the longest infusion period tested and the animals have shown no untoward side effects due to the treatment. Remyelination occurs upon termination of the immunological protocol and, based on MBP immunofluorescence, appears very robust within several days.

The exact basis for remyelination is unknown. However, preliminary data using a transgenic mouse line where oligodendrocytes can be unequivocally identified (due to a *LacZ* reporter gene being coupled to elements of the MBP promotor region) have suggested that the oligodendrocyte cell bodies may survive the complement-mediated attack to a greater degree than the myelin processes (Keirstead et al., unpublished data). Thus, surviving oligodendrocytes could be the source for subsequent remyelination. This suggestion is also supported by the presence of robust MBP mRNA expression after the inhibition of myelination (as determined by Northern analysis; Keirstead et al., 1994). This would not be

a spinal cord injury (i.e., facilitate neuroanatomical regeneration and functional locomotor recovery). (A) The normal number and distribution of reticulospinal neurons in a normally myelinated, unoperated P19 control animal. This pattern of retrograde labeling brainstem-spinal neurons was similar in all normal control animals from E11 onward and represents the adult state of development. The reticulospinal neurons were labeled after an injection of RDA into the caudal thoraco-lumbar spinal cord on P17 with a further 2 days for retrograde transport. (B) Control animal that was subjected to a complete transection of the thoracic cord on P2 without any subsequent demyelination of the cord. Note the complete absence of retrograde labeling. Brainstem-spinal neurons were never labeled in any of the immunological control animals. (C) Experimental hatchling that was transected on P9 and subsequently (within an hour) fitted with an osmotic pump that infused complement plus a GalC monoclonal antibody directly into the thoracic spinal cord (caudal to the transection site) for the next 14 days (i.e., until P23). An RDA injection into the caudal thoraco-lumbar cord was undertaken on P26 and the animal was killed on P28. Retrograde labeling of approximately 10% of the normal number of brainstem-spinal neurons was observed. However, functional locomotor recovery was never observed. Scale bar = 50 μm.

expected if oligodendrocyte cell bodies had been destroyed by the demyelination procedure.

Further experiments are also under way to determine whether an intrathecal (i.e., subdural) administration route is equally effective in producing transient demyelinated states. Intrathecal spinal administration is a well established clinical procedure in patients. It is relatively noninvasive and would be a preferred therapy route if any similar immunological process were contemplated for future trials after a human spinal cord injury.

Delaying the start of the immunological demyelination protocol up to 1 h after a complete thoracic cord transection (later times have not yet been tested) in a (P2–P8) hatchling chick also resulted in equally effective transient demyelination. More important was the observation of axonal regeneration by approximately 5–15% of brainstem-spinal neurons in such demyelinated 'adult' animals (Fig. 10). These preliminary results are based on retrograde labeling of brainstem-spinal neurons from an injection within the lumbar cord, 2–3 weeks after spinal cord injury. The percentage figure for axonal regeneration is based on comparisons with the number of labeled brainstem-spinal neurons observed in untransected or sham operated control animals. Spinal transected hatchling chicks that did not receive the 14 day demyelination treatment showed no evidence of any axonal regeneration.

As encouraging as these preliminary results from adult animals may be, we have yet to observe any functional recovery in those animals displaying the 5–15% brainstem-spinal regeneration. We do not as yet know the explanation for the lack of functional recovery. Perhaps functional recovery requires more than 15% of the available descending projections to regenerate. Perhaps there has been too much muscle wasting during the intervening recovery period. Alternatively, the regenerating brainstem-spinal axons may be unable to make functional synapses with appropriate 'target' neurons in the spinal cord. The latter is considered unlikely due to our preliminary findings of brainstem-evoked motor responses in these experimental animals. In the adult CNS the lack of functional regeneration may be due to the shortage (i.e., the developmental downregulation) of other, as yet unidentified, guidance molecule(s) or trophic factor(s) and/or the presence (i.e., developmental upregulation) of additional unidentified inhibitory factor(s). Further research is under way in several laboratories in an effort to resolve some of these outstanding issues.

Acknowledgements

This work was supported by grants to J.D.S. from the following Canadian agencies: Medical Research Council (MRC), Natural Sciences and Engineering Research Council (NSERC), and Neural Regeneration and Functional Recovery Network (NR Network). H.S.K., S.J.H. and C.B.M. were supported by scholarships from NSERC; G.D.M. was supported by a professional postdoctoral fellowship from MRC; T.J.Z. was supported by a clinical scientist award from MRC. H.S.K. is also a trainee of the NR Network.

References

Armstrong, D. (1986) Supraspinal contributions to the initiation and control of locomotion in the cat. *Prog. Neurobiol.*, 26: 273–361.

Bekoff, A. (1976) Ontogeny of leg motor output in the chick embryo: a neural analysis. *Brain Res.*, 106: 271–291.

Bensted, J.P.M., Dobbing, J., Morgan, R.S., Reid, R.T.W. and Payling-Wright, G. (1957) Neuroglial development and myelination in the spinal cord of the chick embryo. *J. Embryol. Exp. Morph.*, 5: 428–437.

Björklund, A., Katzman, R., Stenevi, U. and West, K.A. (1971) Development and growth of axonal sprouts from noradrenaline and 5-hydroxytryptamine neurons in the rat spinal cord. *Brain Res.*, 31: 21–33.

Caroni, P. and Schwab, M. (1988) Two membrane protein fractions from rat central myelin with inhibitory properties for neurite growth and fibroblast spreading. *J. Cell Biol.*, 106: 1281- 1288.

David, S. and Aguayo, A.J. (1981) Axonal elongation into peripheral nervous system 'bridges' after central nervous system injury in adult rats. *Science*, 214: 931–933.

Dorfman, S.H., Fry, J.M. and Silberberg, D.H. (1979) Antiserum induced demyelination inhibition in vitro without complement. *Brain Res.*, 177: 105-114.

Dow, K.E., Guo, M., Kisilevsky, R. and Riopelle, R.J. (1993) Regenerative neurite modulation associated with astrocyte proteoglycans. *Brain Res. Bull.*, 30: 461–468.

Dow, K.E., Ethell, D.W., Steeves, J.D. and Riopelle, R.J. (1994) Molecular correlates of spinal cord repair in the embryonic chick: heparan sulphate and chondroitin sulphate proteoglycans. *Exp. Neurol.*, in press.

Dubois-Dalcq, M. Niedieck, B. and Buyse, M. (1970) Action of anti-cerebroside sera on myelinated tissue cultures. *Pathol. Eur.*, 5: 331–347.

Dyer, C.A. and Benjamins, J.A. (1990) Glycolipids and transmembrane signalling: antibodies to galactocerebroside cause an influx of calcium in oligodendrocytes. *J. Cell Biol.*, 111: 625–633.

Ethell, D.W. and Steeves, J.D. (1993) Changes in protein expression associated with the developmental transition from permissive to restrictive states of spinal cord repair in embryonic chick. *Dev. Brain Res.*, 76: 163–169.

Ethell, D.W., Cheng, K.W., Jordan, L.M. and Steeves, J.D. (1993) Developmental transition by spinal cord plasma membranes of embryonic chick from permissive to restrictive substrates for the morphological differentiation of neuroblastoma × glioma hybrid NG108–15 cell. *Dev. Brain. Res.*, 72: 1–8.

Ethell, D.W., Steeves, J.D., Jordan, L.M. and Cheng, K.W. (1994a) Increasing in vitro neurite inhibition by plasma membrane substrates isolated at different stages of spinal cord development in the rat. *Dev. Neurosci.*, submitted.

Ethell, D.W., Cheng, K.W. and Steeves, J.D. (1994b) Spinal cord lipid substrates do not inhibit neurite differentiation in vitro. *J. Neurocytol.*, submitted.

Fawcett, J.W. (1992) Intrinsic neuronal determinants of regeneration. *Trends Neurosci.*, 15: 5- 8.

Fry, J.M., Weissbarth, S., Lehrer, G.M. and Bornstein, M.B. (1974) Cerebroside antibody inhibits sulfatide synthesis and myelination and demyelinates in cord tissue cultures. *Science*, 183: 540–542.

Glover, J. (1993) The development of brain stem projections to the spinal cord in the chicken embryo. *Brain Res. Bull.*, 30: 265–272.

Glover J. and Pettursdottir G. (1991) Regional specificity of developing reticulospinal, vestibulospinal, and vestibulo-ocular projections in the chicken embryo. *J. Neurobiol.*, 22: 353–376.

Glover, J.C., Pettursdottir, G. and Jansen, J.K.S. (1986) Fluorescent dextran amines used as axonal tracers in the nervous system of the chicken embryo. *J. Neurosci. Methods*, 18: 243- 254.

Grillner, S. and Dubuc, R. (1988) Control of locomotion in vertebrates: spinal and supraspinal mechanisms. In S.G. Waxman (Ed.), *Functional Recovery in Neurological Disease, Advances in Neurology*, Vol. 47, Raven Press, New York, pp. 425–453.

Hartman, B.K., Agrawal, H.C., Kalmbach, S. and Shearer, W.T. J. (1979) A comparative study of the immunohistochemical localization of basic protein to myelin and oligodendrocytes in rat and chicken brain. *J. Comp. Neurol.*, 188: 273–290.

Hasan, S.J., Nelson, B.H., Valenzuela, J.I., Keirstead, H.S., Schull, S.E., Ethell, D.W. and Steeves, J.D. (1991) Functional repair of transected spinal cord in embryonic chick. *Restor. Neurol. Neurosci.*, 2: 137–154.

Hasan, S.J., Keirstead, H.S., Muir, G.D. and Steeves, J.D. (1993) Axonal regeneration contributes to repair of injured brainstem-spinal neurons in embryonic chick. *J. Neurosci.*, 13: 492–507.

Heimer, L. and Robards, M.J. (1981) *Neuroanatomical Tract-Tracing Methods*, Plenum, New York.

Holder, N. and Clarke, J.D.W. (1988) Is there a correlation between continuous neurogenesis and directed axon regeneration in the vertebrate nervous system. *Trends Neurosci.*, 11: 94–99.

Hruby, S., Alvord, E.C., Jr. and Seil, F.J. (1977) Synthetic galactocerebrosides evoke myelination-inhibiting antibodies. *Science*, 195: 173–175.

Jordan, L.M. (1986) Initiation of locomotion from the mammalian brain stem. In S. Grillner, P.S.G. Stein, D.G. Stuart, H. Forssberg and R.M. Herman (Eds.), *Neurobiology of Vertebrate Locomotion*, MacMillan Press, London, pp. 21–37.

Keirstead, H.S., Hasan, S.J., Muir, G.D. and Steeves, J.D. (1992) Suppression of the onset of myelination extends the permissive period for the functional repair of embryonic spinal cord. *Proc. Natl. Acad. Sci. USA*, 89: 11664–11668.

Keirstead, H.S., Wisniewska, A.B., Muir, G.D., Pataky, D.M. and Steeves, J.D. (1994) Immunological suppression (in vivo) of spinal cord myelin development facilitates the functional repair of brain stem-spinal projections after embryonic transection of chick spinal cord. *Glia*, submitted.

Lawrence, D.G. and Kuypers, H.G.J.M. (1968a) The functional organization of the motor system in the monkey. I. The effects of bilateral pyramidal lesions. *Brain*, 91: 1–14.

Lawrence, D.G. and Kuypers, H.G.J.M. (1968b) The functional organization of the motor system in the monkey. II. The effects of lesions of the descending brain-stem pathways. *Brain*, 91: 15–36.

Macklin, W.B. and Weill, C.L. (1985) Appearance of myelin proteins during development in the chick central nervous system. *Dev. Neurosci.*, 7: 170–178.

Mastiglia, F., Carroll, W. and Jennings, A. (1989) Spinal cord lesions induced by antigalactocerebroside serum. *Clin. Exp. Neurol.*, 26: 33–44.

McClellan, A.D. (1990) Locomotor recovery in spinal-transected lamprey: role of functional regeneration of descending axons from brainstem locomotor command neurons. *Neuroscience*, 37: 781–798.

McConnell, J. and Sechrist, J. (1980) Identification of early neurons in the brainstem and spinal cord. I. An autoradiographic study in the chick. *J. Comp. Neurol.*, 192: 769–783.

Morell, P., Quarles, R.H. and Norton, W.T. (1989) Formation, structure, and biochemistry of myelin. In G.J. Siegel, B.W. Agranoff, R.W. Albers and P.B. Molinoff (Eds.), *Basic Neurochemistry: Molecular, Cellular, and Medical Aspects*, 4th Edn., Raven Press, New York, pp. 109–136.

Noga, B.R., Kettler, J. and Jordan, L.M. (1988) Locomotion produced in mesencephalic cats by injection of putative transmitter substances and antagonists into the medial reticular formation and pontomedullary locomotor strip. *J. Neurosci.*, 8: 2074–2086.

O'Donovan, M., Sernagor, E., Sholomenko, G., Ho, S., Antal, M. and Yee, W. (1992) Development of spinal motor networks in the chick embryo. *J. Exp. Zool.*, 261: 261- 273.

Okado, N. and Oppenheim, R.W. (1985) The onset and development of descending pathways to the spinal cord in the chick embryo. *J. Comp. Neurol.*, 232: 143–161.

Oppenheim, R.W. (1991) Cell death during development of the nervous system. *Annu. Rev. Neurosci.*, 14: 453–501.

Ozawa, K., Saida, T., Saida, K., Nishitani, H. and Kameyama, M. (1989) In vivo CNS demyelination mediated by anti-galactocerebroside antibody. *Acta Neuropathol.*, 77: 621–628.

Ramón y Cajal, S. (1928) *Degeneration and Regeneration of the Nervous System*, (English translation by Raoul M. May), Hafner, New York, 1959.

Ranscht, B., Clapshaw, P.A., Price, J., Noble, M. and Seifert, W. (1982) Development of oligodendrocytes and Schwann cells studied with a monoclonal antibody against galactocerebroside. *Proc. Natl. Acad. Sci. USA*, 79: 2709–2713.

Sarnat, H. and Netsky, M. (1981) *Evolution of the Nervous System*, Oxford University Press, New York.

Schnell, L. and Schwab, M. (1990) Axonal regeneration in the rat spinal cord produced by an antibody against myelin-associated neurite growth inhibitors. *Nature (Lond.)*, 343: 269- 272.

Sergott, R.C., Brown, M.J., Silberberg, D.H. and Lisak, R.P. (1984) Antigalactocerebroside serum demyelinates optic nerve in vivo. *J. Neurol. Sci.*, 64: 297–303.

Shiga, T., Kunzi, R. and Oppenheim, R.W. (1991) Axonal projections and synaptogenesis by supraspinal descending neurons in the spinal cord of the chick embryo. *J. Comp. Neurol.*, 305: 83–95.

Shimizu, I., Oppenheim, R.W., O'Brien, M. and Shneiderman, A. (1990) Anatomical and functional recovery following spinal cord transection in the chick embryo. *J. Neurobiol.*, 21: 918–937.

Sholomenko, G.N. and O'Donovan M. (1994) Development and characterization of pathways descending to the spinal cord in the developing chick. *J. Neurosci.*, submitted.

Sholomenko, G.N. and Steeves, J.D. (1987) Effects of selective spinal cord lesions on hind limb locomotion in birds. *Exp. Neurol.*, 95: 403–418.

Sholomenko, G.N., Funk, G.D. and Steeves, J.D. (1991a) Locomotor activities in the decerebrate bird without phasic afferent input. *Neuroscience*, 40: 257–266.

Sholomenko, G.N., Funk, G.D. and Steeves, J.D. (1991b) Avian locomotion activated by brainstem infusion of neurotransmitter agonists and antagonists. I. Acetylcholine, excitatory amino acids, and substance P. *Exp. Brain Res.*, 85: 659-673.

Sholomenko, G.N., Funk, G.D. and Steeves, J.D. (1991c) Avian locomotion activated by brainstem infusion of neurotransmitter agonists and antagonists. II. Gamma-aminobutyric acid. *Exp. Brain Res.*, 85: 674–681.

Sommer, I. and Schachner, M. (1981) Monoclonal antibodies (O1 and O4) to oligodendrocyte cell surfaces: an immunocytological study in the central nervous system. *Dev. Biol.*, 83: 311-327.

Steeves, J.D. and Jordan, L.M. (1984) Autoradiographic demonstration of the projections from the mesencephalic locomotor region. *Brain Res.*, 307: 263-276.

Steeves, J.D., Sholomenko, G.N. and Webster, D.M.S. (1987) Stimulation of the pontomedullary reticular formation initiates locomotion in decerebrate birds. *Brain Res.*, 401: 205–212.

Steeves, J.D., Hasan, S.J., Keirstead, H.S., Muir, G.D., Ethell, D.W., Pataky, D.M. McBride, C.B., Rott, M.E. and Wisniewska, A.B. (1993) The embryonic chicken as a model for central nervous system injury and repair. *Neuroprotocols*, 3: 35–43.

Tello, F. (1911) La influencia del neurotropismo en la regeneracion de los centros nerviosos. *Trab. Lab. Invest. Biol.*, book 9: 124–159.

Tetzlaff, W., Alexander, S., Miller, F. and Bisby, M. (1991) Response of facial and rubrospinal neurons to axotomy: changes in mRNA expression for cytoskeletal proteins and GAP-43. *J. Neurosci.*, 11: 2528–2544.

Treherne, J.M., Woodward, S.K.A., Varga, Z.M., Ritchie, J.M. and Nicholls, J.G. (1992) Restoration of conduction and growth of axons through injured spinal cord of neonatal opossum in culture. *Proc. Natl. Acad. Sci. USA*, 89: 431–434.

Valenzuela, J.I., Hasan, S.J. and Steeves, J.D. (1990) Stimulation of the brainstem reticular formation evokes locomotor activity in embryonic chicken, in ovo. *Dev. Brain Res.*, 56: 13–18.

Webster, D.M.S. and Steeves, J.D. (1988) Origins of brainstem-spinal projections in the duck and goose. *J. Comp. Neurol.*, 273: 573–583.

Webster, D.M.S. and Steeves, J.D. (1991) Funicular organization of avian brainstem-spinal projections. *J. Comp. Neurol.*, 312: 467–476.

Webster, D.M.S., Rogers, L.J., Pettigrew, J.D. and Steeves, J.D. (1990) Origins of descending spinal pathways in prehensile birds: do parrots have a homologue to the corticospinal tract of mammals? *Brain Behav. Evol.*, 36: 216–226.

F.J. Seil (Ed.)
Progress in Brain Research, Vol 103

CHAPTER 21

Repair of connections in injured neonatal and embryonic spinal cord in vitro

J.G. Nicholls[1], H. Vischer[1], Z. Varga[1], S. Erulkar[1] and N.R. Saunders[2]

[1]*Department of Pharmacology, Biocenter, University of Basel, Klingelbergstrasse 70, CH-4056 Basel, Switzerland and*
[2]*Department of Physiology, University of Tasmania, Hobart, Tas. 7001, Australia*

Introduction

Several lines of evidence suggest that the spinal cord of a neonatal mammal could have greater potential for regeneration than that of an adult. Thus, cellular and molecular mechanisms responsible for growth are still operating; moreover, at early stages of development, oligodendrocytes with their growth inhibiting molecules have not yet differentiated (Aguayo, et al., 1991; Cenci et al., 1993; Schwab et al., 1993). Considerations such as these provided the starting point for our studies on regeneration in the central nervous system (CNS) of the newly born opossum and embryonic rat, which are reviewed here.

Why the South American opossum (*Monodelphis domestica*)? This animal (Fig. 1A) seems to offer real advantages for measuring the outgrowth of fibers across a lesion and for testing whether newly grown fibers can establish synaptic connections. One attractive feature was that we already had background information obtained through collaboration with our colleague, Kjeld Møllgard (in Copenhagen), on the structure of these little creatures which showed how extremely immature they are at birth (Fig. 1B; equivalent to an embryonic day 14 rat in many respects; Saunders et al., 1989). Initial studies of the blood–brain barrier at different stages of development indicated that in spite of their very small size and apparent fragility, they in fact were rather tough experimental preparations. Unlike other marsupials such as kangaroos (which are too large to handle in a usual laboratory setting) and North American opossums (which are violent and ferocious), we showed that *Monodelphis* could be bred in the laboratory for neurobiological studies. Colonies were established in Southampton, Basel and Hobart, allowing one to obtain a regular supply of pups — up to 12 on a mother — that can be compared at different stages of development. Early experiments in Basel showed that the CNS can be removed in its entirety (Fig. 2) and maintained in culture for several days. Thereafter, once the conditions for survival had been established, it became possible to study the events that occur after a lesion has been made. Comparable experiments were also made in Southampton, Basel and Hobart with the CNS isolated from 15-day (E15) rat embryos. In such isolated preparations it became possible to screen for repair by recording electrically from the spinal cord, to test for synapse formation and to observe growth of fibers through and beyond a lesion by microscopy in living preparations (Nicholls et al., 1990; Stewart et al., 1991; Saunders et al., 1992; Treherne et al., 1992; Woodward et al., 1993; Møllgard et al., 1994).

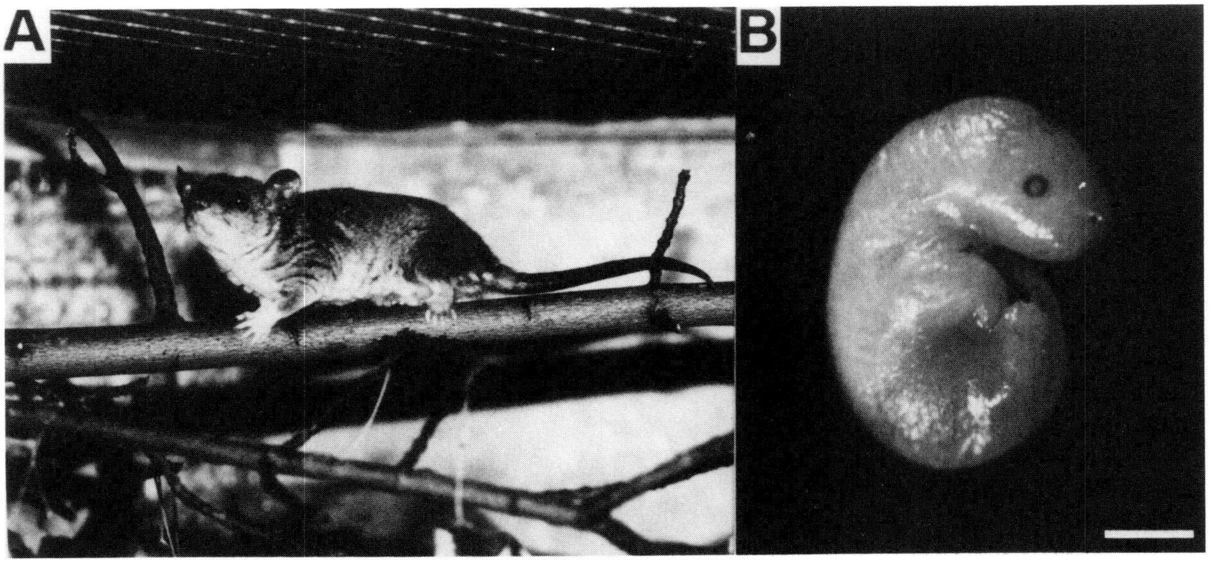

Fig. 1. (A) An adult opossum from our colony, crown to rump length 15 cm. (B) A 2-day-old opossum (bar = 2 mm). An animal such as this can breathe and suck but do little else.

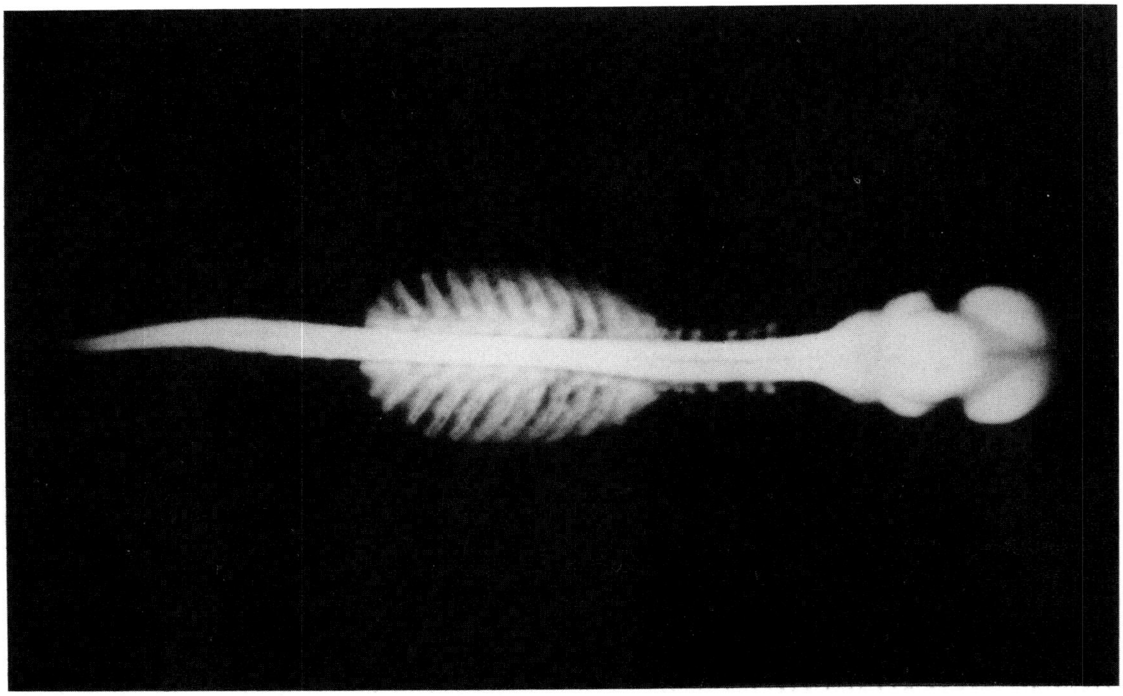

Fig. 2. Central nervous system dissected out of a 4-day-old opossum. In this preparation dorsal root ganglia have been dissected, together with ribs and intercostal muscles. Fictive respiration continues in the dish.

In this brief review we describe the preparation, its survival in culture and the time course of repair after a lesion. We then consider what mechanisms might favor the extensive repair occurring in early life that becomes inhibited at later stages of development.

The CNS of newborn opossum and 15-day rat embryo in culture

The preparations are dissected after anesthetizing the pups with metofane. Spinal cord and brain are removed within a few minutes in oxygenated Krebs's fluid or Eagle's basal medium (BME) equilibrated with 5% CO_2/95% 0_2. BME is the culture medium that we have found to be adequate, if not optimal, for long-term survival. Although the spinal roots are all cut, dorsal root ganglia can be dissected out still attached to the CNS (this dissection is slightly more difficult). The survival in culture is remarkable and, to us, unexpected. After keeping the CNS in 15 ml of BME for several days in culture, one can still record spontaneous electrical activity in ventral roots, as well as conduction and synaptic transmission through the spinal cord. Cells that continue to divide and migrate become labeled by bromodeoxyuridine; differentiation of radial glial cells and neurons continues with surprisingly little cell death. These observations make it possible for an analysis to be made of repair after lesions.

A question that arises is whether culture of an entire nervous system could result in the maintenance of sensations, particularly pain. This can be ruled out by the following observations. First, the newborn opossum pup and the rat embryo cannot walk or even right themselves. Their eyes, cortex, cerebellum, forelimbs and hindlimbs are all rudimentary. The cortex consists of a thin plate of blast cells surrounding the ventricles with no developed neurons and lacking incoming or outgoing connections; the midbrain is still at an early stage of formation. Thus, the key structures that perform higher as well as many lower functions are so poorly developed that the possibility of 'pain' is excluded. In effect, the preparation that we use is 'decerebrate,' as though the appropriate lesion had been made. In addition, preparations are cultured at room temperature.

Experimental procedures and results

Lesions of spinal cord

The spinal cord at the level C5–C7 is still immature, with an abundance of dividing cells migrating from the central canal. We make lesions that extend beyond the midline with fine forceps; alternatively, the cord is transected by compressing with a fine nylon thread. In our experience, it is advantageous to leave the pia mater intact. The following lines of evidence indicate that all fibers are indeed broken by our procedures. (1) If a crush is made acutely and the preparation fixed immediately, light and electron microscopy show no fibers at the crush site, which contains only vesicles and debris. After fixation, fibers labeled with the carbocyanine dye, DiI, are all seen to be broken. (2) Conduction of impulses through the crush becomes abolished immediately, to return only after a delay of 2–4 days.

Re-establishment of conduction and of connections after injury

To test for conduction, brief electrical stimuli are applied to one side of the lesion while recordings are made on the other. In normal unoperated preparations, even after 5–10 days in culture, signals of up to 500 μV are observed to be transmitted, in part by fibers conducting directly and in part by way of synaptic relays. Immediately after crushing, transmission is abolished. Two to four days later, small volleys of the order of 20 μV become apparent. These are not blocked by magnesium (20 mM) applied to the bath. At 5 days after the lesion, the volley may reach 200 μV in amplitude. Experiments made with raised magnesium reveal that although the initial small peak is unaffected, later components become blocked. These results suggest that fibers growing through

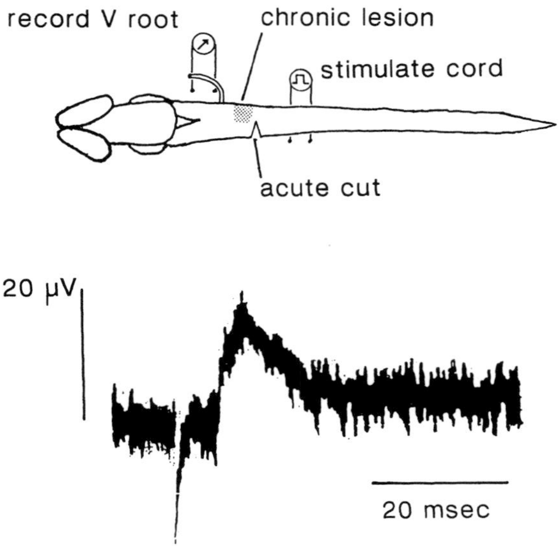

Fig. 3. Evidence for repair and formation of synaptic connections by fibers growing through a chronic lesion. The diagram above illustrates the chronic lesion made 5 days earlier and the acute cut made at the time of the experiment. Both lesions extended beyond the midline. Stimulation of the spinal cord caudal to the lesion gave rise to a volley in the ventral root above the lesion (lower trace).

the crush form connections, a conclusion that is reinforced by our recent experiments. Stimuli applied to the cord below a chronic crush give rise to a discharge in ventral roots above the crush (Fig. 3).

Growth of nerve fibers through lesions

Fibers labeled with DiI can be observed directly in living and in fixed whole-mount preparations (Fig. 4). Three days after a crush has been made, fibers are observed to enter and traverse it. By 5 days fibers can grow for distances of up to 2 mm beyond the crush, in both directions (rostrally or caudally). The features of this outgrowth are that it is (1) abundant, with numerous fibers not just a few; (2) rapid, occurring within 3–5 days and (3) reliable, as about 40% of injured preparations aged 3–7 days show such outgrowth in vitro.

Open questions and work in progress

Of particular interest to us is whether the fibers that grow across a crush are 'regenerating' or entering that region for the first time. One approach is to label identified fibers from dorsal root ganglia with DiI to follow their progress with videomicroscopy, a procedure fraught with technical difficulties. It is also apparent that in most studies by other workers on 'regeneration', it is not known whether the fibers that grow are ones that have been severed or whether they represent new sprouts or collateral sprouting. A second major goal is to determine at what age repair ceases to occur and to analyse the factors responsible. Is it that oligodendrocytes produce inhibitory molecules, that growth factors disappear, or combinations of both? One practical step is to examine the fine structure of the crush site and to label growth promoting and growth inhibitory molecules, as well as assessing the cellular components that invade the lesion. What is clear is that growth across a crush ceases to occur (between 11 and 14 days in the neonatal opossum and probably just before birth in the fetal rat) at the very time that oligodendrocytes and myelin begin to become evident and abundant (Fig. 5). As a long-term goal, we can hope to test whether specific connections are established in neonatal and fetal mammalian central nervous systems after injury and whether functions can be restored.

Summary

A remarkable preparation for studying development and repair is the CNS of the newborn opossum which, removed in its entirety, survives in culture for more than 1 week. In suitable medium, cells continue to divide, mature and reflex activity is maintained. Moreover, nerve fibers grow rapidly, reliably and extensively across lesions made in the spinal cord. Restoration of conduction has been demonstrated by recording electrically; labeled fibres have been observed directly by light and electron microscopy as they

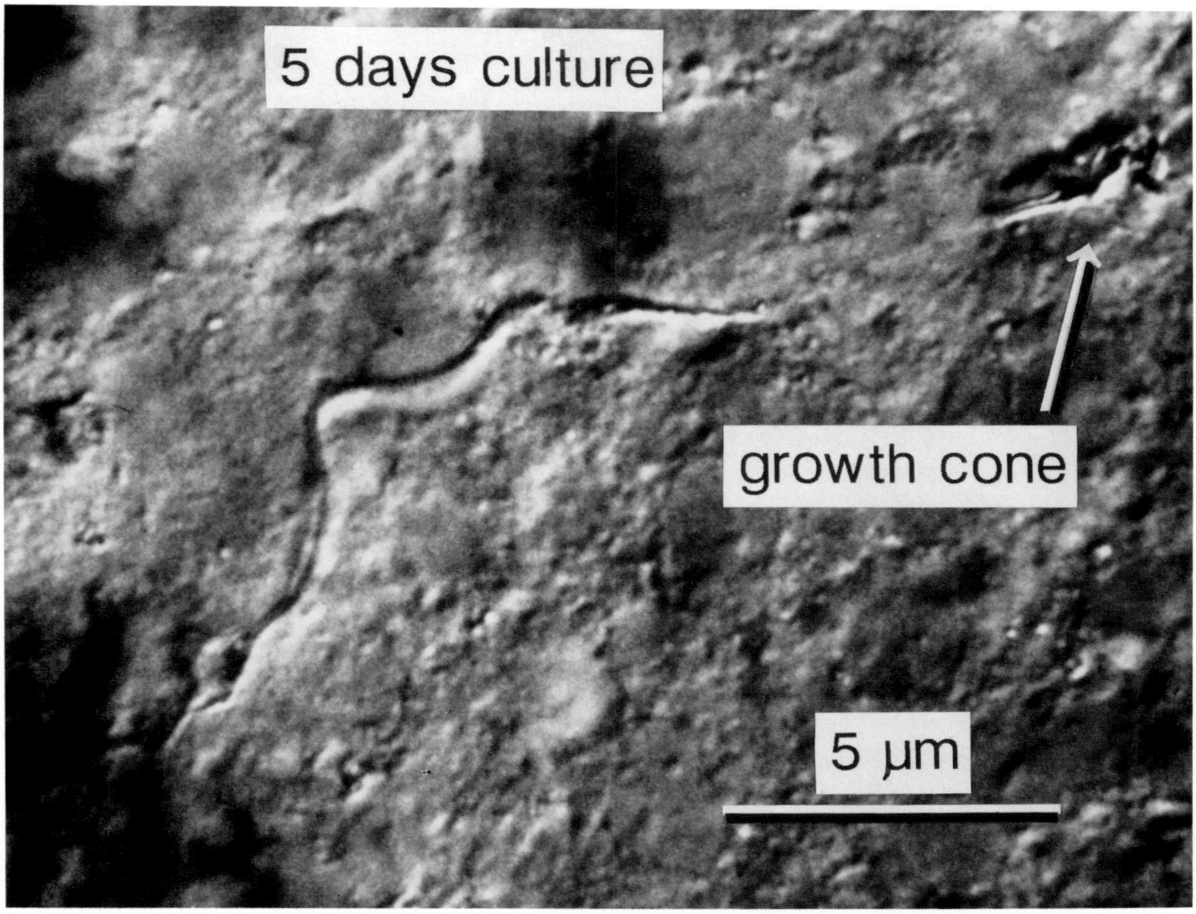

Fig. 4. Fiber growing through the site of a lesion with a growth cone. Fibers were stained with a carbocyanine dye, DiI, applied as fine crystals on the surface of a microelectrode. The fibers are first observed in whole-mounts of living preparations under fluorescent illumination. By photoconversion in the presence of diaminobenzidine, an electron dense product resembling the horseradish peroxidase reaction accumulates. This enables one to observe the same fiber and growth cone by electron microscopy.

traverse the lesion. Similar experiments have also been made in embryonic (E15) rat CNS in culture. Open questions concern the identity of the fibers that traverse the lesion and the specificity of connections that they make with targets. We are now also analysing mechanisms that favor repair in younger opossums and that prevent it in their older siblings. Of particular interest are oligodendrocytes and myelin that start to appear at about 8–9 days after birth.

Acknowledgements

We wish to thank our colleagues who collaborated on work presented in earlier papers and particularly Dr W.B. Adams, who has played a key role at every stage. We thank the Swiss Nationalfond (Grant No. 31-36262.92) and the International Research Program for Paraplegia and the Ramaciotti Foundations for their support.

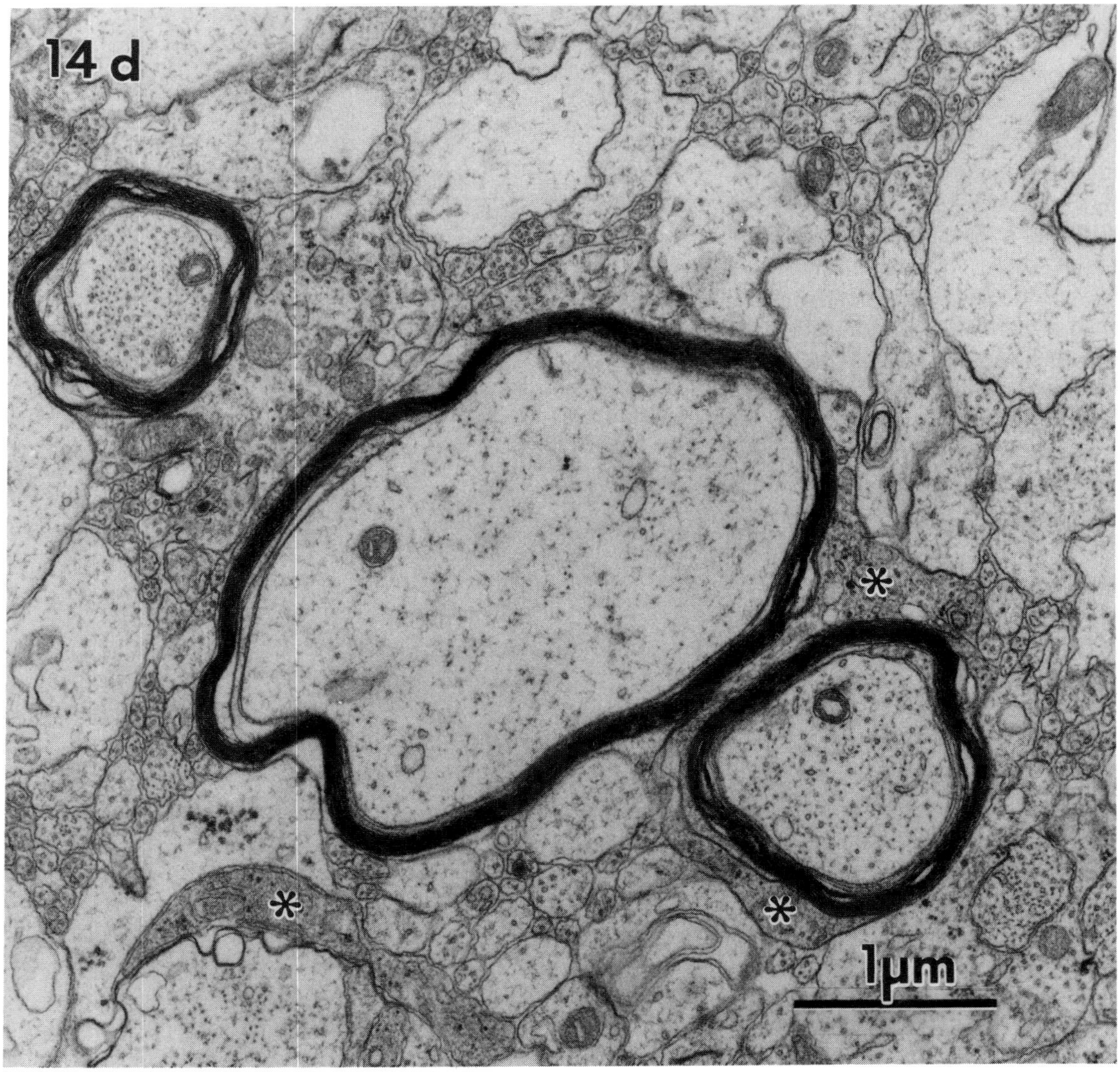

Fig. 5. Electron micrograph of spinal cord in a 14 day old opossum. Myelin and oligodendrocytes (*) are clearly visible. At 7 days of age no oligodendrocytes or myelin are observed; they start to accumulate between 8 and 14 days. This corresponds to the time at which repair ceases to be apparent.

References

Aguayo, A.J., Rasminsky, M., Bray, G.M., Carbonetto, S., McKerracher, L., Villegas-Pérez, M.P., Vidal-Sanz, M. and Carter, D.A. (1991) Degenerative and regenerative responses of injured neurones in the central nervous system of adult animals. *Phil. Trans. R. Soc. Lond. B*, 331: 337–343.

Cenci, M.A., Nilsson, O.G., Kalen, P. and Bjørklund, A. (1993) Characterization of in vivo noradrenaline release from superior cervical ganglia or fetal locus coeruleus transplanted to the subcortically deafferented hippocampus in the rat. *Exp. Neurol.*, 122: 73–87.

Møllgard, K., Balslev, Y., Janas, M.S., Treherne, J.M., Saunders, N.R. and Nicholls, J.G. (1994) Development of spinal cord in the isolated CNS of a neonatal mammal, the opossum *Monodelphis domestica* maintained in long-term culture. *J. Neurocytol.* 23: 151-165.

Nicholls, J.G., Stewart, R.R., Erulkar, S.D. and Saunders, N.R. (1990) Reflexes, fictive respiration and cell division in the brain and spinal cord of the newborn opossum, *Monodelphis domestica*. *J. Exp. Biol.*, 152: 1–15.

Saunders, N.R., Adam, E., Reader, M. and Møllgard, K. (1989) *Monodelphis domestica* (grey, short-tailed opossum): an accessible model for studies of early neocortical development. *Anat. Embryol.*, 173: 81–94.

Saunders, N.R., Balkwill, P., Knott, G., Habgood, M.D., Møllgard, K., Treherne, J.M. and Nicholls, J.G. (1992) Growth of axons through a lesion in the intact CNS of fetal rat maintained in long-term culture. *Proc. R. Soc. Lond. B*, 150: 171–180.

Schwab, M.E., Kapfhammer, J.P. and Bandtlow, C.E. (1993) Inhibitors of neurite growth. *Annu. Rev. Neurosci.*, 16: 565–595.

Stewart, R.R., Zou, D.-J., Treherne, J.M., Møllgard, K., Saunders, N.R. and Nicholls, J.G. (1991) The intact central nervous system of the newborn opossum in long-term culture: fine structure and GABA-mediated inhibition of electrical activity *J. Exp. Biol.*, 161: 25–41.

Treherne, J.M., Woodward, S.K.A, Varga, Z.M., Ritchie, J.M. and Nicholls, J.G. (1992) Restoration of conduction and growth of axons through injured spinal cord of neonatal opossum in culture. *Proc. Natl. Acad. Sci. USA*, 89: 431–434.

Woodward, S.K.A., Treherne, J.M., Knott, G.W., Fernandez, J., Varga, Z.M. and Nicholls, J.G. (1993) Development of connections by axons growing through injured spinal cord of neonatal opossum in culture. *J. Exp. Biol.*, 176: 77–88.

Note added in proof

Important new findings on regeneration and recovery of function in immature rats is provided in Iwashita, Y., Kawaguchi, S. and Murata, M. (1994) Restoration of function by replacement of spinal cord segments in the rat. *Nature* 367, 167–170.

F.J. Seil (Ed.)
Progress in Brain Research, Vol 103

CHAPTER 22

Response of rubrospinal and corticospinal neurons to injury and neurotrophins

W. Tetzlaff, N.R. Kobayashi, K.M.G. Giehl, B.J. Tsui, S.L. Cassar and A.M. Bedard

Department of Physiology and Neuroscience Research Institute, University of Ottawa, Ottawa, Ontario, Canada

Introduction

Evidence is accumulating that the failure of adult mammalian central nervous system (CNS) neurons to regenerate a new axon after injury is due to a combination of factors. These include (1) the microenvironment of the CNS which produces (a) inhibitors to growth cones (for review see Luo et al., 1993; Schwab et al. 1993) and (b) glial scars (for review see Reier et al., 1989); (2) the neuronal death or severe atrophy occurring in many axotomized CNS systems (for review see Barron, 1983, 1989; Villegas-Perez et al., 1988, 1993; Bray et al., 1991), and (3) the failure of CNS neurons to express growth- or regeneration-associated genes, like GAP-43 (Skene 1981, 1989, 1992; Doster et al., 1991; Tetzlaff et al., 1991).

In this chapter we will focus on problems 2 and 3 in rubrospinal and corticospinal neurons, and show that both regeneration-associated gene expression and neuronal atrophy or death are dependent on the distance between the injury and the cell body. First, we test the hypothesis that peripheral nervous system (PNS) neurons and CNS neurons respond differently to axotomy by comparing facial versus rubrospinal motoneurons after axotomy. We show that rubrospinal neurons respond to axotomy with regeneration-associated gene expression after cervical lesions but not after thoracic lesions. This correlates with their regeneration into cervical but not thoracic transplants of peripheral nerve. Second, we demonstrate that the severe atrophy which occurs 2 weeks after injury at the cervical level of the spinal cord can be prevented in full by brain-derived neurotrophic factor (BDNF). In addition, BDNF application stimulates the expression of regeneration-associated genes, like GAP-43. Third, to further analyze the near/far lesion effect, we report that in corticospinal neurons the critical distance to induce GAP-43 is as short as 200 μm; lesions more than 300 μm from the cell body fail to induce GAP-43 expression. These close injuries are followed by death of many of the corticospinal neurons, which can be prevented by neurotrophin-3 (NT-3) application. Together, these results show that CNS neurons can express the propensity to regenerate after injury 'close' to their cell body, and that this can be supported by neurotrophic factors.

Regeneration-associated gene expression in peripheral and central neurons

Neurons projecting into the peripheral nervous system respond to axotomy with a consistent change in cytoskeletal gene expression. These changes have previously been reviewed (Bisby and Tetzlaff, 1992) and only a brief overview is presented here. In earlier studies we have demonstrated that the motoneurons of the facial nucleus of the rat respond with a robust increase in tubulin and actin synthesis and a decrease in neurofilament synthesis after axotomy at the stylomastoid foramen (Tetzlaff et al., 1988). Using in situ hybridization, we have confirmed that these changes were accompanied by neuronal increases in actin and tubulin mRNA expression (Tetzlaff et al., 1991). The tubulin increase after axotomy is partly due to the reexpression of the developmentally regulated Tα1-tubulin isotype (Miller et al., 1989). Similarly, an increased expression of the developmentally regulated class IIβ tubulin has been demonstrated by Hoffman and Cleveland (1988). However, axotomy does not induce a precise reiteration of the developmental pattern of gene expression, as demonstrated by the changes in the microtubule associated protein, tau, after axotomy, which do not show the low molecular weight developmental isotypes (Oblinger et al., 1991).

Another group of cytoskeletal proteins, the intermediate filaments, are differentially regulated after axotomy. All three neurofilament proteins and their mRNAs show a consistent downregulation in facial motoneurons (Tetzlaff et al., 1988, 1991) and other peripheral neurons (Wong and Oblinger, 1987; Hoffman and Cleveland, 1988; Muma et al., 1990, Verge et al., 1990a), while the type III intermediate filament, peripherin, is upregulated after injury (Oblinger et al., 1990). Again, the low expression of neurofilament during regeneration is reminiscent of (Hoffman and Cleveland, 1988) but not identical to early developmental stages (Bates and Meyer, 1993). Similarly, the peripherin response is different from the developmental situation (Oblinger et al., 1990).

In addition to these cytoskeletal protein changes, a marked upregulation of the protein, GAP-43, was observed initially in the fast axonal transport component of axotomized PNS but not CNS neurons (Skene and Willard, 1981; Reh et al., 1987; for review see Skene, 1989, 1992). GAP-43 mRNA is highly expressed during development and is downregulated to very low levels of expression in most but not all neuronal systems (Jacobson et al., 1986; Oestreicher and Gispen, 1986; for review see Kruger et al., 1993). In axotomized peripheral neurons, GAP-43 mRNA increases by more than one order of magnitude; thus, the relative change is considerably larger than for cytoskeletal proteins, which change about 3–5-fold (Verge et al., 1990b; Tetzlaff et al., 1991). The high expression during development and regeneration, and the preferred location in axonal growth cones, led to the hypothesis that GAP-43 is involved in axonal growth cone function (for review see Skene, 1989). More recent data using antisense oligonucleotides (Jap Tjoen San et al., 1992; Aigner and Caroni, 1993) and inhibition with antibodies (Shea et al., 1991) clearly support this notion. In cases of interference with GAP-43 expression or its function, process outgrowth was inhibited in vitro.

In this chapter we refer to the changes in actin, tubulin (Tα1-tubulin) and GAP-43 expression as 'regeneration-associated gene (RAG) expression'. We believe that the expression of these genes is a necessary but not sufficient condition for axonal regeneration in the PNS and CNS. GAP-43 represents the most prominent protein among those that have been associated with axonal growth during development, including SCG-10 (Stein et al., 1988), 33K (Kalil and Perdew, 1988) and pp60c-src (Maness et al., 1988).

The importance of the cell body in axonal regeneration has been emphasized in many studies in vitro and in vivo (Barron, 1989; Skene, 1992). Compelling evidence was provided by Richardson and coworkers (Richardson and Issa, 1984; Richardson and Verge, 1986), who demonstrated that the regeneration of the dorsal column axons into peripheral nerve transplants was seen only when the peripheral axon of the dorsal root ganglion cell was also crushed, inducing a cell body reaction. More recent work demonstrated that injuries to the central dorsal root ganglion (DRG) axon failed to induce GAP-43 expression, unlike axotomy to the distal process (Schreyer and Skene, 1991, 1993). Even more recently, it has been shown that the growth of dorsal column axons into fetal transplants is markedly enhanced by the combination of trophic factors and a peripheral nerve crush (Oudega et al., 1993).

In a previous study (Tetzlaff et al., 1991), we demonstrated that rubrospinal neurons increased their expression of mRNAs coding for actin, total tubulin, Tα1-tubulin and GAP-43 7 days after injury at the cervical spinal cord C3 level. This clearly demonstrated that these spinal cord projection neurons can (initially) respond to injury in a way similar to motoneurons, which regenerate readily. A decrease in neurofilament-M mRNA expression was also observed, consistent with the injury response of motoneurons. The increase in total tubulin and actin mRNA expression, however, lasted only for one week in the rubrospinal neurons and by 14 days after axotomy, actin and total tubulin mRNA levels dropped to about 50% of control. This precipitous drop is not seen in axotomized peripheral neurons, and it parallels the severe rubrospinal neuron atrophy which occurs at the same time (Egan et al., 1977; Barron et al., 1989). The data are expressed as in situ hybridization signals per cell in order to take this shrinkage into account (for details see Tetzlaff et al., 1991). During the second and following weeks after cervical injury, GAP-43 and Tα1-tubulin were still found at elevated levels, which gradually declined as fewer and fewer rubrospinal neurons expressed these genes. However, elevated expression of the latter two genes was observed in some cells as late as 7 weeks after injury. Thus, rubrospinal neurons receive the appropriate 'axotomy signals', but after the first week a second process intervenes which might be caused by a lack of trophic support. This ability of CNS neurons to express RAGs has also been shown for tubulin in the retina (McKerracher et al., 1993) and for GAP-43 in the retina (Doster et al., 1991) and in the spinal cord (Curtis et al., 1993).

Rubrospinal neurons regenerate into cervical but not thoracic nerve transplants

Our finding of RAG expression in axotomized rubrospinal neurons correlated with the earlier finding by Richardson et al. (1984) that rubrospinal neurons are capable of regeneration into peripheral nerve transplants after cervical injury. Peripheral nerve transplants are probably providing these neurons with both a permissive growth environment and trophic support, like nerve growth factor (NGF) and BDNF (Heumann et al., 1987; Meyer et al., 1992). We will show later that rubrospinal neurons are responsive to BDNF. Richardson et al. (1984) did not find regeneration into peripheral nerve transplanted into thoracic injuries. Since this study was performed with horseradish peroxidase (HRP) as a retrograde tracer, this negative finding is difficult to interpret. The greater distance between the thoracic lesion and the rubrospinal cells might have delayed the retrograde arrival of the tracer, which was applied only 2 days prior to killing the animals. Therefore we decided to repeat these experiments using FluoroGold as a retrograde tracer, because this tracer is reliably transported and persists several months, permitting longer survival times (McBride et al., 1989). The rubrospinal tract was injured unilaterally either at cervical level C3 or low thoracic level T10 and a 3–4 cm long piece of the peroneal nerve of the same rat was implanted into the injury site of the cord. Two to 4 months later the distal free end of the peroneal nerve was exposed, cut at about 5 mm from the end and sutured into a polyethylene tube filled with FluoroGold FG (5%). Fourteen days later the animals were killed, and labeled rubrospinal neurons were counted in serial sections through the red nucleus. Four out of five animals with cervical axotomy/peroneal nerve transplant demonstrated between 25 and 73 positive profiles in the red nucleus. This number of regenerating cells represents less than 2% of the rubrospinal neurons (approximately 4,500). The reason for this may be related to glial scar formation, the imperfect positioning of the transplant and other technical problems, such as vascularization of the transplant. Another reason may be neuronal atrophy followed by abortion of sprouting, since the production of BDNF in the Schwann cells of the transplant does not begin before the second week (Meyer et al., 1992). We are currently testing this possibility by using predegenerated nerve transplants.

In contrast to the successful regeneration of some rubrospinal neurons into cervical transplants, none of the thoracic transplantation experiments ($n = 4$) resulted in any positive label in the rubrospinal neurons. Thus, these experiments confirmed the finding of Richardson et al. (1984) that rubrospinal neurons regenerate into cervical but not into thoracic transplants. This negative finding is unlikely to be explained by the smaller number of rubrospinal cells which actually project to the lumbar spinal cord (about 40 to 50% of those present at the cervical level). In both experiments, the rubrospinal neurons had been axotomized at the site of implantation. There is no reason to believe that the scar around the implantation site is different at the thoracic versus cervical spinal cord. Therefore, the failure to regenerate is most likely related to the different distances of the injury from the nerve cell body. Since there is good evidence for the involvement of the cell body in regeneration, we asked if thoracic lesions failed to induce RAGs.

RAG expression is only seen after 'close' but not after 'distant' injuries of rubrospinal neurons

We compared the response of rubrospinal neurons to thoracic versus cervical axotomy (Tetzlaff et al., 1990). At the time of injury, the retrograde tracers FluoroGold or Fast Blue were applied to the injury site to positively identify the cells projecting to and beyond the level of the lesion. In three animals a second tracer injection was placed caudal to the injury site to verify that the axons had been completely severed. This technique was combined with in situ hybridization for RAG expression. Animals were killed at 3, 7, 14, 21 and 28 days post injury. Sections through the red nucleus from a cervically injured animal were mounted next to sections from a thoracically injured animal from the same time point. Thus, sections from cervical and thoracic injury were treated identically with respect to hybridization conditions, autoradiography and quantification. The analysis was restriced to neurons of the lateral portion of the red nucleus which project into the lumbar spinal cord, thus comparing the same population of cells.

The comparison of mRNA expression for GAP-43 (Fig. 1, bottom) clearly reveals increased levels after cervical injury ($P < 0.01$, *t*-test). In contrast, the mean values after thoracic injury were only slightly elevated but not significantly different from uninjured contralateral control slides or from normal unoperated rubrospinal neurons. This minor elevation was due to a few responding neurons. Similar to GAP-43, the expression of Tα1-tubulin mRNA is increased several-fold after cervical injury ($P > 0.01$, *t*-test) but only slightly elevated after thoracic injury (Fig. 1, middle). Total tubulin mRNA does not respond at all to injury at the thoracic level (Fig. 1, top). As mentioned above, the cervical injury induces an increase in total tubulin expression that drops in the second week to subnormal levels (Fig. 1, top). A typical example of GAP-43 mRNA expression 14 days after distal versus proximal injury is given in Fig. 2. The lumbar portion of the red nucleus is shown filled with FluoroGold (Fig. 2, upper panels). Note that most but not all rubrospinal neurons show an increased in situ hybridization signal for GAP-43 after cervical injury (Fig. 2, lower left) but little more than background signal after thoracic injury (Fig. 2, lower right).

Another parameter tested was the immediate early gene, *c-jun*. Jun can dimerize with itself or other immediate early gene products like Fos to form the so-called AP-1 transcription factor (for review see Curran and Franza, 1988; Lamb and McKnight, 1991; Herdegen and Zimmermann, this volume). Jun immunoreactivity is consistently elevated in axotomized peripheral neurons and does not return to normal until the axons reach their targets again (Jenkins and Hunt, 1991; Leah et al., 1991; Herdegen et al., 1992; Rutherford et al., 1992; Haas et al., 1993). The downstream target genes for this AP-1 complex formed after axotomy are unknown; however, a close temporo-spatial relationship exists between Jun and galanin expression (Herdegen et al., 1993) and Jun and GAP-43 expression (W. Tetzlaff, unpublished observation). Similar to GAP-43, the expression of Jun in rubrospinal neurons was elevated after cervical but not after thoracic axotomy (Jenkins et al., 1993).

We have no definite explanation for this 'near/far' difference in response since the molecular mechanism for the regulation of GAP-43 and Tα1-tubulin is not understood (for review see Bisby and Tetzlaff, 1992; Skene, 1992). In fact, two different mechanisms seem to control these two parameters. In the PNS, the increase of GAP-43 mRNA and immunoreactivity are independent of the length of the proximal stump, i.e., the lesion to cell body distance (Tsui et al., 1991; Schreyer and Skene, 1993). In contrast, Tα1-tubulin expression is distance-dependent in spinal motoneurons (Tsui et al., 1991) and superior cervical ganglion cells (Mathew and Miller, 1993). Thus, we will consider the possible axotomy signals for GAP-43 and tubulin independently.

Blockade of axonal transport by vinblastine or colchicine application to the sciatic nerve induced GAP-43 mRNA expression in the DRG (Basi and Skene, 1988; Woolf et al., 1990; Smith and Skene, 1993). These data imply a lack of a factor ('negative signal') in the derepression of GAP-43, rather than a positive inducing signal coming from the injury site or proximal stump. This is further supported by the observation that colchicine, when applied proximal to a nerve cut, fails to prevent a GAP-43 increase (Smith and Skene, 1993); in other words, no positive signal seems to be directly involved. In the case of GAP-43, this negative or repressing factor is most likely derived from the terminal or target cells rather than the sheath cells of the nerve (Schwann cells/fibroblasts) since no 'near/far' distance effect is seen in the sciatic nerve (Tsui et al., 1991; Schreyer and Skene, 1993). NGF is not a likely candidate since it does not reverse the GAP-43 increase after axotomy, despite the fact that there is a good correlation between those DRG neurons which express high affinity NGF receptors and a noticeable baseline level of GAP-43 (Verge et al., 1990b). Insulin-like growth factor 1 appears to prevent the downregulation of GAP-43 during development (Caroni and Becker, 1992), but its role after axotomy is unclear.

The situation appears to be different for Tα1-tubulin. As mentioned above, Tα1-tubulin expression is distance-dependent in sciatic nerve and in the spinal cord. The possibility can therefore not be ruled out that the small Tα1 response in rubrospinal neurons after low thoracic injury is an 'appropriate' response. This is unlikely, since preliminary data suggest that this response is due to a modest increase in a few rubrospinal cells only, rather than a shift of the entire lumbar cell population toward a slightly higher level of expression.

Blockade of axonal transport with a cold block induces Tα1-tubulin expression in facial motoneurons (Wu et al., 1993). This observation is in agreement with the hypothesis that some 'negative' signals are involved in the regulation rather than the entry of a lesion site factor into the nerve (Wu et al., 1993). The 'near/far' difference argues against a factor that is purely target-derived. Since the response increases in proportion to the amount of axon (sheath) removed, the repressing factors most likely originate along the length of the nerve.

It should be added at this point that it is conceivable that Tα1-tubulin or GAP-43 are regulated by intraaxonal signal molecules. These might travel down the axon, become modified along their way or in the terminal, and then

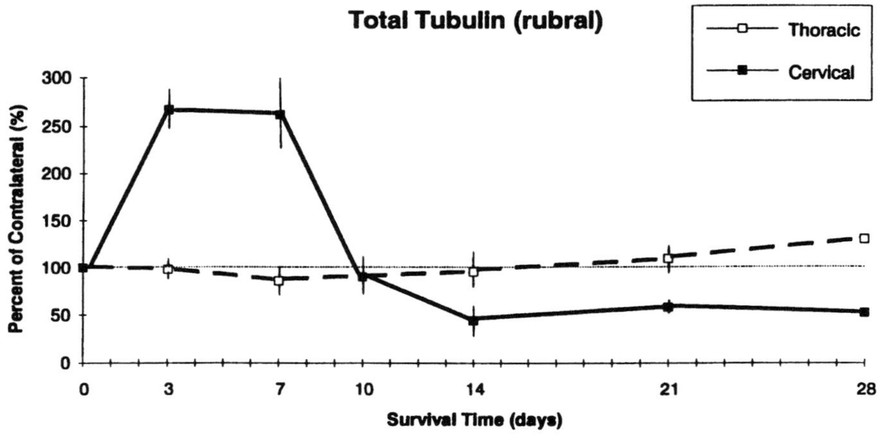
Total Tubulin (rubral)
Thoracic
Cervical
Percent of Contralateral (%)
300
250
200
150
100
50
0
0
3
7
10
14
21
28
Survival Time (days)

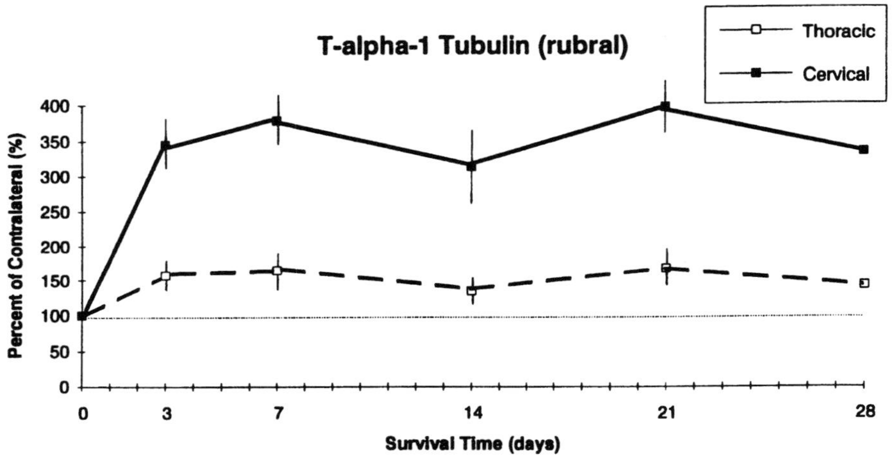
T-alpha-1 Tubulin (rubral)
Thoracic
Cervical
Percent of Contralateral (%)
400
350
300
250
200
150
100
50
0
0
3
7
14
21
28
Survival Time (days)

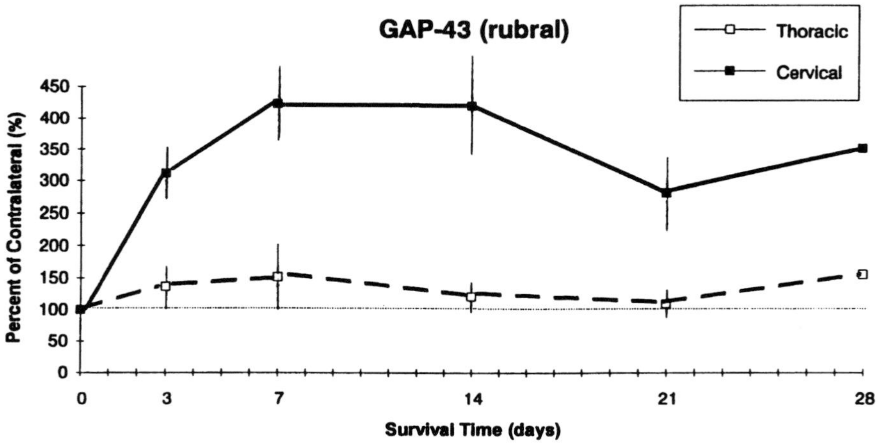
GAP-43 (rubral)
Thoracic
Cervical
Percent of Contralateral (%)
450
400
350
300
250
200
150
100
50
0
0
3
7
14
21
28
Survival Time (days)

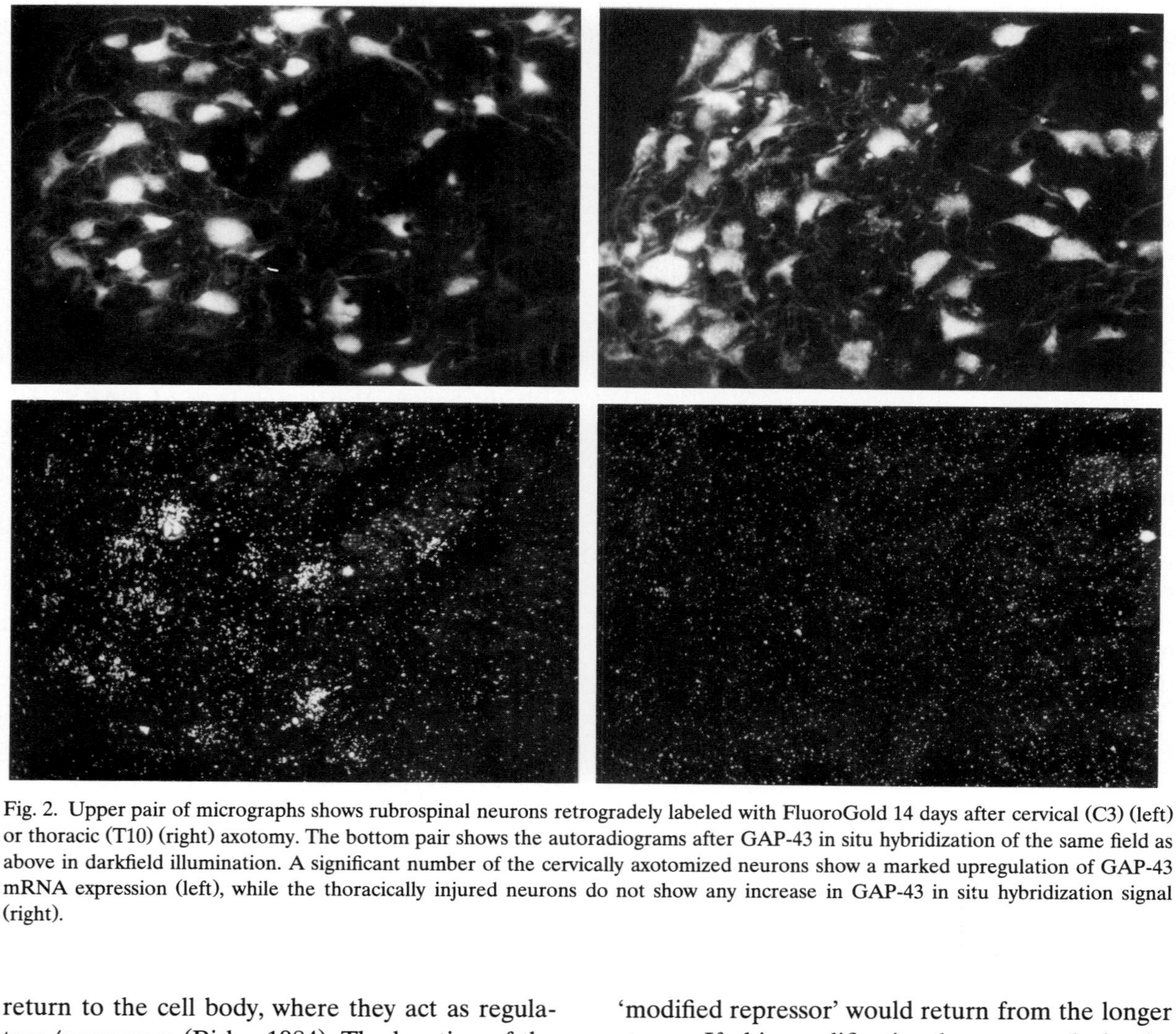

Fig. 2. Upper pair of micrographs shows rubrospinal neurons retrogradely labeled with FluoroGold 14 days after cervical (C3) (left) or thoracic (T10) (right) axotomy. The bottom pair shows the autoradiograms after GAP-43 in situ hybridization of the same field as above in darkfield illumination. A significant number of the cervically axotomized neurons show a marked upregulation of GAP-43 mRNA expression (left), while the thoracically injured neurons do not show any increase in GAP-43 in situ hybridization signal (right).

return to the cell body, where they act as regulators/repressors (Bisby, 1984). The location of the modification would explain the far versus near response. If it happens along the nerve, more 'modified repressor' would return from the longer stump. If this modification happens only in the terminal, a target-dependence would be mimicked. If this modified molecule is a 'stimula-

Fig. 1. Time course of quantitative in situ hybridization for total tubulin, Tα1-tubulin and GAP-43 in rubrospinal neurons after cervical (closed symbols) versus thoracic (open symbols) axotomy. The data are normalized to the unoperated contralateral side. This control side was not different from unoperated normal. Each data point represents the mean of 3 to 6 animals (±S.E.M.) except day 28 ($n = 1$). Upper graph: note the transient increase in total tubulin mRNA during the first week after cervical lesion. This is followed by a precipitous decrease to subnormal levels during the second week. No change in total tubulin expression is seen after thoracic injury at any timepoint. Middle graph: note the sustained expression of Tα1-tubulin after cervical injury. In contrast, the increase after thoracic injury is far less pronounced. Lower graph: pronounced increase in GAP-43 expression after cervical but not after thoracic injury.

tor' generated within the axon at the site of injury or transport block, then it is conceivable that less arrives from a distant lesion than from a proximal lesion. While these latter models are very hypothetical, it is important to note that tubulin monomers have been demonstrated to be involved in posttranscriptional control on β-tubulin synthesis and mRNA expression (Gay et al., 1987, 1989; for review see MacRae and Langdon, 1989). Thus, several levels of control might act in concert. However, a large degree of this Tα1-tubulin increase is regulated at the level of transcription (W. Wu and F.D. Miller, personal communication).

The 'near/far' data in the rubrospinal system are consistent with the hypothesis that the failure to regenerate into peripheral nerve transplants is due to a failure to express RAGs. This hypothesis is further supported by the studies of Aguayo and coworkers in the optic system. Regeneration of retinal ganglion cells into peripheral nerve transplants is only seen with intraorbital transplants but not with intracranial transplants (So and Aguayo, 1985; Vidal-Sanz et al., 1987). Rat retinal ganglion cells express GAP-43 immunoreactivity only when the injury is within 3 mm of the eye (Doster et al., 1991). Axotomies at a 6 mm distance from the eye never generated antibody staining in the retina. Interestingly, Jones and Aguayo (1991) reported an increase in GAP-43 mRNA with both intraorbital as well as intracranial lesions. This finding would imply a translational block in GAP-43 synthesis after intracranial lesions. As in the rubrospinal system, the ability to regenerate into a peripheral transplant is closely paralleled by the expression of GAP- 43. However, the critical distances of an injury which induces GAP-43 are significantly different in the optic (3 mm) and rubrospinal (20 mm) systems. This critical distance is even shorter (200 μm) in corticospinal neurons (Giehl et al., unpublished observations). Corticospinal axotomies below layer VI of the cortex slightly more than 300 μm distant from the cell body fail to induce GAP-43. Similar to the results of Oblinger and coworkers (Mikucki and Oblinger, 1991; Kost and Oblinger, 1993), we find decreases in Tα1-tubulin, total tubulin and neurofilament mRNA expression after injury at the pyramid, which is about 10–12 mm distant from the cell bodies (Tetzlaff and Giehl, 1991). All parameters so far measured by us, including GAP-43, are found to be at approximately 60–70% of uninjured contralateral side measurements 1 week after injury. Since this correlates with the concomitant neuronal atrophy, we believe that this reflects a general atrophic response, rather then a 'novel pattern of cytoskeletal gene expression' (Mikucki and Oblinger, 1991).

If we believe that a repressor of GAP-43 expression (see above) is also acting in the CNS, we have to conclude that in the CNS it is not only target-derived but also obtained from the proximal axonal stump (see also Skene 1989, 1992; Doster et al. 1991). The shorter the stump, the less repressor gets back to the cell bodies, and if it falls below a threshold amount, GAP-43 synthesis becomes derepressed. Should this speculation be correct, then we would expect that the concentration of this repressor would be greatest in the subcortical white matter, high in the optic nerve, and lowest in the lateral funiculus of the spinal cord.

It is also possible that the intracellular concentration of this suppressor would be different in these three types of neurons for reasons that are not yet understood, and perhaps are related to the geometry of the cell (surface to volume ratio). Corticospinal neurons are smaller than retinal ganglion cells and rubrospinal neurons. We cannot rule out the possibility here that this hypothetic 'repressor' is also reaching the cells by terminal uptake via axon collaterals. Corticospinal neurons send out collaterals that leave the main axon at a distance close to the critical distance for GAP-43 induction. Rubrospinal axons that project down to the lumbar cord usually have collaterals at higher thoracic or cervical levels (Huisman et al., 1981). This hypothesis is weakened in the light of the optic nerve situation where no collaterals exist. Thus, the regulatory process might act along the primary axonal stump, as well as via terminals on collaterals.

The importance of an appropriate cell body response for successful regeneration is increasingly recognized. Strategies to overcome the CNS regeneration failure have to focus on these regulatory mechanisms. One avenue for future research will be to identify regulatory elements on the promoters of RAGs, like GAP-43 (Nedivi et al., 1992; Reinhard et al., 1993), or to search for those proteins that are involved in posttranscriptional regulation of the GAP-43 mRNA (Irwin et al., 1993; Kohn and Perrone-Bizzozero, 1993; Perrone-Bizzozero et al., 1993). A second avenue will be to link the known expression of immediate early genes and other transcription factors with RAGs. A third approach will be to test the effects of growth factors and cytokines on the reexpression of RAGs. Local inflammation, presumably via release of cytokines and growth factors, induces GAP-43 mRNA in DRG cells and stimulates their regeneration within the dorsal root (Lu and Richardson, 1991, 1993). This latter approach is further supported by the report of Patterson et al. (1993) that leukemia inhibitory factor-deficient mice lack at least some of their axotomy signals; the changes in neuropeptide expression after injury are not observed.

Rescue of corticospinal neurons by NT-3 and prevention of atrophy of rubrospinal neurons by BDNF

While strategies to induce RAGs will be required for 'distant' axotomies, the problem of neuronal atrophy and/or death dominates after 'close' axotomies. In the rubrospinal system these two problems do not overlap and we face one of two alternatives: (1) after distant axotomy, failure to express RAGs with little atrophy or (2) after close axotomy, expression of RAGs with severe atrophy. The situation is more complicated with the corticospinal neurons since both problems overlap: neuronal death and failure to induce RAGs occur with the same lesion distance. Thus, there is no simple relationship between the lack of trophic support leading to atrophy and death and the induction of RAGs. We have therefore addressed the problem of cell death and atrophy in both rubrospinal and corticospinal systems and subsequently analyzed the effect of neurotrophin application on the expression of RAGs.

The recent discovery of the family of neurotrophins, NGF, BNDF, NT-3 and NT-4/5, provided the tools to address the problem of atrophy and cell death after injury (for review see Ebendal, 1992; Korsching, 1993). While there is still some debate over how the neurotrophins interact with the low- and high-affinity binding sites of their receptors, it is generally accepted that NGF binds to trkA, BDNF and NT-4/5 to trkB , and NT-3 to trkC (for review see Chao, 1992). This identification of the cognate tyrosine kinase receptors prompted us to screen the corticospinal and rubrospinal neurons with in situ hybridization probes specific for trkA, full-length trkB and trkC, as well as the low-affinity neurotrophin receptor, p75.

We found trkC mRNA in retrogradely labeled (thus unequivocally identified) corticospinal neurons, which is in agreement with the localization of the trkC message in layer V cells of the rat cortex (Altar et al., 1993). These data suggested responsiveness of corticospinal neurons to NT-3. To test this hypothesis, we labeled the corticospinal cells via retrograde tracer (Fast Blue, True Blue) injections into the cervical spinal cord. Ten to 14 days later the corticospinal neurons were axotomized in the internal capsule and a second tracer (rhodamine) was injected into the cord. This allowed the positive confirmation of axotomized corticospinal cells, which should only contain the first tracer. NT-3 or saline was applied to the axotomized cortex via an osmotic minipump. In our saline controls, 35% of the corticospinal neurons died within 7 days. This loss was reduced to less than 5% (i.e., 95% survival, $n = 4$) with the application of NT-3 (Giehl and Tetzlaff, unpublished observations). A typical example of a the cell loss in the saline treated cortex and the rescue in the NT-3 treated cortex is given in Fig. 3. This experiment shows for the first time that NT-3 can prevent the axotomy-induced cell death in these upper motoneurons. It also raises the possibility that NT-3 application might rescue corticospinal neurons in neurologic disorders such as amyotrophic lateral sclerosis.

In rubrospinal neurons we found expression of trkB and trkC but not trkA (Tetzlaff et al., 1992; see also Fig. 4). A transient expression of p75 was also observed during the first week after cervical axotomy, which declined at later stages. Similarly, trkB and trkC expression decreased after the second week post injury. The expression of trkB (Middlemas et al., 1991; Soppet et al. 1991) suggested that rubrospinal neurons might respond to BDNF. For BDNF application (Tetzlaff et al., 1993), the rubrospinal tract of male Sprague Dawley rats was injured at cervical level C3 unilaterally and retrogradely labeled with FluoroGold. On day 7 after injury, a 28 gauge application needle was implanted into the vicinity of the red nucleus and connected to an osmotic minipump. This pump was either filled with buffered saline or saline plus 500 ng/μl of BDNF (or NGF or NT-3). The rats were killed on day 14 for histological assessment of cell size and for in situ hybridization for RAG expression. Serial sections from experimental, saline and 'no pump' control

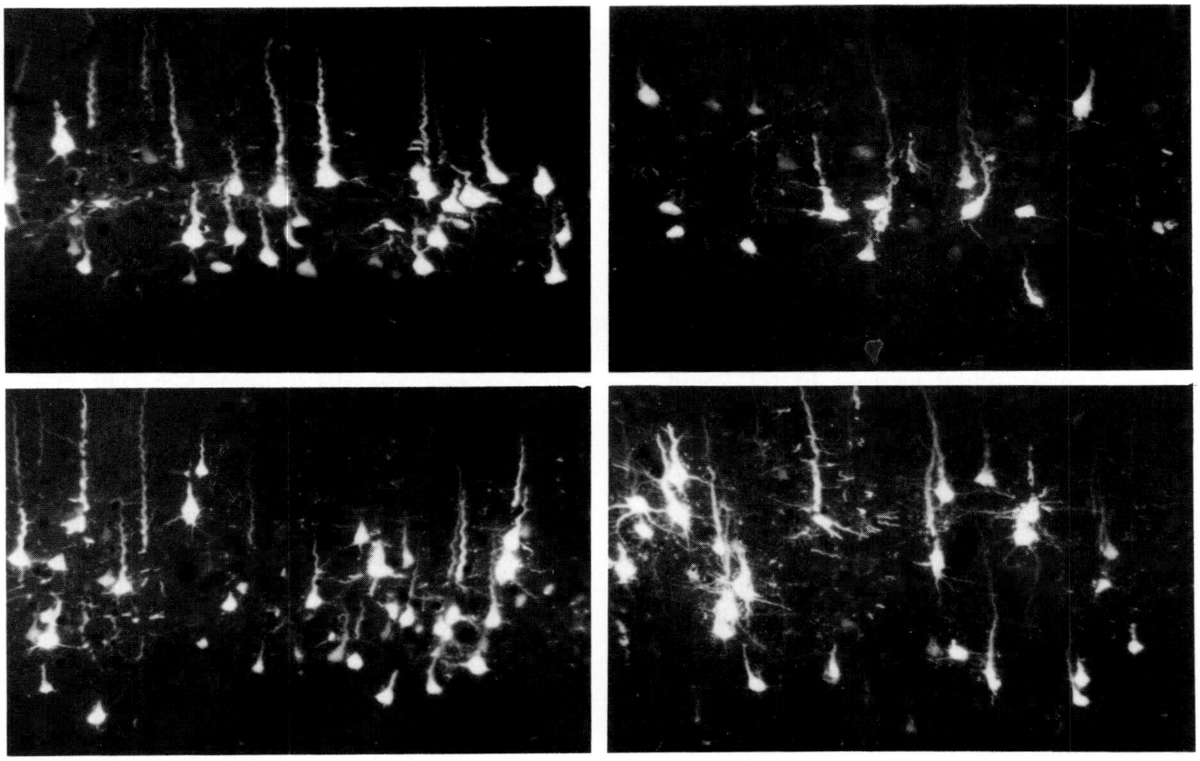

Fig. 3. Corticospinal neurons retrogradely labeled with Fast Blue on the unlesioned (left) and axotomized side at 7 days after lesion (right). Axotomy was performed at the level of the internal capsule. The upper pair of micrographs shows a saline treatment, the lower pair an NT-3 treatment of the lesioned side of the corticospinal neurons (right). A significant number of the axotomized corticospinal neurons died in the saline-treated cortex (top right). In contrast, hardly any death of axotomized neurons occurred under NT-3 treatment (bottom right).

animals were collected on the same slides to ensure equal hybridization conditions.

On day 14 after neuronal injury, neuronal profiles (cross-sectional areas) were 57.5% (S.E.M. = 7.9%) of those of the uninjured contralateral side in 'no pump' controls and 64% (S.E.M. = 3.7%) of those of the uninjured contralateral side in saline-treated animals. This reflects the atrophy which occurs between day 7 and 14 post injury (Barron et al., 1989; Tetzlaff et al., 1991). BDNF treatment fully prevented this atrophy: the mean cell profile area was 98.5% (S.E.M. = 9.5%) of that of the uninjured contralateral side. NGF treatment had no noticeable effect and the NGF-treated cells were 62.4% (S.E.M. = 6.8%) of the unlesioned contralateral side, thus not significantly different from saline control injections (see also Fig. 5). The cell sizes on the contralateral sides used for these comparisons were not significantly different form the contralateral side cell sizes of 'no pump' animals.

The BDNF-treated cells were still chromatolytic in appearance, with eccentric nuclei. This prompted us to ask whether BDNF-treated axotomized rubrospinal neurons still express regeneration-associated genes and, if so, at what level? Was BDNF application 'normalizing', i.e., suppressing RAG expression by substituting for a target or distal stump-derived factor?

We therefore compared saline-treated and BDNF-treated axotomized rubrospinal neurons 14 days post injury, with treatment during the second week. With saline alone, the expression of total tubulin mRNA was 41.5% of the contralateral side at this time, and the contralateral side was not different from unoperated controls. As mentioned above, total tubulin mRNA expression was at 260% of the contralateral side 7 days after injury. Thus, a massive decline occurred during week 2. This decline was still observed with BDNF treatment; however, it was less pronounced and resulted in total tubulin levels of 76.5% of the contralateral side by 14 days post injury. Thus, total tubulin expression is significantly higher in the BDNF-treated group than in the saline-treated group. The expression of GAP-43 was still elevated in 'no pump' and saline-treated animals at 14 days after injury, when compared to uninjured controls. However, when comparing BDNF-treated animals versus saline-treated animals, the number of cells expressing high levels of GAP-43 was larger and the in situ hybridization signal per cell was greater with BDNF treatment. The mean grain counts were 360% of the con-

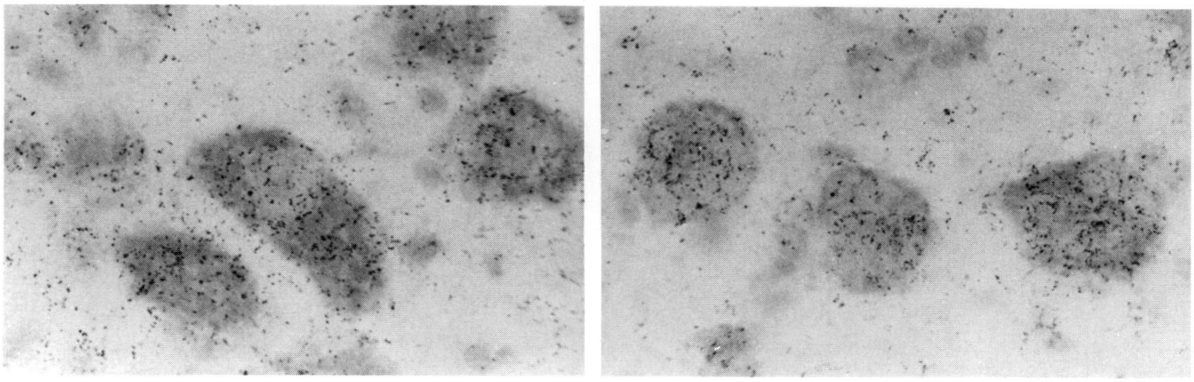

Fig. 4. In situ hybridization for trkB followed by radioautography in unoperated contralateral (left) and axotomized rubrospinal neurons 7 days after injury at the cervical spinal cord (C3) (right). Note that both control and injured rubrospinal neurons express trkB.

tralateral side in the saline group and 536% ($P <$ 0.02) in the BDNF-treated group. This is also illustrated in Fig. 6, which shows GAP-43 mRNA expression revealed by in situ hybridization in a BDNF-treated animal and in a saline control, both 14 days after axotomy. In contrast to total α-tubulin and GAP-43, neurofilament-M expression was not significantly stimulated by BNDF treatment. It was 24.7% of the contralateral control side in saline animals and 31.2% of the uninjured contralateral side with BNDF treatment ($n = 4$); this difference is not significant.

These data suggest that BDNF not only prevents the atrophy of rubrospinal neurons but also stimulates and sustains the expression of RAGs. We therefore hope that BNDF application to the injured rubrospinal neurons will stimulate their growth potential.

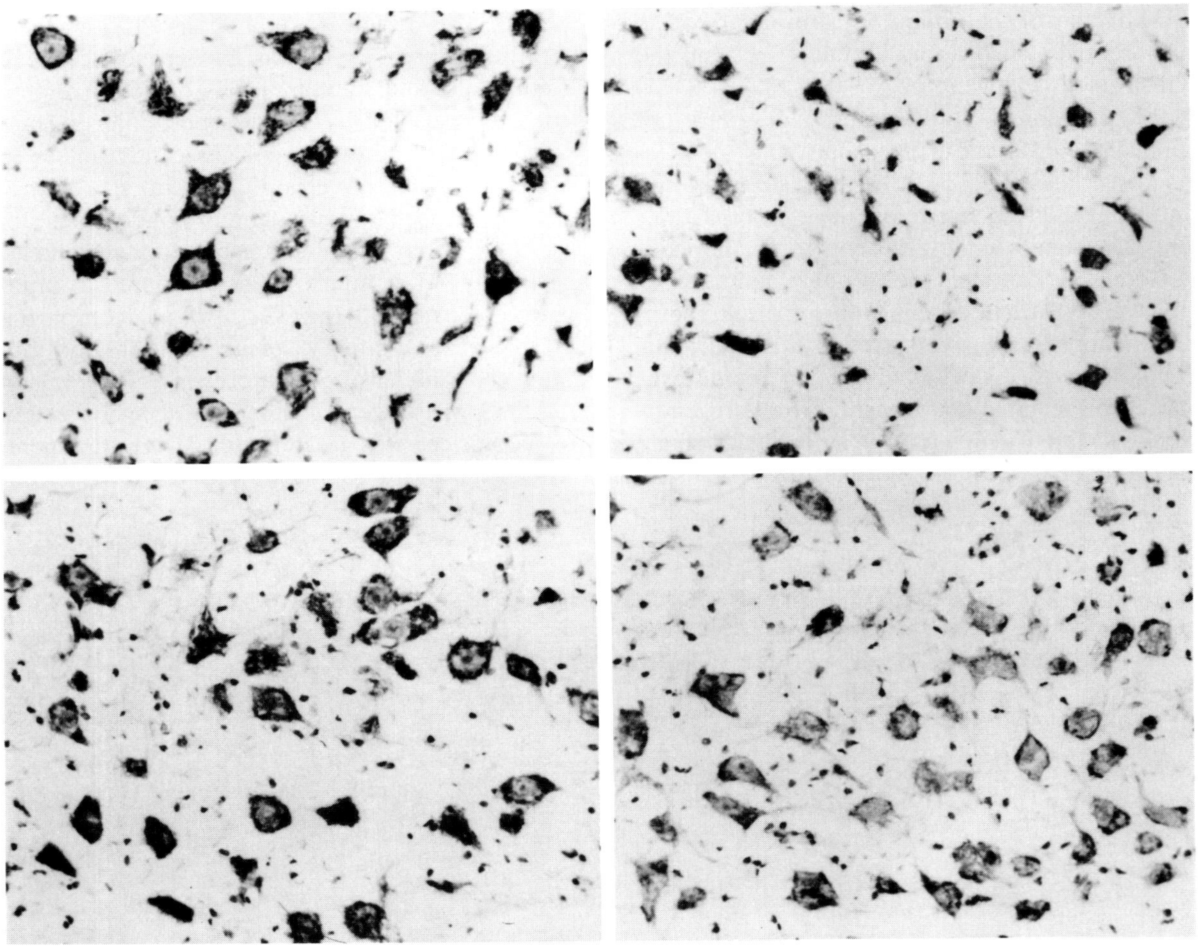

Fig. 5. Micrographs of rubrospinal neurons 14 days after unilateral cervical (C3) axotomy. The upper and lower pictures on the left show the unoperated contralateral control sides while the right pictures display the axotomized neurons. The neurons in the upper right panel were treated with saline between days 7 and 14 after injury and the cells in the bottom right panel were treated with BDNF (500 ng/μl/h). Note the marked atrophy that is normally seen on day 14 after cervical injury. This atrophy is fully prevented by BDNF.

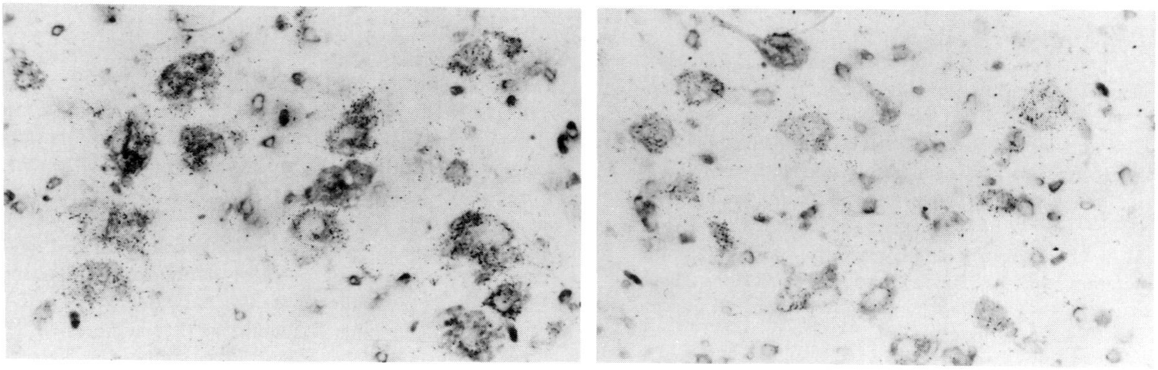

Fig. 6. In situ hybridization for GAP-43 mRNA in axotomized and BDNF-treated (left) and axotomized and saline-treated (right) rubrospinal neurons 14 days after cervical injury. The treatment was given between days 7 and 14. Note that the BDNF-treated cells are significantly larger and display a strong GAP-43 in situ hybridization signal. This signal is much weaker in the saline-treated axotomized cells. Both sections were hybridized in adjacent positions on the same slide and treated identically.

Concluding statement

The application of trophic factors or, even better, small synthetic analogues will become part of a therapeutic concept which addresses the three cardinal problems of CNS regeneration simultaneously: (1) the neutralization of the CNS inhibitors (Keirstead et al., 1992; Schwab et al., 1993; Steeves et al., this volume), (2) trophic support and (3) RAG expression. We believe that the rubrospinal system is a very promising model since the three problems can be dealt with in combination. Future studies will show whether these neurons can regenerate within the spinal cord if (1) the cord is demyelinated or the inhibitory molecules on myelin neutralized, (2) RAGs are induced by cervical injury, and (3) atrophy is prevented with BDNF.

Acknowledgements

We thank Dr. Mark Bisby, Kingston, and Dr. Freda Miller, Montreal, for critical reading of the manuscript and helpful suggestions. Work presented in this chapter was supported by the Medical Research Council of Canada (W.T.), the American Paralysis Association (W.T.), the Spinal Cord Research Foundation (W.T.), Rotary International (N.R.K.), the Deutscher Akademischer Austauschdienst (K.M.G.G.) and the Canadian Network of Centers of Excellence for Neural Regeneration and Functional Recovery. The neurotrophins were provided by Regeneron Pharmaceuticals and Amgen.

References

Aigner, L. and Caroni, P. (1993) Depletion of 43-kD growth-associated protein in primary sensory neurons leads to diminished formation and spreading of growth cones. *J. Cell Biol.*, 123: 417–429.

Altar, C.A., Criden, M.R., Lindsay, R.M. and DiStefano, P.S. (1993) Characterization and topography of high-affinity binding to mammalian brain. *J. Neurosci.*, 13: 733–743.

Barron, K.D. (1983) Axon reaction and central nervous system regeneration. In: F.J. Seil (Ed.), *Nerve, Organ and Tissue Regeneration: Research Perspectives*, Academic Press, New York, pp. 3–36.

Barron, K.D. (1989) Neuronal responses to axotomy: consequences and possibilities for rescue from permanent atrophy or cell death. In: F.J. Seil (Ed.), *Frontiers of Clinical Neuroscience, Vol. 6, Neural Regeneration and Transplantation*, Alan R. Liss, New York, pp. 79–99.

Barron, K.D., Banerjee, M., Dentinger, M.P., Scheibly, M.E. and Mankes, R. (1989) Cytological and cytochemical (RNA) studies on rubral neurons after unilateral rubrospinal tractotomy: the impact of GM1 ganglioside administration. *J. Neurosci. Res.*, 22: 331–337.

Basi, G.S., Jacobson, R.D., Virag, I., Schilling, J. and Skene, J.H.P. (1987) Primary structure and transcriptional regulation of GAP-43, a protein associated with nerve growth. *Cell*, 236: 597- 600.

Basi, G.S. and Skene, J.H.P. (1988) Regulation of GAP-43 gene expression during axonal regeneration in sensory neurons. *Soc. Neurosci. Abstr.*, 14: 408.

Bates, C.A. and Meyer, R.L. (1993) The heavy neurofilament protein is expressed in regenerating adult but not embryonic mammalian optic fibers in vitro. *Exp. Neurol.*, 119: 249–257.

Bisby, M.A. (1984) Retrograde axonal transport and nerve regeneration. In: J. S. Elam and P. Canacalon (Eds.), *Advances in Neurochemistry, Vol. 6, Axonal Transport*, Plenum, New York, pp. 45–67.

Bisby, M.A. and Tetzlaff, W. (1992) Changes in cytoskeletal protein synthesis following axon injury and during axon regeneration. *Mol. Neurobiol.*, 6: 107–123.

Bray, G.M., Villegas-Perez, M.P., Vidal-Sanz, M., Carter, D.A., and Aguayo, A.J. (1991) Neuronal and nonneuronal influences on retinal ganglion cell survival, axonal regrowth, and connectivity after axotomy. *Ann. N.Y. Acad. Sci.*, 633: 214–228.

Caroni, P. and Becker, M. (1992) The downregulation of growth-associated proteins in motoneurons at the onset of synapse elimination is controlled by muscle activity and IGF1. *J. Neurosci.*, 12: 3849–3861.

Chao, M.V. (1992) Neurotrophin receptors: a window into neuronal differentiation. *Neuron*, 9: 583–593.

Curran T., Franza, B.R., Jr. (1988) Fos and Jun: the AP-1 connection. *Cell*, 55: 395–397.

Curtis, R., Green, D., Lindsay, R.M. and Wilkin, G.P. (1993) Up-regulation of GAP-43 and growth of axons in rat spinal cord after compression injury. *J. Neurocytol.*, 22: 51–64.

Doster, S.K., Lozano, A.M., Aguayo, A.J. and Willard, M.B. (1991) Expression of the growth-associated protein GAP-43 in adult rat retinal ganglion cells following axon injury. *Neuron*, 6: 635–647.

Ebendal, T. (1992) Function and evolution in the NGF family and its receptors. *J. Neurosci. Res.*, 32: 461–470.

Egan, D.A., Flumerfelt, B.A. and Gwyn, D.G. (1977) Perikaryal volume changes and the time course of chromatolysis following cervical and thoracic lesions. *Acta Neuropathol.*, 37: 13–19.

Gay, D. A., Yen, T. J., Lau, J. T. Y. and Cleveland, D. W. (1987) Sequences that confer β-tubulin autoregulation through modulated mRNA stability reside within exon 1 of a β-tubulin mRNA. *Cell*, 50: 671–679.

Gay D.A., Sisodia, S.S. and Cleveland, D.W. (1989) Autoregulatory control of β-tubulin mRNA stability is linked to translation elongation. *Proc. Natl. Acad. Sci. USA*, 86: 5763–5767.

Haas, C. A., Donath, C. and Kreutzberg, G.W. (1993) Differential expression of immediate early genes after transection of the facial nerve. *Neuroscience*, 53: 91–99.

Hefti, F. (1991) Nerve growth factor promotes survival of septal cholinergic neurons after fimbrial transsections. *J. Neurosci.*, 6: 2155–2162.

Herdegen, T., Fiallos-Estrada, C. E., Schmid, W., Bravo, R. and Zimmermann, M. (1992) The transcription factors c-JUN, JUN D and CREB, but not FOS and KROX-24, are differentially regulated in axotomized neurons following transection of rat sciatic nerve. *Mol. Brain Res.*, 14: 155–165.

Herdegen, T., Fiallos-Estrada, C.E., Bravo, R. and Zimmermann, M. (1993) Colocalization and covariation of c-JUN transcription factor with galanin in primary afferent neurons and with CGRP in spinal motoneurons following transection of rat sciatic nerve. *Mol. Brain Res.*, 17: 147–154.

Heumann, R., Korsching, S., Bandtlow, C. and Thoenen, H. (1987) Changes of nerve growth factor synthesis in nonneuronal cells in response to sciatic nerve transection. *J. Cell Biol.*, 104: 1623–1631.

Hoffman, P.N. and Cleveland, D.W. (1988) Neurofilament and tubulin expression recapitulates the developmental pattern during axonal regeneration: induction of a specific β-tubulin isotype. *Proc. Natl. Acad. Sci. USA*, 84: 4530–4533.

Huisman, A.M., Kuypers, H.G.J.M. and Verburgh, C.A. (1981) Quantitative differences in collateralization of the descending spinal pathways from red nucleus and other brain stem cell groups in rat as demonstrated with the multiple fluorescent retrograde tracer technique. *Brain Res.*, 209: 271–286.

Irwin, N., Baekelandt, B., Gu, M.F. and Benowitz, L.I. (1993) RNA-protein interactions that may contribute to post transcriptional regulation of GAP-43 expression. *Soc. Neurosci. Abstr.*, 19: 878.

Jap Tjoen San, E.R., Schmidt-Michels, M., Oestreicher, A.B., Gispen, W.H. and Schotman, P. (1992) Inhibition of nerve growth factor-induced B-50/GAP-43 expression by antisense oligomers interferes with neurite outgrowth of PC12 cells. *Biochem. Biophys. Res. Commun.*, 187: 839–846.

Jenkins, R., Tetzlaff, W. and Hunt, S. P. (1993) Differential expression of immediate early genes in rubrospinal neurons following axotomy in rat. *Eur. J. Neurosci.*, 5: 203–209.

Jones, P.J. and Aguayo, A.J. (1991) Axotomy enhances GAP-43 mRNA levels in adult rat retinal ganglion cells. *Soc. Neurosci. Abstr.*, 17: 555.

Kalil, K. and Perdew, M. (1988) Expression of two developmentally regulated brain-specific proteins is correlated with late outgrowth of the pyramidal tract. *J. Neurosci.*, 8: 4797–4808.

Keirstead, H.S., Hasan, S.J., Muir, G.D. and Steeves, J.D. (1992) Suppression of the onset of myelination extends the permissive period for the functional repair of embryonic spinal cord. *Proc. Natl. Acad. Sci. USA*, 89: 11664–11668.

Kohn, D.T. and Perrone-Bizzozero, N.I. (1993) Brain cytosolic proteins specifically bind to a conserved region in the 3′ UTR of GAP-43 mRNA. *Soc. Neurosci. Abstr.*, 19: 878.

Korsching, S. (1993) The neurotrophic factor concept: a reexamination. *J. Neurosci.*, 13: 2739–2748.

Kost, S.A. and Oblinger, M.M. (1993) Immature corticospinal neurons respond to axotomy with changes in tubulin gene expression. *Brain Res. Bull.*, 30: 469–475.

Kruger, L., Bendotti, C., Rivolta, R. and Samanin, R. (1993) Distribution of GAP-43 mRNA in the adult rat brain. *J. Comp. Neurol.*, 333: 417–434.

Lamb, P. and McKnight S.L. (1991) Diversity and specificity in transcriptional regulation: the benefits of heterotypic dimerization. *Trends Biol. Sci.*, 16: 417–422.

Leah, J.D., Herdegen, T. and Bravo, R. (1991) Selective expression of Jun following axotomy and axonal transport block in peripheral nerves in the rat: evidence for a role in the regeneration process. *Brain Res.*, 566: 198–207.

Lu, X. and Richardson, P.M. (1991) Inflammation near the nerve cell body enhances axonal regeneration. *J. Neurosci.*, 11: 972–978.

Lu, X. and Richardson, P.M. (1993) Induction by macrophages of regeneration associated molecules in sensory neurons. *Soc. Neurosci. Abstr.*, 19: 451.

Luo, Y., Raible, D. and Raper, A. (1993) Collapsin: a protein in brain that induces the collapse and paralysis of neuronal growth cones. *Cell*, 75: 217–227.

MacRae, T.H. and Langdon, C.M. (1989) Tubulin synthesis, structure, and function: what are the relationships? *Biochem. Cell Biol.*, 67: 770–790.

Maness, P.F., Aubry, M., Shores, C.G., Frame, L. and Pfenninger, K.H. (1988) C-src gene product in developing rat brain is enriched in nerve growth cone membranes. *Proc. Natl. Acad. Sci. USA.*, 85: 5001–5005.

Mathew, T.C. and Miller, F.D. (1993) Induction of Tα1 α-tubulin mRNA during neuronal regeneration is a function of the amount of axon lost. *Dev. Biol.*, 158: 467–474.

McBride, R.L., Feringa, E.R., Garver, M.K. and Williams, J.K., Jr. (1989) Prelabeled red nucleus and sensorimotor cortex neurons of the rat survive 10 and 20 weeks after spinal cord transection. *J. Neuropathol. Exp. Neurol.*, 48: 568–576.

McKerracher, L., Essagian, C. and Aguayo, A.J. (1993) Temporal changes in beta-tubulin and neurofilament mRNA levels after transection of adult rat retinal ganglion cell axons in the optic nerve. *J. Neurosci.*, 13: 2617–2626.

Meyer, M., Matsuoka, I., Wetmore, C., Olson, L. and Thoenen, H. (1992) Enhanced synthesis of brain derived neurotrophic factor in the lesioned peripheral nerve: different mechanisms are responsible for the regulation of BDNF and NGF mRNA. *J. Cell Biol.*, 119: 45–54.

Middlemas, D.S., Lindberg, R.A. and Hunter, T. (1991) trkB, a neural receptor protein-tyrosine kinase: evidence for a full-length and two truncated receptors. *Mol. Cell. Biol.*, 11: 143–153.

Mikucki, S.A. and Oblinger, M.M. (1991) Corticospinal neurons exhibit a novel pattern of cytoskeletal gene expression after injury. *J. Neurosci. Res.*, 30: 213–225.

Miller, F.D., Tetzlaff, W., Bisby, M.A., Fawcett, J.W. and Milner, R.J. (1989) Rapid induction of the major embryonic α-tubulin mRNA, Tα1, during nerve regeneration in adult rats. *J. Neurosci.*, 9: 1452–1463.

Muma, N.A., Hoffman, P.N., Slunt, H.H., Applegate, M.D., Lieberburg, I. and Price, D.L. (1990) Alterations in levels of mRNAs coding for neurofilament protein subunits during regeneration. *Exp. Neurol.*, 107: 230–235.

Nedivi, E., Basi, G.S., Akey, I.V. and Skene, J.H. (1992) A neural-specific GAP-43 core promoter located between unusual DNA elements that interact to regulate its activity. *J. Neurosci.*, 12: 691–704.

Oblinger, M.M., Wong, J. and Parysek, L.M. (1989) Axotomy-induced changes in the expression of a type III neuronal intermediate filament gene. *J. Neurosci.*, 9: 3766–3775.

Oblinger, M.M., Argasinski, A., Wong, J. and Kosik, K. (1991) *Tau* gene expression in rat sensory neurons during development and regeneration. *J. Neurosci.*, 11: 2453–2459.

Oestreicher, A.B. and Gispen, W.H. (1986) Comparison of immunocytochemical distribution of the phosphoprotein B-50 in the cerebellum and hippocampus of immature and adult rat brain. *Brain Res.*, 375: 267–279.

Oudega, M., Varon, S. and Hagg, T. (1993) Regeneration of adult rat sensory axons into intraspinal peripheral nerve grafts: promoting effects of conditioning lesion, graft degeneration and NGF. *Soc. Neurosci. Abstr.*, 19: 422.

Patterson, P.H., Bugga, I. and Stewart, C.L. (1993) CDF/LIF-deficient mice display an altered complement of neuronal phenotypes in the CNS. *Soc. Neurosci. Abstr.*, 19: 1724.

Perrone-Bizzozero, N.I., Cansino, V.V. and Kohn, D.T. (1993) Posttranscriptional regulation of GAP-43 gene expression in PC12 cells through protein kinase C-dependent stabilization of the mRNA. *J. Cell Biol.*, 120: 1263–1270.

Reh, T.A., Redshaw, J.D. and Bisby, M.A. (1987) Axons of the pyramidal tract do not increase their transport of growth-associated proteins after axotomy. *Mol. Brain Res.*, 2: 1–6.

Reier, P.J., Eng, L.F. and Jakeman, L. (1989) Reactive astrocyte and axonal outgrowth in the injured CNS: Is gliosis really an impediment to regeneration? In: F.J. Seil (Ed.), *Frontiers of Clinical Neuroscience, Vol. 6, Neural Regeneration and Transplantation*, Alan R. Liss, New York, pp. 183–209.

Reinhard, E., Wegner, J. and Skene, J.H.P. (1993) Neural selective activation and downregulation of mammalian GAP-43 promoter sequences in zebrafish. *Soc. Neurosci. Abstr.*, 19: 878.

Richardson, P.M., and Issa, V.M.K. (1982) Peripheral injury enhances regeneration of spinal axons. *Nature (Lond.)*, 284: 264–265.

Richardson, P.M. and Verge V.M.K. (1986) The induction of a regenerative propensity in sensory neurons following peripheral axonal injury. *J. Neurocytol.*, 15: 585–594.

Richardson, P.M., Issa, V.M.K. and Aguayo, A.J. (1984) Regeneration of long spinal axons in the rat. *J. Neurocytol.*, 13: 165–182.

Rutherford, S.D., Louis, W.J. and Gundlach, A.L. (1992) Induction of c-jun expression in vagal motoneurons following axotomy. *NeuroReport*, 3: 465–468.

Schreyer, D.J. and Skene, J.H.P. (1991) Fate of GAP-43 in ascending spinal axons of DRG neurons after peripheral nerve injury; delayed accumulation and correlation with regenerative potential. *J. Neurosci.*, 11: 3738–3751.

Schreyer, D.J. and Skene, J.H.P. (1993) Injury-associated induction of GAP-43 expression displays axon branch specificity in rat dorsal root ganglion neurons. *J. Neurobiol.*, 7: 959–970.

Schwab, M.E., Kapfhammer, J.P. and Bandtlow, C.E. (1993) Inhibitors of neurite growth. *Annu. Rev. Neurosci.*, 16: 565–595.

Shea, T.B., Perrone-Bizzozero, M.L. and Benowitz, L.I. (1991) Phospholipid-mediated delivery of anti-GAP43 antibodies into neuroblastoma cells prevents neuritogenesis. *J. Neurosci.*, 11: 1685- 1690.

Skene, J.H.P. (1989) Axonal growth-associated proteins. *Annu. Rev. Neurosci.*, 12: 127–156.

Skene J.H.P. (1992) Retrograde pathways controlling expression of a major growth cone component in the adult CNS. In: P.C. Letourneau, S.B. Kater and E.R. Macagno, (Eds.), *The Nerve Growth Cone*, Raven Press, New York, pp. 463–475.

Skene, J.H.P. and Willard, M. (1981) Axonally transported proteins associated with axon growth in rabbit central and peripheral nervous system. *J. Cell Biol.*, 89: 96–103.

Smith, D.S. and Skene, J.H.P. (1993) Axotomy-induced transcription is a prerequisite for regenerative axon elongation but not for sprouting. *Soc. Neurosci. Abstr.*, 19: 679.

So, K.F. and Aguayo, A.J. (1985) Lengthy regrowth of cut axons from ganglion cells after peripheral nerve transplantation into the retina of adult rats. *Brain Res.*, 328: 349–354.

Stein, R., Mori, N., Matthews, K., Lo, L.C. and Anderson, D.J. (1988) The NGF-inducible SCG 10 mRNA encodes a novel membrane-bound protein present in growth cones and abundant in developing neurons. *Neuron*, 1: 463–476.

Tetzlaff, W. and Giehl, K.M.G. (1991) Axotomized corticospinal neurons increase GAP-43 mRNA after subcortical lesions but not after pyramidal lesions. *Third IBRO World Congress of Neuroscience*, Aug. 1991, p. 220.

Tetzlaff, W., Bisby, M.A. and Kreutzberg, G.W. (1988) Changes in cytoskeletal proteins in the rat facial nucleus following axotomy. *J. Neurosci.*, 8: 3181–3189.

Tetzlaff, W., Tsui, B.J. and Balfour, J.K. (1990) Rubrospinal neurons increase GAP-43 and tubulin mRNA after cervical but not after thoracic axotomy. *Soc. Neurosci. Abstr.*, 16: 338.

Tetzlaff, W., Alexander, S.W., Miller, F.D. and Bisby, M.A. (1991) Response of facial and rubrospinal neurons to axotomy: changes in mRNA expression for cytoskeletal proteins and GAP-43. *J. Neurosci.*, 11: 2528–2544.

Tetzlaff, W., Leonard, C.A. and Harrington, K.C. (1992) Expression of neurotrophin receptor mRNAs in axotomized facial and rubrospinal neurons. *Soc. Neurosci. Abstr.*, 18: 1294.

Tetzlaff W., Kobasyashi N.R. and Bedard A.M. (1993) BDNF prevents atrophy of rubrospinal neurons after axotomy. *Soc. Neurosci. Abstr.*, 19: 1104

Tsui, B. J., Cassar, S. L. and Tetzlaff, W. (1991) Changes in mRNA levels for GAP-43, tubulin and neurofilament-M in rat spinal motoneurons after proximal versus distal axotomy. *Soc. Neurosci. Abstr.*, 17: 47.

Verge, V.M.K., Tetzlaff, W., Bisby, M.A. and Richardson, P.M. (1990a) Influence of nerve growth factor on neurofilament gene expression in mature primary sensory neurons. *J. Neurosci.*, 10: 2018–2025.

Verge, V.M.K., Tetzlaff, W., Richardson, P.M. and Bisby, M.A. (1990b) Correlation between GAP-43 and nerve growth factor receptors in rat sensory neurons. *J. Neurosci.*, 10: 926–934.

Vidal-Sanz, M., Bray, G.M., Villegas-Perez, M.P., Thanos, S. and Aguayo, A.J. (1987) Axonal regeneration and synapse formation in the superior colliculus by retinal ganglion cells in the adult rat. *J. Neurosci.*, 7: 2894–2909.

Villegas-Perez, M.P., Vidal-Sanz, M., Bray, G.M. and Aguayo, A.J. (1988) Influences of peripheral nerve grafts on the survival and regrowth of axotomized retinal ganglion cells in adult rats. *J. Neurosci.*, 8: 265–280.

Villegas-Perez, M.P., Vidal-Sanz, M., Rasminsky, M., Bray, G.M. and Aguayo, A.J. (1993) Rapid and protracted phases of retinal ganglion cell loss follow axotomy in the optic nerve of adult rats. *J. Neurobiol.*, 24: 23–36.

Wong, J. and Oblinger, M.M. (1987) Changes in neurofilament gene expression occur after axotomy of dorsal root ganglion neurons: an in situ hybridization study. *Metab. Brain Dis.*, 2: 291–303.

Woolf, C.J., Reynolds, M.L., Molander, C., O'Brien, C., Lindsay, R.M. and Benowitz, L.I. (1990) The growth-associated protein GAP-43 appears in dorsal root ganglion cells and in the dorsal horn of the rat spinal cord following peripheral nerve injury. *Neuroscience*, 34: 465–478.

Wu, W., Mathew, T.C. and Miller, F.D. (1993) Evidence that the loss of homeostatic signals induces regeneration-associated alterations in neuronal gene expression. *Dev. Biol.*, 158: 456–466.

SECTION V

Cross-talk Between Nervous and Immune Systems in Response to Injury

F.J. Seil (Ed.)
Progress in Brain Research, Vol 103

CHAPTER 23

Cross-talk between nervous and immune systems in response to injury

Vanda A. Lennon

Departments of Immunology, Neurology and Laboratory Medicine and Pathology, Mayo Clinic, Rochester, MN 55905, USA

Introduction

Potential for cross-talk between the nervous system and the immune system exists at many levels, through anatomical proximity and also by more distant humoral interactions. The growing lay popularity of psychoneuroimmunology implies that there may also be a sociological interaction between the nervous system and immune system (Reichlin, 1993). The two systems have remarkable similarities (Table 1). Both have the unique attribute of memory, and they also share structural motifs in certain key molecules. 'Hard wiring' connections between the nervous system and immune system are inherent in the autonomic innervation of spleen, thymus and other lymphoid tissues, and in the bone marrow derived lymphoid cells that reside in the central nervous system (CNS) in the form of microglia (Steinman, 1993). Examples of structural motifs shared by the immune system and nervous system include integral membrane proteins of the immunoglobulin (Ig) superfamily, which serve as both adhesion and signaling molecules (Table 2).

Cells intrinsic to the immune system and the nervous system are characteristically highly adaptable to environmental stimuli. They can rapidly upregulate and downregulate ion channels and receptors for cytokines, growth factors, hormones and neurotransmitters. Structural and functional analogies between the two systems are illustrated by the complex molecular interactions through which a foreign antigen activates T lymphocytes. After initially processing the antigen, a professional antigen-presenting cell (macrophage, microglia or B lymphocyte) displays peptide fragments of the antigenic protein on its surface major histocompatibility complex molecules (MHC) for recognition by a specific antigen receptor complex on the surface of a T lymphocyte. The ensuing transient formation of intimate cell-cell contacts, reminiscent of synapses, between antigen-presenting cell and responding T cell involves complementary surface molecules of both cells. If the antigen-presenting cell is not 'professionally' specialized to stimulate a T cell effector response (e.g., a tissue cell that expresses MHC molecules but lacks essential costimulatory surface molecules), the resulting signal delivered to the helper T lymphocyte may be inhibitory, again analogous to neuronal interactions.

Molecules that mediate cross-talk

Neuroendocrine factors are known to modulate immune functions. The stress-related hypothalamic and pituitary peptides, corticotrophin releasing factor (CRF) and adrenocorticotropic hormone (ACTH), for example, have direct effects on lymphocytes as well as effecting corticosteroid

TABLE 1

Similar characteristics of the nervous and immune systems

Cellular interactions	(e.g., synaptic transmission; T cell activation)
Molecular interactions	(e.g., cytokines; neurotrophic growth factors)
Homologous structures	(e.g., Ig superfamily; cytokine/neurotrophic growth factor receptors)
Adaptive environmental responses	(e.g., up- and downregulation of receptors and ion channels)
Memory mechanisms	
Excitatory and inhibitory signals	(e.g., receptor agonists/antagonists; anergy, apoptosis)

TABLE 2

Examples of nervous system molecules belonging to the immunoglobulin gene superfamily*

Neural cell adhesion molecules
Fasciclins II and III
Transiently expressed axonal glycoprotein 1
Thy-1 glycoprotein
Myelin associated glycoprotein
Myelin P_0 protein
Myelin/oligodendrocyte glycoprotein

* Reviewed by Steinman, 1993.

secretion through the hypothalamic-pituitary-adrenal pathway. CRF and ACTH, and also the potent immunomodulatory pituitary peptide, prolactin, are produced by lymphoid cells as well as by the hypothalamus/pituitary (Reichlin, 1993). The nature of an injury to the CNS (e.g., trauma, ischemia, anoxia, toxin, infection, neoplasia, autoimmunity, nutritional or trophic factor deficiency) and the age of the individual will influence the CNS response to injury. An emerging theme of the papers presented in this section is that products of leukocytes may facilitate the repair of injured neural tissues. These molecules can be broadly classified as follows.

Cytokines

Multifunctional cytokines are recognized increasingly as the products of and agonists for a wide range of tissues, including the CNS. Furthermore, receptors for certain cytokines and neurotrophic factors have striking homologies (Mallett and Barclay, 1991; Hilton et al., 1992). The unfortunate disciplinary restriction imposed intellectually in the evolution of nomenclature is illustrated in the report by Otten and colleagues (this volume). Their study shows that (i) blood monocytes have functional receptors for nerve growth factor (NGF) and, in response to immunologic activation, a trk receptor mRNA is upregulated, and (ii) mesangial cells in renal glomeruli respond to and release cytokines and NGF.

The endogenous pyrogen factor, interleukin 1 (IL-1), is produced by neural cells as well as by macrophages. This was the first immune product recognized to have specific receptor-mediated actions on the nervous system. Neural activities of IL-1 include elicitation of the hypothalamic fever response and stimulation of neurotrophic factor production (Reichlin, 1993). The theme of cytokines facilitating repair in the injured CNS culminates with recent data of Schwartz and coworkers (this volume) that implicate a role for a product of activated T cells, interleukin 2 (IL-2), in CNS remodeling. In the course of postinjury inflammation, IL-2, or a dimerized related product, acts as an oligodendrocyte-selective cytotoxin, and the nerve-derived transglutaminase that dimerizes IL-2 facilitates CNS axon regrowth. This observation has potential therapeutic implications for clinical situations of demyelination and injury.

Neurotransmitters

Lymphoid cells have functional receptors for neurotransmitters, such as acetylcholine and norepinephrine (Reichlin, 1993). Additionally, lymphocytes secrete neuropeptides (Reichlin, 1993), and lymphocytes, macrophages, microglia and astrocytes have functional receptors for neuropeptides, such as substance P (Lotz et al., 1988; Reichlin, 1993; Mitrovic et al., this volume). Merrill and colleagues (Mitrovic et al., this volume) report that substance P, as well as certain cytokines, induces nitric oxide production in cultured microglia, and that nitric oxide is involved in the microglial-effected lysis of oligodendrocytes in vitro.

Immunoglobulins

The secreted macromolecular products of plasma cells sometimes impair and sometimes repair the nervous system.

Postinfectious / vaccinal antibodies and monoclonal gammopathies . Specific antibodies that neutralize bacteria and viruses are a major defense against infection. Sometimes, however, gastrointestinal and respiratory infections, immunizations, and monoclonal gammopathies associated with plasma cell dyscrasias appear to initiate peripheral neuropathies (Powell et al., 1984; Kornberg et al., 1994; Vallat et al., 1994). Because some of these cases are responsive to therapeutic plasma exchange or intravenous high doses of pooled normal human IgG, an autoimmune basis has been suspected. However, this is not proven. It is conceivable that nonimmunological interactions between heavy chains of certain immunoglobulins and carbohydrate moieties of glycolipids or glycoproteins of myelin, axon or Schwann cell could give rise to a variety of demyelinating neuropathies, with or without inflammation. Binding of oligoclonal (postinfectious/vaccinal) or monoclonal immunoglobulins to neural elements by an interaction with the Fc component of the immunoglobulin molecule might interfere with axonal and myelin maintenance or trigger an inflammatory response by stimulating cytokine secretion. Alternatively, immunoglobulins immobilized by their Fc components could bind circulating antigens and antibodies. If, as suggested by the carbohydrate hypothesis that I have proposed above, neuropathies of this type are not mediated by myelin-specific autoantibodies, immunoglobulins lacking their glycosylated tail segments would not bind to neural tissue. It remains to be determined whether the antiglycolipid and antiglycoprotein 'autoantibodies' associated with certain neuropathies (Kornberg et al., 1994) interact with their target molecules by the immunoglobulins' antigen recognizing Fab components or by glycosylated Fc components.

Pathogenic autoantibodies . The neurological pathogenicity of certain organ-specific autoantibodies is abundantly clear from clinical and experimental observations. Defined targets of these IgG antibodies include NGF (Levi-Montalcini and Angeletti, 1966) and synaptic membrane components, such as ionic channels/neurotransmitter receptors (Lennon, 1979, 1994), exocytotic vesicle proteins (Takamori et al., 1994), and neurotransmitter-degradative enzymes (Brimijoin and Lennon, 1990). Autoantibodies specific for a neurotransmitter-synthetic enzyme are highly associated with the acquired disorder of γ-aminobutyric acid (GABA)ergic synaptic transmission known as 'stiff-man' syndrome (Solimena and De Camilli, 1991; McEvoy and Lennon, 1993), but have not yet been proven to have a pathogenic role. The several defined mechanisms that effect pathogenicity in autoimmune disorders resulting from in vivo interaction of specific autoantibodies with their targets include activation of complement, antigenic modulation, blockade of neurotransmitter binding and deprivation of growth factors at a critical stage of neurogenesis.

CNS reparative autoantibodies . Autoantibodies can function as receptor agonists. This is exemplified clinically by the thyroid-stimulating IgGs that are effectors of Graves' disease, and for which the target is the thyroid-stimulating hormone (TSH) receptor of thyrocytes. Possibly analogous mechanism, pertinent to repair of the injured nervous system, is observed experimentally when IgGs made against a crude mixture of CNS antigens are injected into mice with chronic viral-induced demyelination to promote progenitor glial cell proliferation in situ and remyelination (Rodriquez and Lennon, 1990). Extending this observation, Rodriquez and Miller (this volume) report that a systemically injected monoclonal IgM with CNS specificity is similarly myelin-reparative. Definition of the antigen(s) involved in this phenomenon (possibly an oligodendrocyte receptor for a growth or differentiation factor) may lead to therapeutic applications in demyelinating and traumatic CNS disorders.

References

Brimijoin, S. and Lennon, V.A. (1990) Autoimmune preganglionic sympathectomy induced by acetylcholinesterase antibodies. *Proc. Natl. Acad. Sci. USA*, 87: 9630-9634.

Hilton, D.J., Nicola, N.A. and Metcalf, D. (1992) Distribution and binding properties of receptors for leukemia inhibitory factor. In: *Polyfunctional Cytokines: IL-6 and LIF*, Ciba Foundation Symposium 167, Wiley, Chichester, pp. 227-244.

Kornberg, A.J., Pestronk, A., Bieser, K., Ho, T.W., McKhann, G.M., Wu, H.S. and Jiang, Z. (1994) The clinical correlates of high-titer IgG anti-GM1 antibodies. *Ann. Neurol.*, 35: 234-237.

Lennon, V.A. (1979) Immunological mechanisms in myasthenia gravis - a model of a receptor disease. In: E. Franklin (Ed.), *Clinical Immunology Update: Reviews for Physicians*, Elsevier North Holland, New York, pp. 259-289.

Lennon, V.A. (1994) Serological diagnosis of myasthenia gravis and the Lambert-Eaton myasthenic syndrome. In: R. Lisak (Ed.), *Handbook of Myasthenia Gravis*, Marcel Dekker, New York, pp. 149-164.

Levi-Montalcini, R. and Angeletti, P.U. (1966) Immunosympathectomy. *Pharmacol. Rev.*, 18: 619-628.

Lotz, M., Vaughan, J.H. and Carson, D.A. (1988) Effect of neuropeptides on production of inflammatory cytokines by human monocytes. *Science*, 241: 1218-1220.

Mallett, S. and Barclay, A.N. (1991) A new superfamily of cell surface proteins related to the nerve growth factor receptor. *Immunol. Today*, 12: 220-223.

McEvoy, K.M. and Lennon, V.A. (1993) Stiffman syndrome: clinical aspects and anti-islet cell antibodies as a disease marker. In: G. Piccolo, P. Martinelli (Eds.), *Motor Unit Hyperactivity States,* Raven Press, New York, pp. 45–52.

Powell, H.C., Rodriquez, M. and Hughes, R.A.C. (1984) Microangiopathy of vasa nervorum in dysglobulinemic neuropathy. *Ann. Neurol.*, 15: 386-394.

Reichlin, S. (1993) Neuroendocrine-immune interactions. *N. Engl. J. Med.*, 329: 1246-1252.

Rodriguez, M. and Lennon, V.A. (1990) Immunoglobulins promote remyelination in the central nervous system. *Ann. Neurol.*, 27: 12-17.

Solimena, M. and De Camilli, P. (1991) Autoimmunity to glutamic acid decarboxylase (GAD) in stiff-man syndrome and insulin-dependent diabetes mellitus. *Trends Neurosci.*, 14: 452-457.

Steinman, L. (1993) Connections between the immune system and nervous system. *Proc. Natl. Acad. Sci. USA*, 90: 7912-7914.

Takamori, M., Hamada, T., Komai, K., Takahashi, M. and Yoshida, A. (1994) Synaptotagmin can cause an immune-mediated model of Lambert-Eaton myasthenic syndrome in rats. *Ann. Neurol.*, 35: 74-80.

Vallat, J.M., Leboutet, M.J., Jauberteau, M.O., Tabaraud, F., Couratier, P. and Akani, F. (1994) Widenings of the myelin lamellae in a typical Guillain-Barré syndrome. *Muscle Nerve*, 17: 378-380.

F.J. Seil (Ed.)
Progress in Brain Research, Vol 103

CHAPTER 24

Neurotrophins: signals between the nervous and immune systems

U. Otten, J.L. Scully, P.B. Ehrhard and R.A. Gadient

Department of Physiology, University of Basel, CH-4051 Basel, Switzerland

Introduction

The survival, differentiation and maintenance of neurons depend on the presence of specific neurotrophic factors called the neurotrophins (NTs). Originally defined as retrograde trophic messengers, the concept has had to expand with the realization that anterograde and local actions of neurotrophins are also significant. Beta-nerve growth factor (NGF) is the prototypical example of a target derived NT, and is essential for development and differentiation of peripheral sympathetic and neural crest derived sensory nerve cells (Levi-Montalcini, 1987). In addition to its peripheral actions, NGF plays a physiological role in the mammalian central nervous system (CNS) as a trophic agent for basal forebrain cholinergic neurons (Thoenen et al., 1987; Mobley et al., 1989). Over the last few years additional NGF-like NTs have been molecularly cloned and characterized: brain-derived neurotrophic factor (BDNF, Leibrock et al., 1989), neurotrophin-3 (NT-3; Hohn et al., 1990; Jones and Reichardt, 1990; Maisonpierre et al., 1990; Rosenthal et al., 1990) and neurotrophin-4 (NT-4; Hallböök et al., 1991; Ip et al., 1992), also known as NT-5 (Berkemeier et al., 1991). These factors constitute the NGF-related NT family. The NGF-related NTs display trophic activity on distinct and overlapping neuronal populations within the CNS and the peripheral nervous system (for review see Korsching, 1993).

Increasing evidence indicates that NGF has additional actions that are not neurotrophic. For example, NGF can influence neuroendocrine interactions. Stressful situations, which activate the hypothalamo-pituitary-adrenocortical axis, have been shown to result in a concurrent rise in circulating NGF levels (Aloe et al., 1986). Neutralization of circulating NGF by anti-NGF antibody treatment blocks the stress-induced rise in circulating glucocorticoid levels (Taglialatela et al., 1991). Conversely, the peripheral administration of NGF has been shown selectively to activate the pituitary-adrenocortical axis and increase circulating corticosteroid levels (Otten et al., 1979). NGF deprivation during development has been reported to result in a marked deficit in thyroid and adrenal function (Levi-Montalcini et al., 1990) and steroid hormones, including glucocorticoids (Barbany and Persson, 1992; Lindholm et al., 1992a; Scully and Otten, 1993) and thyroid hormone (Walker et al., 1979, 1980; Figueiredo et al., 1993), have all been shown capable of modulating NGF production in brain.

More recent studies indicate that NGF may have even broader physiological effects, beyond regulating neuronal survival and differentiation and modulating various endocrine systems. There is increasing evidence that NGF also exerts speci-

TABLE I

NGF effects on cells and functions of the immune system

–Rapid shape change of blood cells	(Gudat et al., 1981)
–Increase of vascular permeability	(Otten et al., 1984)
–Chemotaxis for human neutrophils	(Boyle et al., 1985)
–Tissue accumulation of mast cells	(Aloe and Levi-Montalcini, 1977)
–Mast cell degranulation	(Bruni et al., 1982; Pearce and Thompson, 1986; Mazurek et al., 1986)
–Mast cells express trk receptors	(Horigome et al., 1993)
–Modulation of release of inflammatory mediators by human basophils	(Bischoff and Dahinden, 1992)
–T cell-dependent AB synthesis	(Manning et al., 1985)
–Differentiation of granulocytes and macrophages	(Matsuda et al., 1988, 1991)
–Proliferation of human lymphocytes	(Thorpe and Perez-Polo, 1987; Otten et al., 1989)
–Differentiation of human B cells into immunoglobulin secreting plasma cells	(Otten et al., 1989; Kimata et al., 1991)
–Human B cells express functional NGF receptors	(Brodie and Gelfand, 1992)
–Increase in oxidative burst in human monocytes	(Ehrhard and Otten, 1992)
–Human monocytes and activated CD 4-positive T cell clones express functional trk receptors	(Ehrhard et al., 1993a,b)

fic effects on cells of the immune system (Table 1). NGF induces shape changes in platelets (Gudat et al.,1981), enhances vascular permeability in rat skin (Otten et al., 1984), increases the number of mast cells in neonatal rats (Aloe and Levi- Montalcini, 1977) and causes degranulation of rat peritoneal mast cells (Bruni et al., 1982; Mazurek et al., 1986; Pearce and Thompson, 1986), all of which suggest that NGF is involved in antiinflammatory responses. Furthermore, treatment of young rats with NGF prior to and after immunization with sheep erythrocytes results in an enhancement of T lymphocyte dependent antibody synthesis (Manning et al., 1985), suggesting a role for NGF in the modulation of immune responses. In humans NGF promotes colony growth and differentiation of myeloid progenitor cells (Matsuda et al., 1988, 1991), induces proliferation of both B and T lymphocyte populations (Thorpe and Perez-Polo, 1987; Thorpe et al., 1987; Otten et al., 1989; Brodie and Gelfand, 1992), stimulates production of IgG4 (Kimata et al., 1991), and modulates the formation of lipid mediators by mature basophils (Bischoff and Dahinden, 1992).

Studies on the regulatory mechanisms involved in NGF production have revealed that inflammatory stimuli contribute significantly to increased NGF production (Weskamp and Otten, 1987). Inflammatory mediators, in particular interleukin 1 (IL-1), tumor necrosis factor alpha (TNF-α), interleukin 6 (IL-6), and transforming growth factor beta 1 (TGF-β_1) have been described as potent inducers of NGF synthesis in peripheral tissues (Lindholm et al., 1987; Steiner et al., 1991; Hattori et al., 1993), in rat cortical astrocytes (Frei et al., 1989; Gadient et al., 1990; Spranger et al., 1990; Carman-Krzan et al., 1991) and in the CNS (Otten et al., 1990; Spranger et al., 1990; Lindholm et al., 1992b). The observations that, in vitro, activated rat peritoneal macrophages (Otten et al., 1987) and lipopolysaccharide-stimulated rat brain macrophages (Mallat et al., 1989) synthesize NGF, and that conditioned medium from lectin-activated lymphoid cells can maintain sympathetic neurons in culture (Gozes et al., 1983), all suggest that stimulated immune cells release NGF.

The multiple effects of NGF on various target cells depend on the initial binding of NGF to specific cell surface receptors. Two classes of NGF receptors can be distinguished by their low ($K_d \approx 10^{-9}$ M) or high ($K_d \approx 10^{-11}$ M) binding affinities (for review, see Chao, 1992; Meakin and Shooter, 1992). The low-affinity NGF receptor (LNGFR) belongs to a recently recognized superfamily of cytokine receptors, including two tumor necrosis factor receptors, the Fas cell surface antigen, the

T cell antigens OX40, CD27 and 4-1 BB, and B cell antigens CD40 and CD30 (Mallett and Barclay, 1991). However, the binding of NGF to LNGFR alone appears insufficient to mediate NGF signal transduction in contrast to binding to high-affinity NGF receptors (Green et al., 1986). Recent work has demonstrated that the *trk* protooncogene product, a transmembrane tyrosine kinase, is critical for NGF signal transduction. Other closely related tyrosine kinases, trkB and trkC, encode essential components of the receptors for BDNF and NT-3, respectively (for review see Chao, 1992; Meakin and Shooter, 1992). Whether trk constitutes the high-affinity NGF receptor by itself (Klein et al., 1991) or whether the functional receptor represents a complex of the LNGFR and trk (Hempstead et al., 1991; Kaplan et al., 1991) is still unclear.

In this chapter we will summarize the evidence that neurotrophins such as NGF are multifunctional, and that, in addition to their well characterized neurotrophic functions, they also act upon immune cells. NGF involvement in immune function is suggested by our demonstration that functional trk receptors are expressed on monocytes and lymphocytes; our findings that NGF levels are markedly raised in cerebrospinal fluid of patients with multiple sclerosis, in serum of patients with systemic lupus erythematosus, and in joints of patients affected by rheumatoid arthritis, indicate that NGF plays a pathophysiological role in these autoimmune diseases. Finally, we will discuss evidence that the cytokine, IL-6, also has neurotrophic actions, and therefore functions as a signal between the nervous and immune systems.

Role of cytokines in NGF synthesis

Studies on the regulatory mechanisms involved in NGF synthesis revealed that, in addition to neuronally mediated mechanisms, other stimuli, e.g., inflammation, contribute significantly to NGF production. The levels of NGF in damaged or inflamed tissue have been shown to be increased several-fold above normal levels (Weskamp and Otten, 1987; Aloe et al., 1992), and this effect can be detected within hours of the start of inflammation (Weskamp and Otten, 1987). Inflammatory mediators accumulating at sites of inflammation, in particular IL-1, TNF-α and transforming growth factors, are potent stimulators of NGF production by skin and nerve derived fibroblasts (Lindholm et al., 1987; Otten 1991; Hattori et al., 1993). Thus it is very probable that a cytokine cascade, including NGF as a principal component, coordinates immune system regulation, inflammation and specific nerve responses, such as nociception; for example, inflammation-induced increases in NGF in the periphery may be the link between tissue damage and the accompanying hyperalgesia (Lewin and Mendell, 1993). IL-1 and NGF have been found to accumulate at sites of brain injury, and glia, including astrocytes and microglial cells, are known to be potent producers of IL-1. It is therefore very probable that IL-1 also acts as a stimulator of NGF synthesis in brain, and in fact intrastriatal and intraventricular application of IL-1β has been shown to induce NGF synthesis (Otten et al., 1990; Spranger et al., 1990), implicating IL-1 as a physiological regulator of NGF synthesis in rat brain. Additional in vitro studies have shown that inflammatory cytokines, including IL-1 and TNF-α, which are produced by activated microglia following injury (see Perry et al., 1993), cooperatively enhance NGF secretion by astrocytes (Gadient et al., 1990).

To characterize cytokine-induced NGF expression we have introduced a new cellular model, the rat mesangial cell, allowing us to analyze in detail the mechanisms involved in cytokine-induced NGF synthesis that may play a crucial role in the modulation of kidney immune function (see Steiner et al., 1991). We found that simultaneous addition of IL-1β and TNF-α elicited within 24 h a marked (13-fold) increase in NGF protein release by cultured rat glomerular mesangial cells, whereas IL-1α in combination with TNF-α, or each cytokine alone, did not promote NGF synthesis. The synergistic IL-1β/TNF-α effect was dose dependent and caused a maximal 5-fold increase in NGF mRNA within 8 h. Stimulation of NGF synthesis was abolished by mepacrine or dexamethasone, indicating that phospholipase A_2 may be involved in NGF regulation. In addition, pretreatment of the cells with the lipoxygenase inhibitor, nordihydroguaiaretic acid, abolished induction of NGF by cytokines in a dose dependent fashion, but indomethacin and diclofenac at concentrations that completely inhibit cyclooxygenase activity failed to influence NGF synthesis. Our data suggest that phospholipase A_2 activation, and possibly lipoxygenase metabolites produced in response to cytokines, is involved in mesangial cell NGF expression. Studies are in progress to elucidate the physiological and pathophysiological role of mesangial cell derived NGF. Since recent data suggest that a phospholipase-lipoxygenase pathway mediates IL-1 stimulation of NGF release from astrocytes (Carman-Krzan and Wise, 1993), it appears rather probable that similar mechanisms are involved in cytokine-induced NGF synthesis in astroglial cells as well. The recent finding that isolated rat glomeruli synthesize NGF mRNA (Steiner et al., 1991) clearly documents the physiological relevance of our data. Since renal mesangial cells are considered central to the pathogenesis of immune mediated glomerulonephritis (Schlondorff, 1987; Radeke and Resch, 1992), our findings could indicate that a cytokine cascade is a significant part of the pathophysiology of inflammatory renal diseases.

Expression of functional NGF receptors in cells of the immune system

Monocytes

Given the evidence that NGF might act in the immune system, it was of interest to investigate whether monocytes/macrophages, which are known to be essential to immune responses and repair mechanisms (Perry et al., 1993), are influenced by neurotrophins such as NGF. We analyzed the expression of the trk protooncogene in human monocytes by reverse transcription combined with the polymerase chain reaction (RT/PCR). PCR amplification with primers specific for trk yielded a single band of the size expected for the amplified fragment. The identity of the PCR product was confirmed both by digestion with appropriate restriction enzymes (*Bam*HI and *Pst*I) and by hybridization to a trk-specific probe. As an external control, primers specific for a constitutively expressed control mRNA encoding the ribosomal protein S12 were used (Ehrhard et al., 1993a).

Using highly purified populations of human peripheral blood monocytes (purity $> 98\%$ as assessed by M3 + surface marker analysis, morphology, nonspecific esterase staining, and latex bead phagocytosis), we found that human monocytes express trk (Ehrhard et al., 1993a). This receptor is functional, since interaction of NGF with monocytes triggered respiratory burst activity, the major component of monocyte cytotoxic activity. During differentiation in vitro of human blood monocytes to macrophages (monitored by expression of maturation markers MAX-1 and α_2-macroglobulin), trk expression declined, indicating a maturation dependent trk regulation. Conversely, treatment of monocytes with *Staphylococcus aureus* Cowan I, a potent stimulator of monocyte activation, caused a marked upregulation of trk mRNA levels and of functional receptors. This suggests that NGF-trk interactions may be particularly relevant during immune responses. Our finding that dibutyryl cAMP induced expression of trk in a time dependent way in monocytes and in phorbol ester-differentiated U937 cells suggests that adenylate cyclase is involved in the mechanism of monocyte trk expression (Ehrhard et al., 1993a).

Surprisingly, monocytes did not express detectable levels of LNGFR message. This is in contrast to previous studies using immunofluorescence and radioimmunobinding techniques (Morgan et al., 1989; Otten et al., 1989) that indicated the presence of low-affinity surface membrane receptors for NGF on lymphocytes/monocytes. However, the techniques used in these studies did not permit an unequivocal discrimination between LNGFR and potential crossreactive molecules such as tumor necrosis factor receptor, OX40, CD40, the Fas antigen and CD30, which are all expressed on hematopoietic cells (Itoh et al., 1991; Mallet and Barclay, 1991; Dürkop et al., 1992).

Our data provide evidence that trk alone is sufficient to mediate biological activity in hematopoietic cells such as human monocytes. This is consistent with results from rat peritoneal mast cells which express trk at both the mRNA and protein levels, but not LNGFR (Horigome et al., 1993). Further confirmation that LNGFR may not be required for NGF signal transduction is provided by studies using neuronal cells showing that (1) PC12 cells are able to respond to NGF in the presence of a blocking antibody to LNGFR (Weskamp and Reichardt, 1991), (2) a mutant NGF molecule lacking a LNGFR binding site is still biologically active in PC12 cells (Ibáñez et al., 1992), and (3) developing neurons expressing trk but not LNGFR can still respond functionally to NGF (Birren et al., 1992).

NGF-trk interactions may be involved in nerve regeneration, since macrophages and cytokines recruited at sites of lesion have been shown to modulate neuronal survival as well as neurite fiber outgrowth, and cytokines, including IL-1, can potently upregulate the production of NGF at sites of injury (Lindholm et al., 1987). Moreover, injection of monocytes/macrophages near sensory nerve cell bodies in rat dorsal root ganglia significantly enhances axonal regeneration in the dorsal root (Lu and Richardson, 1991). Since NGF and monocytes colocalize at sites of inflammation and axonal injury, it is possible that NGF-monocytic trk interactions may by some mechanism be favorable to axonal regeneration. Under all conditions of brain injury, microglial cells activate and convert into active macrophages. Activated and reactive microglia participate in inflammatory processes, removal of cellular debris and wound healing (for review see Thomas, 1992). A key question is therefore whether a CNS injury that results in degeneration of neurons, their axons or cell bodies, causes changes in microglial trk expression similar to those seen in monocytes, if indeed trk is transcribed at all in these cells. In any case, the results presented here show that NGF has the potential to act as a signaling molecule mediating cross-talk between the immune and nervous systems.

Lymphocytes

A sensitive immunoprecipitation assay for the quantification of human NGF receptors was able to detect functional receptors on human B and T lymphocytes (Otten et al., 1989). Interaction of NGF with these receptors induced a proliferative response as well as the differentiation of B cells into antibody secreting cells. Given the evidence that NGF promotes T lymphocyte proliferation (Otten et al., 1989; Thorpe and Perez-Polo, 1989), we wanted to see whether NGF exerts its specific effects on T cells by interaction with LNGFR or trk, either alone or in combination. The synthesis of NGF-like neuronal maintenance activity by lymphoid cells (Gozes et al., 1983) also prompted us to see whether T cells release NGF. Using RT/PCR and flow cytometry, we have analyzed murine $CD4^+$ T cell clones for expression of LNGFR, trk and NGF mRNA (Ehrhard et al., 1993b). The generation, maintenance and functional characterization of $CD4^+$ murine keyhole limpet hemocyanin (KLH)-specific T cell clones 8/37 [T helper (Th) O type] 9/6 and 9/9 (both Th1 type), and of conalbumin-specific T cell clone D10.G4.1 (Th2 type) have been previously described (Kaye et al., 1983; Erb et al., 1991).

Activation of 8/37 T cells by a mitogenic stimulus (Con A) induced trk mRNA expression within 24 h, detectable by RT/PCR (Fig. 1, lane 2). T cell receptor-mediated activation by antigen and antigen presenting cells (KLH/A20.2J) also induced trk mRNA in 8/37 T cells, although induction was less pronounced than with Con A (Fig. 1, lane 3). In contrast, A20.2J cells cultured with KLH did not contain detectable trk mRNA (Fig. 1, lane 4), confirming that activated 8/37 T cells rather than the antigen-presenting cells are the site of trk synthesis. The expression of trk in activated 8/37 T cells is specific since neither mitogenic nor antigenic stimulation significantly changed ribosomal protein S12 mRNA levels (Fig. 1). In contrast to trk, no LNGFR mRNA was detected in 8/37 T cells after stimulation with mitogen or with antigen and antigen-presenting cells (APC) (Fig. 1). Analysis of other $CD4^+$ T cell clones revealed that stimulation with mitogen or by the T cell receptor pathway (with antigen and APC) induced the expression of trk in Th2-type clone D10.G4.1 and Th1-type clone 9/6 (Ehrhard et al., 1993b; Table 2). Furthermore, trk protein could be detected on the surface of the clones by flow cytometry, indicating that trk mRNA was translated. The expressed receptors were functional since interaction of these clones with NGF induced the transcription of the *c-fos* gene, a marker for NGF signal transduction. Expression of trk on activated murine $CD4^+$ T cells is consistent with data showing that NGF induces proliferation in human peripheral blood T lymphocytes (Otten et al., 1989), and in rat spleen lymphocytes (Thorpe and Perez-Polo, 1987) and stimulates the expression of IL-2 receptors on cultured human lymphocytes (Brodie and Gelfand, 1992). Con A, the most potent inducer of trk mRNA expression, also stimulated the transcription, synthesis and secretion of NGF by clones 8/37 and D10.G4.1 (Table 2). NGF and trk were both induced to a similar extent and over a similar time course in activated 8/37 T cells, raising the possibility that NGF and trk genes are under coordinate control (Ehrhard et al., 1993b). The finding that the Th1-type clone 9/9, a non-specific killer clone expressing natural killer surface markers, failed to express detectable NGF or trk transcripts after stimulation indicates that such expression is not a universal property of all activated $CD4^+$ T cells (Table 2). None of the activated $CD4^+$ T cell clones analyzed expressed detectable LNGFR transcripts, regardless of the stimulus used. We conclude that LNGFR is not involved in NGF signal transduction in $CD4^+$ T cells under these conditions.

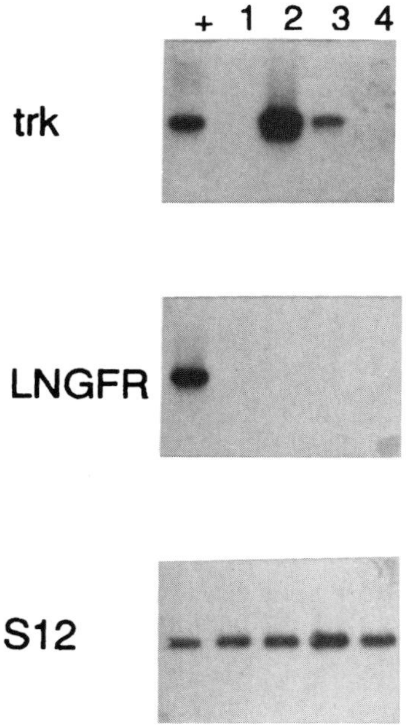

Fig. 1. Expression of trk and LNGF mRNA in T cell clone 8/37. T cells (5×10^6) were either untreated (lane 1) or activated with ConA (5 mg/ml) (lane 2) or with KLH (50 mg/ml) and 5×10^6 A20.2J cells (lane 3). Control cultures included KLH and A20.2J cells only (lane 4). After 24 h, total RNA was isolated, reverse-transcribed, and PCR-amplified using primers specific for trk (upper), for LNGFR (middle) and for ribosomal protein S12 (lower.). Lane + shows RNA that was extracted from PC12 cells used as a positive control.

The cooexpression of neurotrophins and neurotrophin receptors in the same cell population has been described for a wide variety of different cell types, including glial cells, keratinocytes and neurons. For example, enhanced synthesis of both NGF and LNGFR occurs in Schwann cells after rat sciatic nerve transection (Heumann et al., 1987; Lindholm et al., 1987) and primary cultures of rat astrocytes have been shown to produce NGF (Gadient et al., 1990) and to express LNGFR and trk mRNA (Hutton et al., 1992). Moreover, in situ hybridization experiments have shown that neurons, including sensory, sympathetic and hippocampal neurons, coexpress neurotrophins with cognate receptors (Schecterson and Bothwell, 1992). Thus NGF and other neurotrophins may support neuron survival by an autocrine mode of action. Our finding that activated $CD4^+$ T cell clones not only express trk but also synthesize and release biologically active NGF implicates

TABLE II

Expression of NGF and NGF receptor mRNAs in different CD4$^+$ T cell clones. T cells were stimulated for 24 h either with ConA (5 mg/ml), or with keyhole limpet hemocyanin (KLH) or conalbumin (100 mg/ml) and 5 × 10^6 irradiated (3000 rad) antigen-presenting cells (APC) in Iscove's medium containing 10% fetal calf serum and 50 mM 2-mercaptoethanol. The major histocompatibility complex class II-positive B lymphoma A20.2J was used as the APC for T cell clones 8/37, 9/6 and 9/9, and TA3 cells were used for clone D10.G4.1. Using reverse transcription combined with polymerase chain reaction (RT/PCR), CD4$^+$ T cell clones were analyzed for expression of trk, LNGFR and NGF mRNA (Modified from Ehrhard et al., 1993b.)

CD 4 + T cell clone	Subset		Activation	mRNA expression		
	Lymphokine Secretion	Effector Function		trk	LNGFR	NGF
9/6	Th 1	Killer and Suppressor	KLH/A20.2J	+	–	–
			Con A	–	–	–
8/37	Th 0	Helper	KLH/A20.2J	+	–	+
			Con A	+	–	+
D10.G4.1	Th 2	Helper	Conalbumin/TA3	+	–	–
			Con A	+	–	+
9/9	Th 1	Nonspecific Killer	KLH/A20.2J	–	–	–
			Con A	–	–	–

NGF as an autocrine and/or paracrine factor in the development and regulation of the immune response. The fact that this expression is part of a response to activation provides a functional connection between the nervous and immune systems. It should be borne in mind, however, that although T cells express trk and NGF, it has not yet been shown that NGF is required either for the survival of T (and B) cells, perhaps by suppression of apoptotic cell death (Rabizadeh et al., 1983), or for modulation of T cell functions such as cytotoxicity, delayed-type hypersensitivity or help with antibody formation. The involvement of NGF-related NTs in immune responses is also an open question. As a first step, we need to know whether T or B lymphocytes or monocytes express trkB or trkC and/or their cognate NTs.

Involvement of neurotrophins in neurodegenerative diseases

Neurodegenerative diseases which involve inflammation may provide valuable data about the pathophysiological role of NGF-cytokine interactions. Multiple sclerosis (MS) is a chronic recurrent inflammatory disease of the CNS which may be an autoimmune disorder. It is characterized by a patchy destruction of the myelin sheath, during which lymphocytes infiltrate white matter and release cytokines when stimulated. We have used a specific sandwich immunoassay (ELISA) to measure NGF content in the cerebrospinal fluid (CSF) of MS patients compared to CSF from age-matched normal subjects (Bracci-Laudiero et al., 1992). We found that during acute attacks patients exhibit a significant increase in NGF content compared to controls. In contrast, during remission the mean NGF level in CSF markedly declines. Thus, there is a good correlation between the inflammatory episodes of the disease and increased NGF production. Although the mechanisms controlling NGF expression are unclear, increased levels of inflammatory cytokines such as IL-1, IL-6 and TNGF-α, which are known to accumulate in the CSF of MS patients, could contribute to enhanced NGF production.

Systemic lupus erythematosus (SLE) is a multisystem autoimmune disease characterized by B cell hyperactivity, aberrant immune regulation and an excessive production of immunoglobulins and autoantibodies. We found a significant increase in NGF levels in the sera of SLE patients, and again a good correlation between inflammatory episodes of the disease and increase in NGF levels (Bracci-Laudiero et al., 1993) In addition, elevated NGF levels have been found in the synovial fluid of patients with rheumatoid arthritis. Typically, synovial fluid NGF correlates with the degree of apparent inflammation (Otten and Schilter, unpublished observations).

Since NGF accumulates at sites of inflammation, in the joints of patients affected by rheumatoid arthritis and in the CSF of MS patients, it is suggested that NGF is involved in the pathogenesis of autoimmune disorders. In line with this hypothesis are recent findings demonstrating high titers of autoantibodies to NGF in sera from patients with SLE, autoimmune thyroiditis and rheumatoid arthritis (Dicou et al., 1993).

IL-6: a candidate for a new neurotrophic factor

Cytokines initially identified as signals in the immune system have also been shown to exert specific effects on neurons (reviewed in Patterson and Nawa, 1993). These include a family comprising ciliary neurotrophic factor (CNTF), leukemia inhibitory factor (LIF, also known as cholinergic differentiation factor - CDF), oncostatin M and IL-6. Although the amino acid sequence homology of these molecules is quite low, they share a common receptor system consisting of a specific ligand binding subunit and a signal transducing receptor subunit, gp 130, which is shared by all receptors (Kishimoto et al., 1992). The extensive overlap between the cellular targets and neuron-specific activities of CNTF and LIF/CDF have led them to be considered as 'neurokines' or 'neuropoietic factors' (see Hall and Rao, 1992; Patterson and Nawa, 1993).

In the past few years it has become evident that the multifunctional cytokine, IL- 6, which has a key role in the regulation of hematopoiesis, immune responses, inflammation and the acute-phase reaction (Hirano et al., 1990), also exerts specific effects in the CNS. It promotes neuronal survival (Hama et al., 1989, 1991) and differentiation (Satoh et al., 1988) and modulates NGF production in astrocytes (Frei et al., 1989). Elevated IL-6 levels were detected in the CSF of patients with human immunodeficiency virus (HIV) infection (Laurenzi et al., 1990) and SLE (Hirohata and Miyamoto, 1990), and IL-6 immunoreactive material was found in amyloid plaques of Alzheimer's patients (Strauss et al., 1992). In addition, elevated IL-6 protein and mRNA levels have been found in the CNS of animals during neurodegeneration (Gijbels et al., 1990; Grau et al., 1990; Minami et al., 1991).

However, the cellular origin or site of action of this cytokine in the brain is not clear. Using RT/PCR, the expression of IL-6 and IL-6 receptor in various brain regions was analyzed. Our findings that IL-6 and IL-6 receptor are expressed in various brain regions, such as neocortex, hippocampus, hypothalamus, neostriatum, pons/medulla and cerebellum, and are developmentally regulated in a region-specific manner, strongly implicate the IL-6 system in the differentiation and maintenance of different neuronal subpopulations in the CNS (Gadient and Otten, 1993, 1994). Our results are in agreement with other recent studies showing IL-6 and IL-6 receptor message expression in various brain areas (Schöbitz et al., 1992, 1993).

Concluding remarks

Neurotrophins including NGF are clearly multifunctional (see Fig. 2), and increasing evidence indicates that NGF, in addition to its neurotrophic actions, regulates and is regulated by components of the immune system. In support of this we have found expression of functional trk protooncogene, constituting the signal transducing receptor for NGF, on monocytes and lymphocytes. In addition, a possible pathophysiological role for NGF in autoimmune disorders is suggested by our findings that NGF levels are

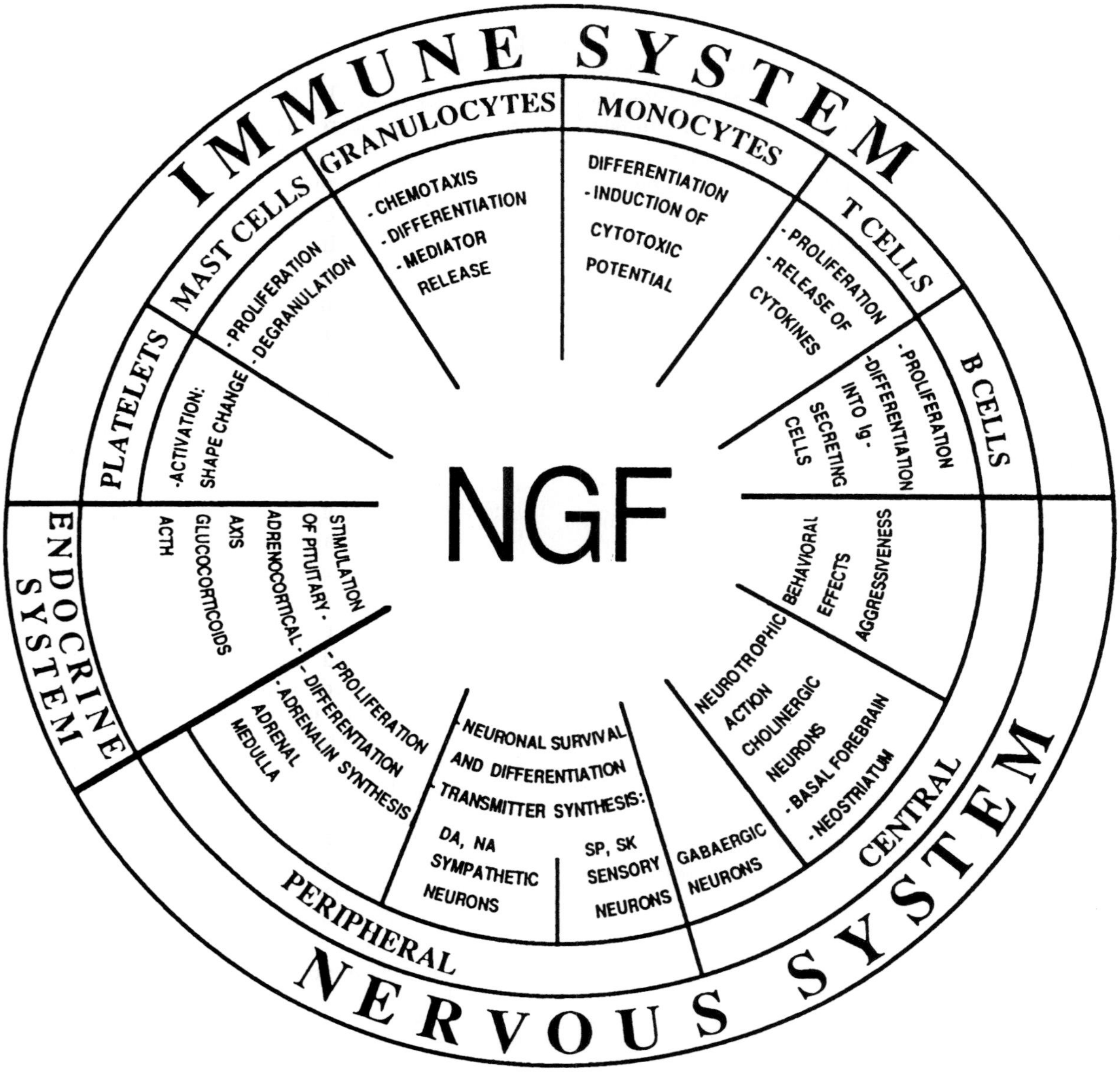

Fig. 2. Multiple biological effects of NGF.

markedly raised in cerebrospinal fluid of patients with MS and in serum of patients with SLE. As yet, it is completely unknown whether other members of the NGF-like NT family such as BDNF, NT-3, and NT-4/5 are also involved in modulation of immune system responses.

We have reviewed the evidence that IL-6, a major promoter of immune and inflammatory responses, also exerts specific effects in the CNS. Our findings that IL-6 and IL-6 receptor transcripts are coexpressed and developmentally regulated in a region-specific manner in rat brain strongly supports the suggestion that the cytokine, IL-6, also has neurotrophic actions.

Our experiments and others provide evidence for a significant degree of interaction between the nervous and immune systems. If such communication is physiologically important, then disturbances in homeostasis and in cross-talk between these systems would conceivably effect pathological changes leading, eventually, to neurodegenerative and autoimmune disorders. The idea has obvious clinical implications; but a clearer understanding of the mechanisms involved is essential as a basis for any possible therapeutic intervention.

Acknowledgements

This study was supported by the Swiss National Foundation for Scientific Research (Grant 31-29954.90), by the Deutsche Forschungsgemeinschaft (SFB 325), the Bundesministerium für Forschung und Technologie/BMFT (Grant 01KL89046) and by grants of the Roche Research Foundation and Stiftung E. Guggenheim-Schnurr, Basel, Switzerland.

References

Aloe, L. and Levi-Montalcini, R. (1977) Mast cell increase in tissues of neonatal rats injected with the nerve growth factor. *Brain Res.*, 133: 358–366.

Aloe, L., Alleva, E., Bohm, A. and Levi-Montalcini, R. (1986) Nerve growth factor mRNA and protein increase in hypothalamus in a mouse model of aggression. *Proc. Natl. Acad. Sci. USA*, 86: 8555–8559.

Aloe, L., Tuveri, M., Carcassi, U. and Levi-Montalcini, R. (1992) Nerve growth factor in the synovial fluid of patients with chronic arthritis. *Arthritis Rheum.*, 35: 351–355.

Barbany, G. and Persson, H. (1992) Regulation of neurotrophin mRNA expression in the rat brain by glucocorticoids. *Eur. J. Neurosci.*, 4: 404- 410.

Berkemeier, L.R., Winslow, J.W., Kaplan, D.R., Nikolics, K., Goeddel, D.V. and Rosenthal, A. (1991) Neurotrophin-5: a novel neurotrophic factor that activates trk and trkB. *Neuron*, 7: 857–866.

Birren, S.J., Verdi, J.M. and Anderson, D.J. (1992) Membrane depolarization induces p140trk and NGF responsiveness, but not p75LNGFR, in MAH cells. *Science*, 257: 395–397.

Bischoff, S.C. and Dalhinden, C.A. (1992) Effect of nerve growth factor on the release of inflammatory mediators by mature human basophils. *Blood*, 79: 2662–2669.

Bracci-Laudiero, L., Aloe, L., Levi-Montalcini, R., Buttinelli, C., Schilter, D., Gillessen, S. and Otten, U. (1992) Multiple sclerosis patients express increased levels of β-nerve growth factor in cerebrospinal fluid. *Neurosci. Lett.*, 147: 9–12.

Bracci-Laudiero, L., Aloe, L., Levi-Montalcini, R., Galeazzi, M., Schilter, D., Scully, J.L and Otten, U. (1993) Increased levels of NGF in sera of systemic lupus erythematosus patients. *NeuroReport*, 4: 563–565.

Brodie, C. and Gelfand, E.W. (1992) Functional nerve growth factor receptors on human B lymphocytes – Interaction with IL-2. *J. Immunol.*, 148: 3492–3497.

Bruni, A., Bigon, E., Boarato, E., Mietto, L., Leon, A. and Toffano, G. (1982) Interaction between nerve growth factor and lysophosphatidylserine on rat peritoneal mast cells. *FEBS Lett.*, 138: 190–192.

Carman-Krzan, M. and Wise, B.C. (1993) Arachidonic acid lipoxygenation may mediate interleukin-1 stimulation of nerve growth factor secretion in astroglial cultures. *J. Neurosci. Res.*, 34: 225–232.

Carman-Krzan, M., Vigé, X. and Wise, B.C. (1991) Regulation by interleukin-1 of nerve growth factor secretion and nerve growth factor mRNA expression in rat primary astrocyte cultures. *J. Neurochem.*, 56: 636–643.

Chao, M.V. (1992) Neurotrophin receptors: a window into neuronal differentiation. *Neuron*, 9: 583–593.

Dicou, E., Hurez, D. and Nerrière, V. (1993) Natural autoantibodies against the nerve growth factor in autoimmune diseases. *J. Neuroimmunol.*, 47: 159–168.

Dürkop, H., Latza, U., Hummel, M., Eitelbach, F., Seed, B. and Stein, H. (1992) Molecular cloning and expression of a new member of the nerve growth factor receptor family that is characteristic of Hodgkin's disease. *Cell*, 68: 421–427.

Ehrhard, P.B., Ganter, U., Bauer, J. and Otten, U. (1993a) Expression of functional trk protooncogene in human moncytes. *Proc. Natl. Acad. Sci. USA*, 90: 5423–5427.

Ehrhard, P.B., Erb, P., Graumann, U. and Otten, U. (1993b) Expression of nerve growth factor and nerve growth factor receptor for tyrosine kinase Trk in activated CD4-positive T cell clones. *Proc. Natl. Acad. Sci. USA*, 90:10984–10988.

Erb, P., Troxler, M., Fluri, M., Grogg, D. and Alkan, S.S. (1991) Functional heterogeneity of CD4-positive T cell subsets: the correlation between effector functions and lymphokine secretion is limited. *Cell. Immunol.*, 135: 232–244.

Figueiredo, B.C., Otten, U., Strauss, S., Volk, B. and Maysinger, D. (1993) Effects of perinatal hypo- and hyperthyroidism on the levels of nerve growth factor and its low-affinity receptor in cerebellum. *Dev. Brain Res.*, 72: 237–244.

Frei, K., Malipiero, U.V., Leist, T.P., Zinkernagel, R.M., Schwab, M.E. and Fontana, A. (1989) On the cellular source and function of interleukin-6 produced in the central nervous system in viral diseases. *Eur. J. Immunol.*, 19: 689–694.

Gadient, R.A. and Otten, U. (1993) Differential expression of interleukin-6 and interleukin-6 receptor mRNAs in rat hypothalamus. *Neurosci. Lett.*, 153: 13- 16.

Gadient, R.A. and Otten, U. (1994) Expression of interleukin-6 and interleukin-6 receptor mRNAs in rat brain during postnatal development. *Brain Res.*, 637: 10–14.

Gadient, R.A., Cron, K.C. and Otten, U. (1990) Interleukin-1 β and tumor necrosis factor-α synergistically stimulate nerve growth factor release from cultured astrocytes. *Neurosci. Lett.*, 117: 335–340.

Gijbels, K., van Damme, J., Proost, P., Put, W., Carton, H. and Billiau, A. (1990) Interleukin-6 production in the central nervous system during experimental autoimmune encephalomyelitis. *Eur. J. Immunol.*, 20: 233–235.

Gozes, Y., Moskowitz, M.A., Strom, T.B. and Gozes, I. (1983) Conditioned media from activated lymphocytes maintain sympathetic neurons in culture. *Dev. Brain Res.*, 6: 93–97.

Grau, G.E., Frei, K., Pigues, P., Fontana, A., Heremans, H., Billiau, A., Vasalli, P. and Lambert, P. (1990) Interleukin 6 production in experimental cerebral malaria: modulation by anticytokine antibodies and possible role in hypergammaglobulinemia. *J. Exp. Med.*, 172: 1505–1508.

Green, S.H., Rydel, R.E., Conolly, J.L. and Greene, L.A. (1986) PC12 cell mutants that possess low- but not high-affinity nerve growth factor receptors neither respond to nor internalize nerve growth factor. *J. Cell Biol.*, 102: 830–843.

Gudat, F., Laubscher, A., Otten, U. and Pletscher, A. (1981) Shape changes induced by biologically active peptides and nerve growth factor in blood platelets of rabbits. *Br. J. Pharmacol.*, 74: 533–538.

Hall, A.K. and Rao, M.S. (1992) Cytokines and neurokines: related ligands and related receptors. *Trends Neurosci.*, 15: 35–37.

Hallböök, F., Ibáñez, C.F. and Persson, H. (1991) Evolutionary studies of the nerve growth factor family reveal a novel member abundantly expressed in *Xenopus* ovary. *Neuron*, 6: 845–858.

Hama, T., Miyamoto, M., Tsukui, H., Nishio, C. and Hatanaka, H. (1989) Interleukin-6 as a neurotrophic factor for promoting the survival of cultured basal forebrain cholinergic neurons from postnatal rats. *Neurosci. Lett.*, 104: 340–344.

Hama, T., Kushima, Y., Miyamoto, M., Kubota, M., Takei, N. and Hatanaka, H. (1991) Interleukin-6 improves the survival of mesencephalic catecholaminergic and septal cholinergic neurons from postnatal two-week-old rats in cultures. *Neuroscience*, 40: 445–452.

Hattori, A., Tanaka, E., Murase, K., Ishida, N., Chatani, Y., Tsujimoto, M., Hayashi, K. and Kohno, M. (1993) Tumor necrosis factor stimulates the synthesis and secretion of biologically active nerve growth factor in non-neuronal cells. *J. Biol. Chem.*, 268: 2577–2582.

Hempstead, B.L., Martin-Zanca, D., Kaplan, D.R., Parada, L.F. and Chao, M.V. (1991) High-affinity NGF binding requires coexpression of the trk protooncogene and the low-affinity NGF receptor. *Nature (Lond.)*, 350: 678–683.

Heumann, R., Lindholm, D., Bandtlow, C., Meyer, M., Radeke, M.J., Misko, T.P., Shooter, E.M. and Thoenen, H. (1987) Differential regulation of mRNA encoding nerve growth factor and its receptor in rat sciatic nerve during development, degeneration and regeneration, role of macrophages. *Proc. Natl. Acad. Sci. USA*, 84: 8735–8739.

Hirano, T., Akira, S., Taga, T. and Kishimoto, T. (1990) Biological and clinical aspects of interleukin-6. *Immunol. Today*, 11: 443–449.

Hirohata, S. and Miyamoto, T. (1990) Elevated levels of interleukin-6 in cerebrospinal fluid from patients with systemic lupus erythematosus and central nervous system involvement. *Arthritis Rheum.*, 33: 644–649.

Hohn, A., Leibrock, J., Bailey, K. and Barde, Y.A. (1990) Identification and characterization of a novel member of the nerve growth factor/brain-derived neurotrophic factor family. *Nature (Lond.)*, 344: 339–341.

Horigome, K., Pryor, J.C., Bullock, E.D. and Johnson, E.M. (1993) Mediator release from mast cells by nerve growth factor. *J. Biol. Chem.*, 268: 14881–14887.

Hutton, L.A., de Vellis, J. and Perez-Polo, J.R. (1992) Expression of p75NGFR, trkA and trkB mRNA in rat C6 glioma and type I astrocyte cultures. *Neurosci. Res.*, 32: 375–383.

Ibáñez, C.F, Ebendal, T., Barbany, G., Murray Rust, J., Blundell, T.L. and Persson, H. (1992) Disruption of the low affinity receptor-binding site in NGF allows neuronal survival and differentiation by binding to the trk gene product. *Cell*, 69: 329–341.

Ip, N.Y., Ibáñez, C.F., Nye, S.H., McClain, J., Jones, P.F., Gies, D.R., Belluscio, L., LeBeau, M.M., Espinosa, R., III, Squinto, S.P., Persson, H. and Yancopoulos, G.D. (1992) Mammalian neurotrophin-4: structure, chromosomal localization, tissue distribution and receptor specificity. *Proc. Natl. Acad. Sci. USA*, 89: 3060- 3064.

Itoh, N., Yonehara, S., Ishii, A., Yonehara, M., Mizushima, S.I., Sameshima, M., Hase, A., Seto, Y. and Nagata, S. (1991) The polypeptide encoded by the cDNA for human cell surface antigen Fas can mediate apoptosis. *Cell*, 66: 233–243.

Jones, K.R. and Reichardt, L.F. (1990) Molecular cloning of the human gene that is a member of the nerve growth factor family. *Proc. Natl. Acad. Sci. USA*, 87: 8060- 8064.

Kaplan, D.R., Hempstead, B.L., Martin-Zanca, D., Chao, M.V. and Parada, L.F. (1991) The trk protooncogene product: a signal transducing receptor for nerve growth factor. *Science*, 252: 554–558.

Kaye, J., Porcelli, S., Tite, J., Jones, B. and Janeway, C.A. (1983) Both a monoclonal antibody and antisera specific for determinants unique to individual cloned helper T cell lines can substitute for antigen and antigen-presenting cells in the activation of T cells. *J. Exp. Med.*, 158: 836–856.

Kimata, H., Yoshida, A., Ishioka, C., Kusunoki, T., Hosoi, S. and Mikawa, H. (1991) Nerve growth factor specifically induces human IgG4 production. *Eur. J. Immunol.*, 21: 137–141.

Kishimoto, T., Akira, S. and Taga, T. (1992) Interleukin-6 and its receptor: a paradigm for cytokines. *Science*, 258: 593–597.

Klein, R., Jing, S., Nanduri, V., O'Rourke, E. and Barbacid, M. (1991) The trk proto-oncogene: a receptor for nerve growth factor. *Cell*, 65: 189–197.

Korsching, S. (1993) The neurotrophic factor concept: a reexamination. *J. Neurosci.*, 13: 2739–2748.

Laurenzi, M.A., SidÄn, A., Persson, M.A.A., Norkrans, G., Hagberg, L. and Chiodi, F. (1990) Cerebrospinal fluid interleukin-6 activity in HIV infection and inflammatory and noninflammatory diseases of the nervous system. *Clin. Immunol. Immunopathol.*, 57: 233–241.

Leibrock, J., Lottspeich, F., Hohn, A., Hofer, M., Hengerer, B., Masiakowski, P., Thoenen, H. and Barde, Y.A. (1989) Molecular cloning and expression of brain-derived neurotrophic factor. *Nature (Lond.)*, 341: 149–152.

Levi-Montalcini, R. (1987) The nerve growth factor 35 years later. *Science*, 237: 1154–1162.

Levi-Montalcini, R., Aloe, L. and Alleva, E. (1990) A role for nerve growth factor in nervous, endocrine and immune systems. *Prog. Neuroendocrinimmunol.*, 3: 1- 10.

Lewin, G.R. and Mendell, L.M. (1993) Nerve growth factor and nociception. *Trends Neurosci.*, 16: 353–359.

Lindholm, D., Heumann, R. and Thoenen, H. (1987) Interleukin-1 regulates synthesis of nerve growth factor in nonneuronal cells of rat sciatic nerve. *Nature (Lond.)*, 330: 658–659.

Lindholm, D., Castrén, E., Hengerer, B., Zafra, F., Berninger, B. and Thoenen, H. (1992a) Differential regulation of nerve growth factor synthesis in neurons and astrocytes by glucocorticoid hormones. *Eur. J. Neurosci.*, 4: 396–403.

Lindholm, D., Castrén, E., Kiefer, R., Zafra, F. and Thoenen, H. (1992b) Transforming growth factor-β1 in the rat brain: increase after injury and inhibition of astrocyte proliferation. *J. Cell Biol.*, 117: 395–400.

Lu, X. and Richardson, P.M. (1991) Inflammation near the nerve cell body enhances axonal regeneration. *J. Neurosci.*, 11: 972–978.

Maisonpierre, P.C., Belluscio, L., Squinto, S.P., Ip, N.Y., Furth, M.E., Lindsay, R.M. and Yancopoulos, G.D. (1990) Neurotrophin-3: a neurotrophic factor related to NGF and BDNF. *Science*, 247: 1446–1451.

Mallett, S. and Barclay, A.N. (1991) A new superfamily of cell surface proteins related to the nerve growth factor receptor. *Immunol. Today*, 12: 220- 223.

Mallat, M., Houlgatte, R., Brachet, P. and Prochiantz, A. (1989) Lipopolysaccharide-stimulated rat brain macrophages release NGF in vitro. *Dev. Biol.*, 133: 309–311.

Manning, P.T., Russell, J.H., Simmons, B. and Johnson, E.M. (1985) Protection from guanethidine-induced neuronal destruction by nerve growth factor: effects of NGF on immune function. *Brain Res.*, 340: 61–69.

Matsuda, H., Coughlin, M.D., Bienenstock, J. and Denburg, J. (1988) Nerve growth factor promotes human hemopoietic colony growth and differentiation. *Proc. Natl. Acad. Sci. USA*, 85: 6508–6512.

Matsuda, H., Kannan, Y., Ushio, H., Kiso, Y., Kanemoto, T., Suzuki, H. and Kitamura, Y. (1991) Nerve growth factor induces development of connective tissue-type mast cells in vitro from murine bone marrow cells. *J. Exp. Med.*, 174: 7–14.

Mazurek, N., Weskamp, G., Erne, E. and Otten, U. (1986) Nerve growth factor induces mast cell degranulation without changing intracellular calcium levels. *FEBS Lett.*, 198: 315–320.

Meakin, S.O. and Shooter, E.M. (1992) The nerve growth factor family of receptors. *Trends Neurosci.*, 15: 323–331.

Minami, M., Kuraishi, Y. and Satoh, M. (1991) Effects of kainic acid on messenger RNA levels of IL-1β, IL-6, TNF-α and LIF in the rat brain. *Biochem. Biophys. Res. Commun.*, 176: 593–598.

Mobley, W.C., Woo, J.E., Edwards, R.H., Riopelle, R.J., Longo, F.M., Weskamp, G., Otten, U., Valetta, J.S. and Johnston, M.V. (1989) Developmental regulation of nerve growth factor and its receptor in the rat caudate putamen. *Neuron*, 3: 655–664.

Morgan, B., Thorpe, L.W., Marchetti, D. and Perez-Polo, J.R. (1989) Expression of nerve growth factor receptors by human peripheral blood mononuclear cells. *J. Neurosci. Res.*, 23: 41–45.

Otten, U. (1991) Nerve growth factor: a signaling protein between the nervous and the immune systems. In: A. Basbaum and J. Besson (Eds.), *Toward a new pharmacotherapy of pain*, J. Wiley and Sons, New York, pp. 353–363.

Otten, U., Baumann, J.B. and Girard, J. (1979) Stimulation of the pituitary-adrenocortical axis by nerve growth factor. *Nature (Lond.)*, 282: 413- 414.

Otten, U., Baumann, J.B. and Girard, J. (1984) Nerve growth factor induces plasma extravasation in rat skin. *Eur. J. Pharmacol.*, 106: 199–201.

Otten, U., Weskamp, G., Hardung, M. and Meyer, D.K. (1987) Synthesis and release of nerve growth factor by rat macrophages. *Soc. Neurosci. Abstr.*, 13: 184.

Otten, U., Ehrhard, P and Peck, R. (1989) Nerve growth factor induces growth and differentiation of human B lymphocytes. *Proc. Natl. Acad. Sci. USA*, 86: 10059–10063.

Otten, U., Boeckh, C., Ehrhard, P., Gadient, R.A. and Frankenberg, M. (1990) Molecular mechanisms of nerve growth factor biosynthesis in rat central nervous system. In:

H. Kewitz, T. Thomson and U. Bickel (Eds.), *Pharmacological interventions on central cholinergic mechanisms in senile dementia (Alzheimer's disease)*, Zuckschwerdt Verlag, München, pp. 20–27.

Patterson, P.H. and Nawa, H. (1993) Neuronal differentiation factors/cytokines and synaptic plasticity. *Neuron*, 10: 123–137.

Pearce, F.L. and Thompson, H.L. (1986) Some characteristics of histamine secretion from rat peritoneal mast cells stimulated with nerve growth factor. *J. Physiol.*, 372: 379–393.

Perry, V.H., Andersson, P.B. and Gordon, S. (1993) Macrophages and inflammation in the central nervous system. *Trends Neurosci.*, 16: 268–273.

Rabizadeh, S., Oh, J., Zhong, L.-T., Yang, J., Bitler, C.M., Butcher, L.L. and Bredesen, D.E. (1993) Induction of apoptosis by the low-affinity NGF receptor. *Science*, 261: 345–348.

Radeke, H.H. and Resch, K. (1992) The inflammatory function of renal glomerular mesangial cells and their interaction with the cellular immune system. *Clin. Invest.*, 70: 825–842.

Rosenthal, A., Goeddel, D.V., Nguyen, T., Lewis, M., Shih, A., Laramee, G.R., Nikolics, K. and Winslow, J.W. (1990) Primary structure and biological activity of a novel human neurotrophic factor. *Neuron*, 4: 767–773.

Satoh, T., Nakamura, S., Taga, T., Matsuda, T., Hirano, T., Kishimoto, T. and Kaziro, Y. (1988) Induction of neuronal differentiation in PC12 cells by B-cell stimulatory factor 2/interleukin-6. *Mol. Cell. Biol.*, 8: 3546–3549.

Schecterson, L.C. and Bothwell, M. (1992) Novel roles for neurotrophins are suggested by BDNF and NT3 mRNA expression in developing neurons. *Neuron*, 9: 449–463.

Schlondorff, D. (1987) The glomerular mesangial cell: an expanding role for a specialized pericyte. *FASEB J.*, 1: 272–281.

Schöbitz, B., De Kloet, E.R., Sutanto, W. and Holsboer, F. (1993) Cellular localization of interleukin 6 mRNA and interleukin 6 receptor mRNA in rat brain. *Eur. J. Neurosci.*, 5: 1426–1435.

Schöbitz, B., Voorhuis, D.A.M. and De Kloet, E.R. (1992) Localization of interleukin 6 mRNA and interleukin receptor mRNA in rat brain. *Neurosci. Lett.*, 136: 189–192.

Scully, J.L. and Otten, U. (1993) Glucocorticoid modulation of neurotrophin expression in immortalized mouse hippocampal neurons. *Neurosci. Lett.*, 155: 11–14.

Spranger, M., Lindholm, D., Bandtlow, C., Heumann, R., Gnahn, H., Näher-Noe, M. and Thoenen, H. (1990) Regulation of nerve growth factor synthesis in the rat central nervous system: comparison between the effects of interleukin-1 and various growth factors in astrocyte cultures and in vivo. *Eur. J. Neurosci.*, 2: 69–76.

Steiner, P., Pfeilschifter, J., Boeckh, C., Radeke, H. and Otten, U. (1991) Interleukin-1β and tumor necrosis factor-α synergistically stimulate nerve growth factor synthesis in rat mesangial cells. *Am. J. Physiol.*, 261: F792–798.

Strauss, S., Bauer, J., Ganter, U., Jonas, U., Berger, M. and Volk, B. (1992) Detection of interleukin-6 and α_2-macroglobulin immunoreactivity in cortex and hippocampus of Alzheimer's disease patients. *Lab. Invest.*, 66: 223–230.

Taglialatela, G., Angelucci, L., Scaccianoce, S., Foreman, P.J. and Perez-Polo, J.R. (1991) Nerve growth factor modulates the activation of the hypothalamo-pituitary-adrenocortical axis during the stress response. *Endocrinology*, 129: 2212–2218.

Thoenen, H., Bandtlow, C. and Heumann, R. (1987) The physiological function of nerve growth factor in the central nervous system: comparison with the periphery. *Rev. Physiol. Biochem. Pharmacol.*, 109: 145–178.

Thomas, W.E. (1992) Brain macrophages: evaluation of microglia and their functions. *Brain Res. Rev.*, 17: 61–74.

Thorpe, L.W. and Perez-Polo, J.R. (1987) The influence of nerve growth factor on the in vitro proliferative response of rat spleen lymphocytes. *J. Neurosci. Res.*, 18: 134–139.

Thorpe, L.W., Stack, R.W., Hashim, G.A., Marchetti, D. and Perez-Polo, J.R. (1987) Receptors for nerve growth factor on rat spleen mononuclear cells. *J. Neurosci. Res.*, 17: 128–134.

Walker, P., Weichsel, M.E., Fisher, D., Guo, S.M. and Fisher, D.A. (1979) Thyroxine increases nerve growth factor concentration in adult mouse brain. *Science*, 204: 427–429.

Walker, P., Wil, M.L., Weichsel, M.E. and Fisher, D.A. (1981) Effect of thyroxine on nerve growth factor concentration in neonatal mouse brain. *Life Sci.*, 28: 1777–1787.

Weskamp, G. and Otten, U. (1987) An enzyme-linked immunoassay for nerve growth factor: a tool for studying regulatory mechanisms involved in NGF production in brain and peripheral tissues. *J. Neurochem.*, 48: 779–1786.

Weskamp, G. and Reichardt, L.F. (1991) Evidence that biological activity of NGF is mediated through a novel subclass of high affinity receptors. *Neuron*, 6: 649–663.

F.J. Seil (Ed.)
Progress in Brain Research, Vol 103

CHAPTER 25

Class I and II MHC expression and its implications for regeneration in the nervous system

L.A. Lampson, A. Grabowska and J.P. Whelan

Center for Neurologic Diseases, Department of Medicine, Division of Neurology, Brigham and Women's Hospital, and Department of Neurology, Harvard Medical School, Boston MA 02115, USA

Introduction

The major histocompatibility complex (MHC) is a multigene family whose products play an essential role in the cell-mediated immune response (Lampson, 1987; Armstrong and Lampson, 1994). It is thought that MHC proteins may participate in nonimmunologic cell-cell interactions as well (Lampson, 1984). In this chapter we review neural MHC expression under a variety of developmental, pathological, and experimental conditions. Ways in which the predominant patterns of neural MHC expression are most likely to influence neural regeneration are discussed.

Functions that may be served by MHC$^+$ cells

Antigen presentation to T cells

T lymphocytes do not recognize free antigen. Rather, they recognize antigen that is expressed on a cell surface in association with an MHC protein. In other words, antigen is presented to T cells as an antigen/MHC complex, and T cells are restricted by the requirement to recognize antigen/MHC rather than free antigen (Lampson, 1987; Armstrong and Lampson, 1994). Two major families of MHC proteins can present antigen to T cells. The class I MHC proteins consist of a highly polymorphic heavy chain and an invariant light chain, β2-microglobulin. The class I molecules are called 'HLA-A,B,C' and 'H-2' in humans and mice, respectively.

Typically, the class I MHC proteins present antigen that is synthesized within the antigen-expressing cell itself. Viral or tumour-associated antigens are examples. Nascent viral protein or tumor antigen is broken down within the cytosol. Fragments then become complexed to class I molecules within the endoplasmic reticulum, and the antigen/MHC complex is transported to the cell surface (Fig. 1, top).

The second major class of MHC proteins, the class II MHC proteins, consist of two highly polymorphic chains, the α and β chains. The class II molecules are called 'HLA-D' in humans, and 'Ia' in mice. Typically, the class II MHC proteins present ingested antigen. The ingested protein is broken down, its fragments are complexed to class II MHC proteins within intracellular vesicles, and the antigen/MHC complex is then transported to the cell surface. Secreted or released products of infected, transformed or damaged cells may be presented to T cells in this way (Fig. 1, bottom).

Functions of MHC-restricted T cells

Traditionally, different functions have been assigned to class I-restricted and class II-restricted T cells. Cytotoxic T lymphocytes (CTL), which

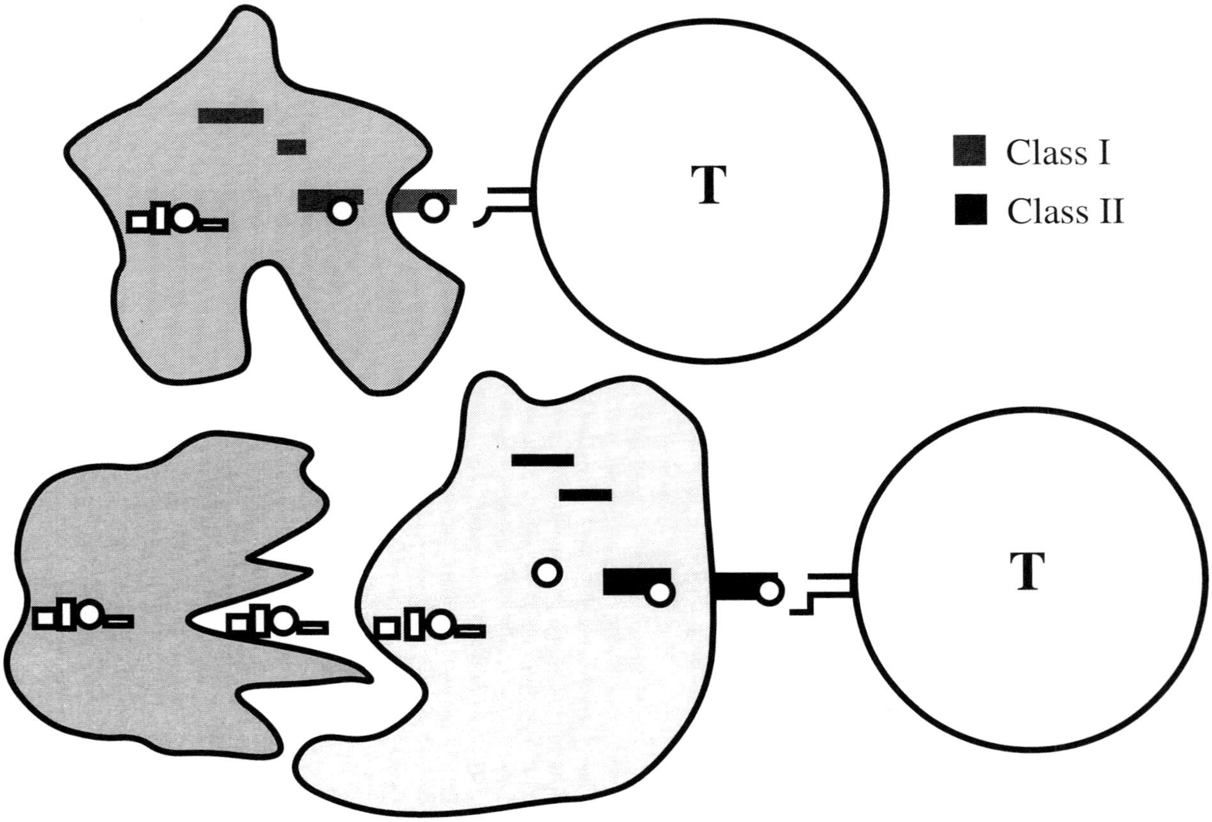

Fig. 1. Antigen presentation to T cells. The two major pathways of MHC-restricted antigen presentation are illustrated. (Top) A foreign protein (small white shapes) is broken down within the cell that synthesized it. An antigenic fragment (small white circle) is complexed to a two-chain class I MHC protein (dark grey rectangles) within the cell. The antigen/class I complex is presented at the cell surface, where it can be recognized by an appropriate T cell. This is the major pathway by which cytotoxic T lymphocytes (CTL) recognize antigen on their targets. The result is the direct attack of the antigen-bearing target cell. (Bottom) The cell that synthesized the foreign protein (small white shapes) has released or secreted it. The protein has been ingested by an antigen-presenting cell (APC) (the central cell). The protein is broken down within the APC. An antigenic fragment (small white circle) is complexed to a two-chain class II MHC protein (black rectangles) within the APC. The antigen/class II complex is presented at the cell surface, where it can be recognized by an appropriate T cell. This is the major pathway by which helper/inducer T lymphocytes (Th) recognize antigen on APC. Th help to initiate and regulate the CTL response (top of figure). Antigen presentation to Th can also lead to the DTH (delayed-type hypersensitivity) response, a cascade that results in accumulation of additional inflammatory cells, and their secreted cytokines (see Fig. 2). As part of the DTH response, the original antigen-bearing cell may be damaged as a bystander, even if it is not itself directly recognized by the T cell. By this mechanism, damaged or regenerating neural cells that express foreign antigen may be subject to T cell-mediated attack, even if they are not directly recognized by the T cells.

directly lyse their targets, are often class I-restricted. Helper T cells (Th), which secrete immunoactive cytokines, are often class II-restricted. Cells that process ingested antigen and present it to class II-restricted Th are called 'antigen-presenting cells (APC)'. Th play several different regulatory roles in the immune system, including initiation and regulation of CTL responses. Cytokines secreted by Th can initiate the delayed-type hypersensitivity (DTH) cascade, bringing additional inflammatory cells and their secreted cytokines to the site.

More recently, the traditional demarcations between CTL and Th have given way to a more complex picture. Although CTL can lyse their targets in vitro, this need not be the only way, or even the major way, that they influence their targets in vivo. CTL can also secrete immunoactive cytokines, including many of those secreted by Th. Conversely, Th can directly lyse targets, as well as secreting cytokines (reviewed in Armstrong and Lampson, 1994).

For a cell expressing antigen/MHC complexes, the consequences of recognition by a given T cell depend upon the cell's susceptibility to several factors: the direct lytic mechanism used by the T cell, the cytokines secreted by the T cell, and the lytic mechanism or secreted cytokines of other cells that may be attracted to the site. A cell that is adjacent to the cell expressing the antigen/MHC complex may also be affected, even if it does not itself express antigen or MHC proteins (Mason, 1988). The effect on the adjacent or bystander cell will depend upon its susceptibility to the cytokines secreted by the T cell, and to the lytic mechanism or secreted cytokines of secondary cells that are attracted to the site.

The complexity of interaction among cells expressing antigen/MHC complexes, responding T cells, bystander cells, secondary cells and secreted cytokines means that MHC expression must be evaluated at the level of the whole tissue rather than at the single cell level. The role of secondary or bystander effects is of particular interest in tissues, including neural tissue, with restricted patterns of MHC expression (Fig. 2).

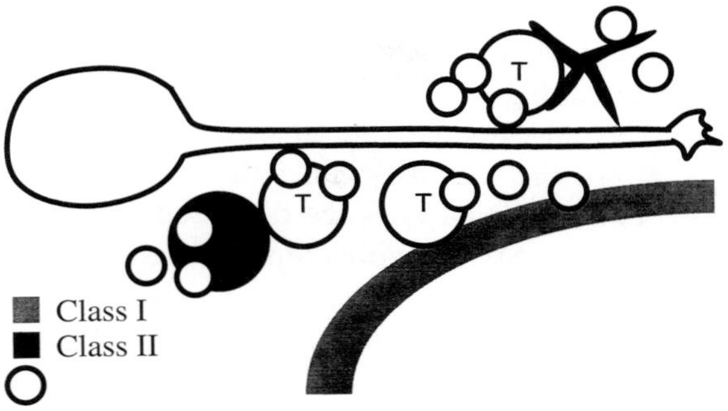

Fig. 2. MHC$^+$ and cytokine-secreting cells in the CNS. The predominant pattern of MHC expression, found under a variety of experimental and pathological conditions, is illustrated. The strongest class I expression is in the walls of the blood vessels (grey arc), within the endothelial cells. The strongest class II expression is in blood-borne monocytes (round black cell) and microglia (stellate black cell). Neural cells themselves (neurons, astrocytes, oligodendrocytes) do not show detectable MHC expression. T cells can recognize antigen/MHC complexes on the different MHC$^+$ cells. Cytokines may be secreted into the environment by the T cells, or by the MHC$^+$ cells. Adjacent neural cells may be exposed to the secreted cytokines, even if they are not directly recognized by the T cells.

MHC expression, T cell function, and secreted cytokines: summary and implications

A cell's susceptibility to direct T cell surveillance depends upon its MHC repertoire. If the cell can display appropriate complexes between antigen and MHC proteins, this permits direct recognition by antigen-specific, MHC-restricted T cells (Fig. 1, top).

At the level of the whole tissue, the situation is more complex. Once T cells have recognized antigen/MHC and begun to secrete cytokines, it is possible that adjacent cells can also be affected, even if they themselves do not express either antigen or MHC molecules (Fig. 1, bottom; Fig. 2). The importance of such a bystander effect is only now being defined. It is of particular interest in neural tissue because of the characteristic pattern of neural MHC expression, as described in succeeding sections.

Regenerating neural tissue offers several potential sources of antigen. Damaged cells, regenerating cells, and adjacent cells may all express molecules that are not found in normal adult neural tissue, and so may potentially be recognized by T cells as 'foreign'. The pattern of MHC expression within the regenerating tissue will determine which T cell populations can be stimulated, and whether direct or indirect recognition of regenerating cells can occur. Although MHC$^+$ cells play an essential role in stimulating T cells, this is not the way they can influence regeneration. Two additonal ways are discussed below.

Increased MHC expression is indicative of metabolic activation in a variety of cells, including endothelial cells, microglia and mononuclear phagocytes (Lapierre et al., 1988). Where MHC expression is changed, the repertoire and levels of secreted cytokines are also likely to be changed, even if the cell does not present antigen to T cells. The relevance to regeneration following tissue damage is implied by studies of degenerated neural tissue in amyotrophic lateral sclerosis (ALS). In the damaged white manner, mononuclear phagocytes with strong MHC class II expression are seen in the tissue and packing the perivascular spaces. These activated cells themselves are likely to affect the surrounding tissue, even though few T cells are seen (Lampson et al., 1990).

It has often been proposed that MHC proteins mediate cell-cell interactions in nonimmunologic contexts, perhaps including neural development or regeneration (Lampson, 1984). If neural MHC proteins play a direct role in regeneration, this would limit one's freedom to manipulate MHC expression as a way of influencing T cell stimulation or cytokine secretion by MHC$^+$ cells.

In the following sections, the patterns of class I and class II MHC expression in different neural tissues are reviewed. The findings are interpreted in terms of each of the three potential functions for MHC$^+$ cells in neural regeneration: the potential for MHC-restricted T cell activity, for cytokine secretion by metabolically activated MHC$^+$ cells, and for MHC-mediated non-immunologic functions in neural tissue.

Expression of MHC proteins in situ

The method of choice for defining MHC expression in neural tissue in situ has been monoclonal antibody immunocytochemistry. Often, MHC$^+$ cells appear to be filled with stain in microscopic assays. This is not surprising, since if the proteins are made within the cell they should be expressed internally (Lampson, 1990). Evaluation of cell surface vs. internal MHC expression can be difficult when tissue is examined by light microscopy. For this reason, we speak of MHC expression by or within cells, rather than on cells, in neural tissue.

When a single antibody is used to identify a molecule, there is always the possibility of cross-reaction with a different molecule, even an unrelated one (Lampson, 1984). One way of confirming the staining interpretation in tissue sections is to show the same pattern with multiple antibodies, directed against different determinants on the molecule of interest (Lampson et al., 1983; Lampson and Fisher, 1984; Lampson, 1987). Complementary analysis of tissue homogenates can confirm that the molecule of interest is present (Lampson et al., 1983; Lampson and Fisher, 1984; Lampson and Hickey, 1986). Analysis of mRNA in tissue homogenates or by in situ hybridization can confirm the potential to synthesize the protein of interest (Lampson and George, 1986), but cannot reveal whether the native protein is actually present and functional (Main et al., 1985, 1988; Lampson, 1990). Most of the reports in the literature have used immunocytochemistry alone; unfortunately, often with only one antibody to each MHC protein class.

MHC expression in normal neural tissue

In the normal adult CNS, the strongest MHC expression is concentrated in nonneural cells. Class I MHC expression is seen as a continuous, cell-filling stain in endothelial cells of the human brain and spinal cord (Lampson and Hickey, 1986; Lampson et al., 1990). Endothelial class I stain may be much weaker in the rodent brain (Sethna and Lampson, 1991), and may reflect soluble class I protein adsorbed from serum (Whelan et al., 1986a). In some cases, particularly with antibody to β_2-microglobulin (the invariant class I light chain), there is an overall light blush of stain that is specific, but cannot be localized to individual cell types. This may result from protein that has been released from internal vesicles (Lampson, 1990).

In human and rodent brain, Class II MHC expression is seen as a strong cell-filling stain in individual cells in the perivascular space, meninges and choroid plexus (Lampson and Hickey, 1986; Sethna and Lampson, 1991). The class II$^+$ cells are most likely to be different kinds of mononuclear phagocytes. In the human brain, strong class II stain is also seen in occasional cells with the characteristic dendritic morphology of microglia. These may indicate areas of local insult (Lampson and Hickey, 1986). Greater numbers of strongly stained class II$^+$ microglia are seen in the human spinal cord (Lampson et al., 1990). More sensitive assay conditions may reveal additional MHC expression by microglia (Mattiace et al., 1990).

The same assays that reveal MHC class I and II in nonneural cells do not reveal MHC expression by neurons, astrocytes or oligodendrocytes. This is true for the normal human brain and spinal cord, and also for the rodent brain. Complementing the low baseline MHC expression in normal brain and spinal cord is the rarity of T cells or other leukocytes (Lampson et al., 1990; Sethna and Lampson, 1991). The lack of both MHC$^+$ cells and MHC-restricted T cells contributes to the brain's normal state of immune quiescence (Lampson, 1987; Armstrong and Lampson, 1994). We prefer the term 'immune quiescence' to 'immune privilege' because in the brain, as in other tissues, both MHC expression and leukocyte entry are under regulatory control. Yet, even when MHC expression is upregulated, the strongest expression remains concentrated in nonneural cells, as described below.

Direct injection of MHC-upregulating cytokine

Of the drugs known to upregulate MHC expression in vitro, gamma interferon (IFN-γ) is one of the most efficient at increasing class I expression, and one of the few that can upregulate class II expression. Class I expression can be increased on most cell types in vitro, including neuroblastoma cell lines (Lampson and Fisher, 1984; Lampson and George, 1986). Class II can be upregulated only on a more limited number of cell types, including cells and cell lines of glial origin, but not neuroblastoma cells.

To assess the potential of neural cells to express MHC protein in situ, IFN-γ was injected stereotactically into the rat brain (Sethna and Lampson, 1991). Following a single focal injection, MHC class I expression was increased on endothelial cells and ependymal cells. The most dramatic change was seen in MHC class II expression. Strong class II staining was seen in microglia throughout both hemispheres, and class II$^+$ microglia were seen as long as a month after the IFN injection. Class II staining was also seen on ependymal cells lining the ventricles in both hemispheres. The IFN injection increased the number of MHC$^+$ cells in the brain in another way as well, by causing increased entry of MHC$^+$ inflammatory cells. In the same sections, no MHC class I or II expression was detected in neurons, astrocytes or oligodendrocytes.

The IFN-γ injections define a pattern of regulation that draws attention to the potential importance of bystander effects against neural cells. Even though neural cells themselves do not show increased MHC expression, MHC$^+$ cells are widespread in the brain after IFN injection. MHC$^+$ cells directly adjacent to neural cells include endothelial cells, inflammatory cells, microglia and ependymal cells. T cells also enter the brain after the IFN injection, so that MHC-restricted T cells and MHC$^+$ cells are both present (Fig. 2). The way is open for MHC-restricted recognition of antigen expressed by nonneural cells, with neural cells potentially damaged as bystanders. This pathway of neural damage would be independent of MHC expression or function in the neural cells themselves.

MHC expression in other clinical or experimental settings

The importance of bystander effects against neural cells is implied by findings in other contexts as well. An example from human tissue comes from analysis of degenerated human spinal cord from patients with ALS, discussed above. In the damaged areas, strong MHC class II expression is seen in mononuclear phagocytes, which may be derived from either microglia or blood-borne monocytes. In the same sections, increased MHC expression is not seen in neural cells themselves (Lampson et al., 1990).

Studies of neural transplants again point to the relevance of bystander effects against neural targets. When neural tissue is grafted into the brain, MHC upregulation is often seen, but the identity of the MHC^+ cells has been difficult to establish. To avoid ambiguity, host and donor MHC expression were examined after human neural cell lines had been grafted into the rat brain. Grafted cells with different baseline MHC levels were compared. During the course of graft rejection, strong host MHC class II expression was seen in microglia and blood-borne monocytes. The MHC^+ cells, and also T cells, were seen surrounding and within the graft. The MHC expression of the grafted cells themselves did not change, and the grafts disappeared with the same time course regardless of their MHC levels (Armstrong and Lampson, 1994). Studies of central nervous system (CNS) viral infections have also increased interest in indirect and bystander responses to neural targets (reviewed in Armstrong and Lampson, 1994).

Neural MHC expression, T cells and secreted cytokines: summary and implications

Neural cells themselves do not usually show detectable MHC expression. While alternative techniques may yet reveal neural MHC expression or function (reviewed in Armstrong and Lampson, 1994), even complete absence of MHC expression does not provide protection against T cell attack. Foreign antigen that is expressed in the course of neural damage or regeneration can be presented to MHC-restricted T cells by MHC^+ nonneural cells that have ingested the antigen (Fig. 1, bottom). In the brain, potential APCs include endothelial cells, microglia, ependymal cells, and blood-borne monocytes (Fig. 2). The ultimate effect on regenerating neurons will depend upon their susceptibility to cytokines secreted by the T cells, or by secondary cells that have been attracted to the site. Even where T cell responses are not activated, the metabolically activated MHC^+ cells at sites of damage can secrete cytokines that are likely to influence regenerating neural cells.

The effects of immunoactive cytokines on regenerating neurons are just now being defined. An intriguing possibility is that some cytokines may promote, rather than impede, regeneration (Unsicker et al., 1992; Schwartz et al., this volume). This means that proposed alterations in cytokine secretion or function must take into account the possible effects on both leukocytes and regenerating neural cells.

Manipulating cytokine expression may directly or indirectly involve changing MHC expression. Reducing MHC expression on potential target cells or APC would impede antigen presentation to T cells, and consequent cytokine secretion. Immunoactive cytokines are also secreted by other cells. For many cells, increased MHC expression is indicative of metabolic activation. Manipulations designed to alter cytokine secretion in these cells may concomitantly affect MHC expression. Conversely, manipulation designed to alter MHC expression may concomitantly change the repertoire or levels of secreted cytokines. Finally, since many immunocative cytokines can affect MHC expression, as cytokine production is altered, MHC expression may be further modified.

Given the close links between cytokine secretion and MHC expression, it is important to know whether altering MHC expression might itself influence neural regeneration. The question of whether MHC molecules might play a nonimmunologic role during regeneration is discussed below.

MHC expression in neural tissue: seeking evidence of a nonimmunologic role

In the normal adult brain, MHC expression is not seen in neural cells. If stronger expression were seen at any stage during normal development or regeneration, this would provide evidence for the nonimmunologic MHC role that has been proposed in other contexts (Lampson, 1984). Accordingly, MHC expression in developing and regenerating neural tissue was examined.

MHC expression in developing neural tissue

MHC class I expression was evaluated in the developing mouse embryo. To optimize morphology, paraffin embedded tissue was studied. To optimize staining, a rabbit antiserum to β_2-m, the invariant light chain of all class I molecules, was used. Staining was seen in expected locations in maternal tissues. In the same assays, no stain was seen in neural cells of the developing neural tube, or of the developing brain or spinal cord (Whelan, 1986; Lampson and Whelan, 1987).

To expand the analysis, nonlymphoid tissues of the developing rat were analyzed (Grabowska and Lampson, 1994). In addition to conventional antiserum to β_2-m, monoclonal antibodies to class I and II MHC molecules were used. To increase the sensitivity of staining, frozen sections as well as paraffin sections were evaluated, and assay conditions were included that increased the exposure of internal antigen (Lampson, 1990). Expected strong expression was seen in adult tissues, and in developing lymphoid and hematopoietic tissues. The strongest MHC expression in most tissues of the developing rat embryo was in individual cells. Ubiquitous expression was seen in only a few locations, including class I staining of epithelial cells lining developing gut villi. It was not seen in neural tissue (Grabowska and Lampson, 1994).

Apart from the lymphoid and hematopoietic tissues, the strongest staining for class I and class II MHC molecules was seen in individual cells in the skin, lung, gut and interorgan connective tissue. The strongest class I and class II expression was in different cells, with different morphologies and distributions, and with different expression of antigens characteristic of mononuclear phagocytes. Individual class I^+ cells were most abundant in the deeper layers of the skin and its invaginations, and surrounding other structures. Class II^+ cells were most abundant in the gut wall and villi. A mixture of class I^+ and class II^+ cells was seen in the developing lung.

On the same slides, MHC expression was not detected in neural cells of the developing neural tube, brain or spinal cord. MHC^+ cells were seen in the developing skin of the scalp, and in the band of connective tissue that invaginates the developing head. MHC expression was not seen in neural cells themselves. MHC^+ cells were seen in the skin overlying the spinal cord, but not in the neural tissue (Grabowska and Lampson, 1994).

Olfactory epithelium

Unlike most mammalian CNS tissue, the olfactory epithelium turns over even in the adult. The olfactory epithelium has a well-defined layered structure, including layers of new olfactory neurons, developing neurons, and dying neurons. The major nonneuronal cell of the olfactory epithelium is the sustentacular cell.

MHC class I expression was evaluated in olfactory epithelium of the mouse. Class I staining was seen in cells of the adjacent respiratory epithelium, and in endothelial cells of the underlying connective tissue. No neural cells or layers of the olfactory epithelium showed positive staining. The same pattern was seen in the sensory epithelium and adjoining structures of the vomeronasal organ (Whelan et al., 1986b).

Neuroblastoma cell lines

To complement studies of neural tissue in situ, human neuroblastoma cell lines growing in vitro were examined. Two lines were found to have a heterogeneous MHC expression within the population, such that strong class I expression was seen on fewer than 1% of the cells (Lampson, 1990). Unequal MHC distribution among mitotic sisters showed that the minority population was a regulatory population, rather than a contaminating cell type (Fig. 3, panels 1C, D). In these circumstances, it was of interest to ask whether the cells with strong class I expression showed a different spectrum of morphologies or cell-cell

1

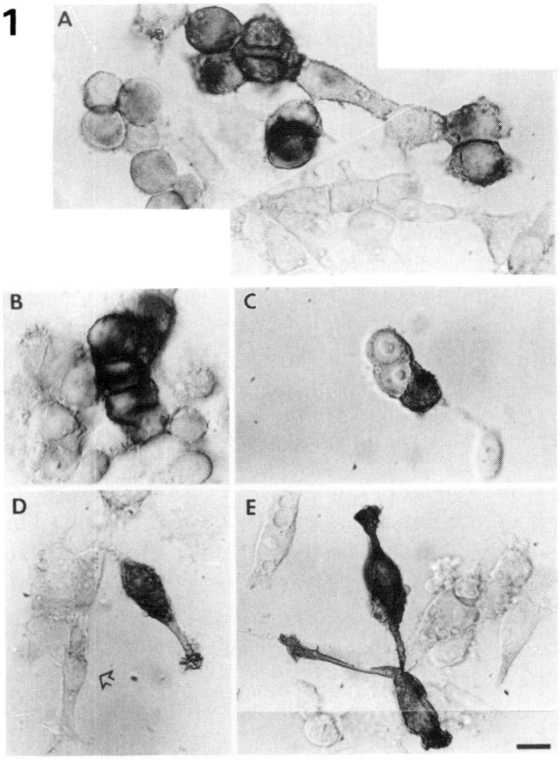

2

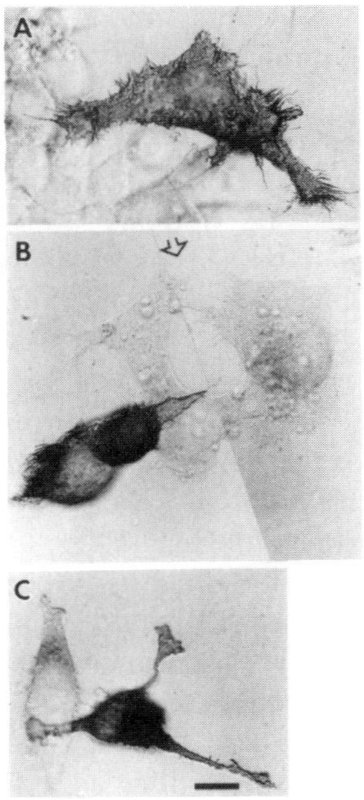

3

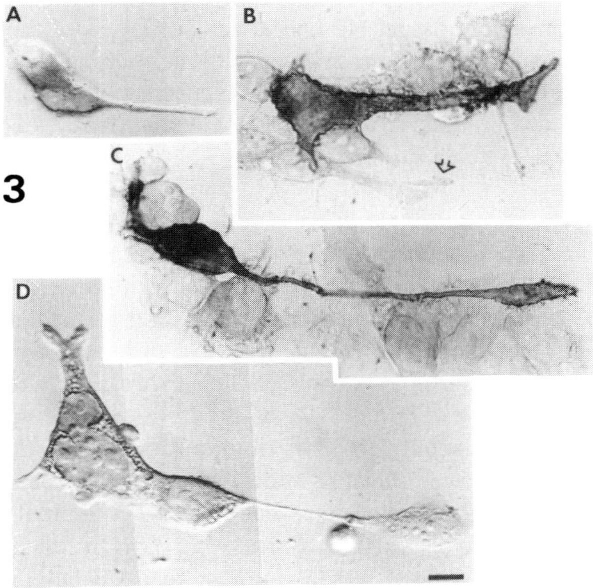

4

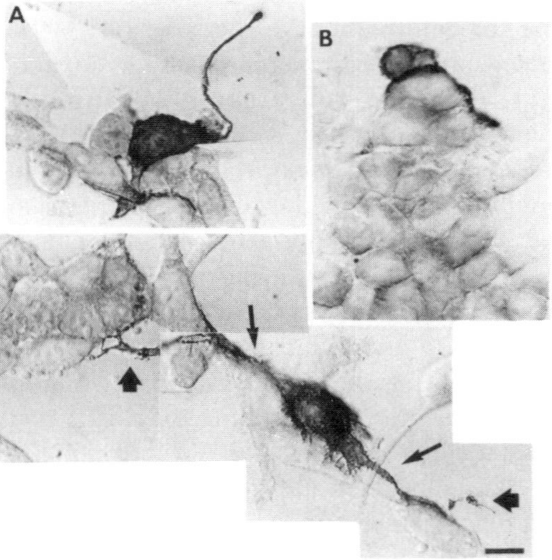

interactions from the majority population. In practice, no difference was seen. The cells were found over each other, under each other, and intertwined in all possible combinations, and no morphologies were found to be unique to either population (Fig 3; Lampson, 1990).

Implications for regenerating neural tissue

Manipulation of MHC levels is a logical way of controlling T cell-mediated responses to foreign antigen in regenerating tissue. A concern has been whether changing MHC levels might, of itself, affect neuronal outgrowth. Our findings provide no evidence for a requirement for MHC expression by developing or regenerating neural cells. This suggests that manipulation of MHC expression need not itself impede neural regeneration or repair.

Although MHC expression is not detected in most neural cells, MHC^+ cells are found directly adjacent to neural cells in many circumstances. The available body of evidence suggests that MHC^+ cells are most likely to influence regeneration by secretion of cytokines that can affect T cells, attract inflammatory cells, or influence neural cells directly. The pleiotrophic effects of the cytokines raise intriguing questions about regulation of their effects in situ, as discussed below.

Evaluating and manipulating differential cytokine regulation in situ

There are now abundant examples of neurotransmitters and neuromodulators affecting leukocytes, and of immunoactive cytokines affecting neural cells (Unsicker et al., 1992; Merrill et al., Schwartz et al.,; Otten et al., this volume). It may be most useful to think in terms of a single pool of regulatory molecules with multiple potential targets, rather than tissue-specific regulators (Lampson, 1984). Once the pleiotrophic effects of regulatory molecules are appreciated, it becomes important to understand how differential regulation can be achieved in situ.

In normal tissue in situ, anatomic barriers can provide one basis for differential regulation. Where normal anatomic barriers are disrupted, as in damaged and degenerating neural tissue, other bases for specificity may assume greater importance. Differences in the baseline levels of cytokine receptors on different cell types are an example of what may be thought of as physiologic factors. The combinations of regulatory factors at particular sites define what may be termed the pharmacologic basis of differential regulation.

The importance of anatomic and pharmacologic factors helps to explain why different cytokine effects are observed in vitro and in situ (Wen et al., 1992). We have been working to develop a model that permits quantitative evaluation of cytokine effects on neural cells in situ. Homogeneous cell lines with characteristic patterns of growth in the brain are used as antigenic targets. To facilitate identification of individual target cells, the lines are made to express the *lacZ* reporter gene (Lampson et al., 1992, 1993). Cytokines are injected stereotactically into selected sites in the brain. The relationships among target cells, inflammatory cells, cells with altered MHC expression, and neural cells are defined by a combination of histochemistry, immunocytochemistry and conventional histological stains

Fig. 3. Morphology and interactions of β_2-m$^+$ and β_2-m$^-$ variants of a neuronal cell line. A human neuroblastoma cell line was grown on glass coverslips and stained for β_2-m, the invariant light chain of MHC class I molecules. The majority of the cells appear β_2-m$^-$, but a subpopulation is strongly stained. The β_2-m$^+$ and β_2-m$^-$ cells appear to be regulatory subpopulations. Mitotic sisters with different levels of β_2-m expression can be seen (panel 1C, D). The β_2-m$^+$ and β_2-m$^-$ cells display the same spectrum of morphologies (panels 1; 2A, B, arrow; 3). Multiple interactions between β_2-m$^+$ and β_2-m$^-$ cells are seen: The β_2-m$^+$ cells can be seen on top of or underneath the β_2-m$^-$ cells (panel 2B and C, respectively), and β_2-m$^+$ and β_2-m$^\phi$ processes can be intertwined (panel C). Strong β_2-m expression does not appear to be required for any observed morphology or type of interaction, nor does it appear to be required for any observed morphology or type of interaction, nor does it appear to prevent any. (From Lampson, 1990).

on single slides. Computer-assisted image analysis is used to obtain quantitative information about numbers of affected cells, their relationship to each other, and their distribution in the brain. Simple three-dimensional reconstructions are used to complement the analysis of single sections (Lampson et al., 1992, 1993; Lampson, 1993).

Quantitative analysis of cytokine effects in situ should help to reveal how individual regulatory molecules affect regenerating neural tissue, and the extent to which differential regulation occurs, or can be achieved. For example, is it possible to enhance neuronal growth without increasing inflammation? Is it possible to reduce inflammation without impeding regeneration? If differential regulation can be achieved in regenerating tissue, it should be possible in other contexts, such as antitumor responses, as well (Lampson, 1993).

Conclusion

Neural tissue displays a consistent pattern of MHC expression under a variety of conditions. MHC^+ cells, including endothelial cells, mononuclear phagocytes, microglia and ependymal cells, can be in direct contact with neural cells. Neural cells themselves, including neurons, astrocytes and oligodendrocytes, do not show detectable MHC expression. While alternative techniques may yet reveal neural MHC expression or function, the predominant pattern itself offers multiple opportunities for MHC-mediated effects (Fig. 3).

Given the predominant pattern of MHC expression, MHC-mediated effects that can affect neural cells as bystanders are of particular interest. Two kinds of bystander effects are stressed, both mediated by secreted cytokines. T cells that have recognized antigen/MHC on nonneural cells may affect adjacent neural cells through their secreted cytokines. Proteins that are newly expressed during the process of tissue damage or repair may serve as the source of 'foreign' antigen in this case. Even in the absence of 'foreign' antigen or responding T cells, MHC expression on nonneural cells may be a sign of metabolic activation and cytokine secretion.

Evidence for a nonimmunologic role for MHC proteins in neural tissues was sought, but not found. This implies that modulating MHC expression need not itself interfere with neural regeneration. A more subtle question concerns the effects of modulating cytokine secretion. Neural cells and leukocytes may be affected by the same cytokines, and individual cytokines may enhance rather than inhibit regeneration. Defining the optimal cytokine environment, and defining ways of obtaining it in situ, are foci of current research.

Direct and indirect regulatory links between MHC expression and cytokine secretion are described. Fuller understanding of MHC regulation and function is likely to be an important part of optimizing the regulatory environment to favor regeneration of neural cells.

References

Armstrong, W.S. and Lampson, L.A. (1994) Direct cell-mediated responses in the nervous system: CTL vs. NK activity, and their dependence upon MHC expression and modulation. In: R.W. Keane and W.F. Hickey (Eds.), *Immunology of the Nervous System*, Oxford, in press.

Grabowska, A. and Lampson, L.A. (1994) MHC expression in nonlymphoid tissues of the developing embryo: strongest β_2-m or class II expression in distinct populations of potential antigen-presenting cells in the skin, lung, gut and inter-organ connective tissue. *Dev. Comp. Immunol.*, in press.

Lampson, L.A. (1984) Molecular bases of neuronal individuality: lessons from anatomical and biochemical studies with monoclonal antibodies. In: R.H. Kennett, T.J. McKearn and K.B. Bechtol (Eds.), *Monoclonal Antibodies and Functional Cell Lines: Progress and Applications*, Plenum Press, New York, pp. 153–189.

Lampson, L.A. (1987) Molecular bases of the immune response to neural antigens. *Trends Neurosci.*, 10: 211–216.

Lampson, L.A. (1990) MHC regulation in neural cells. Distribution of peripheral and internal b2-microglobulin and class I molecules in human neuroblastoma cell lines. *J. Immunol.*, 144: 512–520.

Lampson, L.A. (1993). Cell-mediated immunotherapy directed against disseminated tumour in the brain. In: P.M. Black, W.C. Schoene, L.A. Lampson (Eds.), *Astrocytomas: Diag-*

nois, Treatment and Biology, Blackwell Scientific, London, pp. 261–289.

Lampson, L.A. and Fisher, C.A. (1984) Weak HLA and β_2-microglobulin expression of neuronal cell lines can be modulated by interferon. *Proc. Natl. Acad. Sci. USA*, 81: 6476–6480.

Lampson, L.A. and George, D.L. (1986) IFN-mediated induction of class I MHC products in human neuronal cell lines: analysis of HLA and β_2-m RNA, and HLA-A and HLA-B proteins and polymorphic specificities. *J. Interferon Res.*, 6: 257–265.

Lampson, L.A. and Hickey, W.F. (1986) Monoclonal antibody analysis of MHC expression in human brain biopsies: tissue ranging from 'histologically normal' to that showing different levels of glial tumor involvement. *J. Immunol.*, 136: 4054–4062.

Lampson, L.A. and Levy, R. (1980) Two populations of Ia-like molecules on a human B cell line. *J. Immunol.*, 125: 293–299.

Lampson, L.A. and Whelan, J.P. (1987) A role for the major histocompatibility complex in normal differential of non-lymphoid tissues. Proceedings of the 19th Miami Winter Symposium. Advances in Gene Technology: The Molecular Biology of Development. *ICSU Short Reports, Vol.7*, Cambridge University Press, Cambridge, p. 125.

Lampson, L.A., Fisher, C.A., and Whelan J.P. (1983) Striking paucity of HLA-A,B,C and β_2-microglobulin on human neuroblastoma cell lines. *J. Immunol.*, 130: 2471–2478.

Lampson, L.A., Kushner, P.D. and Sobel, R.A. (1990) Major histocompatibility antigen expression in the affected tissues in amyotrophic lateral sclerosis. *Ann. Neurol.*, 28: 365–372.

Lampson, L.A., Wen, P., Roman, V.A., Morris, J.H. and Sarid, J.A. (1992) Disseminating tumor cells and their interactions with leukocytes visualized in the brain. *Cancer Res.*, 52: 1018–1025.

Lampson, L.A., Lampson, M.A. and Dunne, A.D. (1993) Exploiting the *lacZ* reporter gene for quantitative analysis of disseminated tumor growth within the brain: use of the *lacZ* gene product as a tumor antigen, for evaluation of antigenic modulation, and to facilitate image analysis of tumor growth in situ. *Cancer Res.*, 53: 176–182.

Lapierre, L.A., Fiers, W. and Pober, J.S. (1988) Three distinct classes of regulatory cytokines control endothelial cell MHC antigen expression. *J. Exp. Med.*, 167: 794–804.

Main, E.K., Lampson, L.A., Hart M.K., Kornbluth, J. and Wilson D.B. (1985) Human neuroblastoma cell lines are susceptible to lysis by natural killer cells but not by cytotoxic T lymphocytes. *J. Immunol.*, 135: 242–246.

Main E.K., Monos D.S. and Lampson L.A. (1988). IFN-treated neuroblastoma cell lines remain resistant to T cell-mediated allo-killing, and susceptible to non-MHC-restricted cytotoxicity. *J. Immunol.*, 141: 2943–2950.

Mason, D. (1988) The roles of T cell subpopulations in allograft rejection. *Transpl. Proc.*, 20: 239–242.

Mattiace, L.A., Davies, P. and Dickson, D.W. (1990) Detection of HLA-DR on microglia in the human brain is a function of both clinical and technical factors. *Am. J. Pathol.*, 136: 1101–1114.

Sethna, M.P. and Lampson, L.A. (1991) Immune modulation within the brain: recruitment of inflammatory cells and increased major histocompatibility antigen expression following intracerebral injection of IFN-γ. *J. Neuroimmunol.*, 34: 121–132.

Turner, W.J.D., Chatten J. and Lampson L.A. (1990) Human neuroblastoma cell growth in xenogeneic hosts: comparison of T cell-deficient and NK-deficient hosts, and subcutaneous or intravenous injection routes. *J. NeuroOncol.*, 8: 121–132.

Unsicker, K., Grothe, C., Westermann, R. and Wewetzer, K. (1992) Cytokines in neural regeneration. *Curr. Opin. Neurobiol.*, 2: 671–678.

Wen, P.Y., Lampson, M.A. and Lampson, L.A. (1992) Effects of γ-interferon on major histocompatibility complex expression and lymphocytic infiltration in the 9L gliosarcoma brain tumor model: implications for strategies for immunotherapy. *J. Neuroimmunol.*, 36: 57–68.

Whelan, J.P. (1986) Major histocompatibility complex (MHC) class I expression in normal, neoplastic, and developing neural tissues. University of Pennsylvania (Thesis).

Whelan, J.P., Eriksson, U. and Lampson, L.A. (1986a) Expression of mouse β_2-microglobulin in frozen and formaldehyde-fixed central nervous tissues: comparison of tissue behind the blood-brain barrier and tissue in a barrier-free region. *J. Immunol.*, 137: 2561–2566.

Whelan, J.P., Wysocki, C.J. and Lampson, L.A. (1986b) Distribution of β_2-microglobulin in olfactory epithelium: a proliferating neuroepithelium not protected by a blood-tissue barrier. *J. Immunol.*, 137: 2567–2571.

F.J. Seil (Ed.)
Progress in Brain Research, Vol 103

CHAPTER 26

Neurotransmitters and cytokines in CNS pathology

Branislava Mitrovic, Fredricka C. Martin, Andrew C. Charles, Louis J. Ignarro, Peter A. Anton, Fergus Shanahan and Jean E. Merrill

UCLA School of Medicine, Los Angeles, CA 90024, USA

Introduction

There is growing evidence that two molecules produced by neurons in the central nervous system (CNS) may play a role in inflammation. One of these molecules is substance P (SP), a neuropeptide involved in peripheral pain perception and vasodilation peripherally and centrally. The other is nitric oxide (NO). In physiological concentrations, NO regulates homeostatic signaling in blood vessels and within the CNS through its activation of guanylate cyclase and cyclic GMP (reviewed in Murphy et al., 1993). SP participates in inflammation and is elevated in the arthritis model (Colpaert, 1983), autoimmune skin disorders (Wallengren et al., 1986), and inflammatory bowel disease (Mantyh et al., 1988). Kostyk et al. (1989) demonstrated colocalization of SP with gliotic astrocytes in multiple sclerosis (MS) plaques. SP also causes inflammation by inducing mast cell release of histamine which results in edema (Shanahan et al., 1985) and leukocyte production of the proinflammatory cytokines, interleukin 1 (IL-1), interleukin 6 (IL-6) and tumor necrosis factor alpha (TNF-α). SP stimulates production of superoxide anion (O_2^-), chemotaxis, and phagocytosis (Bar-Shavit et al., 1980; Ruff et al., 1985; Lotz et al., 1987, 1988; Peck, 1987).

Likewise, NO participates in inflammation in that NO from activated microglia causes damage to normal cells in the CNS such as neurons and oligodendrocytes (Boje and Arora, 1992; Merrill et al., 1993). SP induces IL-1 and TNF-α (Lotz et al., 1988; Martin et al., 1992, 1993); IL-1 and TNF-α contribute to the induction of NO synthase and NO production (Stuehr and Marletta, 1987; Welsh et al., 1991; Merrill et al., 1993). Damage in cells exposed to NO varies from the crippling of the mitochondrial electron transport chain, forcing cells to alternative energy pathways such as glycolysis (Drapier and Hibbs, 1988), to interference with DNA replication or even induction of DNA fragmentation and apoptosis (Albina et al., 1993; Sarih et al., 1993). Formation of nitroso-sulfur-iron complexes in iron-containing enzymes or production of peroxynitrite when combined with O_2^- are two mechanisms by which NO injures or kills cells (reviewed in Nussler and Billiar, 1993; Lipton et al., this volume).

Since both of these molecules are of interest in CNS inflammation, we have hypothesized a role for them in CNS white matter pathology in MS and in CNS acquired immunodeficiency syndrome (AIDS). Performing in vitro experiments with glial cells to assess their response to and production of cytokines and these two neurotransmitters, we have designed two model systems to explain a role for SP and NO in CNS inflammatory diseases.

SP receptors on glial cells

While receptors for SP have been well characterized on astrocytes in vitro, they are not well characterized on microglial cells. We have characterized the binding of Bolton-Hunter ^{125}I-radiolabeled SP to primary rat microglial cells in vitro and found the SP receptor to be different from that on astrocytes and, in fact, a nonclassical neurokinin 1 (NK-1) receptor. There are two types of SP receptors on rat microglia, one with a high affinity K_d of 8×10^{-8} M and one with a low affinity with a K_d of 2×10^{-6} M. There are 35,000 ± 3,500 receptors (mean ± SE) per cell, of which 5–10% are of high affinity (Martin et al., 1993). Studies were run to determine specificity, the tachykinin receptor subtype, and the portion of the SP molecule facilitating binding activity. Only SP, the antagonists ([D-Pro^4, D-Trp^{1,9}] SP[4-11] > SP > spantide > CP 96,345) and the NK-1 agonist, SP methylester, competed strongly with ^{125}I-SP, while the other NK-1 agonist, physalaemin, did not (Regoli et al., 1989). CP 96,345 incompletely displaced ^{125}I-SP from its receptor. This suggests the receptor is not a classical NK-1 receptor (McLean et al, 1991; Snider et al., 1991). In addition, agonists for the NK-2 (neurokinin A [NKA], eledoisin) (Regoli et al., 1989) and NK-3 receptor subtypes (kassinin and [pGlu^5,MePhe^8,Sar^9]-Substance P[5-11]) (Torrens et al., 1985; Regoli et al., 1989) had little effect on SP binding even at 1×10^{-5} M concentration. SP(1-4) also had little effect on binding, while SP(4-11) competed moderately, indicating the C-terminal mediates SP binding to this receptor (Martin et al., 1993). The SP receptor on microglia does have similarities with SP receptors seen on other immune cells. In particular, macrophages have a low-affinity SP receptor (K_d of 1.9×10^{-8} M), which, just like the microglia receptor, binds SP > SP methylester with no binding by physalaemin or NKA (Hartung et al., 1986). SP receptors with low binding affinities have also been reported on T cells (Payan et al., 1984). These characteristics (low-affinity, binding for SP methylester but not for physalaemin or NKA) may indicate an SP receptor is present on some immune cells which is different from the NK-1, NK-2, and NK- 3 tachykinin receptors described in the literature (Table 1).

Astrocytes acquire functional SP receptors during inflammation in vivo or when activated in vitro by culturing (Torrens et al., 1986; Mantyh et al., 1989). Binding of SP to such receptors induces phospholipase C activation (Torrens et al., 1989), prostaglandin E (PGE) production (Hartung et

TABLE 1

Nonclassical neurokinin-1 receptor (NK-1R) for substance P on rat microglia. The similarity in affinity and peptide or nonpeptide antagonists for the NK-1-like receptor on microglia and NK-1R on macrophages distinguishes these cells from other NK-1R-bearing cells in the brain (astrocytes) and elsewhere in the body. SP = substance P; SPM.ester = substance P methylester; NKA, B = neurokinins A or B.

Cell type	Affinity K_d(M)	Hierarchy of peptide displacement of SP	Non competitor peptides
rat microglia	8×10^{-8} 2×10^{-6}	(D-pro, D-tryp) SP (4–11) > SP > spantide > CP-96,345 > SP m.ester > SP (4–11)	SP (1–4); SP (5–11) eledoisin; kassinin physalaemin; NKA
g.pig macrophages	2×10^{-8}	SP > SP m.ester	physalaemin; NKA
rat astrocytes	3×10^{-10}	SP > physalaemin > SP m.ester > NKA > kassinin > NKB	
g.pig brain striatal membranes	7×10^{-10}	CP-96,345 > SP = physalaemin > spantide = SP m.ester > (D-pro, D-trp) SP (4–11) = NKA = NKB = eledoisin	

al., 1988), and changes in membrane potential (Weinrich and Kettenmann, 1989). Astrocytes may also participate in immune mediated inflammation by production of IL-1 and TNF-α (Lieberman et al., 1989), and expression of major histocompatibility molecules (MHC II) (Frank et al., 1986). Under normal circumstances, astrocytes may have too few SP receptors to respond to SP in an inflammatory fashion. However, under abnormal conditions, where astrocytes are expressing large numbers of SP receptors, they may contribute to inflammatory and proliferative responses associated with the presence of SP by production of inflammatory cytokines such as IL-1 and TNF-α (Fig. 1).

While the receptor on microglia is distinct from NK-2 and NK-3 receptors, though similar to the NK-1 receptor, the NK-1 receptor on astrocytes looks like the NK-1 receptor seen on other cells. The astrocyte NK- 1 receptor has a binding hierarchy of SP > physalaemin > SP methylester > NKA, with 1×10^{-6} NKA strongly displacing 1×10^{-10} M SP (Torrens et al., 1986). The microglia SP receptor has a hierarchy of SP > SP methylester with essentially no displacement of 10^{-10} M SP by even 10^{-5} M of NKA or physalaemin. The microglia SP receptor also has a lower binding affinity of 8×10^{-8} M compared to the NK1 receptor binding affinities of $1–6 \times 10^{-10}$ M reported for SP on astrocytes (Torrens et al., 1986), smooth muscle (Burcher and Buck, 1986), and pituitary gland (Larsen et al., 1989) (Table 1).

SP induction of cytokines in glial cell cultures

We have previously demonstrated intercellular signaling in glial cells by calcium waves and oscillations in response to glutamate or mechanical stimulation (Table 1; Charles et al., 1991, 1993). This intercellular signaling is regulated both by Ca^{2+}-induced as well as inositol-1,4,5-tris-phos-

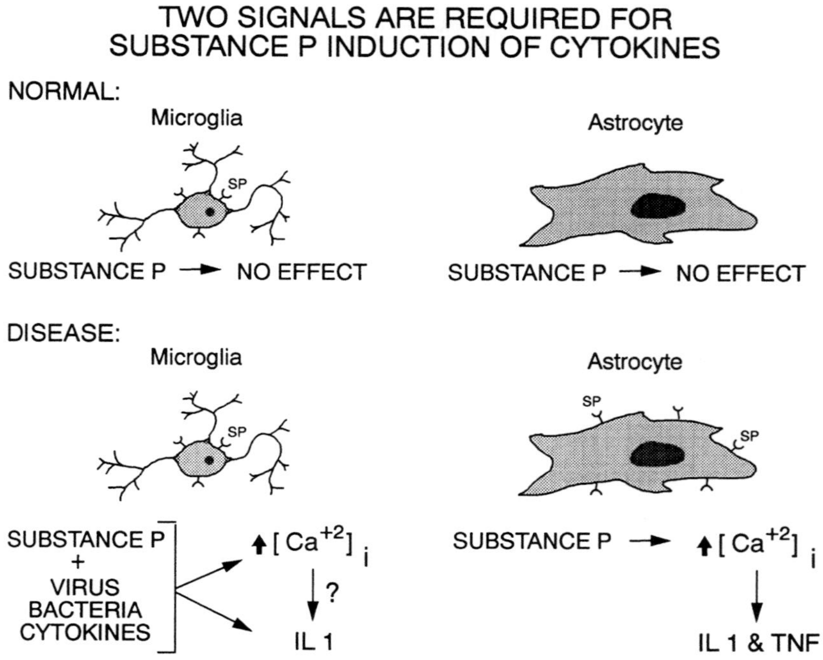

Fig. 1. Two signals are required for substance P (SP) induction of cytokines. The SP receptors on resting microglia in normal brain tissue are hypothetical. As with astrocytes, they may need to be induced. $[Ca^{2+}]_i$ = intracellular calcium.

phate (IP3)-induced Ca^{2+} release (Charles et al., 1993). Cooperative glial cell function at local sites of injury as well as parts of the CNS remote from the traumatic stimulus (Graeber et al., 1990; Woodroofe et al., 1991) and tandem signaling by factors such as cytokines which cannot cross the blood-brain barrier (Hashimoto et al., 1991) may possibly be explained by calcium-mediated communication. Astrocyte cultures exposed to 10^{-8}–10^{-6} M SP responded with an abrupt (within seconds) increase in $[Ca^{2+}]_i$ to levels of nearly 1 μM from a baseline of 40–75 nM. Asynchronous oscillations were also seen. Cells exposed to SP in Ca^{2+}-free conditions responded similarly, indicating that the $[Ca^{2+}]_i$ response to SP was generated primarily by Ca^{2+} release from intracellular stores (Martin et al., 1992). In contrast, the effects of both SP and lipopolysaccharide (LPS) on intracellular calcium in the microglia were small or nonexistent, similar to the effects of LPS on intracellular calcium in peripheral monocytes and macrophages (Conrad and Rink, 1986; Prpic et al, 1987). We inconsistently saw that when LPS and SP did induce $[Ca^{2+}]_i$ increases, the lag time was up to 5 min. Even then, neither SP nor LPS alone induced $[Ca^{2+}]_i$; both SP and LPS were required for any increase to occur (Martin et al., unpublished observations). LPS induces IL-1 production in macrophages via protein kinase C and a calmodulin binding protein that is activated by LPS without increased calcium levels (Conrad and Rink, 1986). It appears microglia may function in the same manner. Contrary to our expectations based on the literature (Shinomiya and Nakano, 1987), SP increases IL-1 production in response to LPS with little or no effect on intracellular calcium, possibly by somehow amplifying the pathways already in use. Other possibilities are that SP prolongs the half-life of IL-1 mRNA, improves translation efficiency for the mRNA, or enhances the cellular release of already synthesized IL-1 into the medium.

Studies were performed to test the ability of SP to stimulate astrocyte production of IL-1 and TNF-α. The possible role of calcium as a second messenger for inflammatory cytokine production was examined. Astrocytes stimulated with SP produced significant amounts of IL-1 and some TNF-α. SP had no effect on IL-1 induction by LPS. Even though the K_d for the astrocyte SP receptor is 3.3×10^{-10} M (Torrens et al., 1986), astrocytes responded to SP at concentrations of 10^{-7}–10^{-8} M, which are similar to those concentrations seen during inflammation (Wallengren et al., 1986; Tissot et al., 1988). The effect of SP on $[Ca^{2+}]_i$ suggested that an increase in $[Ca^{2+}]_i$ might mediate IL-1 production. Stimulating astrocytes with the calcium ionophore A23187 raised $[Ca^{2+}]_i$ and stimulated significant IL-1 production but did not induce TNF-α (Martin et al., 1992). This has been shown in macrophages (Shinomiya and Nakano, 1987). A role for Ca^{2+} as a second messenger for SP-induced IL-1 production by astrocytes was demonstrated when increases in $[Ca^{2+}]_i$ were inhibited by the intracellular calcium chelator, 1,2-bis(2 aminophenoxy)ethane-*N*,*N*,*N'*,*N'*-tetraacetic acid (di-bromo BAPTA/AM). Pretreatment with di-bromo BAPTA/AM completely blocked IL-1 production by SP-treated astrocytes, without blocking IL-1 production by astrocytes stimulated with LPS (Martin et al., 1992).

Astrocytes are thus capable of producing IL-1 in response to SP-dependent Ca^{2+} release from intracellular stores. Increased $[Ca^{2+}]_i$ may be the second messenger for IL-1 production in this system. Both SP (Hartung et al., 1988) and A23187 (Pearce and Murphy, 1988) rapidly induce PGE production by astrocytes, and PGE is known to inhibit IL-1 production if present early or during IL-1 induction (Brandwein, 1986). Excessive PGE secretion in response to overly strong stimulation with A23187 or SP may thus have inhibited subsequent IL-1 production.

It has been demonstrated that SP and SP methylester augment LPS induction of IL-1 but not TNF-α in rat microglial cultures at 1×10^{-8} M to 1×10^{-6} M, which stimulate IL-1 production by monocytes/macrophages (Kimball et al., 1988; Lotz et al., 1988; Laurenzi et al., 1990). Unlike human peripheral blood, microglia do not respond to SP alone (Martin et al., 1992). SP receptors on cells of monocyte-macrophage lineage may respond only after priming (in this case by endotoxin) and only to high levels of SP to avoid triggering inflammation in response to low levels of SP normally present during smooth muscle contraction and other CNS functions (Bailey et al., 1986). SP is known to be released during the course of peripheral inflammatory disorders (Wallengren et al., 1986; Tissot et al., 1988; Marshall et al., 1990). This would be equivalent to in vivo where SP would induce local IL-1 production, alteration in vasodilation, increased infiltration of leukocytes and tissue destruction (Fig. 1).

Cytokines in MS tissue

MS is a demyelinating disease of the CNS in which myelin sheaths and the myelin-producing cells, oligodendrocytes, are destroyed (Prineas, 1985). There is an accumulation of activated microglia and inflammatory macrophages as well as presence of proinflammatory cytokines such as TNF-α and interferon gamma (IFN-γ) at the lesion edge (Hofman et al., 1986, 1989; Merrill et al., 1989). The asymmetry of the pathology of these lesions with myelin loss and oligodendrocyte death in the wake or trailing edge of the growing lesion, but not at the leading edge of the lesion, suggests that the plaque formation is cell-mediated. Indeed, proliferation of oligodendrocytes is seen just beyond the plaque margin (Prineas, 1985). Were the lesion being created by significant diffusion of toxic molecules or proteins from cells at the lesion edge, there would be damage to myelin and oligodendrocytes beyond the leading edge of the growing plaque as well. Since macrophages in MS patients are activated (Merrill et al., 1989), cytokines like IFN-γ, TNF-α, and IL-1 are associated with worsening of disease (Panitch et al., 1987; Beck et al., 1988), and since IL-1 and TNF-α have been demonstrated in vitro to inhibit or kill oligodendrocytes (Robbins et al., 1987; Merrill et al., 1991), it seems plausible that these events are linked in causing pathology in vivo. Indeed, it appears that blood macrophages and brain microglia are responsible for disease pathology.

IFN-γ is elevated in some but not all patients with MS, as assessed by serum and cerebrospinal fluid (CSF) levels, or produced by cells in situ in lesions in brain tissue or in vitro by lymphocytes. This has been postulated to result in expression of MHC II molecules (HLA-DR) on macrophages and astrocytes in lesions which could then perpetuate the autoimmune cycle if these cells act as antigen-presenting cells (reviewed in Merrill et al., 1992). In any case, HLA-DR is a sign of macrophage activation in vitro. IFN-γ treatment of MS patients leads to upregulation of MHC II on peripheral monocyte/macrophages and to exacerbation of disease (Panitch et al., 1987). MS patients may even show an increase in IFN-γ preceding clinical symptoms; this may parallel an increase in TNF-α (Beck et al., 1988). Sharief et al. (1991) have also shown a correlation with disease progression and TNF-α levels in CSF in MS patients. Measurement of TNF-α in MS has not always been definitive, with some reports finding it elevated, the same, or not detectable in serum and CSF. Likewise IL-1 and IL-6 have been examined in CSF and serum with the same variable results. More consistently, IL-1 and TNF-α production by MS macrophages in culture has been shown to be elevated (Beck et al., 1988; Merrill et al., 1989, 1992).

There is evidence for toxic oxygen metabolite production and lipid peroxidation in MS patients (Hunter et al., 1985). In addition, TNF-α and IL-1 production are elevated both in situ in the lesions (Fig. 2) as well as in vitro by peripheral blood and cerebrospinal fluid macrophages (Hofman et al., 1986, 1989; Merrill et al., 1989). Primed macrophages can be induced by phorbol myristate acetate (PMA) to undergo oxygen burst and to lyse susceptible targets, while LPS and IFN-γ typically induce TNF-α-mediated cytotoxicity. Nevertheless, the production of free radicals and that of TNF-α may be related to each other in that reactive oxygen species have been implicated in both the production of TNF-α as well as in the actual mechanism of TNF-α tumoricidal activity. IL-1 and TNF-α both occur as membrane components of effector cells and, in such form, TNF-α has been shown to mediate killing in the absence of released cytokine (Decker et al., 1987). In some cases it is a more efficient mechanism of lysis by macrophages than is the soluble form (Peck et al., 1989).

Two other cytokines may be important in inflammation because of their dual regulatory effects on the immune system. TGF-β is a powerful chemotactic agent and may induce cells to cross the blood-brain barrier. TGF-β is a natural antagonist of TNF-α and IL-1β. TGF-β has also been shown to induce mRNA for IL-1β and TNF-α, though it may inhibit their release as proteins. TGF-β can downregulate both oxygen burst and NO-mediated cytotoxicity (Chantry et al., 1989; Wahl et al., 1990). Thus, early in the immune response and formation of MS plaques, TGF-β may be proinflammatory; later, it may inhibit IL-2 responses by T cells and the cytolytic function of activated macrophages. Interestingly, TGF-β is one of the earliest cytokines seen in MS lesions, usually in association with the blood-brain barrier and at the lesion edge. It is also seen produced by resident glia in 'burned out' lesions, in normal-appearing white matter, and at the plaque edge where there are few if any inflammatory leukocytes (Fig. 2). Interleukin 6 (IL-6) may also behave as a proinflammatory cytokine, possibly altering the blood-brain barrier permeability and inducing immunoglobulin production in early acute lesions. IL-6 may also downregulate cytotoxicity by inhibiting IL-1 and TNF-α transcription (Schindler et al., 1990). IL-6 is present in the same regions of acute lesions as TGF-β and presumably is the product of macrophage activation and IL-1 and TNF-α production. In burned-out plaques, it is associated with the blood-brain barrier, while TGF-β is seen at the lesion margin (Fig. 2).

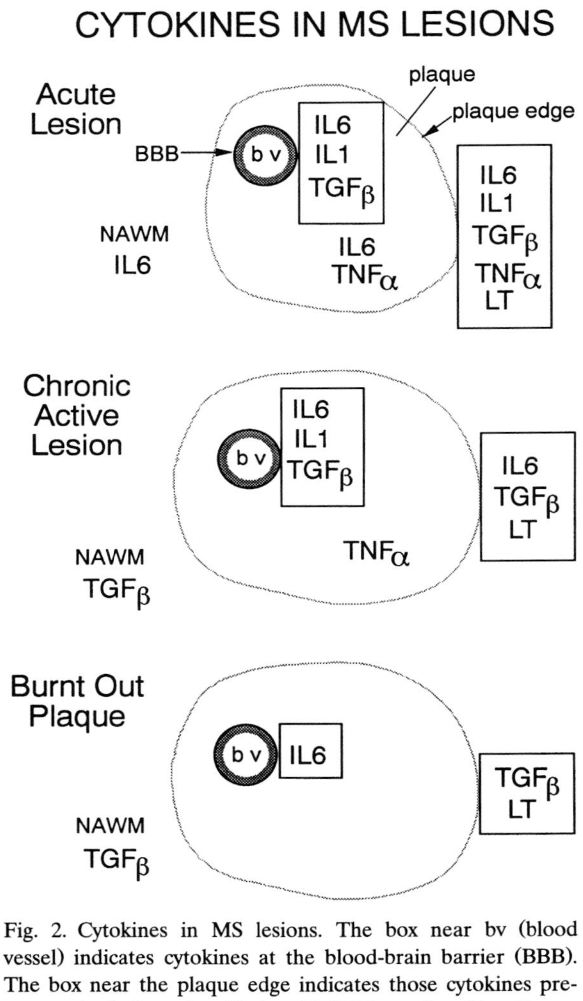

Fig. 2. Cytokines in MS lesions. The box near bv (blood vessel) indicates cytokines at the blood-brain barrier (BBB). The box near the plaque edge indicates those cytokines present at the lesion edge. IL-6 and TGF-β produced by glia are also found in normal-appearing white matter (NAWM) at various plaque stages.

Role of adhesion molecules, TNF-α, IFN-γ and neurotransmitters in NO cytotoxicity

IL-1, TNF-α and IFN-γ all increase intercellular adhesion molecule-1 (ICAM-1) and/or leukocyte functional antigen-1 (LFA-1), which leads to enhanced vulnerability of target cells to macrophage-mediated lysis (Dustin et al., 1986; Mentzer et al., 1986; Webb et al., 1991). TNF-α and IFN-γ synergize to induce L-arginine dependent cytotoxicity by macrophages (Green et al., 1990; Kilbourn et al., 1990). While early work concentrated on NO production by rodent macrophages, recently human macrophages have been shown to produce cytotoxic NO in response to TNF-α and granulocyte-macrophage colony stimulating factor (GM-CSF) (Denis, 1991). Thus, a precedent for studying NO in human macrophages has been established. These cytokines have also been implicated in oxygen burst and reactive oxygen intermediates in macrophages which can be toxic to target cells. Interestingly, NO and O_2^- may be injurious if they react to form stable peroxynitrite anion (Shingu et al., 1989; Beckman et al., 1990). Thus, oxygen reduction and nitrogen oxidation may cooperate to render the effector more lethal. Furthermore, inactivation of NO by superoxide anion increases leukocyte adherence to endothelial cells, another indicator of interactions of these two metabolic pathways (Kubes et al., 1991).

Microglial cells can produce NO (Zielasek et al., 1992; Merrill et al., 1993). NO production in macrophages requires induction. NO production in macrophages is predominantly regulated by a calcium,calmodulin-independent inducible enzyme, NO synthase (iNOS), which has recently been cloned (Xie et al., 1992). iNOS is inducible by LPS or IFN-γ alone. When used together, LPS and IFN-γ induce the majority of primary macrophages from the mouse to produce NOS and NO (Fig. 3). The inducibility of NO by single agents or cytokines or the requirement for combinations of stimuli appears to be dependent on the source of the macrophages, as well as on effector mechanisms and targets being examined. While LPS and IFN-γ induction of NO are additive, other cytokines and neurotransmitters also activate NO production in microglia. IL-1β, glutamate, and SP cause significant increases in NO production in vitro. IL-6, on the other hand, does not induce NO (Fig. 3). In our recent study demonstrating microglial cell (effectors) killing of oligodendrocytes (targets), we noticed that the targets induced increased NO production in the presence of the effectors (Merrill et al., 1993). Both NO production and cytotoxicity are upregulated by cytokines and inhibited by monomethyl-

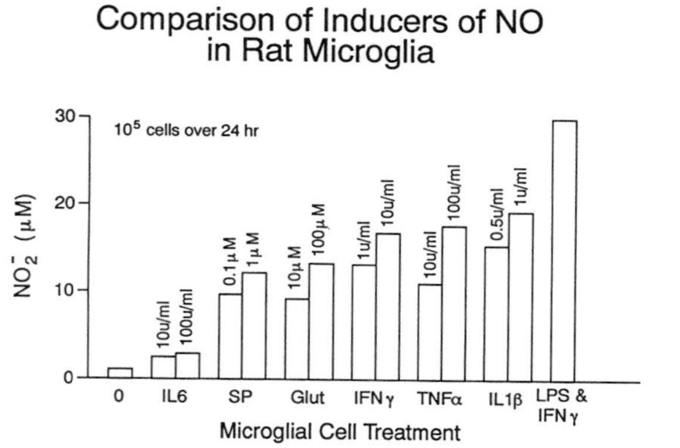

Fig. 3. Comparison of inducers of NO in rat microglia. Glut = glutamate. Lipopolysaccharide (LPS) was used at 10 $\mu g/ml$. Recombinant murine IFN-γ, when used with LPS, was used at 1 U/ml. Microglia at $10^5/ml$ were incubated for 24 h with cytokines or neurotransmitters.

L-arginine in a dose- and time-related fashion (Fig. 4).

Studies examining the suppression by TGF-β have demonstrated 1 to 10 ng/ml of TGF-β to be adequate to prevent NO production and cytotoxic effector functions by activated peritoneal murine macrophages (Ding et al., 1990; Nelson et al., 1991). We had previously demonstrated TGF-β-inhibitable spontaneous and induced cytotoxicity of oligodendrocytes by ameboid microglia (Fig. 5;

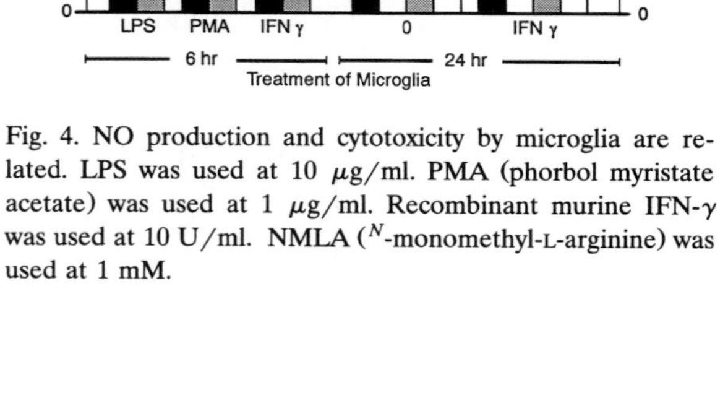

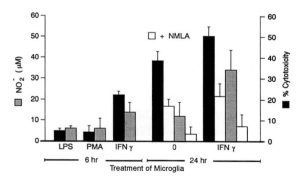

Fig. 4. NO production and cytotoxicity by microglia are related. LPS was used at 10 $\mu g/ml$. PMA (phorbol myristate acetate) was used at 1 $\mu g/ml$. Recombinant murine IFN-γ was used at 10 U/ml. NMLA (^{N}-monomethyl-L-arginine) was used at 1 mM.

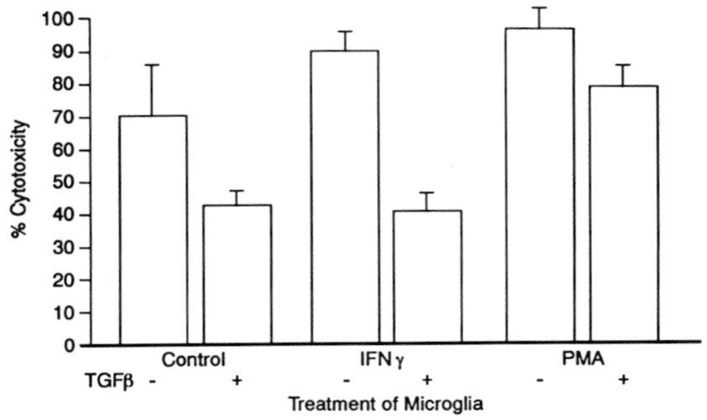

Fig. 5. Microglial cell cytotoxicity of oligodendrocytes is inhibited by TGF-β. Primary rat microglia effectors were mixed with rat oligodendrocyte targets at a ratio of 25:1. TGF-β (100 ng/ml), IFN-γ (10 U/ml) and PMA (1 μg/ml) were added separately or together to microglia 24 h prior to addition of oligodendrocyte targets.

Merrill and Zimmerman, 1991) and recently have demonstrated that stimulated microglia produce TGF-β-inhibitable NO_2^-. In addition, 50–60% of the spontaneous and IFN-γ-induced microglial cell cytotoxicity of oligodendrocytes is inhibitable by L-arginine analogues (NMLA, NAME) (Merrill et al., 1993). In vivo activation of microglia to produce O_2^- from O_2 and NO from N may account for the spontaneous cytotoxicity seen in vitro (Giulian et al., 1986) and a role for free radicals in modeling of the CNS during development (Boje et al., 1991; Chao et al., 1992).

Antibody treatment of ameboid microglia demonstrated a role for TNF-α in the killing of oligodendrocytes. Soluble TNF-α has been implicated in oligodendrocyte cell death and myelin destruction in vitro (Robbins et al., 1987; Selmaj and Raine 1988). We have been unable to demonstrate cytotoxic effects of soluble TNF-α on oligodendrocytes in vitro (Merrill, 1991). The role of TNF-α in microglia killing is probably due to its presence on the surface of the effector macrophage or microglia cell. Such ameboid microglia should have been present in the fetal spinal cord explant cultures studied by Selmaj and Raine (1988). The TNF-α molecule exists in two membrane-bound forms: a 17 kDa molecule bound to its receptor and a 26 kDa molecule which is an integral membrane protein. The transmembrane form is cytotoxic for tumor and virus-infected targets. Indeed, target cells resistant to killing by soluble TNF-α are sensitive to macrophage surface TNF-α (Peck et al., 1989). Cell-borne TNF-α acting as a cytotoxin or mediator could therefore account for directed inflammatory responses in vivo in tissues. It remains to be determined in our system whether TNF-α is acting by being bound to its receptor or as the transmembrane protein. In addition, the fact that inhibition of NO reduces killing by 60%, but inhibition of TNF-α reduces killing by 100%, suggests that TNF-α could be contributing to cell death in several ways. Membrane TNF-α could be directly cytotoxic but preliminary data from this lab suggest this is a nonapoptotic or necrotic lysis (Mitrovic et al., unpublished observations). This type of cell death in vitro resembles the pathology of the MS lesion, where there is evidence of cytoplasmic swelling of oligodendrocytes as well as membrane damage and lipid peroxidation (Prineas, 1985).

In addition to its induction of NO or direct cytotoxic activity, TNF-α may also act as a biological glue. Since TNF-α is active as a trimer and could bind more than one receptor at a time, it could bring enough effectors together with targets bearing TNF receptors to allow for membrane damage as well as induction or transmission of cytotoxins like NO or peroxynitrite to occur. Requirements for lysis include an effector to target ratio of 25:1 or 50:1, cell surface TNF-α, and viable cells in contact. Target and effector cell contact improves nitrite (NO_2^-) production, albeit through as yet undetermined mechanisms (Merrill et al., 1993). IL-1, TNF-α, and IFN-γ will increase expression of ICAM-1 and/or LFA-1, two cell surface adhesion molecules which lead to enhanced vulnerability of target cells to macrophage-mediated lysis (Dustin et al., 1986; Mentzer et al., 1986; Webb et al., 1991). Ameboid microglia express both ICAM-1 and LFA-1 in

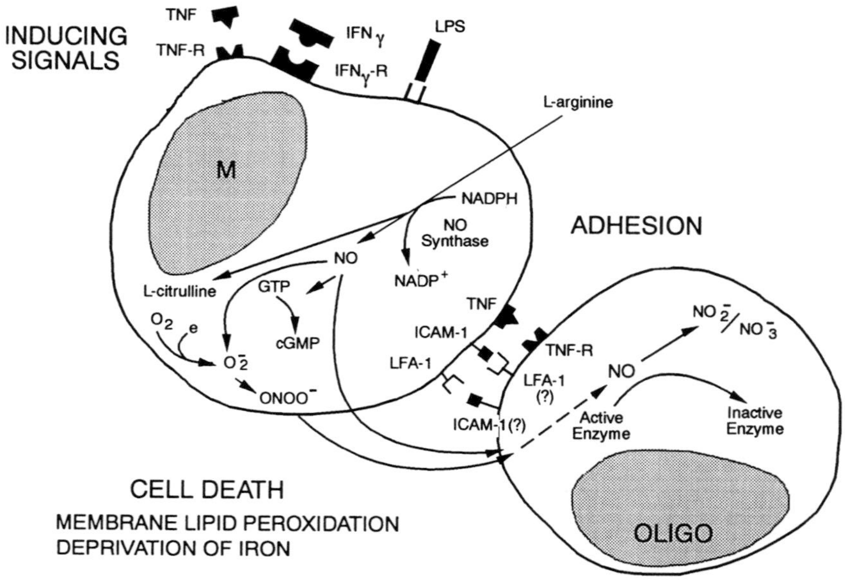

Fig. 6. Nitric oxide as a cytotoxic mediator. M = microglia; oligo = oligodendrocyte; $ONOO^-$ = peroxynitrite.

vitro and in vivo in experimental allergic encephalomyelitis (EAE) lesions (Raine et al., 1990). Such an interaction among microglia effectors themselves may facilitate aggregation of effectors for more efficient killing. Since anti-LFA-1 and anti-ICAM-1 antibodies inhibited cytotoxicity, this suggests that the stoichiometric requirements for cytotoxicity and numbers of cells required for production of NO_2^- in cultures of unstimulated ameboid microglia may be facilitating crosslinking and signaling through ICAM-1 (Fig. 6).

Summary

In summary, we have demonstrated an in vitro model for oligodendrocyte cell death that may be relevant to events in formation of lesions in MS. It involves cell contact to oligodendrocytes with activated, viable microglia (or inflammatory macrophages), surface TNF-α, surface adhesion molecules, and production of NO. Precise mechanisms of TNF-α and ICAM-1/LFA-1 participation and the nature of the susceptibility of the oligodendrocyte are currently being studied.

Acknowledgements

This research was partially funded by the UCLA Psychoneuroimmunology Task Force and an NIH Fogarty International AIDS Fellowship (BM), the Conrad N. Hilton Foundation, the Joe Gheen Fund, and National Institutes of Health grants NS26983 and NS30768 (JEM). The authors wish to thank Richard Burger (text, tables) and Carol A. Gray and Sharon Belkin (figures).

References

Albinia, J.E., Cui, S., Mateo, R.B. and Reichner, J.S. (1993) Nitric oxide-mediated apoptosis in murine peritoneal macrophages. *J. Immunol.*, 150: 5080–5085.

Bailey, S.J., Featherstone, R.L., Jordan, C.C. and Morton, I.K.M. (1986) An examination of the pharmacology of two substance P antagonists and the evidence for tachykinin receptor subtypes. *Br. J. Pharmacol.*, 87: 79–89.

Bar-Shavit, Z., Goldman. R., Stabinski, Y., Gottlieb, P., Fridkin, M., Teichberg, V.I. and Blumberg, S. (1980) Enhancement of phagocytosis – a newly found activity of substance P residing in its N-terminal tetrapeptide sequence. *J. Immunol.*, 130: 89–97.

Beck, J., Rondot, P., Catinot, L., Falcoff, E., Kirchner, H. and Wietzerbin J. (1988) Increased production of interferon gamma and tumor necrosis factor precedes clinical manifestation in multiple sclerosis: do cytokines trigger off exacerbations? *Acta Neurol. Scand.*, 78: 318–330.

Beckman, J., Beckman, T.W., Chen, J., Marshall, P.A. and Freeman, B.A. (1990) Apparent hydroxyl radical production by peroxynitrite: implications for endothelial injury from nitric oxide and superoxide. *Proc. Natl. Acad. Sci. USA*, 87: 1620–1624.

Boje, K.M. and Arora, P.K. (1992) Microglia-produced nitric oxide and reactive nitrogen oxides mediate neuronal cell death. *Brain Res.*, 587: 250–261.

Brandwein, S.R. (1986) Regulation of interleukin 1 production by mouse peritoneal macrophages. Effects of arachidonic acid metabolites, cyclic nucleotides, and interferons. *J. Biol. Chem.*, 261: 8624–8631.

Burcher, E. and Buck, S.H. (1986) Multiple tachykinin binding sites in hamster, rat, and guinea pig urinary bladder. *Eur. J. Pharmacol.*, 128: 165–178.

Chantry, D., Turner, M., Abney, E. and Feldmann, M. (1989) Modulation of cytokine production by transforming growth factor-β. Comparative study of cytotoxicity, tumor necrosis factor, and prostaglandin. *J. Immunol.*, 142: 4295–4300.

Chao, C.C., Hu, S., Molitor, T.W., Shaskan, E.G. and Peterson, P.K. (1992) Activated microglia mediated neuronal cell death injury via a nitric oxide mechanism. *J. Immunol.*, 149: 2736–2741.

Charles, A.C., Merrill, J.E., Dirksen, E.R. and Sanderson, M.J. (1991) Intercellular signaling in glial cells: calcium waves and oscillations in response to mechanical stimulation and glutamate. *Neuron*, 6: 983–992.

Charles, A.C., Dirksen, E.R., Merrill, J.E. and Sanderson, M.J. (1993) Mechanisms of intercellular calcium signaling in glial cells studied with dantrolene and thapsigargin. *Glia*, 7: 134–145.

Colpaert, F.C., Donnerer, J. and Lembeck, F. (1983) Effects of capsaicin on inflammation and on the substance P content of nervous tissue in rats with adjuvant arthritis. *Life Sci.*, 32: 1827–1832.

Conrad, G.W. and Rink, T.J. (1986) Platelet activating factor raises intracellular calcium ion concentration in macrophages. *J. Cell Biol.*, 103: 439–444.

Decker, T., Lohmann-Matthes, M.-L. and Gifford, G.E. (1987) Cell associated tumor necrosis factor (TNF) as a killing mechanism of activated cytotoxic macrophages. *J. Immunol.*, 138: 957–962.

Denis, M. (1991) Tumor necrosis factor and granulocyte-macrophage colony stimulating factor stimulate human macrophages to restrict growth of virulent mycobacterium and to kill avirulent *M. avium*. *J. Leuko. Biol.*, 94: 380–387.

Dustin, M.L., Rothlein, R., Bhan, K.A., Dinarello, C.A. and Springer, T.A. (1986) Induction by IL1 and interferon gamma: tissue distribution, biochemistry, and function of natural adherence molecule (ICAM-l). *J. Immunol.*, 137: 245–253.

Drapier, J.-C. and Hibbs, J.B. (1988) Differentiation of murine macrophages to express nonspecific cytotoxicity for tumor cells results in L-arginine-dependent inhibiton of mitochondrial iron sulfur enzymes in the macrophage effector cells. *J. Immunol.*, 140: 2829–2838.

Giulian, D. and Baker, T.J. (1986) Characterization of ameboid microglia isolated from developing mammalian brain. *J. Neurosci.*, 6: 2163- 2169.

Graeber, M.B., Streit, W.J., Kiefer, R., Schoen, S.W. and Kreutzberg, G.W. (1990) New expression of myelomonocytic antigens by microglia and perivascular cells following lethal motor neuron injury. *J. Neuroimmunol.*, 27: 121–127.

Green, S.J., Mellouk, S., Hoffman, S.L., Meltzer, M.S. and Nacy, C.A. (1990) Cellular mechanisms of nonspecific immunity to intracellular infection: cytokine-induced synthesis of toxic nitrogen oxides from L-arginine by macrophages and hepatocytes. *Immunol. Lett.*, 25: 15–19.

Hartung, H.-P., Wolters, K. and Toyka, K.V. (1986) Substance P: binding properties and studies on cellular responses in guinea pig macrophages. *J. Immunol.*, 136: 3856–3864.

Hartung, H.-P., Heininger, K., Schafer, B. and Toyka, K.V. (1988) Substance P and astrocytes: stimulation of the cyclooxygenase pathway of arachidonic acid metabolism. *FASEB J.*, 2: 48–53.

Hashimoto, M., Ishikawa, Y., Yokota, S., Goto, F., Bando, T., Sakakibara, Y. and Iriki, M. (1991) Action site of circulating Interleukin-1 on the rabbit brain. *Brain Res.*, 540: 217–223.

Hofman, F.M., von Hanwehr, F.I., Dinarello, C.A., Mizel, S.B., Hinton, D. and Merrill, J.E.. (1986) Immunoregulatory molecules and IL2 receptors identified in multiple sclerosis brain. *J. Immunol.*, 136: 3239–3245.

Hofman, F.M., Hinton, D.R., Johnson, K. and Merrill, J.E. (1989) Tumor necrosis factor identified in multiple sclerosis brain. *J. Exp. Med.*, 170: 607–612.

Hunter, M.I.S., Nlemadim, B.C. and Davidson, D.L.W. (1985) Lipid peroxidation production and antioxidant proteins in plasma and cerebrospinal fluid from multiple sclerosis patients. *Neurochem. Res.*, 10: 1645–1652.

Kilbourn, R.G., Gross, S.S., Jubran, A., Adams, J., Griffith, O.W., Levi, R. and Lodato, R.F. (1990) N^G-methyl-L-arginine inhibits tumor necrosis factor induced hypotension: implications for the involvement of nitric oxide. *Proc. Natl. Acad. Sci. USA*, 87: 3629–3632.

Kimball, E.S., Persico, F.J. and Vaught, J.L. (1988) Substance P, Neurokinin A, and Neurokinin B induce generation of

IL-1-like activity in P388D1 cells. *J. Immunol.*, 141: 3564–3572.

Kostyk, S.K., Kowall, N.W. and Hauser, S.L. (1989) Substance P immunoreactive astrocytes are present in multiple sclerosis plaques. *Brain Res.*, 504: 284–289.

Kubes, P., Suzuki, M. and Granger, D.N. (1991) Nitric oxide: an endogenous modulator of leukocyte adhesion. *Proc. Natl. Acad. Sci. USA*, 88: 4651- 4655.

Larsen, P.J., Mikkelsen, J.D. and Saermak, T. (1989) Binding of an iodinated substance P analog to an NK1 receptor on isolated cell membranes from rat anterior pituitary. *Endocrinology*, 124: 2548- 2552.

Laurenzi, M.A., Persson, M.A.A., Dalsgaard, C.-J. and Haegerstrand, A. (1990) The neuropeptide substance P stimulates production of interleukin 1 in human blood monocytes: activated cells are preferentially influenced by the neuropeptide. *Scand. J. Immunol.*, 31: 529–535.

Lieberman, A.P., Pitha, P.M., Shin, H.S. and Shin, M.L. (1989) Production of tumor necrosis factor and other cytokines by astrocytes stimulated with lipopolysaccharide or a neurotrophic virus. *Proc. Natl. Acad. Sci. USA*, 86: 6348–6351.

Lotz, M., Carson, D. and Vaughan, J.H. (1987) Substance P activation of rheumatoid synoviocytes: neural pathway in pathogenesis of arthritis. *Science*, 238: 893–895.

Lotz, M., Vaughan, J.H. and Carson, D.A. (1988) Effect of neuropeptides on production of inflammatory cytokines by human monocytes. *Science*, 241: 1218–1220.

Mantyh, C.R., Gates, T.S., Zimmerman, R.P., Welton, M.L., Passaro, E.P., Vigna, S.R., Maggio, J.E., Kruger, L. and Mantyh, P.W. (1988) Receptor binding sites for substance P, but not substance K or neuromedin K, are expressed in high concentrations by arterioles, venules, and lymph nodes in surgical specimens obtained from patients with ulcerative colitis and Crohn disease. *Proc. Natl. Acad. Sci. USA*, 85: 3235–3239.

Mantyh, P.W., Johnson, D.J., Boehmer, C.G., Catton, M.D., Vinters, H.V., Maggio, J.E., Too, H.-P. and Vigna, S.R. (1989) Substance P receptor binding sites are expressed by glia in vivo after neuronal injury. *Proc. Natl. Acad. Sci. USA*, 86: 5193–5196.

Martin, F.C., Charles, A.C., Sanderson, M.J. and Merrill, J.E. (1992) Substance P stimulates IL1 production by astrocytes via intracellular calcium. *Brain Res.*, 599: 13–18.

Martin, F.C., Anton, P.A., Gornbein, J.A., Shanahan, F. and Merrill, J.E. (1993) Production of ILl by microglia in response to substance P: role for a nonclassical NKl receptor. *J. Neuroimmunol.*, 42: 53–60.

McLean, S., Ganong, A.H., Seeger,. J.F., Bryce, D.K., Pratt, K.G., Reynolds, L.S., Siok, C.J., Lowe, J.A., III and Heym, J. (1991) Activity and distribution of binding sites in brain of a nonpeptide substance P (NK) receptor antagonist. *Science*, 251: 437–439.

Mentzer, S.J., Faller, D.V. and Burakoff, S.S. (1986) Interferon γ induction of LFA-1 mediated homotypic adhesion of human monocytes. *J. Immunol.*, 137: 108–114.

Merrill, J.E. (1991) The effect of IL1 and TNFα on astrocytes, microglia, oligodendrocytes, and glial precursors in vitro. *Dev. Neurosci.*, 13: 130–137.

Merrill, J.E. and Zimmerman, R.P. (1991) Natural and induced cytotoxicity of oligodendrocytes by microglia is inhibitable by TGFβ. *Glia*, 4: 327- 331.

Merrill. J.E., Strom, S.R., Ellison, G.W. and Myers, L.W.. (1989) In vitro study of mediators of inflammation in multiple sclerosis. *J. Clin. Immunol.*, 9: 84–96.

Merrill, J.E., Graves, M.C. and Mulder, D.G. (1992) Autoimmune disease and the nervous system: biochemical, molecular, and clinical update. *West. J. Med.*, 156: 639–6461.

Merrill, J.E., Ignarro, L.J., Sherman, M.P., Melinek, J. and Lane, T.E. (1993) Microglial cell cytotoxicity of oligodendrocytes is mediated through nitric oxide. *J. Immunol.*, 151: 2132–2141.

Murphy, S., Simmons, M.L., Aguillo, L., Garcia, A., Feinstein, D.L., Galea, E., Reis, D.J., Ninc-Golomb, D. and Schwartz, J.P. (1993) Synthesis of nitric oxide in CNS glial cells. *Trends Neurosci.*, 16: 323-328.

Nussler, A.K. and Billiar, T.R. (1993) Review. Inflammation, immunoregulation, and inducible nitric oxide synthase. *J. Leuko. Biol.*, 54: 171–178.

Panitch, H.S., Hirsch, R.L., Schindler, J. and Johnson, K.P. (1987) Treatment of multiple sclerosis with gamma interferon: exacerbations associated with activation of the immune system. *Neurology* , 37: 1097–1100.

Payan, D.G., Brewster, D.R., Missirian-Bastian, A. and Goetzel, E.J. (1984) Substance P recognition by a subset of human T lymphocytes. *J. Clin. Invest.*, 74: 1532–1537.

Pearce, B. and Murphy, S. (Eds.) (1983) *Neurotransmitter Receptors Coupled to Inositol Phospholipid Turnover and Ca^{2+} Flux: Consequences for Astrocyte Function*, Raven Press, New York.

Peck, R. (1987) Neuropeptides modulating macrophage function. *Science*, 239: 264–267.

Peck, R., Brockhaus, M. and Frey, J.R. (1989) Cell surface tumor necrosis factor (TNF) accounts for monocyte and lymphocyte-mediated killing of TNF resistant target cells. *Cell. Immunol.*, 122: 1–10.

Prineas, J.W. (1985) The neuropathology of multiple sclerosis. In: J.C. Kostzier (Ed.) *Handbook of Clinical Neurology*, Elsevier Science Publishers, Amsterdam, pp. 213–257.

Prpic, V., Weiel, J.E., Somers, S.D., DiGuiseppi, J., Gonias, S.L., Pizzo, S.V., Hamilton, T.A., Herman, B. and Adams, D.O. (1987) Effects of bacterial lipopolysaccharide on the hydrolysis of phosphatidylinositol-4,5-bisphosphate in murine peritoneal macrophages. *J. Immunol.*, 139: 526-534.

Raine, C.S., Cannella, B., Duijvestijn, A.M. and Cross, A.H. (1990) Homing to central nervous system vasculature by antigen-specific lymphocytes. II. Lymphocyte/endothelial cell adhesion during the initial stages of autoimmune demyelination. *Lab. Invest.*, 63: 476–488.

Regoli, D., Drapeau, G., Dion, S. and D'Orleans-Juste, P. (1989) Receptors for substance P and related neurokinins. *Pharmacology*, 38: 1–11.

Robbins, D.S., Shirazi, Y., Drysdale, B.-E., Lieberman, A., Shin, H.S. and Shin, M.L. (1987) Production of cytotoxic factors for oligodendrocytes by stimulated astrocytes. *J. Immunol.*, 139: 2593–2597.

Ruff, M.R., Wahl, S.M. and Pert, C.B. (1985) Substance P receptor-mediated chemotaxis of human monocytes. *Peptides*, 6 (Suppl 2): 107.

Sarih, M., Souvannavong, V. and Adam, A. (1993) Nitric oxide synthase induces macrophage death by apoptosis. *Biochem. Biophys. Res. Commun.*, 191: 503–508.

Schindler, R., Mancilla, J., Endres, S., Ghorhani, R., Clark, S.C. and Dinarello, C.A. (1990) Correlations and interactions in the production of interleukin 6 (IL6), IL1 and tumor necrosis factor (TNF) in human blood mononuclear cells: IL6 suppresses IL1 and TNF. *Blood*, 75: 40- 47.

Selmaj, K.W. and Raine, C.S. (1988) Tumor necrosis factor mediates myelin and oligodendrocyte damage in vitro. *Ann. Neurol.*, 23: 339–343.

Shanahan, F., Denburg, J.A., Fox, J., Bienenstock, J. and Befus, D. (1985) Mast cell heterogeneity: effects of neuroenteric peptides on histamine release. *J. Immunol.*, 135: 1331–1339.

Sharief, M.K. and Hentges, R. (1991) Association between tumor necrosis factor-α and disease progression in patients with multiple sclerosis. *N. Engl. J. Med.*, 25: 467–472.

Shingu, M., Nonaka, S., Nobunaga, M. and Ahamadzadeh, N. (1989) Possible role of H_2O_2-mediated complement activation and cytokine-mediated fibroblast superoxide generation on skin inflammation. *Dermatology*, 179: 107–112.

Shinomiya, H. and Nakano, M. (1987) Calcium ionophore A23187 does not stimulate lipopolysaccharide nonresponsive CSH/HeJ peritoneal macrophages to produce interleukin 1. *J. Immunol.*, 139: 2730–2738.

Snider, R.M., Constantine, J.W., III, Longo, K.P., Lebel, W.S., Woody, H.A., Drozda, S.E., Desai, M.C., Vinick, F.J., Spencer, R.W. and Hess, H.-J. (1991) A potent nonpeptide antagonist of the substance P (NK1) receptor. *Science*, 251: 435–437.

Stuehr, D.J. and Marletta, M. (1987) Induction of nitrite/nitrate synthesis in murine macrophages by BCG infection, lymphokines, or interferon-γ. *J. Immunol.*, 139: 518–522.

Tissot, M., Pradelles, P. and Giroud, J.P. (1988) Substance-P-like levels in inflammatory exudates. *Inflammation*, 12: 25–35.

Torrens, Y., Beaujouan, J.C. and Glowinski, J. (1985) Pharmacological characterization of two tachykinin binding sites in the rat cerebral cortex. *Neuropeptides*, 6: 59–64.

Torrens, Y., Beaujouan, J.C., Saffray, M., Daguet de MonTety, M.C., Bergstrom, L. and Glowinski, J. (1986) Substance P receptors in primary cultures of cortical astrocytes from the mouse. *Proc. Natl. Acad. Sci. USA*, 83: 9216–9219.

Torrens, Y., Daguet De Montety, M.C., El Etr, M., Beaujouan, J.C. and Glowinski, J. (1989) Tachykinin receptors of the NK1 type (substance P) coupled positively to phospholipase C on cortical astrocytes from the newborn mouse in primary culture. *J. Neurochem.*, 52: 1913-1920.

Wahl, S.M., Allen, J.B., Wong, H.L., Dougherty, S.F. and Ellingsworth, L.R. (1990) Antagonistic and agonistic effects of transforming growth factor-β and IL-1 in rheumatoid synovium. *J. Immunol.*, 145: 2514- 2519.

Wallengren, J., Ekman, R. and Moller, H. (1986) Substance P and vasoactive intestinal peptide in bullous and inflammatory skin disease. *Acta Derm. Venereol.*, 66: 23–28.

Webb, D.S., Mostowski, H.W. and Gerrard, T.L. (1991) Cytokine-induced enhancement of ICAM-1 expression results in increased vulnerability of tumor cells to monocyte-mediated lysis. *J. Immunol.*, 146: 3682- 3687.

Welsh, N., Eizirik, D.L., Bendtzen, K. and Sandler, S. (1991) Interleukin 1β-induced nitric oxide production in isolated rat pancreatic islets requires gene transcription and may lead to inhibition of the Krebs cycle enzyme aconitase. *Endocrinology*, 129: 3167–3172.

Wienrich, M. and Kettenmann, H. (1989) Activation of substance P receptors leads to membrane potential responses in cultured astrocytes. *Glia*, 2: 155–160.

Woodroofe, M.N., Sarna, G.W., Wadhwa, M., Hayes, G.M., Loughlin, A.J., Tinker, A. and Cuzner, M.L. (1991) Detection of interleukin 1 and interleukin 6 in adult rat brain following mechanical injury by in vivo microdialysis: evidence of a role for microglia in cytokine production. *J. Neuroimmunol.*, 33: 227–233.

Xie, Q-W., Cho, H.J., Calaycay, J., Mumford, R.A., Swiderek, K.M., Lee, A.D., Ding, A., Troso, T. and Nathan, C. (1992) Cloning and characterization of inducible nitric oxide synthase from mouse macrophages. *Science*, 256: 225- 227.

Zielasek, J. M., Tausch, M., Toyka, K.V. and Hartung, H.-P. (1992) Production of nitrite by neonatal rat microglia cells/brain macrophages. *Cell. Immunol.*, 141: 111–120.

F.J. Seil (Ed.)
Progress in Brain Research, Vol 103

CHAPTER 27

Cytokines and cytokine-related substances regulating glial cell response to injury of the central nervous system

Michal Schwartz, Tomer Sivron, Shoshana Eitan, David L. Hirschberg, Mirit Lotan and Anat Elman-Faber

Department of Neurobiology, The Weizmann Institute of Science, 76100 Rehovot, Israel

Introduction

Axons of the central nervous system (CNS) of mammals do not normally regenerate after injury, unlike those of phylogenetically lower vertebrates, such as fish and amphibians, or the peripheral nerves of mammals (Ramón y Cajal, 1928; Sperry, 1948; Reier and Webster, 1974; Murray, 1976; Kiernan, 1979; Grafstein, 1986). Because injured mammalian CNS axons can, under certain conditions, grow for considerable distances (David and Aguayo, 1981; Lavie et al., 1990; Schnell and Schwab, 1990), it is generally believed today that the ability or inability of nerves to regenerate their injured axons depends on the cellular milieu surrounding the axons and its response to axonal injury.

Among the components of the cellular milieu are oligodendrocytes, astrocytes, resident microglia and invading macrophages. Recent research has shed more light on the nature of these cells and their associated soluble and insoluble substances in the mature nerve in the resting state and after injury. Several studies have helped to elucidate key cellular processes and substances in regeneration, and have demonstrated the involvement of regeneration-related cross-talk between the immune and the nervous systems. These findings are based on two independent lines of research, one involving studies of the fish optic nerve, and the other studies of mammalian sciatic nerves. Both systems regenerate readily after injury.

Postinjury acquisition of growth-supportive characteristics

The ability of nerves to regenerate has been correlated with the ability of sections of these nerves to support neuronal attachment and axonal growth in vitro. Thus, sections of rat sciatic nerve and fish optic nerve, both of which are capable of regeneration, support neuronal attachment and axonal growth of neuroblastoma cells or embryonic neurons, while sections of the non-regenerative rat optic nerve do not (Carbonetto et al., 1987; Savio and Schwab, 1989). This by itself might lead one to conclude that fish CNS and mammalian peripheral nervous systems (PNS) differ constitutively from mammalian CNS. However, recent data accumulated by Bedi et al. (1992) and in our laboratory (Sivron et al., 1994a) point to the possibility that the postinjury response is critical for acquisition of regeneration-supportive properties. Thus, for example, fish optic nerve sections which support the growth of embryonic neurons did not support neuritic outgrowth from adult neurons, i.e., regenerating retina (Sivron et al., 1994a). Once injured, however, both the fish optic nerve and the rat sciatic nerve became permissive to growth of adult neurons (Bedi et al., 1992; Sivron et al., 1994a). The nonpermissive character of the normal (i.e. uninjured) nerve could result from a deficiency in growth-supportive elements or the presence of growth-inhibitory molecules, or from both. These results imply that: (i) even a system that regenerates might, like nonregenerating systems, contain inhibitors; and (ii) the response to injury plays a crucial role in conferring growth-supportive properties on a nervous system.

Further studies demonstrated that fish optic nerve and spinal cord myelin contain growth inhibitors similar to those of rat CNS myelin (Sivron et al., 1994a). Thus, antibodies directed against rat myelin inhibitors (IN-1 antibodies) (Caroni and Schwab, 1988) were also able to neutralize the inhibitors of fish myelin (Fig. 1). These findings appear to contradict the claim of Bastmeyer et al. (1991) that fish oligodendrocyte-like cells are supportive of axonal growth. In that study, however, the oligodendrocyte-like cells were positive for glial fibrillary acidic protein (GFAP), an astrocyte marker, which might imply that they were immature oligodendrocytes or even progenitor cells (Sivron et al., 1992, 1994b). Since even rat oligodendrocytes, when immature, do not inhibit axonal growth (Schwab and Caroni, 1988), it should not be surprising that the fish cells in

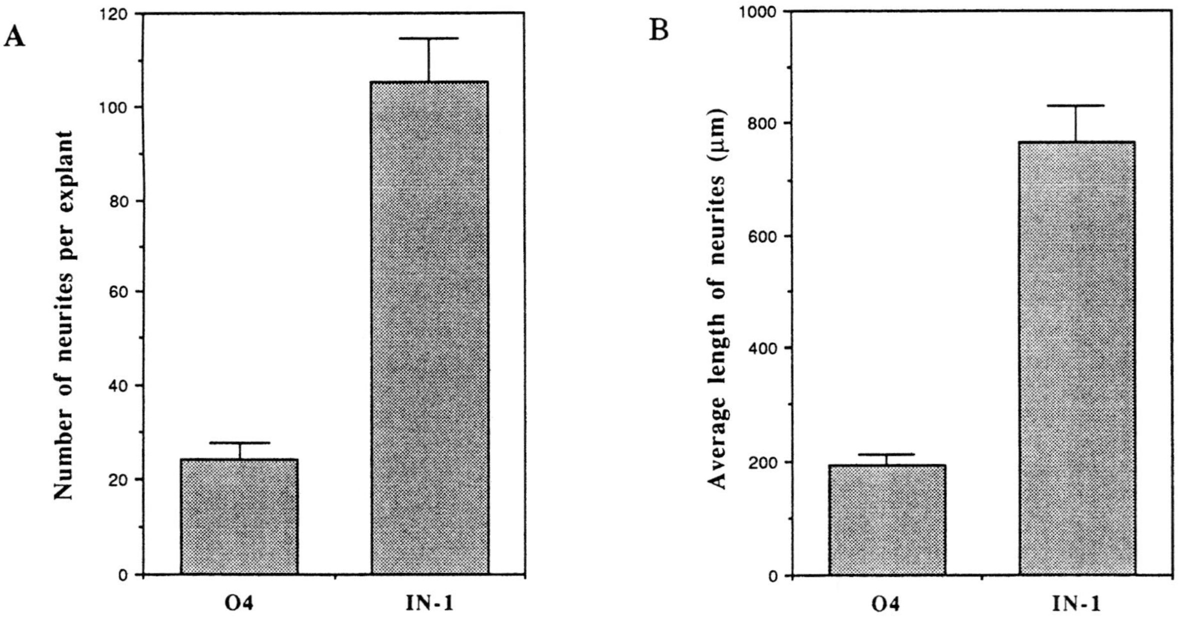

Fig. 1. Neutralization of the fish myelin growth inhibitors by the IN-1 antibodies. Fish optic nerve myelin was coated on poly-L-lysine (PLL)-coated Petri dishes and then incubated either with the IN-1 antibodies or with 04 antibodies as control. After washing off the antibodies, fish retinal explants were placed onto the myelin. Neuritic outgrowth was assessed 48 h after explanting, and the number of neurites per explant and their lengths were determined. The figure gives results of three different experiments, each carried out in quadruplicate. Incubation with IN-1 antibodies increased both the number of neurites (A) and their lengths (B) by a factor of 4. (From Sivron et al., 1994b.)

Bastmeyer's study were found to support axonal growth. It thus seems that both fish and rat optic nerves, representative of regenerating and nonregenerating nervous systems, respectively, contain similar myelin-associated growth inhibitors, and that in both of these systems the uninjured nerves are nonpermissive to the growth of adult axons. What, then, makes the two systems behave differently after injury?

Firstly, in the regenerating system there is probably a lower level of growth-inhibitory molecules, as indicated by the weaker inhibition exhibited by fish myelin than by rat myelin (Fig. 2). This, however, is not enough to explain their differences in ability to regenerate (Sivron et al., 1994a). A second major difference between the two systems has to do with their response to injury. Thus, the injury-induced increase in permissiveness in the fish optic nerve could be the result of elimination of inhibitory molecules and/or increase of growth-supportive molecules.

Involvement of interleukin 2 or related compounds in the posttraumatic glial cell response to injury of the fish optic nerve

The postinjury changes in permissiveness to neuronal growth observed in the fish optic nerve

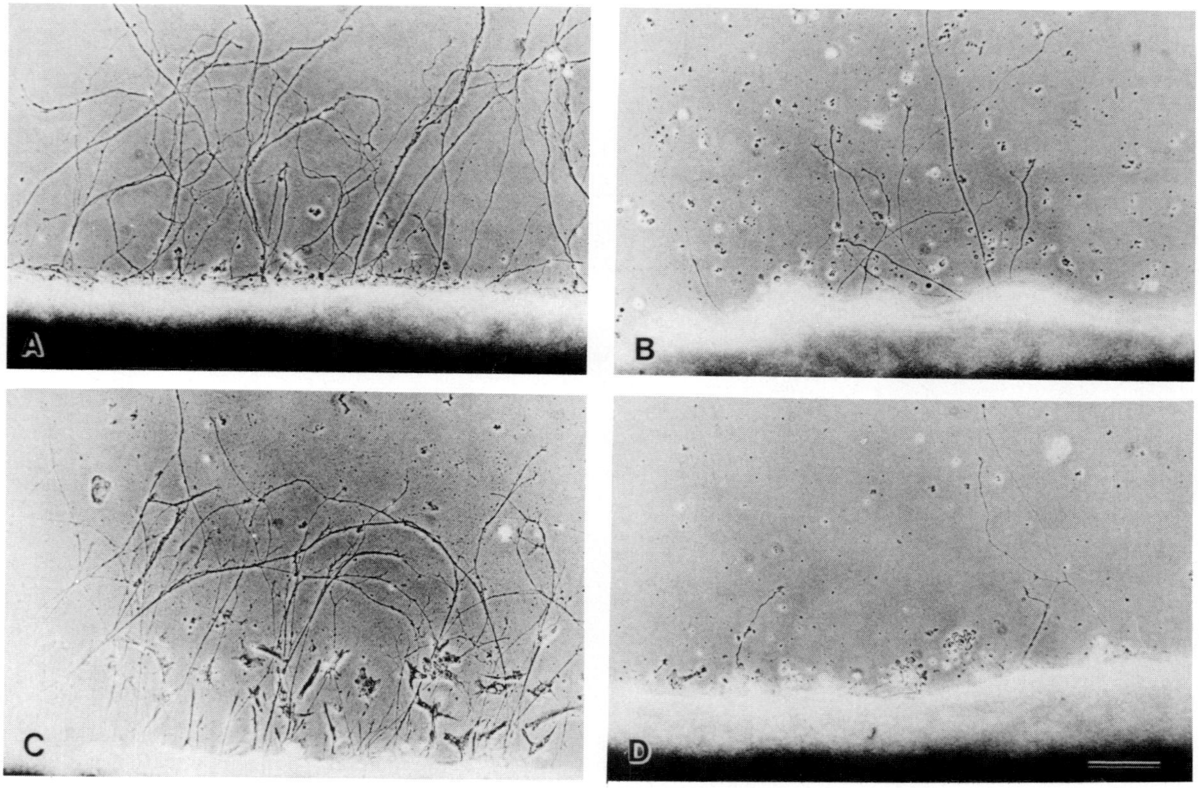

Fig. 2. Retinal explants on fish optic nerve myelin, fish optic nerve membranes and rat optic nerve myelin. PLL-coated coverslips were coated with fish optic nerve myelin (B), fish optic nerve membranes (C), or rat optic nerve myelin (D). After washing, retinal explants were placed on the coverslips and allowed to grow for 48h. While many neurites can be seen growing on the PLL (A) and fish membranes (C), only a few grew on fish optic nerve myelin (B) and even fewer on rat myelin (D). Scale bar is 100 μm. (From Sivron et al., 1994b.)

suggest that, as a result of the injury, the axonal milieu undergoes cellular and molecular changes. Previous studies have indicated that, following injury, there is a change in the repertoire of soluble substances originating from the regenerating fish optic nerve (Schwartz et al., 1985; Harel et al., 1989, 1990). We postulated that these soluble substances include those that are actively involved in making the nerve permissive to growth; in other words, they regulate the glial response to injury in such a way that inhibition is eliminated and supportive elements are acquired or enhanced. Application of a preparation containing such substances to injured rabbit optic nerves in vivo resulted in regenerative growth, which significantly exceeded the growth occurring spontaneously after injury in untreated nerves (Schwartz et al., 1985; Lavie et al., 1990). On the basis of this finding we proposed that the preparation might contain glia-modulating factors, and we examined this possibility in vitro in cultures of dissociated adult rat optic nerve. The most pronounced effect was found to be on the number of mature oligodendrocytes (Fig. 3) (Cohen et al., 1990). Application of the preparation to cultures of mixed glial cells verified that its effect was specific for oligodendrocytes. Further studies revealed that the active molecule within the preparation is an interleukin 2 (IL-2)-like compound, as its activity was neutralized by antibodies directed against IL-2 (Fig. 4) (Eitan et al., 1992). However, it was found to be twice the molecular weight of IL-2 (Eitan et al., 1992). The same preparation was also found to contain an

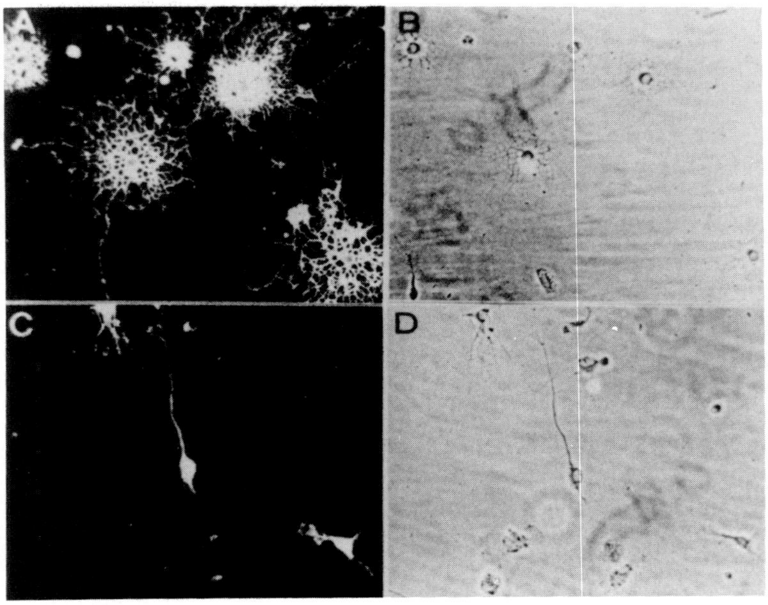

Fig. 3. Effect of fish soluble substances derived from regenerating nerves on adult 04-positive cells in cultures of injured adult rat optic nerves dissected out 3 days after injury. Each experiment involved cells from five adult rat optic nerves, crushed 3 days before excision, that were seeded on PLL-coated coverslips in defined medium. Cultures were stained for 04 immunoreactivity at 96 h in vitro by an indirect immunofluorescent method. Panels A and B show, respectively, fluorescent and phase micrographs of the control cells in defined medium without any treatment. Panel C shows 04-positive cells in cultures which were treated with the soluble substances derived from the regenerating fish optic nerves (12 μg protein/ml) for 48 h prior to the staining. Panels C and D represent fluorescent and phase micrographs of the same cells. Pictures were taken from one experiment, the results of which were reproduced in two additional experiments. (From Cohen et al., 1990.)

enzyme which is capable of dimerizing IL-2 and is present in increased amounts in the regenerating fish optic nerve (Eitan and Schwartz, 1993). The resulting dimer was cytotoxic to oligodendrocytes. The enzyme was identified as a nerve-derived transglutaminase (TG_N) and was purified to homogeneity (Eitan and Schwartz, 1993). Dimeric IL-2 produced in the presence of the purified enzyme and Ca^{2+} was found to be cytotoxic to oligodendrocytes (Fig. 5). Taken together, the above findings suggest that oligodendrocytes may be prevented from inhibiting axonal growth after injury of the fish optic nerve by being eliminated. It follows that the presence in the injured nerve of a factor cytotoxic to oligodendrocytes may be crucial for regeneration. It is possible that mammals lack the mechanism for eliminating oligodendrocytes, or at least that the mechanism does not operate at the right time. One should, however, bear in mind that the increase in growth-permissiveness following fish optic nerve injury might also involve at least one other phenomenon in addition to the elimination of inhibitory molecules, namely, the increase of growth-supportive elements.

Interestingly, the discovery of the IL-2-like factor and TG_N points to the likelihood that, contrary to the widely held view, the rules and principles determining response to injury in other systems may apply to the nervous system as well. In addition, the data suggest a mechanism by which an external cytokine derived from the immune system is converted by a CNS element, namely TG_N, to an active cytotoxic factor. This cascade of events, if it occurs also in vivo, indicates that the cross-talk between the immune system and the nervous system in response to axonal injury has beneficial implications for regeneration. Such cross-talk could be mediated by invading inflammatory cells and/or their products. Such invading inflammatory cells may participate in the remodeling of the tissue by: (i) removal of degradation products; (ii) secretion of growth factors and cytokines; and (iii) recycling of lipid degradation products needed for reconstruction.

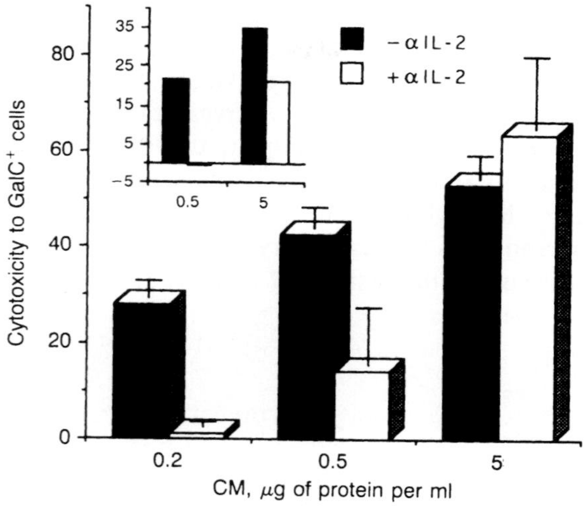

Fig. 4. Neutralization of the cytotoxic effect of fish soluble substances on oligodendrocytes by rabbit polyclonal antibodies directed against recombinant human IL-2 antibodies: assessment by immunofluorescence. The highest concentration of the soluble substances derived from regenerating fish optic nerves (5 μg protein) resulted in about 60% cytotoxicity and no neutralization with anti-IL-2 antibodies; 0.5 μg of conditioned medium caused 42% cytotoxicity, half of which could be neutralized by the antibodies; complete neutralization with the same amount of antibodies could be obtained when only 0.2 μg of the conditioned medium was applied. Results are expressed as percent cytotoxicity, in relation to cytoxocity-free control cultures treated with antibodies only (100% survival, no cytotoxicity). All experiments were repeated three times and were carried out using 0.1 μg of anti-IL-2 antibodies (IgG). The results of one experiment are given in this figure; CM designates conditioned medium. The absolute total number of galactocerebroside (galC)-positive cells counted in each coverslip ranged from 300 to 500 in the various experiments. The inset shows basically the same experiments carried out with 10-fold more anit-IL-2 antibodies, i.e., 1 μg IgG. (From Eitan et al., 1992.)

Cross-talk between the immune and the nervous system

Cross-talk between the immune and nervous systems has already been implicated from other studies, mainly those related to peripheral nerve regeneration or involving the postinjury comparison of macrophage invasion in mammalian CNS and PNS.

A few years ago, Perry et al. (1987) showed that, after crush injury of the sciatic or optic nerve in mouse or rat, large numbers of macrophages enter sciatic nerves containing degenerating axons. In contrast, the degenerating optic nerve attracts few macrophages. These results highlighted the different responses of macrophages to nerve injury in the PNS and CNS. In view of the ability of the sciatic nerve to regenerate, the massive invasion of macrophages in the injured sciatic nerve supports the assumption that macrophages may be an important component of postinjury neuronal repair. Further insight into the relationship between macrophages and regeneration comes from a series of studies with C57BL/6/Ola mice, in which leukocyte invasion into injured peripheral nerves is slow and sparse (Lunn et al., 1989). In these mice, the

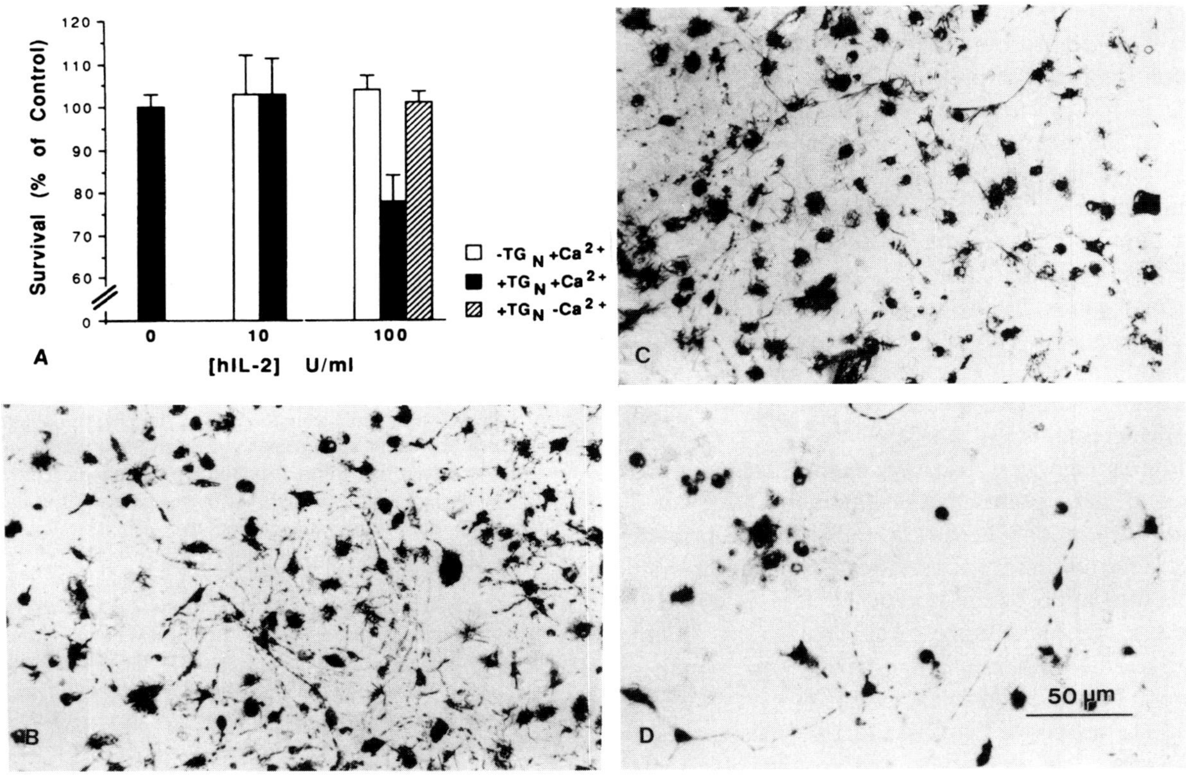

Fig. 5. Cytotoxic effect of dimeric IL-2 on oligodendrocytes. Oligodendrocyte cultures derived from neonatal rat brains were prepared as previously described (Cohen et al., 1990) and seeded in wells coated with PLL (20 $\mu g/\mu l$; Sigma). After 72 h, the seeded cells were treated for 48 h with various preparations containing IL-2, TG_N or both. (A) Human IL-2 (hIL-2)(10 U/ml and 100U/ml) was incubated with a constant amount of TG_N. Cytotoxic activity was assessed by the colorimetric MTT [3-(4,5-dimethylthiazol-2-y1)-2,5-diphenyltetrazolium bromide] assay (Sigma). MTT was added for 3 h, and the medium was then removed and 100 μl of 0.04 M HC1 in isopropanol was added. Absorbance of the cells was recorded at 540 nm and compared to absorbance at 630 nm. Oligodendrocytes were incubated as described with IL-2 or TG_N alone, or with IL-2 incubated with TG_N in the presence and absence of Ca^{2+}; results are expressed as percentage survival (mean $\pm$ SE) relative to that of untreated cells. The group treated with IL-2 incubated with TG_N in the presence of CA^{2+} is significantly different from all others ($n = 3$, $P = 0.02$, $F = 7.83$; ANOVA). (B) Cultures treated with hIL-2 only (100 U/ml). The micrographs show the various treated cultures after MTT staining. (C) Cultures treated with TG_N only. (D) Cultures treated with a mixture of hIL-2 (100 U/ml) and TG_N in the presence of Ca^{2+} (i.e., containing the dimeric hIL-2). (From Eitan and Schwartz, 1993.)

myelinated sensory axons regenerated slowly and incompletely, while the regeneration of motor axons was only slightly slowed as compared to normal mice.

Further support of the notion that mammals may suffer, at least temporarily, from a deficiency of macrophages and/or their products (in terms of amount of invading macrophages or the specific repertoire of factors that they produce) comes from studies carried out in mammalian CNS. For example, David et al. (1990), using an in vitro assay to investigate the role of macrophages in influencing axonal growth, showed that soon after transection of adult rat optic nerve, the normally nonpermissive nerve becomes growth-permissive near the lesion. This injury-associated change in the axonal growth-promoting properties of the CNS near the lesion may be induced by mononuclear phagocytes.

The spatial and temporal relationships between regeneration and postinjury macrophage invasion suggest that the inability of mammalian CNS to regenerate may be at least partly due to a deficiency (even temporary) of macrophages and/or their products. This impairment of macrophage invasion in the mammalian CNS might result from a defect in a critical signal that comes from the injured nerves and is needed for macrophage recruitment. In addition, the invading macrophages might be receiving an inappropriate stimulus for production of the needed factors. This possible bidirectional interaction between the nervous and the immune systems is summarized schematically in Fig. 6. Support for this notion comes from our work, in which we compared the ability of macrophages to migrate in vitro toward gradients created by sciatic nerves and by optic nerves. In this study, segments of adult rat sciatic or optic nerves were placed at the bottom of a Boyden chamber containing medium, and a filter (Sartorius) was placed over the top. The upper part of the chamber contained leukocytes in medium. At various times after the sealing of the chamber the filters were removed, fixed, visualized and quantified. Our preliminary results revealed that migration of leukocytes toward a gradient created by the sciatic nerves was far more efficient, in terms of time and number, as compared with a gradient created by optic nerves. This finding implies the possible presence in vivo of factors that recruit leukocytes more efficiently in sciatic than in optic nerves and that possibly trigger these cells differently (D.L. Hirschberg and M. Schwartz, unpublished observations).

Injured nerves --------> Macrophages
Migration (invasion)
Activation (cytokines)

Nerve <------------------ Invading activated macrophages
Permissiveness for axonal growth
Astrocytes (motility, protease
activity, production
of GF, ECM and CAM)
Oligodendrocytes (elimination)

Fig. 6. Schematic representation of the bidirectional relationship between injured nerve and invading inflammatory cells.

Enhanced macrophage recruitment and growth permissiveness

To further address the possibility that injured CNS axons of mammals are deficient with respect to macrophage invasion, two cytokines, tumor necrosis factor-α (TNF-α) and colony stimulating factor-1 (CSF-1), the latter alternatively defined as macrophage-colony stimulating factor (M-CSF), were chosen as agents likely to augment inflammation in vivo and stimulate macrophage proliferation in vitro, respectively. Each of these cytokines was injected locally into injured rat optic nerves. The resulting effect was examined by assessment of the ability of the excised nerve to support neuronal adhesion and neurite extension in vitro. Both TNF-α and CSF-1 when injected locally into injured rat optic nerves, caused an increase in the number of macrophages within the nerve shortly after the injury (Lotan et al., 1994). We therefore were further interested in finding out whether this increase would result in an increased permissiveness of the nerve to axonal growth, as assessed in vitro. We also examined the effect of IL-1, which resembles TNF-α

in some of its biological activities, on the recruitment of macrophages into the injured nerve. No significant effect was observed (data not shown).

Unfixed longitudinal cryostat sections of TNF-α-treated, CSF-1-treated and control injured adult rat optic nerves were obtained at various times after injury and plated on round coverslips coated with poly-D-lysine (PDL). The nerve sections were prepared for tissue culture (Carbonetto et al., 1987; David et al., 1990) and seeded with pheochromocytoma (PC12) cells. Significantly more PC12 cells were attached to the nerve sections near the site of the lesion than in regions distal to the lesion, as previously described (David et al., 1990). However, the number of PC12 cells that became attached to the site of the injury was higher in TNF-α-treated nerves than in either the CSF-1-treated group or the control group. This difference was observed at all time points examined (2 days, 1 week and 3 weeks), but was most pronounced 3 weeks after injury and treatment (Lotan et al., 1994). The borders of the injury site were delineated by GFAP staining, as described previously (Blaugrund et al., 1992). As shown in Fig. 7A, 3 weeks after injury only a few PC12 cells were attached to tissue sections from the control group, while in the TNF-α-treated nerves a very large number of cells were attached, especially at the injury site itself and at the proximal part of the nerve, but also at the distal portion of the nerve near the lesion (Fig. 7A). Within the site of injury, adherent PC12 cells appeared to be spatially correlated with astrocytes, as determined immunohistochemically using anti-GFAP antibodies. Surprisingly, although our results indicated that CSF-1 recruited a large number of macrophages into the nerve, it had no effect on the ability of the injured nerve to support PC12 cell adhesion, as can be seen in Fig. 7B. Thus the CSF-1-treated injured nerves behaved like the control group with respect to neuronal adhesion at both time points measured, i.e., 1 day after injury (data not shown) and 3 weeks after injury.

It thus appears from our results that although CSF-1 increases the number of macrophages in the nerve, it did not affect the nerve's nonpermissiveness to neuronal adhesion, or at least not within the time frame of this study. One possible explanation of these seemingly contradictory results is that only appropriately stimulated macrophages can influence neuronal regeneration. According to this interpretation, CSF-1 is able to recruit large numbers of macrophages but apparently does not provide them with the proper stimulus needed to support regeneration. Presumably, TNF-α not only recruits macrophages but also activates them properly.

The nature of 'proper' stimulation is not yet clear, but it might be related to the ability of TNF-α to stimulate astrocytes in such a way that they become active participants in the inflammatory response and hence might indirectly affect the recruited macrophages. In line with this observation are our recent observations that TNF-α causes, in vitro, an increase in fibronectin expression and a reduction in chondroitin sulphate proteoglycan (CSPG) expression by astrocytes (O. Spiegler, M. Lotan and M. Schwartz, unpublished data). It was also shown to increase the production of collagenase type-4 and to decrease the overall activity of plasminogen activator (PA) in astrocytes by reducing PA and increasing plasminogen activator inhibitor (PAI) production (A. Elman-Faber, R. Miskin and M. Schwartz, unpublished observations). It was also suggested that TNF-α mediates myelin and oligodendrocyte damage in vitro (Selmaj and Raine, 1988). CNS myelin and oligodendrocytes were shown to be inhibitory to neuronal growth (Caroni and Schwab, 1988). It remains to be determined whether TNF-α in vivo accelerates the elimination of these potential growth-inhibitory cells from the system and modulates the level of supportive elements by astrocytes, thus contributing to the nerve's increased permissiveness to growth.

The possibility that TNF-α itself directly mediates the adhesion of PC12 cells to the nerve sections is very unlikely, since the adhesion 3 weeks after TNF-α administration was significantly higher than after 2 days, when presumably

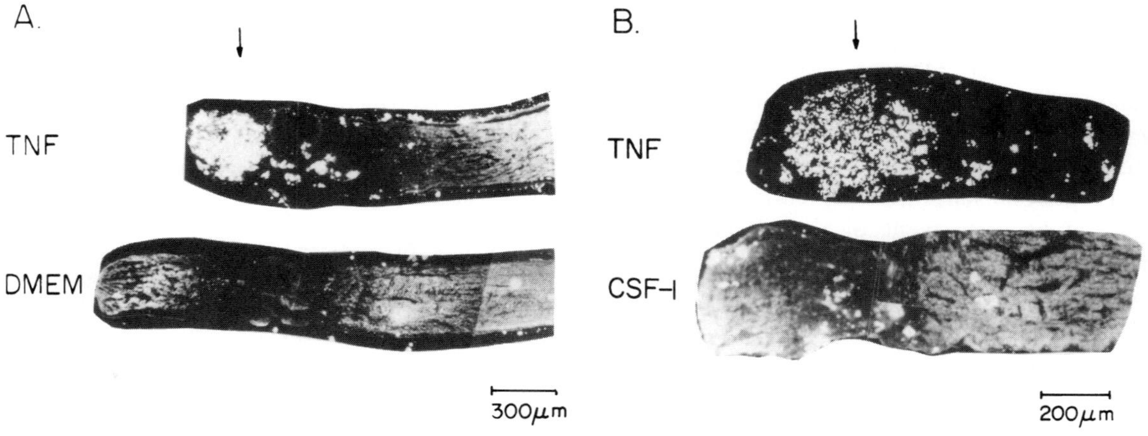

Fig. 7. Adhesion of PC12 cells to sections obtained from injured nerves treated with TNF-α, CSF-1 or Dulbecco's modified Eagle's medium (DMEM). Pc12 cells were prestained with the fluorescent dye DiI and plated on unfixed cryostat sections of each of the excised nerves. (A) Large numbers of PC12 cells are attached to the TNF-α-treated nerve, predominantly at the lesion site (arrow) and its vicinity. Very few cells have become attached to the control DMEM-treated nerve. (B) A very small number of PC12 cells adhere to CSF-1-treated cells, as compared to the number adhering to TNF-α-treated nerves. The arrow indicates the injury site. (From Lotan et al., 1994.)

the levels of residual TNF-α in the tissue were higher.

The results of this study are in line with previous work in which we showed that application of TNF-α to injured rabbit optic nerves results in the appearance of abundant newly growing axons which traverse the site of injury (Schwartz et al., 1991). The beneficial effect of TNF-α on axonal regeneration could result from an effect on the neurons themselves or from an indirect influence on the surrounding glial environment. The present study demonstrates that TNF-α brings about a marked increase in the permissiveness of the injured CNS nerve to axonal growth, and allows this change to occur in synchrony with the response of the cell body to injury (i.e., its conversion to a mode of growth).

Postinjury regulation of astrocyte behavior

Astrocytes have been viewed as the cells which, following injury, form a scar that acts as a mechanical barrier. In fish and amphibians no scar is formed, unless regeneration is artificially prevented. In an attempt to elucidate the relationship between absence of scar formation and regeneration ability, we compared the astrocytic response to axonal injury in fish and rodent optic nerves. Immediately after injury in both species, astrocytes disappeared from the injury site and densely packed astrocytes were seen at the interfaces between the proximal stump of the nerve and the site of injury and between the injury site and the distal stump. In fish, the site of injury was repopulated soon afterwards by astrocytes, in temporal and spatial correlation with axonal growth across it. In rodents, however, astrocytes did not repopulate the injury site and axons did not traverse it (Blaugrund et al., 1992, 1993; Cohen et al., 1993). Although we do not yet know whether the axonal growth or the astrocyte repopulation comes first, it appears that the two phenomena are interdependent and accordingly that the failure of astrocytes to cross the injury site, or to cross it at the right time, is a reason for the failure of mammalian axons to regenerate. Moreover, it seems likely that the astrocytes, being highly motile cells, exist in a growth state that expresses molecules needed for growth support, such as the appropriate extracellular matrix (ECM) and cellular adhesion molecules (CAM) associated with developing glial cells. The motility of the astrocytes and their migratory ability might be a reflection of their interaction with the invading macrophages. This issue is currently being investigated by assessment of the effect of cytokines such as TNF-α and IL-1β on astrocytic motility.

Concluding remarks

The results outlined above suggest that macrophages and/or their products (cytokines) at the site of the injury affect local glial cells in a way that benefits regeneration. Such effects presumably include elimination of oligodendrocytes and proper activation of astrocytes. Taken together, the observations that inflammation is beneficial for regeneration and that anti-inflammatory agents promote posttraumatic rescue of fibers from secondary degeneration (Hirschberg et al., 1994) lead us to propose that inflammation has dissimilar effects on axonal rescue and regeneration.

Acknowledgements

This work was supported in part by Farmitalia Carlo Erba, Milano, by the Alan T. Brown Foundation of Nerve Paralysis, and by the Daniel Heumann Fund for Spinal Cord Research. M. S. is an incumbent of the Maurice and Ilse Katz Professorial Chair in Neuroimmunology.

References

Bastmeyer, M., Beckmann, M., Schwab, M.E. and Stuermer, C.A.O. (1991) Growth of regenerating goldfish axons is inhibited by rat oligodendrocytes and CNS myelin but not by goldfish optic nerve tract oligodendrocyte-like cells and fish CNS myelin. *J. Neurosci.*, 11: 626–640.

Bedi, K.S., Winter, J., Berry, M. and Cohen, J. (1992) Adult rat dorsal root ganglion neurons extend neurites on predegenerated but not on normal peripheral nerves in vitro. *Eur. J. Neurosci.*, 4: 193–200.

Blaugrund, E., Sharma, S. and Schwartz, M. (1992) L1 immunoreactivity in the developing fish visual system. *Brain Res.*, 574: 244–250.

Blaugrund, E., Lavie, V., Cohen, I., Schreyer, D.Y. and Schwartz, M. (1993) Axonal regeneration is associated with glial migration: comparison between the injured optic nerves of fish and rats. *J. Comp. Neurol.*, 330: 105–112.

Carbonetto, S., Evans, D. and Cochard, P. (1987) Nerve fiber growth in culture on tissue substrata from central and peripheral nervous systems. *J. Neurosci.*, 7: 610–620.

Caroni, P. and Schwab, M.E. (1988) Antibody against myelin-associated inhibitor of neurite growth neutralizes non-permissive substrate properties of CNS white matter. *Neuron*, 1: 85–96.

Cohen, A., Sivron, T., Duvdevani, R. and Schwartz, M. (1990) Oligodendrocyte cytotoxic factor associated with fish optic nerve regeneration: implications for mammalian CNS regeneration. *Brain Res.*, 537: 24–32.

Cohen, I., Shani, Y. and Schwartz, M. (1993) Cloning and characteristics of fish glial fibrillary acidic protein: implications for optic regeneration. *J. Comp. Neurol.*, 334: 431–443.

David, S. and Aguayo, A.J. (1981) Axonal elongation into peripheral nervous system 'bridges' after central nervous system injury in adult rats. *Science*, 214: 931–933.

David, S., Bouchard, C., Tsatas, O. and Giftochristos, N. (1990) Macrophages can modify the nonpermissive nature of the adult mammalian central nervous system. *Neuron*, 5: 463–469.

Eitan, S. and Schwartz, M. (1993) A novel nerve-regeneration-associated transglutaminase that converts interleukin-2 to a factor cytotoxic to oligodendrocytes. *Science*, 261: 106–108.

Eitan, S., Zisling, R., Cohen, A., Belkin, M., Hirschberg, D.L., Lotan, M. and Schwartz, M. (1992) Identification of an interleukin-2-like substance as a factor cytotoxic to oligodendrocytes and associated with central nervous system regeneration. *Proc. Natl. Acad. Sci. USA*, 89: 5442–5446.

Grafstein, B. (1986) The retina as a regenerating organ. In: R. Adler and D. Farber (Eds.), *The Retina: A Model for Cell Biology Studies, Part II*, Academic Press, New York, pp. 275–323.

Harel, A., Fainaru, M., Shafer, Z., Hernández, M. and Schwartz, M. (1989) Optic nerve regeneration in adult fish and apolipoprotein-A-I. *J. Neurochem.*, 52: 1218–1228.

Harel, A., Fainaru, M., Rubinstein, M., Tal, N. and Schwartz, M. (1990) Fish apolipoprotein-A-I has heparin binding activity: implication for nerve regeneration. *J. Neurochem.*, 55: 1237–1243.

Hirschberg, D.L., Yoles, E., Belkin, M. and Schwartz, M. (1994) Inflammation after axonal injury has conflicting consequences for recovery of function by rescue of spared axons and by regeneration. *J. Neuroimmunol.*, in press.

Kiernan, J.A. (1979) Hypotheses concerned with axonal regeneration in the mammalian nervous system. *Biol. Rev.*, 54: 155–197.

Lavie, V., Murray, M., Solomon, A., Ben-Bassat, S., Belkin, M., Rumelt, S. and Schwartz, M. (1990) Growth of injured rabbit optic axons within their degenerating optic nerve. *J. Comp. Neurol.*, 298: 293–314.

Lotan, M., Solomon, A., Ben-Bassat, S. and Schwartz, M. (1994) Cytokines modulate the inflammatory response and change permissiveness to neuronal adhesion in injured mammalian central nervous system. *Exp. Neurol.*, in press.

Lunn, E.R., Perry, V.H., Brown, M.L., Rosen, H. and Gordon, S. (1989) Absence of Wallerian degeneration does not hinder regeneration in peripheral nerve. *Eur. J. Neurosci.*, 1: 27–33.

Murray, M. (1976) Regeneration of retinal axons into the goldfish optic tectum. *J. Comp. Neurol.*, 168: 175–196.

Perry, V.H., Brown, M.C. and Gordon, S. (1987) The macrophage response to central and peripheral nerve injury: a possible role for macrophages in regeneration. *J. Exp. Med.*, 165: 1218–1223.

Ramón y Cajal, S. (1928) *Degeneration and Regeneration of the Nervous System*, Vol. 1 (R.M. May, Ed.), Hafner, New York.

Reier, P.J. and Webster, H.F. (1974) Regeneration and remyelination of *Xenopus* tadpole optic nerve fibers following transection or crush. *J. Neurocytol.*, 3: 591–618.

Savio, T. and Schwab, M.E. (1989) Rat CNS white matter, but not grey matter, is nonpermissive for neuronal cell adhesion and fiber outgrowth. *J. Neurosci.*, 9: 1126–1129.

Schnell, L. and Schwab, M.E. (1990) Axonal regeneration in the rat spinal cord produced by an antibody against myelin-associated neurite growth inhibitors. *Nature (Lond.)*, 343: 269–272.

Schwab, M.E. and Caroni, P. (1988) Oligodendrocytes and CNS myelin are nonpermissive substrates for neurite growth and fibroblast spreading in vitro. *J. Neurosci.*, 8: 2381–2393.

Schwartz, M., Belkin, M., Harel, A., Solomon, A., Lavie, V., Hadani, M., Rachailovich, I. and Stein-Izsak, C. (1985) Regenerating fish optic nerves and a regeneration-like response in injured optic nerves of adult rabbits. *Science*, 228: 601–603.

Schwartz, M., Solomon, A., Lavie, V., Ben-Bassat, S., Belkin, M. and Cohen, A. (1991) Tumor necrosis factor facilitates regeneration of injured central nervous system axons. *Brain Res.*, 545: 334–338.

Selmaj, K.W. and Raine, C.S. (1988) Tumor necrosis factor mediates myelin and oligodendrocyte damage in vitro. *Ann. Neurol.*, 23: 339–346.

Sivron, T., Jeserich, G., Nona, S. and Schwartz, M. (1992) Characteristics of fish glial cells in culture: possible implications as to their lineage. *Glia*, 6: 52–66.

Sivron, T., Schwab, M.E. and Schwarz, M. (1994a) Postinjury elevation of growth permissiveness of fish optic nerve: association with myelin inhibitors. *J. Comp. Neurol.*, in press.

Sivron, T., Cohen, I. and Schwartz, M. (1994b) Intermediate filaments reminiscent of immature cells expressed by goldfish (*Carassius auratus*) astrocytes and oligodendrocytes in vitro. *Cell Tissue Res.*, in press.

Sperry, R.W. (1948) Patterning of central synapses in regeneration of the optic nerve in teleosts. *Physiol. Zool.*, 23: 351–361.

F.J. Seil (Ed.)
Progress in Brain Research, Vol 103

CHAPTER 28

Immune promotion of central nervous system remyelination

Moses Rodriguez and David J. Miller

Departments of Neurology and Immunology, Mayo Clinic, Rochester, MN 55905, USA

Introduction

An important question in multiple sclerosis (MS) research is why there is absence of full remyelination and recovery following demyelinating disease. Morphologic studies suggest that central nervous system (CNS) remyelination by oligodendrocytes (Raine et al., 1981; Ghatak et al., 1989; Prineas et al., 1989, 1993) and Schwann cells (Ghatak et al., 1973; Itoyama et al., 1983) can occur in MS lesions. CNS remyelination by oligodendrocytes, manifested by abnormally thin myelin sheaths relative to axon diameter, occurs primarily at the edge of demyelinated plaques, whereas the center of most chronic lesions remains devoid of myelin and oligodendrocytes. Our own electron microscopic studies of eleven acute MS lesions analyzed following stereotaxic biopsy (Rodriguez et al., 1993; Rodriguez and Scheithauer, 1994) revealed extensive attempts at myelin repair, suggesting that some oligodendrocytes are preserved in the early events of the evolving MS lesion. In addition, oligodendrocytes appear to proliferate in areas of remyelination and contain abundant microtubules as well as endoplasmic reticulum, indicating a state of activation (Raine et al., 1981). Therefore, the human CNS is capable of myelin repair.

Remyelination by oligodendrocytes has been demonstrated in CNS in a number of model systems of demyelination (Ludwin, 1988). Remyelination can be observed following acute virus-induced demyelination using JHM virus, a coronavirus (Arenella and Herndon, 1984). CNS remyelination and the proliferation of glial cells has been studied in detail using cuprizone, a toxin that injures the oligodendrocyte, in which the timing of the onset of remyelination can be controlled by placing the animals on a normal diet (Ludwin, 1978). Oral ingestion of ethidium bromide (Yajima and Suzuki, 1979) or intraspinal injection of lysolecithin (Blakemore et al., 1977) results in remyelination following toxic damage to myelin sheaths. Simple mechanical trauma of spinal cord produces demyelination followed by remyelination (Ludwin, 1984, 1985). These observations suggest that there is the potential for full remyelination and recovery from injuries to CNS.

Factors implicated to inhibit full CNS remyelination in multiple sclerosis

A number of factors have been implicated to explain the absence of full remyelination in immune-mediated demyelinating diseases such as MS (Ludwin, 1987, 1989). These include: (1) irreversible damage to oligodendrocytes, (2) poor mitotic activity of oligodendrocytes, (3) scar formation by astrocytes, (4) alteration in surface components of axons which prevents oligodendroglia-axonal contact, and (5) immune factors which interfere with repair. Each of these will be addressed.

(1) There is controversy whether the oligodendrocyte or the myelin sheath is the primary target of the MS lesions. Some investigators (Raine et al., 1981) have proposed that oligodendrocytes survive during the earliest MS insult whereas others view the cell as particularly vulnerable (Rodriguez et al., 1993; Rodriguez and Scheithauer, 1994). Morphologic and immunocytochemical data have indicated that oligodendrocytes are destroyed in the acute phase of disease but this is followed by a phase of oligodendrocyte proliferation (Prineas et al., 1989). Our electron microscopic experiments (Rodriguez et al., 1993) in acute lesions have indicated degeneration of the inner glial loops, the most distal extension of the oligodendrocyte, as has been proposed in 'dying back oligodendrogliopathies' (Ludwin and Johnson, 1981; Rodriguez, 1985). However, many oligodendrocytes in the acute lesion appear morphologically normal, suggesting that these cells are not permanently injured but have the capacity to myelinate. As the disease progresses, newly generated oligodendrocytes may be preferentially destroyed and are permanently lost from the lesion. This raises the possibility that failed remyelination in MS may be the result of an immune response directed against a developmentally restricted oligodendrocyte-specific antigen (Prineas et al., 1990).

(2) Experimental studies in rodents indicate that mature adult nervous system oligodendrocytes divide and proliferate after white matter injury (Ludwin, 1984; Ludwin and Bakker, 1988). Remyelination appears to be dependent on the new generation of oligodendrocytes. Most studies indicate that at least one cell division is required prior to remyelination (Ludwin, 1979). The process is quite rapid (days to weeks) in most models of demyelination followed by remyelination. However, the potential for adult human oligodendrocytes to divide in vivo is unknown (Armstrong et al., 1992). The experiments in animals as well as the extensive remyelination seen in acute MS lesions would argue against the possibility that oligodendrocytes or their progenitors cannot divide.

(3) Classically, astrocytes have been considered a determinant for failure of myelin repair (Ludwin, 1987). Many chronic MS lesions without remyelination show extensive gliosis. However, experiments using various models of demyelination (Blakemore, 1978; Dal Canto and Barbano, 1984; Rodriguez, 1991) argue against the inhibitory role of the astrocyte. By contrast, some experiments suggest that astrocytes are prerequisite for remyelination (Keilhauer et al., 1985; Franklin et al., 1991). Astrocytes are seen in intimate association with oligodendrocytes and remyelinated axons in the Theiler's murine encephalomyelitis virus (TMEV) model of demyelination. Tissue culture experiments indicate that astrocytes secrete essential growth factors (Raff et al., 1987), including platelet derived growth factors (Hart et al., 1989; Wolswijk and Noble, 1992) and fibroblast growth factors (McKinnon et al., 1990, 1991) necessary for the maintenance and proliferation of oligodendrocytes.

(4) Morphologically, MS is considered to be a 'primary' demyelinating disease with the relative preservation of axons. This is in contrast to 'secondary' demyelinating disorders in which myelin destruction follows injury to the axon. However, most pathologic studies indicate that as MS progresses, axons are injured (Rodriguez and Scheithauer, 1994). Using quantitative magnetic resonance imaging and electron microscopy, studies have documented progressive axonal loss in lesions as they age (Barnes et al., 1991). This raises the possibility that alterations in the surface component of naked axons may prevent contact of oligodendrocytes for myelination.

(5) The MS lesion is characterized by a prominent inflammatory response containing primarily macrophages, but also $CD4^+$ and $CD8^+$ T cells (Prineas and Wright, 1978). In immune-mediated disorders such as experimental allergic encephalomyelitis (EAE) or TMEV infection, spontaneous remyelination is much less compared to

lesions induced by cuprizone or by mouse hepatitis virus in which immune mechanisms are not implicated. A similar relationship exists between the degree of inflammation and the failure of remyelination in humans has been proposed but not proven (Ghatak et al., 1989).

Hypotheses to explain failure of full myelin repair in MS

We have considered two hypotheses to explain the absence of full remyelination in MS (Rodriguez and Lindsley, 1992). Hypothesis I is that CNS remyelination is the normal consequence of primary myelin injury, but there are factors which prevent its full expression (Ludwin, 1980). The determinants interfering with CNS remyelination may be local, possibly immune factors, within the demyelinated lesions. This hypothesis would predict that removing inhibitory factors would allow for spontaneous remyelination. Hypothesis II is that there are factors within some demyelinated lesions which, when present, promote new synthesis of myelin by oligodendrocytes or promote proliferation of progenitor glia which then differentiate to myelin-producing cells. We envision these local factors to be present in demyelinated lesions where there is remyelination (i.e., shadow plaques of MS) but not in those lesions that remain demyelinated.

Theiler's virus model of MS

We have used a model induced by TMEV to understand the mechanisms of demyelination and the extent of CNS remyelination following demyelination in vivo (Rodriguez et al., 1987a). TMEV is a picornavirus which persists in the CNS and induces immune-mediated demyelination. Intracerebral injection of Daniel's (DA) strain of virus into SJL mice (Lehrich et al., 1976) results in extensive areas of demyelination with relative absence of remyelination in spinal cord (Dal Canto and Lipton, 1975). Therefore, the model provides the unique opportunity to examine the role of virus and of the inflammatory response in development of new myelin synthesis. Chronic infection with TMEV results in chronic demyelination which is indistinguishable pathologically from MS (Dal Canto and Lipton, 1977). The histology is that of primary demyelination, i.e., destruction of myelin sheaths with relative preservation of axons. Lesions contain many lymphocytes, plasma cells and macrophages which are intimately involved in demyelination. After an incubation period of 1–3 months, mice develop spasticity, weakness of the lower extremities and bladder incontinence. In addition, recurrent episodes of acute demyelination are superimposed on the chronic progressive disease (Dal Canto and Lipton, 1979). The model is particularly attractive because of the possibility that MS may result from an immune-mediated response triggered by virus infection in the CNS (Rodriguez, 1989).

The extent of remyelination observed following intracerebral infection with TMEV depends on the genetics of the host as well as the viral strain used. Experiments using the DA strain of TMEV in SJL mice demonstrate abortive attempts at CNS remyelination beginning as early as 21 days following infection (Dal Canto and Lipton, 1975). However, the observed extent of remyelination by oligodendrocytes is small, with only 2 to 3% of demyelinated lesions showing CNS remyelination. This contrasts with observations in outbred Swiss mice infected with more attenuated strains of TMEV, including the WW strain (Dal Canto and Barbano, 1984), in which the course of demyelination is slower and the severity of inflammation is less. The result is demyelinated lesions which show remyelination, both by oligodendrocytes and by Schwann cells. This indicated that components of the inflammatory response may inhibit remyelination.

Immunosuppression using monoclonal antibodies promotes CNS remyelination

To test hypothesis I that there are immune factors which interfere with remyelination, we used cyclophosphamide and/or monoclonal antibodies (mAbs) directed against T cell subsets or against immune response gene products to interfere with components of the immune response (Rodriguez and Lindsley, 1992). SJL/J mice were chronically infected for 5 to 10 months with the DA strain of TMEV. Mice then received various immunosuppressive regimens and the animals were killed 5 weeks later. Prior to death, mice received twice-daily injections of [^{3}H]thymidine for 5 days to detect proliferating cells by in vivo autoradiography.

Immunosuppression using cyclophosphamide or anti-T cell mAbs directed against CD4 or CD8 promoted remyelination of CNS axons in spinal cords of mice infected chronically with TMEV (Fig. 1). Quantitative morphometry revealed a 5–7-fold increase in the level of new myelin synthesis. Of interest, treatment with mAbs directed against Ia (class II MHC antigens) did not increase the extent of CNS remyelination. In addition, we demonstrated the presence of glial cells incorporating [^{3}H]thymidine in areas of remyelination. Remyelination occurred in mice depleted of T cells despite local persistence of virus antigen. These studies indicated that helper and cytotoxic T cells impair the extent of remyelination, because interference with the function of immune T cells resulted in enhanced CNS remyelination by oligodendrocytes. These results have particular relevance to MS because it indicates that similar depletion of immune T cells may allow for enhanced remyelination in CNS of patients with chronic demyelination.

Promotion of remyelination with polyclonal immunoglobulins directed from mice immunized with normal spinal cord

We considered the possibility that differences in the extent of remyelination observed using various models of TMEV infection may be determined by the immune response to autoantigens. We tested hypothesis II that certain immune factors, possibly serum factors, may stimulate myelinogenesis after myelin injury. Previous experiments had indicated that CNS remyelination could be enhanced in guinea pigs with chronic EAE by treatment with emulsions of myelin components in incomplete Freund's adjuvant (IFA) (Traugott et al., 1982; Raine and Traugott, 1983; Raine et al., 1988a,b). We performed similar experiments in SJL mice chronically infected with the DA strain of TMEV and demonstrated extensive remyelination in mice treated with emulsions of spinal cord homogenate (SCH) with IFA (Lang et al., 1984). To test further whether the humoral immune response was important in mediating this repair, we directly transferred serum from uninfected hyperimmunized donor mice (syngeneic SJL) by subcutaneous injection with SCH in IFA into the flanks of recipient mice which had been infected with TMEV for as long as 9 months (Rodriguez et al., 1987b). Detailed morphometric analysis was performed on plastic embedded spinal cord sections of TMEV-infected mice following 5 weeks of serum treatment. CNS remyelination was extensive in TMEV-infected SJL mice treated with sera from SCH/IFA donors, in contrast to mice treated with sera from phosphate-buffered saline or IFA control groups. We then purified the immunoglobulin G (IgG) fraction of SCH sera (SCH/IgG) and showed a 6-fold increase in the extent of new myelin synthesis in TMEV-infected mice treated with SCH/IgG compared to mice receiving control IgG (Rodriguez and Lennon, 1990). These experiments indicated that immunoglobulins directed

Fig. 1. Demyelinated lesions with minimal CNS remyelination in the spinal cord of an SJL/J mouse injected with the DA strain of TMEV for 6 months (×400). (B) Extensive CNS remyelination in a chronically infected mouse treated for 5 weeks with cyclophosphamide. Myelin debris is seen at the edge of the remyelinated area (×720). (C) Remyelination in a chronically infected mouse treated with mAb GK1.5 which depletes helper CD4$^+$ T cells (×720). (D) Remyelination in a chronically infected mouse treated with mAb 2.43 which depletes cytotoxic CD8$^+$ T cells (×720). Mice were injected with [^{3}H]thymidine for 5 days prior to being killed. Cells incorporating DNA (silver grains) are shown by the arrows. One-μm-thick Araldite-embedded plastic sections were stained with paraphenylenediamine.

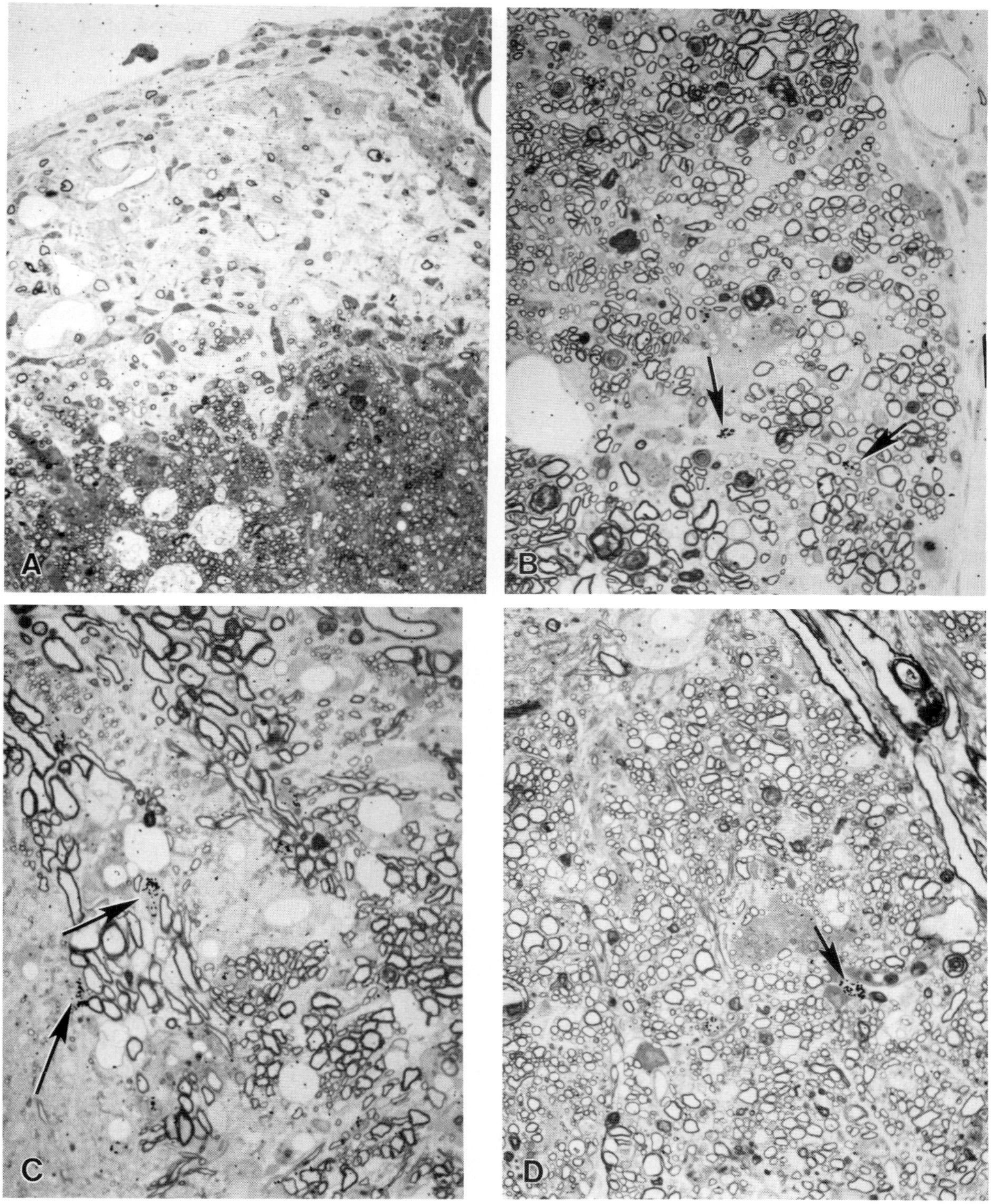
A
B
C
D

against normal CNS autoantigens promote remyelination.

We measured levels of infectious virus, virus antigen, and virus-specific antibodies to determine whether treatment which promotes CNS remyelination modulates infection (Patick et al., 1991). The levels of virus-specific antibody were higher in mice treated with SCH/IgG than in controls. Although the number of virus antigen-positive cells in spinal cord was lower in mice treated with SCH/IgG than in mice treated with controls, there was, by regression analysis, only a modest negative correlation with the extent of remyelination. Titers of infectious virus isolated 3 to 6 months following initial inoculation were not different among the treatment groups. These experiments demonstrated that CNS remyelination induced by SCH/IgG can occur in the continued presence of infectious virus.

Immunoglobulins directed against spinal cord antigens promote proliferation of cells of the oligodendroglial lineage

We performed a quantitative analysis to determine the type and extent of proliferating cells in the CNS following treatment of SCH/IgG using in vivo autoradiography (Prayoonwiwat and Rodriguez, 1993). The phenotypic characteristics of cells proliferating in CNS were determined using simultaneous immunocytochemistry and in vivo autoradiography. Anti-glial fibrillary acidic protein (GFAP) antibodies were used as a marker for astrocytes, GSA-IB4 lectin was used as a marker for microglia, antibodies to myelin basic protein (MBP), proteolipid protein (PLP), CNPase, and galactocerebroside (GC) were used as markers for oligodendroglia, and antibody to CD3 was used as a marker for T lymphocytes. An extensive study of spinal cord sections (counting an average of 26,000 to 34,000 labeled cells per experimental group) demonstrated that approximately one-third of all proliferating cells within areas of demyelination and remyelination were of the oligodendroglial lineage and had differentiated to express MBP or PLP, approximately 10% were astrocytes, 40% were microglia, and 10% were T lymphocytes. Of interest, cells of the oligodendroglial lineage proliferated both in remyelinated and in demyelinated areas, but in remyelinated areas more proliferating cells had differentiated to express late myelin antigens (PLP). The extent of astrocyte proliferation in demyelinated vs. remyelinated areas was not different and the extent of positive reactivity for GFAP did not correlate with incorporation of [^{3}H]thymidine. This indicated that astrocytes did not inhibit remyelination. These experiments support the hypothesis that factors (possibly autoantibodies) within a demyelinated lesion promote the proliferation and differentiation of cells within the oligodendroglial lineage.

Immunoglobulins induce upregulation of proteolipid protein mRNA in spinal cord

We tested whether promotion of remyelination by SCH/IgG induced the differentiation of progenitor glial cells into cells which produce myelin (Rodriguez et al., 1994). Using simultaneous in situ hybridization and immunocytochemistry, we studied PLP antigen and mRNA in spinal cord of adult normal mice and of mice infected with TMEV. Downregulation of PLP mRNA was observed within 3 days and persisted for as long as 367 days following infection. However, treatment of chronically infected SJL/J mice with SCH/sera resulted in a 3–4-fold increase in PLP mRNA expression in cells expressing PLP antigen. Actin mRNA expression in PLP antigen-positive cells was unchanged following TMEV-induced demyelination or remyelination. These experiments support the hypothesis that early regulation of myelin gene expression may be an important determinant in demyelination and in subsequent promotion of remyelination by immune factors.

Generation of remyelination promoting mAbs from mice hyperimmunized with spinal cord antigens

We made a panel of mAbs derived from splenocytes of SJL/J mice injected with homogenized spinal cord and screened them for their autoantigen binding capacity. These mAbs showed binding to SCH by both ELISA and protein dot blots, and immunostained glial cells in cell culture. Monoclonal IgM antibodies from two clones, designated SCH 94.03 and SCH 94.32, promoted 4-fold more CNS remyelination than mice receiving control IgM mAbs (Fig. 2). By electron microscopy, the majority of axons in lesions from mice treated with mAb SCH 94.03 or SCH 94.32 showed morphologic evidence of repair, with abnormally thin myelin sheaths relative to axonal diameter (Fig. 3). The generation of these mAbs may allow us to eludicate the mechanism of CNS repair by antibodies.

The concept of immunoglobulin as a stimulatory molecule

The concept that immunoglobulins may be important in promotion of remyelination is novel. Most investigators have tested the hypothesis that the immunoglobulins (autoantibodies) present in the

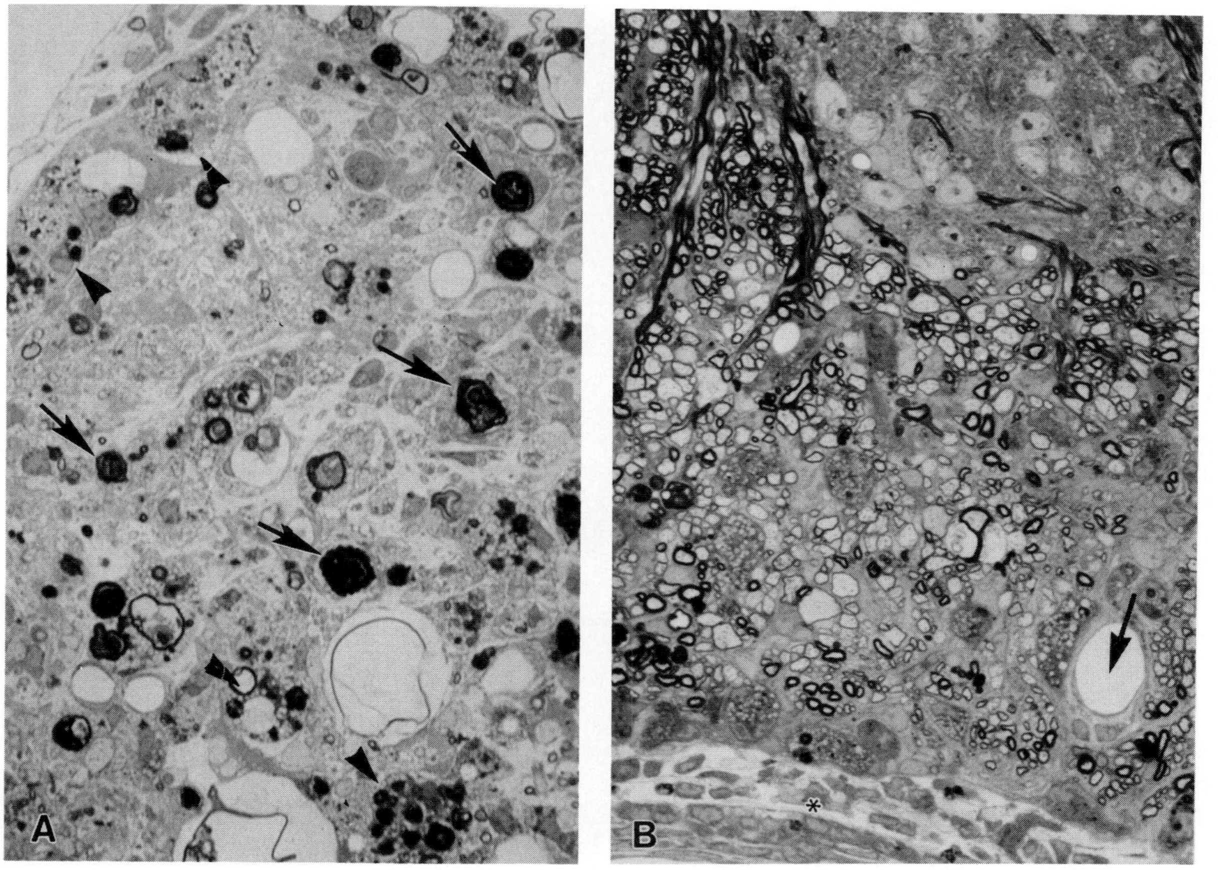

Fig. 2. (A) Extensive demyelination with myelin debris (arrows) and macrophages (arrowheads) in an SJL/J mouse infected chronically with TMEV and treated with phosphate-buffered saline (×720). (B) Almost complete CNS remyelination by oligodendrocytes in the spinal cord of a SJL/J mouse infected with TMEV and treated for 5 weeks with mAb SCH 94.03 (total dose 100 μg). Inflammatory cells (asterisk) are seen in the meninges. Note that many of the remyelinated axons surround a blood vessel (arrow) (×720).

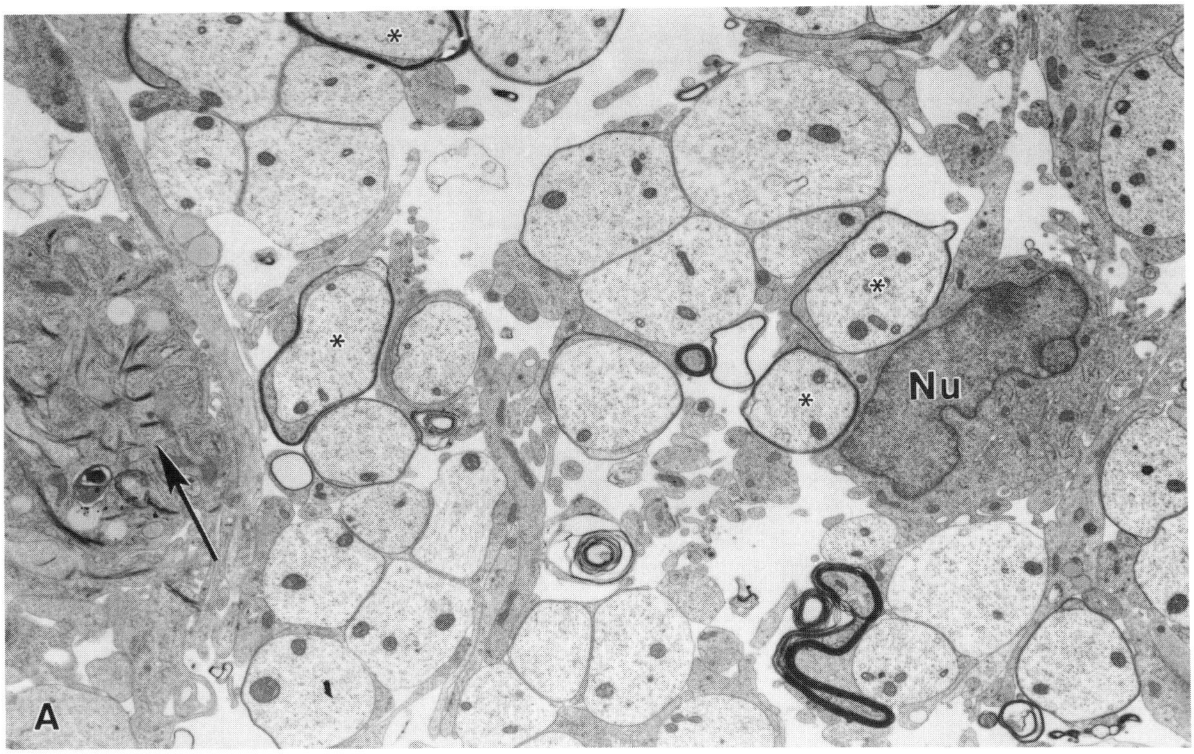
*
*
*
*
Nu
A

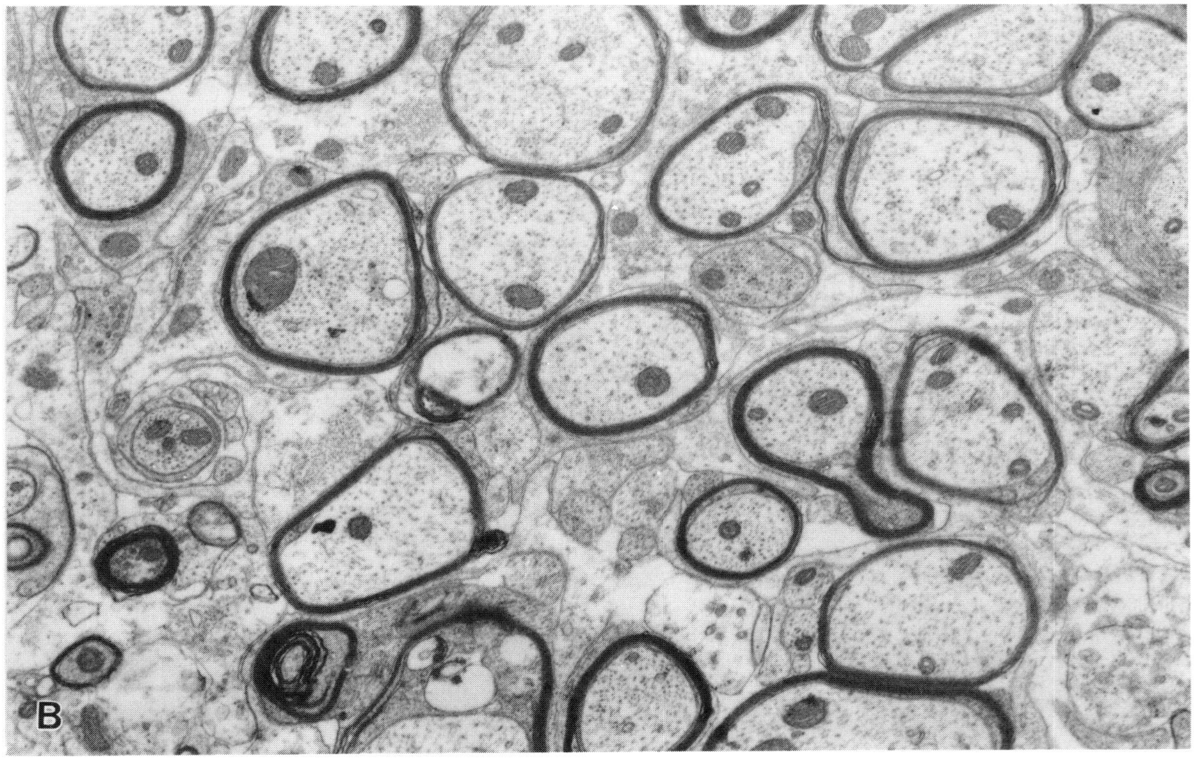
B

lesions may play a pathogenic role in demyelination (Link et al., 1989; Warren and Catz, 1993). To date, there is minimal evidence that immunoglobulins play a role in destroying myelin (Farrell et al., 1985). However, there are precedents for immunoglobulins performing agonist functions (Clark and Ledbetter, 1986). In autoimmune disorders, antibodies reacting to hormonal receptors on the cell surface may mimic the effect of trophic hormones. This includes Graves' disease, in which anti-thyroglobulin antibodies are directed to the thyroid stimulating hormone (TSH) receptor (Fukue et al., 1987). Stimulatory antibodies have been described in patients with hypersecretory duodenal ulcers (Dobi and Lewkey, 1982). Immunoglobulins may mimic the function of cellular mediators such as interleukins (Ohta et al., 1988). MRL/Lpr mice, which spontaneously develop a lupus-like autoimmune disease, contain immunoglobulins in their sera which support the growth of interleukin 3 (IL-3) dependent cell lines (Hirsch et al., 1989). Immunoglobulins may also affect the function of T cells (Hirsch et al., 1988, 1989). For example, mAbs against the CD3 receptor on T cells may stimulate the function of T cells at low concentrations (Hirsch et al., 1989), but may be immunosuppressive at high concentrations (Hirsch et al., 1988).

In vitro experiments supporting the role of immunoglobulins in promoting remyelination

Tissue culture studies have suggested that immunoglobulins directed against CNS components may promote oligodendroglial differentiation. Anti-oligodendroglial or anti-myelin antibodies have been shown to induce myelinogenesis. Myelinogenesis in tissue culture has been reported using heat-inactivated anti-white matter serum (Diaz et al., 1978). An antiserum from animals with EAE induced by inoculation with CNS white matter stimulates synthesis of galactocerebroside and sulfatides in tissue cultures, possibly reflecting an attempt at remyelination (Lehrer et al., 1979). A mAb that reacts with sulfatide, seminolipid, and an undefined lipid, has been shown to stimulate myelinogenesis in culture (Bansal et al., 1988). Antibodies to glycolipids can trigger transmembrane signaling in oligodendroglia (Benjamins and Dyer, 1990). An anti-reovirus receptor antibody has been shown to accelerate the developmental program of optic nerve oligodendrocytes (Cohen et al., 1991). Phorbol ester can enhance morphologic differentiation of oligodendrocytes in culture (Yong et al., 1988). It is possible that components on the surface of oligodendrocytes may function as receptors or components of receptors. Antibodies could mimic endogenous ligands, therefore, inducing the proliferation or differentiation of these cells. Antibodies could also act on other glial cells, promoting through some other factor the proliferation or differentiation of oligodendrocytes.

Relevance to multiple sclerosis

The results of these experiments may have practical applications to MS and related human demyelinating disorders. High-dose intravenous gamma globulin (IVIg) has been used as an effective therapy for a number of autoimmune diseases (Dwyer, 1992). In the nervous system, recent clinical trials have shown encouraging results in patients with myasthenia gravis, chronic inflammatory neuropathy (Cook et al., 1990; Dyck, 1990; Van Doorn et al., 1990) and Guillain-Barré syndrome (Kleuweg et al., 1988). In addition, successful results with IVIg have been reported in adrenoleukodystrophy, a dysmyelinating disease of children which has a superimposed inflammatory component (Miike et al., 1989). Preliminary

Fig. 3. (A) Multiple demyelinated axons, some with early attempts at remyelination (asterisks) in the spinal cord of a chronically infected SJL mouse treated with phosphate-buffered saline. Nu, nucleus of a presumed glial cell. Note macrophages (arrow) with intracytoplasmic myelin debris (×9,500). (B) CNS remyelination characterized by abnormal myelin thickness compared to axon diameter in the spinal cord of a mouse chronically infected with TMEV and treated with mAb SCH94.03 (×20,000).

studies suggest IVIg may be beneficial in MS (Schuller and Govaerts, 1983; Soukop and Tschabitscher, 1986; Cook et al., 1992). The potential of IVIg treatment to promote remyelination in MS was tested in an open-labeled, unblinded study (van Engelen et al., 1992). In the study, five MS patients with nonrecovering static, steroid-unresponsive optic neuritis (8 eyes, optic neuritis duration of 7 months to 4 years) received repeated administration of IVIg. Within 1 to 2 months, improvement was observed in visual acuity and color vision (5 eyes), light brightness (3 eyes), and visual evoked responses (5 eyes). Improvement was temporarily related to administration of IVIg and persisted for 1.2 to 1.7 years. The timing for onset of clinical improvement was similar to the time course for antibody-mediated remyelination in the TMEV model.

Summary and conclusion

Remyelination by oligodendrocytes is the normal response to injury of the central nervous system following experimental demyelination by toxins and viruses in rodents. By contrast, in immune-mediated myelin disorders such as human MS, Theiler's virus-induced demyelination or EAE, remyelination is incomplete. We have considered two hypotheses to explain why myelin repair is incomplete in these disorders. Hypothesis I is that myelin repair is the normal consequence of primary myelin injury but there are immune factors which prevent its full expression. To test hypothesis I, we depleted T cells in Theiler's virus infected mice with cyclophosphamide or with monoclonal antibodies to CD4, CD8, or immune response gene products (Ia). Enhanced remyelination and proliferation of glial cells was observed in mice depleted of $CD4^+$ or $CD8^+$ T cells. Hypothesis II is that there are immune factors within some demyelinated lesions which, when present, promote new myelin synthesis. We envision these factors to be present in those lesions showing remyelination but absent in those lesions that remain demyelinated. To test hypothesis II, we generated polyclonal immunoglobulins directed against normal CNS antigens. Transfer of immunoglobulins from mice immunized repeatedly with spinal cord homogenate resulted in 4–5-fold enhancement of remyelination in Theiler's virus infected mice. We have also generated a series of monoclonal antibodies directed against normal autoantigens which also promote CNS remyelination.

These experiments support the concept that full CNS remyelination is possible in human demyelinating diseases such as MS. Manipulation of the immune response either by inhibiting the function of T cells or by treatment with immunoglobulins (possibly normal autoantibodies) appears to promote remyelination. These experiments provide hope for patients with fixed neurological deficits for whom there are currently no available therapies.

References

Arenella, L.S. and Herndon, R.M. (1984) Mature oligodendrocytes. Division following experimental demyelination in adult animals. *Arch. Neurol.*, 41: 1162-1165.

Armstrong, R.C., Dorn, H.H., Kufta, C.V., Friedman, E. and Dubois Dalcq, M.E. (1992) Pre-oligodendrocytes from adult human CNS. *J. Neurosci.*, 12: 1538-1547.

Bansal, R., Gard, A.L. and Pfeiffer, S.E. (1988) Stimulation of oligodendrocyte differentiation in culture by growth in the presence of a monoclonal antibody to sulfated glycolipid. *J. Neurosci. Res.*, 21: 260-267.

Barnes, D., Munro, P.M., Youl, B.D., Prineas, J.W. and McDonald, W.I. (1991) The longstanding MS lesion. A quantitative MRI and electron microscopic study. *Brain*, 114: 1271-1280.

Benjamins, J.A. and Dyer, C.A. (1990) Glycolipids and transmembrane signaling in oligodendroglia. *Ann. N.Y. Acad. Sci.*, 605: 90-100.

Blakemore, W.F. (1978) Observations on remyelination in the rabbit spinal cord following demyelination induced by lysolecithin. *Neuropathol. Appl. Neurobiol.*, 4: 47-59.

Blakemore, W.F., Eames, R.A., Smith, K.J. and McDonald, W.I. (1977) Remyelination in the spinal cord of the cat following intraspinal injections of lysolecithin. *J. Neurol. Sci.*, 33: 31-43.

Clark, E.A. and Ledbetter, J.A. (1986) Amplification of the immune response by agonistic antibodies. *Immunol. Today*, 7: 267-270.

Cohen, J.A., Williams, W.V., Geller, H.M. and Greene, M.I. (1991) Anti-reovirus receptor antibody accelerates expression of the optic nerve oligodendrocyte developmental program. *Proc. Natl. Acad. Sci. USA*, 88: 1266-1270.

Cook, C., Dalakas, M., Galdi, A., Biondi, D. and Porter, H. (1990) High-dose intravenous immunoglobulin in the treatment of demyelinating neuropathy associated with monoclonal gammopathy. *Neurology*, 40: 212-214.

Cook, S.D., Troiano, R., Rohowsky-Kochan, C., Jotkowitz, A., Bielory, L., Mehta, P.D., Oleske, J., Bansil, S. and Dowling, P.C. (1992) Intravenous gamma globulin in progressive MS. *Acta. Neurol. Scand.*, 86: 171-175.

Dal Canto, M.C. and Barbano, R.L. (1984) Remyelination during remission in Theiler's virus infection. *Am. J. Pathol.*, 116: 30-45.

Dal Canto, M.C. and Lipton, H.L. (1975) Primary demyelination in Theiler's virus infection. An ultrastructural study. *Lab. Invest.*, 33: 626-637.

Dal Canto, M.C. and Lipton, H.L. (1977) Multiple sclerosis. Animal model: Theiler's virus infection in mice. *Am. J. Pathol.*, 88: 497-500.

Dal Canto, M.C. and Lipton, H.L. (1979) Recurrent demyelination in chronic central nervous system infection produced by Theiler's murine encephalomyelitis virus. *J. Neurol. Sci.*, 42: 391-405.

Diaz, M., Bornstein, M.B. and Raine, C.S. (1978) Disorganization of myelinogenesis in tissue culture by anti-CNS antiserum. *Brain Res.*, 154: 231-239.

Dobi, S. and Lewkey, B. (1982) Role of secretogogue immunoglobulins in gastric acid secretion. *Acta. Physiol. Acad. Sci. Hungary*, 69: 9-25.

Dwyer, J.M. (1992) Manipulating the immune system with immune globulin. *N. Engl. J. Med.*, 326: 107-116.

Dyck, P.J. (1990) Intravenous immunoglobulin in chronic inflammatory demyelinating polyradiculoneuropathy and in neuropathy associated with IgM monoclonal gammopathy of unknown significance. *Neurology*, 40: 327-328.

Farrell, M.A., Kaufmann, J.C., Gilbert, J.J., Noseworthy, J.H., Armstrong, H.A. and Ebers, G.C. (1985) Oligoclonal bands in multiple sclerosis: clinical-pathologic correlation. *Neurology*, 35: 212-218.

Franklin, R.J., Crang, A.J. and Blakemore, W.F. (1991) Transplanted type-1 astrocytes facilitate repair of demyelinating lesions by host oligodendrocytes in adult rat spinal cord. *J. Neurocytol.*, 20: 420-430.

Fukue, U., Uchimura, H., Mitsuhasthi, T., Okano, S., Kanaji, U. and Takaku, F. (1987) Thyroglobulin release-stimulating activity in immunoglobulin G from patients with Graves' disease studied by human thyroid cells in vitro. *J. Clin. Endocrinol. Metab.*, 64: 261-265.

Ghatak, N.R., Hirano, A., Doron, Y. and Zimmerman, H.M. (1973) Remyelination in multiple sclerosis with peripheral type myelin. *Arch. Neurol.*, 29: 262-267.

Ghatak, N.R., Leshner, R.T., Price, A.C. and Felton, W.L.,III (1989) Remyelination in the human central nervous system. *J. Neuropathol. Exp. Neurol.*, 48: 507-518.

Hart, I.K., Richardson, W.D., Bolsover, S.R. and Raff, M.C. (1989) PDGF and intracellular signaling in the timing of oligodendrocyte differentiation. *J. Cell Biol.*, 109: 3411-3417.

Hirsch, R., Eckhaus, M., Auchincloss, H., Sachs, D.H. and Bluestone, J.A. (1988) Effects of in vivo administration of anti-T3 monoclonal antibody on T cell function in mice. I. Immunosuppression of transplantation responses. *J. Immunol.*, 140: 3766-3772.

Hirsch, R., Gress, R.E., Pcuznik, D.H., Eckhau, S.M. and Bluestone, J.A. (1989) Effects of in vivo administration of anti CD3 monoclonal antibody on T cell function in mice. II. In vivo activities of T cells. *J. Immunol.*, 142: 737-743.

Itoyama, Y., Webster, H.D., Richardson, E.P.,Jr. and Trapp, B.D. (1983) Schwann cell remyelination of demyelinated axons in spinal cord multiple sclerosis lesions. *Ann. Neurol.*, 14: 339-346.

Keilhauer, G., Meier, D.H., Kuhlmann-Krieg, S., Nieke, J. and Schachner, M. (1985) Astrocytes support incomplete differentiation of an oligodendrocyte precursor cell. *EMBO J.*, 4: 2499-2504.

Kleuweg, R.P., Van der Meche, F.G.A. and Meulstee, J. (1988) Treatment of Guillain-Barré syndrome with high dose gammaglobulin. *Neurology*, 38: 1639-1641.

Lang, W., Rodriguez, M., Lennon, V.A. and Lampert, P.W. (1984) Demyelination and remyelination in murine viral encephalomyelitis. *Ann. N.Y. Acad. Sci.*, 436: 98-102.

Lehrer, G.M., Maker, S., Silides, D.J., Weiss, C. and Bornstein, M.B. (1979) Stimulation of myelin lipids synthesis in vitro by white matter antiserum in the absence of complement. *Brain Res.*, 172: 557-560.

Lehrich, J.R., Arnason, B.G. and Hochberg, F.H. (1976) Demyelinative myelopathy in mice induced by the DA virus. *J. Neurol. Sci.*, 29: 149-160.

Link, H., Baig, S., Jiang, Y.P., Olsson, O., Hojeberg, B., Kostulas, V. and Olsson, T. (1989) B cells and antibodies in MS. *Res. Immunol.*, 140: 219-226.

Ludwin, S.K. (1978) Central nervous system demyelination and remyelination in the mouse: an ultrastructural study of cuprizone toxicity. *Lab. Invest.*, 39: 597-612.

Ludwin, S.K. (1979) An autoradiographic study of cellular proliferation in remyelination of the central nervous system. *Am. J. Pathol.*, 95: 683-696.

Ludwin, S.K. (1980) Chronic demyelination inhibits remyelination in the central nervous system. An analysis of contributing factors. *Lab. Invest.*, 43: 382-387.

Ludwin, S.K. (1984) Proliferation of mature oligodendrocytes after trauma to the central nervous system. *Nature (Lond.)*, 308: 274-275.

Ludwin, S.K. (1985) Reaction of oligodendrocytes and astrocytes to trauma and implantation. A combined autoradiographic and immunohistochemical study. *Lab. Invest.*, 52: 20-30.

Ludwin, S.K. (1987) Remyelination in demyelinating diseases of the central nervous system. *Crit. Rev. Neurobiol.*, 3: 1-28.

Ludwin, S.K. (1988) Remyelination in the central nervous system and the peripheral nervous system. In: S.G. Waxman (Ed.), *Functional Recovery in Neurological Disease. Advances in Neurology*, Vol. 47, Raven Press, New York, pp. 215-254.

Ludwin, S.K. (1989) Evolving concepts and issues in remyelination. *Dev. Neurosci.*, 11: 140-148.

Ludwin, S.K. and Bakker, D.A. (1988) Can oligodendrocytes attached to myelin proliferate? *J. Neurosci.*, 8: 1239-1244.

Ludwin, S.K. and Johnson, E.S. (1981) Evidence for a 'dying-back' gliopathy in demyelinating disease. *Ann. Neurol.*, 9: 301-305.

McKinnon, R.D., Matsui, T., Dubois Dalcq, M. and Aaronson, S.A. (1990) FGF modulates the PDGF-driven pathway of oligodendrocyte development. *Neuron*, 5: 603-614.

McKinnon, R.D., Matsui, T., Aranda, M. and Dubois Dalcq, M. (1991) A role for fibroblast growth factor in oligodendrocyte development. *Ann. N.Y. Acad. Sci.*, 638: 378-386.

Miike, T., Taku, K., Tamura, T., Ohta, J., Ozaki, M., Yamamoto, C., Sakai, T., Antoku, Y. and Yadomi, C. (1989) Clinical improvement of adrenoleukodystrophy following intravenous gammaglobulin therapy. *Brain Dev.*, 11: 134-137.

Ohta, Y., Tamura, S., Tezuka, E., Sugawara, M., Imai, S. and Tanaka, H. (1988) Autoimmune MRL/LPR mice sera contain IgG with interleukin 3-like activity. *J. Immunol.*, 140: 520-525.

Patick, A.K., Thiemann, R.L., OBrien, P.C. and Rodriguez, M. (1991) Persistence of Theiler's virus infection following promotion of central nervous system remyelination. *J. Neuropathol. Exp. Neurol.*, 50: 523-537.

Prayoonwiwat, N. and Rodriguez, M. (1993) The potential for oligodendrocyte proliferation during demyelinating disease. *J. Neuropathol. Exp. Neurol.*, 52: 55-63.

Prineas, J.W. and Wright, R.G. (1978) Macrophages, lymphocytes, and plasma cells in the perivascular compartment in chronic multiple sclerosis. *Lab. Invest.*, 38: 409-421.

Prineas, J.W., Kwon, E.E., Goldenberg, P.Z., Ilyas, A.A., Quarles, R.H., Benjamins, J.A. and Sprinkle, T.J. (1989) Multiple sclerosis. Oligodendrocyte proliferation and differentiation in fresh lesions. *Lab. Invest.*, 61: 489-503.

Prineas, J.W., Kwon, E.E., Goldenberg, P.Z., Cho, E.S. and Sharer, L.R. (1990) Interaction of astrocytes and newly formed oligodendrocytes in resolving multiple sclerosis lesions. *Lab. Invest.*, 63: 624-636.

Prineas, J.W., Barnard, R.O., Kwon, E.E., Sharer, L.R. and Cho, E.S. (1993) Multiple sclerosis: remyelination of nascent lesions. *Ann. Neurol.*, 33: 137-151.

Raff, M.C., ffrench-Constant, C. and Miller, R.H. (1987) Glial cells in the rat optic nerve and some thoughts on remyelination in the mammalian CNS. *J. Exp. Biol.*, 132: 35-41.

Raine, C.S. and Traugott, U. (1983) Chronic relapsing experimental autoimmune encephalomyelitis. Ultrastructure of the central nervous system of animals treated with combinations of myelin components. *Lab. Invest.*, 48: 275-284.

Raine, C.S., Scheinberg, L. and Waltz, J.M. (1981) Multiple sclerosis. Oligodendrocyte survival and proliferation in an active established lesion. *Lab. Invest.*, 45: 534-546.

Raine, C.S., Hintzen, R., Traugott, U. and Moore, G.R. (1988a) Oligodendrocyte proliferation and enhanced CNS remyelination after therapeutic manipulation of chronic relapsing EAE. *Ann. N.Y. Acad. Sci.*, 540: 712-714.

Raine, C.S., Moore, G.R., Hintzen, R. and Traugott, U. (1988b) Induction of oligodendrocyte proliferation and remyelination after chronic demyelination. Relevance to multiple sclerosis. *Lab. Invest.*, 59: 467-476.

Rodriguez, M. (1985) Virus-induced demyelination in mice: 'dying back' of oligodendrocytes. *Mayo Clin. Proc.*, 60: 433-438.

Rodriguez, M. (1989) Multiple sclerosis: basic concepts and hypothesis. *Mayo Clin. Proc.*, 64: 570-576.

Rodriguez, M. (1991) Immunoglobulins stimulate central nervous system remyelination: electron microscopic and morphometric analysis of proliferating cells. *Lab. Invest.*, 64: 358-370.

Rodriguez, M. and Lennon, V.A. (1990) Immunoglobulins promote remyelination in the central nervous system. *Ann. Neurol.*, 27: 12-17.

Rodriguez, M. and Lindsley, M.D. (1992) Immunosuppression promotes CNS remyelination in chronic virus-induced demyelinating disease. *Neurology*, 42: 348-357.

Rodriguez, M. and Scheithauer, B. (1994) The ultrastructure of multiple sclerosis. *Ultrastruct. Pathol.*, 18: 3–13.

Rodriguez, M., Oleszak, E. and Leibowitz, J. (1987a) Theiler's murine encephalomyelitis: a model of demyelination and persistence of virus. *Crit. Rev. Immunol.*, 7: 325-365.

Rodriguez, M., Lennon, V.A., Benveniste, E.N. and Merrill, J.E. (1987b) Remyelination by oligodendrocytes stimulated by antiserum to spinal cord. *J. Neuropathol. Exp. Neurol.*, 46: 84-95.

Rodriguez, M., Scheithauer, B.W., Forbes, G. and Kelly, P.J. (1993) Oligodendrocyte injury is an early event in lesions of multiple sclerosis. *Mayo Clin. Proc.*, 68: 627-636.

Rodriguez, M., Prayoonwiwat, N., Howe, C. and Sandborn, K. (1994) Proteolipid protein gene expression in demyelination and remyelination of the central nervous system: a model for multiple sclerosis. *J. Neuropathol. Exp. Neurol.*, 53: 136–143.

Schuller, E. and Govaerts, A. (1983) First results of immunotherapy with immunoglobulin G in multiple sclerosis patients. *Eur. Neurol.*, 22: 205-212.

Soukop, W. and Tschabitscher, H. (1986) Gammaglobulintherapie bei multipler sklerose (MS). *Wien. Med. Wochenschr.*, 136: 477-480.

Traugott, U., Stone, S.H. and Raine, C.S. (1982) Chronic relapsing experimental autoimmune encephalomyelitis. Treatment with combinations of myelin components promotes clinical and structural recovery. *J. Neurol. Sci.*, 56: 65-73.

Van Doorn, P.A., Brand, A., Strengers, P.F.W., Meulstee, J. and Vermeulen, M. (1990) High dose intravenous immunoglobulin treatment in chronic inflammatory demyelinating polyneuropathy. A double-blind placebo-controlled, crossover study. *Neurology*, 40: 209-212.

van Engelen, B.G., Hommes, O.R., Pinckers, A., Cruysberg, J.R., Barkhof, F. and Rodriguez, M. (1992) Improved vision after intravenous immunoglobulin in stable demyelinating optic neuritis. *Ann. Neurol.*, 32: 834-835.

Warren, K.G. and Catz, I. (1993) Autoantibodies to myelin basic protein within multiple sclerosis central nervous system tissue. *J. Neurol. Sci.*, 115: 169-176.

Wolswijk, G. and Noble, M. (1992) Cooperation between PDGF and FGF converts slowly dividing O-2A adult progenitor cells to rapidly dividing cells with characteristics of O-2A perinatal progenitor cells. *J. Cell Biol.*, 118: 889-900.

Yajima, K. and Suzuki, K. (1979) Demyelination and remyelination in the rat central nervous system following ethidium bromide injection. *Lab. Invest.*, 41: 385-392.

Yong, V.W., Sekiguchi, S., Kim, M.W. and Kim, S.U. (1988) Phorbol ester enhances morphological differentiation of oligodendrocytes in cultures. *J. Neurosci. Res.*, 19: 187-194.

SECTION VI

Nitric Oxide in the Central Nervous System

F.J. Seil (Ed.)
Progress in Brain Research, Vol 103

CHAPTER 29

Nitric oxide in the central nervous system

Stuart A. Lipton[1], David J. Singel[3] and Jonathan S. Stamler[2]

Departments of [1]Neurology, [2]Respiratory, and [2]Cardiovascular Medicine, Harvard Medical School and the [3]Department of Chemistry, Harvard University, Boston, MA 02115, USA

Introduction

In the central nervous system (CNS), nitric oxide or closely related molecules have been reported to be both neurodestructive and neuroprotective. In this brief review we attempt to resolve this apparent paradox, at least in part, by showing that there are different redox states of nitrogen oxides (NO), and these distinct states can display opposing effects on neurons as well as on other cell types.

Nitric oxide was originally considered to be a gaseous pollutant of the atmosphere. Subsequently, nitric oxide, or a closely related molecule, was identified in biological systems as an endothelium relaxing factor (EDRF), mediating vasodilatation via production of cyclic guanosine monophosphate (cGMP) (reviewed by Moncada and Higgs, 1993). In the CNS, Garthwaite et al. (1988) first demonstrated that cerebellar granule cells produce nitric oxide in response to stimulation of their *N*-methyl-D-aspartate (NMDA) subtype of glutamate receptors. In this neuronal system, a constitutive form of the enzyme, nitric oxide synthase, is activated by the influx of Ca^{2+} via NMDA receptor operated ion channels (Bredt et al., 1990). The resulting increase in nitric oxide activates soluble guanylate cyclase with the consequent formation of cGMP.

That nitric oxide production in neurons is triggered by stimulation of NMDA receptors is particularly intriguing because of the importance of this receptor type in neuronal plasticity, including roles in neurite outgrowth, synaptic transmission, and long-term potentiation (LTP, thought to represent a cellular correlate of learning and memory). However, excessive activation of NMDA receptors has also been associated with a wide range of acute neurologic disorders and chronic neurodegenerative diseases, including hypoxic-ischemic brain injury, trauma, epilepsy, Parkinson's disease, Huntington's disease, amyotrophic lateral sclerosis, and acquired immunodeficiency syndrome (AIDS) dementia (Lipton and Rosenberg, 1994). A number of NMDA receptor subunits have been cloned that, together with their electrophysiological and pharmacological properties, have facilitated the characterization of several sites of drug interaction (Seeburg, 1993). These include coagonist binding sites for glutamate (or NMDA) and glycine, and a redox modulatory site(s) defined by the existence of critical thiol group(s) (Aizenman et al., 1989). This latter site controls the frequency of opening of the receptor coupled ion channel: when oxidized (apparently in disulfide form), channel activity is downregulated and when chemically reduced, the channel opens more frequently, allowing additional permeation of Ca^{2+} following agonist binding. The influx of Ca^{2+} leads to several biochemical events that are associated with neurotoxicity (Lip-

ton and Rosenberg, 1994). In one proposed mechanism, excessive rises in neuronal Ca^{2+} lead to an increase in constitutive nitric oxide synthase activity, in turn leading to release of nitric oxide which damages surrounding neurons (Dawson et al., 1991). Notwithstanding these findings, several groups have been unable to demonstrate toxicity of nitric oxide on cortical neurons and have even found that NO donor compounds protect against NMDA neurotoxicity (Lei et al., 1992). Similar discordant effects of nitric oxide have been reported in other tissues. In this light, we have attempted to expand the perspective of NO action by considering its various redox related states and their distinctive chemistries: NO^+ (nitrosonium ion), $NO^{\cdot}$ (nitric oxide), and NO^- (nitroxyl anion), each respective species (or NO group) containing one additional electron (Stamler et al., 1992). To address specifically the present paradox, we examined the effects of several NO congeners on neurotoxicity and neuroprotection. Here, we describe the effects of $NO^{\cdot}$ and NO^+ equivalents; the actions of NO^- in this system are currently under investigation.

Nitric oxide ($NO^{\cdot}$), superoxide ($O_2^{\cdot-}$),
peroxynitrite ($OONO^-$) and neurotoxicity

The addition of *S*-nitrosocysteine (cys-NO) to cerebrocortical cultures caused dose-dependent neuronal cell killing (confirmed by trypan blue exclusion and lactate dehydrogenase (LDH) leakage) at concentrations $\geq 100\ \mu M$. The toxicity of cys-NO was inhibited by pre-incubation or coaddition of superoxide dismutase (SOD, 50 U/ml), whereas the rate of $NO^{\cdot}$ generation was unaffected or slightly increased (as demonstrated by a nitric oxide sensor electrode, WPI, Inc.). Such superoxide-dependent toxicity was confirmed with several other NO donor compounds including 3-morpholinosydnonimine (SIN-1) and several *N*-hydroxy nitrosamines (NONOates). These events are best rationalized as follows: *S*-nitrosocysteine undergoes rapid homolytic fission to liberate nitric oxide ($NO^{\cdot}$) which in turn reacts with superoxide ($O_2^{\cdot-}$) to form peroxynitrite ($OONO^-$). At the specific concentrations used, the addition of SOD scavenges $O_2^{\cdot-}$, limiting peroxynitrite formation and consequent cell death (Lipton et al., 1993) :

$$NO^{\cdot} + O_2^{\cdot-} \rightarrow OONO^-$$

$$OONO^- \text{ or degradation products} \rightarrow \text{neuronal cell death}$$

The above chemical pathways are supported by the demonstration of direct neurotoxic effects of $OONO^-$ on neurons (Lipton et al., 1993). Predictably, SOD does not limit $OONO^-$-mediated cell killing.

Nitrosonium (NO^+), NMDA receptor thiol groups, and neuroprotection

We next examined the effects of several NO donor compounds on NMDA receptor-mediated neurotoxicity. As assessed in assays of neuronal viability, sodium nitroprusside (SNP) significantly protected against NMDA-induced neurotoxicity, whereas the drug had no significant affect when added to cultures alone (Fig. 1). These findings are rationalized as follows. Nitroprusside contains an NO group coordinated to the metal with strong nitrosonium (NO^+) character. The tendency for nitroprusside is not to liberate $NO^{\cdot}$ spontaneously, but to react with thiolate anion (RS^-) on the NMDA redox site(s) to form a complex in which sulfur is bound to nitrogen (this reaction is best rationalized in terms of *S*-nitrosation):

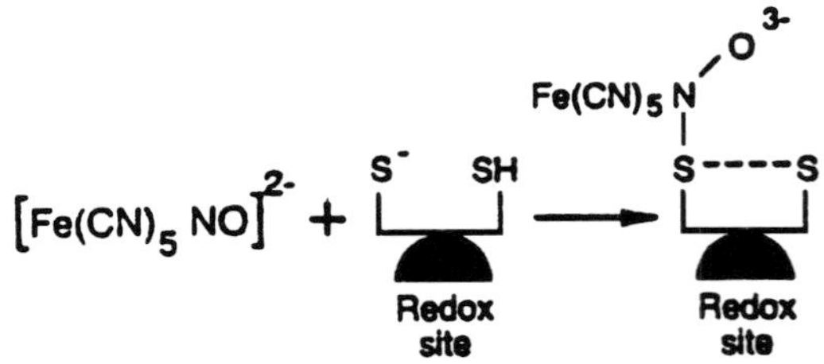

(mechanism of SNP neuroprotection)

Downregulation of NMDA receptor activity may occur directly (through formation of the

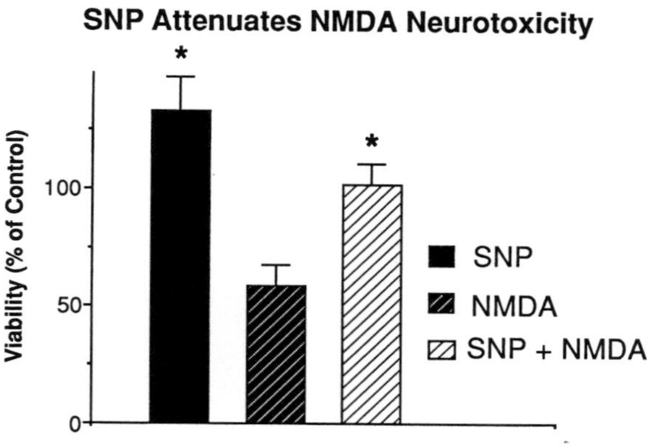

Fig. 1. Sodium nitroprusside (SNP) attenuates NMDA receptor-mediated neurotoxicity. Overnight incubation of SNP (300 μM) in cerebrocortical cultures, prepared as in Lei et al. (1992), resulted in slightly increased neuronal viability, although this increase was not significantly different from control cultures. A 5 min incubation in 100 μM NMDA followed by washout resulted in significant neurotoxicity by the next day. However, a 5 min pretreatment of the cultures in 300 μM SNP, followed by washout, significantly attenuated the neurotoxicity observed subsequent to a similar exposure of NMDA. Asterisk indicates $P < 0.01$ from value for the degree of neuronal cell death following NMDA exposure. Neurotoxicity was assessed by counting neurons that excluded trypan blue and by lactate dehydrogenase (LDH) leakage into the culture medium.

above complex) or by way of subsequent oxidation of the redox site to disulfide (represented by a dashed line in the chemical structure).

Likewise, neuroprotective effects could be observed in the case of *S*-nitrosocysteine (cys-NO). Application of cys-NO attenuated NMDA-evoked Ca^{2+} influx, a prerequisite for NMDA receptor-mediated neurotoxicity. In these experiments, Ca^{2+} influx was monitored by whole cell recording with a patch electrode or by digital calcium imaging with the dye fura-2 (Lei et al., 1992; Lipton et al., 1993). Further, in the presence of SOD, cys-NO ameliorated NMDA receptor-mediated neurotoxicity. These findings are explained as follows: Under these conditions, any $NO^{\cdot}$ produced from homolytic cleavage of cys-NO (vide supra) is prevented from entering the neurotoxic pathway with $O_2^{\cdot-}$ by the presence of SOD. Cys-NO (or possibly another RS-NO) can also react heterolytically to transfer NO^+ to thiol(s) of the NMDA receptor's redox modulatory site(s), resulting in a nitrosothiol derivative. This statement should not be construed to imply the existence of free nitrosonium ions under our conditions at pH 7.4. Rather, a transnitrosation reaction is envisioned to occur that downregulates NMDA receptor activity, possibly through facilitation of disulfide formation, as follows:

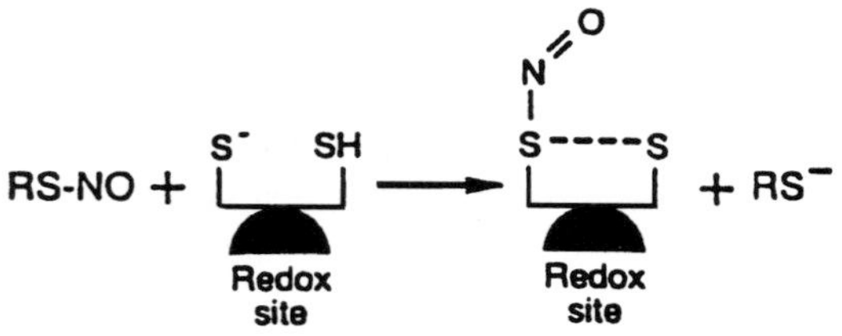

(mechanism of RSNO neuroprotection)

Interconversion of NO redox states with electron donors

Nitric oxide ($NO^{\cdot}$) itself is not primarily responsible for downregulation of NMDA receptor activity, as we found no correlation between rates of $NO^{\cdot}$ release from NO donor compounds, as measured by the $NO^{\cdot}$ sensor electrode, and the magnitude of NMDA-evoked responses. For example, ascorbate, acting as a chemical reducing agent to donate electrons, markedly enhanced the rate of release of $NO^{\cdot}$ from cys-NO (Fig. 2). Yet, at the same time such reducing agents markedly diminished the inhibitory effect of cys-NO on NMDA-evoked currents (Lipton et al., 1993), presumably by eliminating NO^+ equivalents ($NO^+ \xrightarrow{e^-} NO^{\cdot}$) and thus preventing transnitrosation of NMDA receptor thiol.

To emphasize further that ambient redox conditions will dictate the potential neuroprotective or neurotoxic effects of a given nitroso-compound, we incubated nitroprusside with excess ascorbate or thiol (cysteine or *N*-acetylcysteine) to show that we can convert nitroprusside to a neurotoxin. Under conditions in which ascorbate

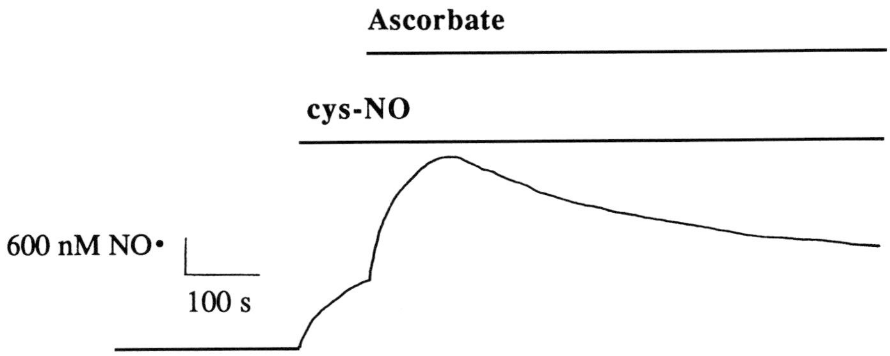

Fig. 2. Reducing agents increase the generation of NO˙ from *S*-nitrosocysteine (cys-NO). The production of NO˙ was monitored with a specific electrode, as described in Lipton et al. (1993). All incubations were carried out in a Hepes buffered solution of physiological Hanks' salts. Addition of reducing equivalents, in the form of 100 μM ascorbate, resulted in the generation of substantially increased amounts of NO˙ from cys-NO (200 μM).

or thiol are not neurotoxic by themselves, these substances act as reducing agents to donate electrons ($NO^+ \overset{e^-}{\rightarrow} NO^{\cdot}$). This reaction promotes the evolution of NO˙ from nitroprusside, which in turn leads to neurotoxicity by reaction with $O_2^{\cdot-}$ (Lipton et al., 1993):

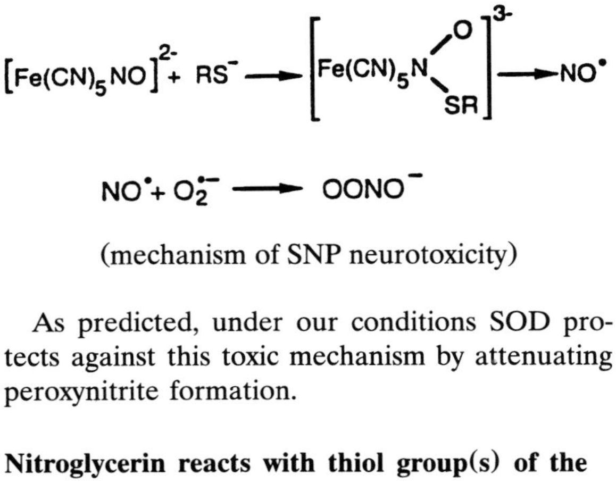

(mechanism of SNP neurotoxicity)

As predicted, under our conditions SOD protects against this toxic mechanism by attenuating peroxynitrite formation.

Nitroglycerin reacts with thiol group(s) of the NMDA receptor

Based on the above findings, we rationalized that the ideal NO donor drug would be one that does not rapidly generate NO˙, but rather would react readily with thiol group(s) on the NMDA receptor to inhibit Ca^{2+} influx. We therefore studied nitroglycerin (NTG) as an exemplary compound. Specifically, this drug does not spontaneously liberate nitric oxide to any significant extent, and it is known to react readily with thiol groups, forming derivative thionitrites (RS-NO) or thionitrates ($RS\text{-}NO_2$) (Lei et al., 1992; Lipton et al., 1993):

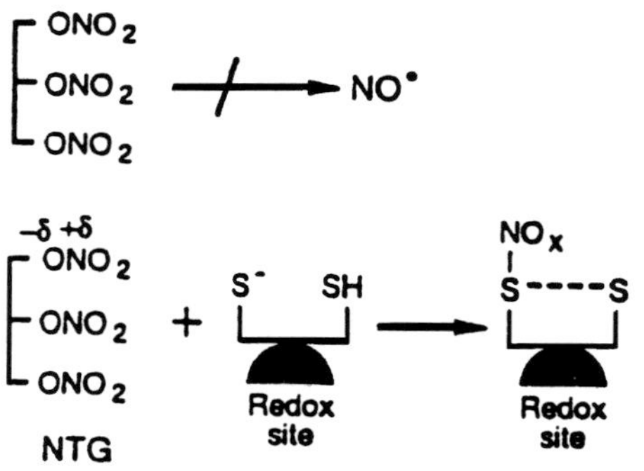

(mechanism of NTG neuroprotection)

Using whole cell recordings with patch-clamp electrodes and digital calcium imaging with fura-2, we found that nitroglycerin inhibits NMDA-evoked currents and Ca^{2+} influx (Lei et al., 1992; Lipton et al., 1993). Strong evidence that this effect of nitroglycerin is mediated by its reactions with thiol in the above-illustrated manner came from a series of chemical experiments. These studies showed that specific alkylation of thiol groups with *N*-ethylmaleimide (NEM) completely abrogates the inhibitory effect of nitroso-compounds, such as nitroglycerin, on subsequent NMDA-evoked responses (Lei et al., 1992).

The finding that nitroglycerin could inhibit NMDA-evoked responses was corroborated by the demonstration that nitroglycerin also significantly ameliorates NMDA-induced neuronal killing in cerebrocortical cultures (Lei et al., 1992; Lipton et al., 1993). Moreover, preliminary data suggest that high doses of nitroglycerin are neuroprotective in rat models of focal ischemia under conditions of constant systemic blood pressure and cerebral blood flow (Sathi et al., 1993). These parameters are held stable by inducing tolerance to these systemic effects of nitroglycerin by chronic transdermal application, or by intravenous infusion of a pressor agent concurrently with acute nitroglycerin administration.

Summary

1. The reactions of nitric oxide with superoxide can lead to neurotoxicity through formation of peroxynitrite, and not by $NO^{\cdot}$ alone, at least under our conditions.

2. Transfer of NO^{+} groups to thiol(s) on the NMDA receptor can lead to neuroprotection by inhibiting Ca^{2+} influx. These findings suggest that cell function can be controlled by, or through, protein *S*-nitrosylation, and raise the possibility that the NO group may initiate signal transduction in or at the plasma membrane.

3. The local redox milieu of a biological system is of critical importance in understanding NO actions as disparate chemical pathways involving distinct redox related congeners of NO may trigger neurotoxic or neuroprotective pathways. These claims are highlighted in the CNS by the recent finding that tissue concentrations of cysteine approach 700 μM in settings of cerebral ischemia (Slivka and Cohen, 1993); these levels of thiol would be expected to influence the redox state of the NO group.

4. Finally, our findings suggest novel therapeutic strategies. For example, downregulation of NMDA receptor activity via *S*-nitrosylation with NO^{+} donors could be implemented in the treatment of focal ischemia, AIDS dementia, and other neurological disorders associated, at least in part, with excessive activation of NMDA receptors.

Acknowledgements

This invited review, as well as those to be published by the New York Academy of Sciences and by the Taniguchi Foundation in Japan, summarizes work in the authors' laboratories and is closely adapted from our presentation in the Proceedings of the Third International Meeting on Nitric Oxide Biology; all of these meetings were held essentially concurrently.

References

Aizenman, E., Lipton, S.A. and Loring, R.H. (1989) Selective modulation of NMDA responses by reduction and oxidation. *Neuron*, 2: 1257–1263.

Bredt, D.S., Hwang, P.M. and Snyder, S.H. (1990) Localization of nitric oxide synthase indicating a neural role for nitric oxide. *Nature (Lond.)*, 347: 768–770.

Dawson, V.L., Dawson, T.M., London, E.D., Bredt, D.S. and Snyder, S.H. (1991) Nitric oxide mediates glutamate neurotoxicity in primary cortical cultures. *Proc. Natl. Acad. Sci. USA*, 88: 6368–6371.

Garthwaite, J., Charles, S.L. and Chess, W.R. (1988) Endothelium-derived relaxing factor release on activation of NMDA receptors suggests role as intercellular messenger in the brain. *Nature (Lond.)*, 336: 385–388.

Lei, S.Z., Pan, Z.-H., Aggarwal, S.K., Chen, H.-S.V., Hartman, J., Sucher, N.J. and Lipton, S.A. (1992) Effect of nitric oxide production on the redox modulatory site of the NMDA receptor-channel complex. *Neuron*, 8: 1087–1099.

Lipton, S.A. and Rosenberg, P.A. (1994) Excitatory amino acids as a final common pathway for neurologic disorders. *N. Engl. J. Med.*, 330: 613–622.

Lipton, S.A., Choi, Y.-B., Pan, Z.-H., Lei, S.Z., Chen, H.-S.V., Sucher, N.J., Loscalzo, J., Singel, D.J. and Stamler, J.S. (1993) A redox-based mechanism for the neuroprotective and neurodestructive effects of nitric oxide and related nitroso-compounds. *Nature (Lond.)*, 364: 626–632.

Moncada, S. and Higgs, A. (1993) The L-arginine-nitric oxide pathway. *N. Engl. J. Med.*, 329: 2002–2012.

Sathi, S., Edgecomb, P., Warach, S., Manchester, K., Donaghey, T., Stieg, P.E., Jensen, F.E. and Lipton, S.A. (1993)

Chronic transdermal nitroglycerin (NTG) is neuroprotective in experimental rodent stroke models. *Soc. Neurosci. Abstr.*, 19: 849.

Seeburg, P.H. (1993) The TINS/TiPS Lecture. The molecular biology of mammalian glutamate receptor channels. *Trends Neurosci.*, 16: 359–365.

Slivka, A. and Cohen, G. (1993) Brain ischemia markedly elevates levels of the neurotoxic amino acid, cysteine. *Brain Res.*, 608: 33–37.

Stamler, J.S., Singel, D.J. and Loscalzo, J. (1992) Biochemistry of nitric oxide and its redox activated forms. *Science*, 258: 1898–1902.

F.J. Seil (Ed.)
Progress in Brain Research, Vol 103

CHAPTER 30

Nitric oxide: cellular regulation and neuronal injury

Ted M. Dawson[1,4] Jie Zhang[1], Valina L. Dawson[4,5] and Solomon H. Snyder[1,2,3]

[1]Department of Neuroscience, [2]Department of Pharmacology and Molecular Sciences, [3]Department of Psychiatry and Behavioral Sciences, [4]Department of Neurology, and [5]Department of Physiology, Johns Hopkins University School of Medicine, 725 North Wolfe Street, Baltimore, MD 21205, U.S.A.

Introduction

Nitric oxide (NO) is a recently identified neuronal messenger molecule that increases cyclic guanosine monophosphate (cGMP) levels in response to glutamate receptor activation. It regulates blood vessel relaxation, serves as a neurotransmitter, and mediates macrophage killing of tumor cells and bacteria (Ignarro et al., 1984; Moncada et al., 1991; Nathan, 1992; Marletta, 1993; Dawson and Snyder, 1994). When excessive amounts of NO are formed in response to the actions of the excitatory neurotransmitter, glutamate, acting at *N*-methyl-D-aspartate (NMDA) receptors, NO mediates components of neuronal killing (Dawson and Snyder, 1994). NMDA toxicity acting via NO may account for neural damage associated with acquired immunodeficiency syndrome (AIDS) dementia as well as neural damage in cerebral infarction (Dawson and Snyder, 1994). A variety of mechanisms have been proposed for NO neurotoxicity, including inhibition of mitochondrial enzymes such as *cis*-aconitase, inhibition of the mitochondrial electron transport chain, inhibition of ribonucleotide reductase, DNA damage, mono-adenosine diphosphate (ADP)-ribosylation, and *S*-nitrosylation of glyceraldehyde-3-phosphate dehydrogenase (Dawson et al., 1992; Dawson and Snyder, 1994).

NO neurotoxicity

DNA damage may be central to neurotoxicity elicited by NO and other free radicals as DNA damage activates poly(ADP-ribose)synthetase (PARS), a nuclear enzyme which ADP-ribosylates nuclear protein, such as histones and PARS itself, by adding up to 100 ADP-ribose units per molecule (Zhang et al., 1994). NO activates PARS indirectly by damaging DNA. Activation of PARS may lead to cell death due to the depletion of the energy stores, nicotinamide-adenine dinucleotide (NAD) and adenosine triphosphate (ATP) (Berger, 1985; Gaal et al., 1987).

PARS activity is elevated several-fold by adding DNA that has been treated with authentic NO gas or the NO releasers, 3-morpholinosylnonimine (SIN-1) and sodium nitroprusside (SNP). Selective PARS inhibitors — 4-amino-1,8-naphthalimide, 1,5-dihydroxyisoquinoline and benzamide — completely prevent PARS activation by NO damaging DNA (Fig. 1). NO also enhances PARS activity in intact neuronal cells, which is inhibited by benzamide (data not shown). PARS activation directly participates in NMDA neurotoxicity as NMDA-mediated injury of primary cortical neurons is attenuated by benzamide and 1,5-dihydroxyisoquinoline (Table 1). A variety of benzamide derivatives exist with different potencies as PARS inhibitors. Benzamide is the most active PARS inhibitor and it provides the greatest amount of protection against NMDA toxicity. 3-Aminobenzamide is about half as potent as benzamide in inhibiting PARS and it is also less effective in preventing NMDA neurotoxicity. 4-Aminobenzamide and benzoic acid are relatively inactive as PARS inhibitors, and they are also ineffective as potential neuroprotective agents (Table 1). A structurally unrelated PARS inhibitor, 1,5-dihydroxyisoquinoline, is also neuroprotective.Neurotoxicity elicited by the NO releasers, SNP and *S*-nitroso-*N*-acetyl-penicillamine (SNAP), is prevented by benzamide, thus establishing that NO toxicity is mediated by activation of PARS. It is unlikely that inhibition of mono-ADP-ribosylation plays a role in neuroprotection as the selective mono-ADP-ribosylation inhibitor, novobiocin, was ineffective against NMDA toxicity (Zhang et al., 1994).

The protection against NMDA neurotoxicity

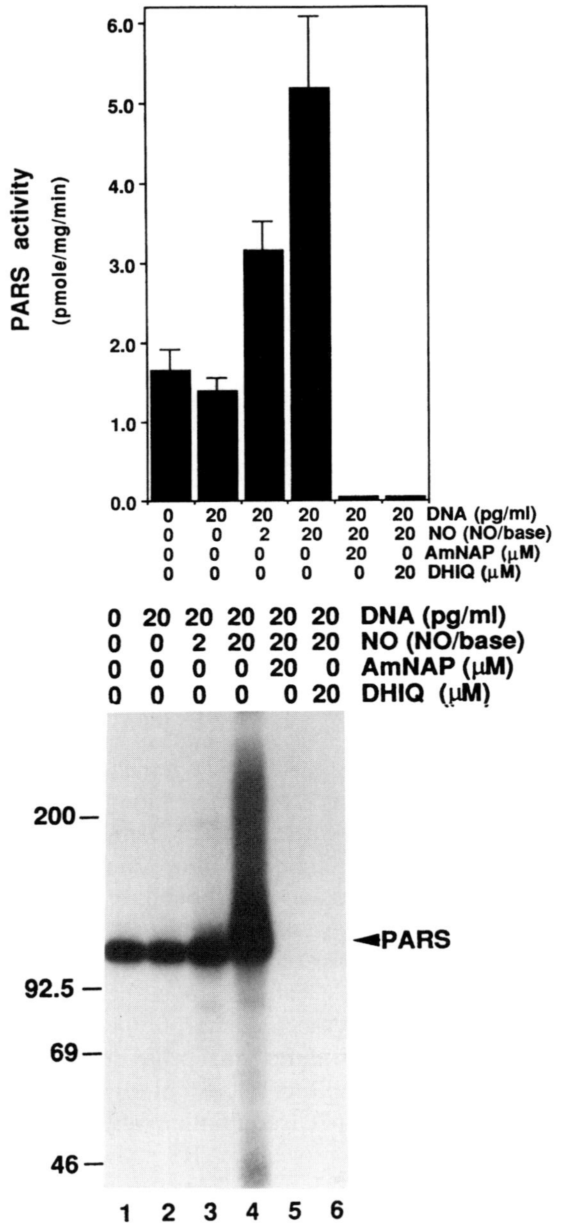

Fig. 1. Activation of PARS by NO damaged DNA. (A) PARS activity, (mean ± S.E.M., $n = 3$), after different treatments. (B) Autoradiography of PARS auto-poly(ADP-ribosyl)ation of 7.5% SDS-PAGE. *Abbreviations:* AmNAP, 4-amino-1,8-naphthalimide; DHIQ, 1,5-dihydroxyisoquinoline. (From Zhang et al., 1994.)

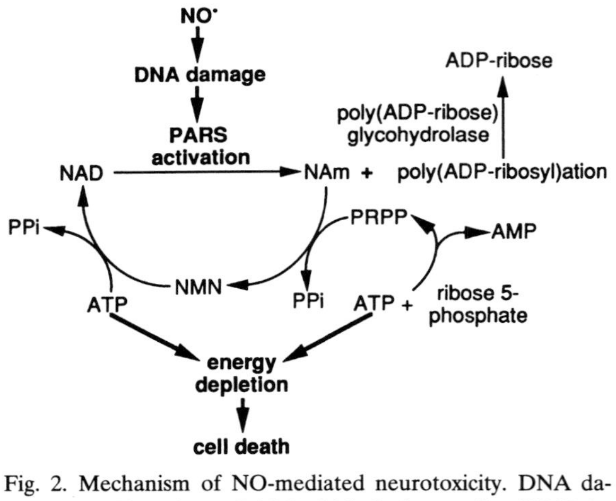

Fig. 2. Mechanism of NO-mediated neurotoxicity. DNA damaged by NO activates PARS which depletes cells of NAD by poly-ADP-ribosylating nuclear proteins. Poly(ADP-ribose) is rapidly degraded by poly(ADP-ribose) glycohydrolase. This futile cycle continues during the prolonged PARS activation. It takes an equivalent of four ATPs to resynthesize NAD from nicotinamide (NAm) via nicotinamide mononucleotide (NMN), a reaction that requires phosphoribosyl pyrophosphate (PRPP) and ATP. The depletion of energy ultimately leads to cell death. (From Zhang et al., 1994.)

TABLE 1

PARS inhibitors protect against NMDA neurotoxicity

Treatment	Percent cell death (± S.E.M.)
500 μM NMDA	57 ± 4.7
+50 μM benzamide	60.1 ± 12.1
+100 μM benzamide	39.5 ± 5.0*
+500 μM benzamide	21.9 ± 4.1*
+100 μM 3-aminobenzamide	45.9 ± 5.1*
+100 μM 4-aminobenzamide	55.8 ± 7.6
+1 mM benzoic acid	58.9 ± 5.7
+10 μM 1.5-dihydroxyisoquinoline	39.0 ± 4.5*
+1 mM novobiocin	62.4 ± 8.9

PARS inhibitors were applied 30 min before and during NMDA application. Data are the means ± S.E.M. ($n \geq 8$). Each data point represents 4000–12,000 neurons counted. *$P < 0.001$ Student's t-test. (From Zhang et al., 1994.)

TABLE 2

FK506 attenuates NMDA neurotoxicity

Drug % Cell Death (± S.E.M.)	
500 μM NMDA	82.8 ± 4.3
+500 pM FK506	78.3 ± 4.7
+1 nM FK506	77.1 ± 4.0
+10 nM FK506	68.5 ± 11.2
+25 nM FK506	67.2 ± 4.1*
+50 nM FK506	61.9 ± 5.8*
+100 nM FK506	40.0 ± 9.1*
+500 nM FK506	29.7 ± 5.8**
+1 μM FK506	29.2 ± 4.1**
+500 nM FK506 + 1 μM RAPA	82.4 + 3.3
+1 μM CsA	56.7 + 4.8*
500 μM Glutamate	76.0 + 5.2
+500 nM FK506	40.6 + 3.9*
+500 nM FK506 + 1 μM RAPA	61.7 + 5.4
500 μM Quisqualate	85.9 + 6.0
+500 nM FK506	90.5 + 4.4
100 μM Kainate	83.2 + 6.3
+500 nM FK506	88.1 + 3.8

Data are the means ± S.E.M. ($n \geq 8$). Cell death was determined by 0.4 % trypan blue exclusion by viable cells. Significance was determined by Student's t-test for independent means. *$P \leq 0.05$, 0.05, **$P \leq 0.0001$. CsA, cyclosporin A; RAPA, rapamycin. (From Dawson et al., 1993.)

afforded by PARS inhibition supports a mechanism of cell death in which DNA damage overwhelms repair mechanisms, leading to energy depletion by activation of PARS (Zhang et al., 1994). PARS activation rapidly leads to energy depletion, since for each ADP-ribose unit transferred by PARS, one molecule of NAD is consumed and an equivalent of 4-ATP are required to regenerate NAD from nicotinamide (Berger, 1985; Gaal et al., 1987) (Fig. 2).

Neuroprotection by NOS manipulation

Another potential means of influencing NO-mediated neurotoxicity elicited by activation of NMDA receptors is through manipulation of the regulatory sites of NO synthase (NOS). NOS is a phosphoprotein whose catalytic activity is inhibited by phosphorylation by protein kinase C (PKC), cAMP-dependent protein kinase, calcium calmodulin-dependent kinase and cGMP-dependent protein kinase (J.L. Dinerman, J. P. Steiner, T.M. Dawson and S.H. Snyder, unpublished data). Cyclophilins and FK506 binding proteins (FKBPs) are highly concentrated in the brain in discrete neuronal structures, where they are colocalized with the calcium activated phosphatase, calcineurin (Steiner et al., 1992). Very low concentrations of FK506 and cyclosporin A, which bind to FKBP and cyclophilin, respectively, inhibit calcineurin and enhance the phosphorylation of a number of proteins in brain. The immunosuppressants, FK506 and cyclosporin A, inhibit the neurotoxicity elicited by NMDA and glutamate in primary cortical cultures, while having no effect on quisqualate- and kainate-mediated neurotoxicity (Dawson et al., 1993). Rapamycin, an antagonist of FK506, completely reverses the neuroprotective effect of FK506 (Table 2). FK506 and cyclosporin A inhibit NMDA-elicited NO-mediated increases in cGMP levels in cortical cultures, while FK506 has no effect on SNP-induced increases in cGMP. FK506 also inhibits the Ca^{2+} ionophore, A23187, stimulates increases in nitrite

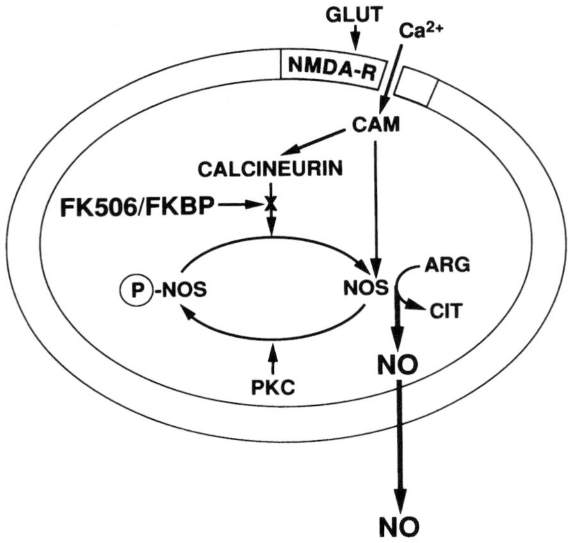

Fig. 3. Proposed mechanism for the regulation of the phosphorylation state and catalytic activity of NOS. Glutamate released from nerve terminals from adjacent neurons activates the NMDA subclass of glutamate receptors to increase intracellular Ca^{2+}. Ca^{2+} binds to calmodulin (CAM), activating NOS. The generated NO diffuses to adjacent cells to activate guanylate cyclase and increase intracellular cGMP levels. If sufficient quantities of NO are produced, adjacent cells die via undefined mechanisms, whereas neurons which produce NO are uniquely resistant. NOS catalytic activity is inhibited by PKC-mediated phosphorylation. Ca^{2+} entry activates calcineurin, which dephosphorylates and activates NOS. FK506, complexed to FKBP, binds to calcineurin, inhibiting its phosphatase activity. This prevents the dephosphorylation of NOS, thus decreasing NOS catalytic activity. With lowered NO production, adjacent neurons remain viable. (From Dawson et al., 1993.)

(a breakdown product of NO) and potentiates PKC-mediated inhibition of nitrite formation. FK506-mediated inhibition of NO formation is completely reversed by rapamycin. Furthermore, NOS is a calcineurin substrate whose PKC-mediated phosphorylation is dephosphorylated by calcineurin. FK506 prevents the calcineurin-mediated dephosphorylation of NOS and thereby diminishes NOS catalytic activity. Thus, NOS catalytic activity is regulated by the phosphorylation state of NOS. Enhanced phosphorylation of NOS diminishes catalytic activity and dephosphorylation through activation of calcinuerin enhances catalytic activity. The neuroprotective effects of FK506 and cyclosporin A presumably involve the inhibition of calcineurin, preventing the dephosphorylation of NOS and its subsequent activation (Fig. 3).

Conclusion

Derangements in glutamatergic neurotransmission are thought to contribute to pathogenetic mechanisms in a number of neurodegenerative disorders, including Huntington's disease, Alzheimer's disease and amyotrophic lateral sclerosis, and also in epilepsy and cerebral infarction. Excessive stimulation of NMDA by glutamate leads to excess production of NO, which is toxic to neurons under a variety of experimental paradigms and pathological conditions. Strategies aimed at decreasing the formation of NO or identifying targets of NO's action may have clinical relevance for the development of agents which can prevent or reverse these degenerative disorders.

Acknowledgements

T.M.D. is supported by the USPHS grant C.I.D.A. NS-01578. V.L.D. is supported by Intramural Research Training Award from the N.I.H. S.H.S. is supported by Research Scientist Award DA-00074 and USPHS grant DA-00266. We thank Dawn C. Dodson for excellent secretarial assistance.

References

Berger, N.A. (1985) Poly(ADP-ribose) in the cellular response to DNA damage. *Radiat. Res.*, 101: 4–15.

Dawson, T.M. and Snyder, S.H. (1994) Gases as biological messengers: nitric oxide and carbon monoxide in the brain. *J. Neurosci.*, in press.

Dawson T.M., Dawson, V.L. and Snyder, S.H. (1992) A novel neuronal messenger molecule in brain: the free radical, nitric oxide. *Ann. Neurol.*, 32: 297–311.

Dawson, T.M., Steiner, J.P., Dawson, V.L., Dinerman, J.L., Uhl, G.R. and Snyder, S.H. (1993) Immunosuppressant, FK506, enhances phosphorylation of nitric oxid protects against glutamate neurotoxicity. *Proc. Natl. Acad. Sci. USA*, 90: 9808–9812.

Gaal, J.C., Smith, K.R. and Pearson, C.K. (1987) Cellular euthanasia mediated by a nuclear enzyme: a central role for nuclear ADP-ribosylation in cellular metabolism. *Trends Biol. Sci.*, 12: 129–130.

Ignarro, L.J., Wood, K.S. and Wolin, M.S. (1984) Regulation of purified soluble guanylate cyclase by porphyrins and metalloporphyrins: a unifying concept. In: P. Greengard (Ed.), *Advances in Cyclic Nucleotide and Protein Phosphorylation Research*, Vol. 17, Raven Press, New York, pp. 267–274.

Marletta, M.A. (1993) Nitric oxide synthase structure and mechanism. *J. Biol. Chem.*, 268: 12231–12234.

Moncada, S., Palmer, R.M.J. and Higgs, E.A. (1991) Nitric oxide: physiology, pathophysiology and pharmacology. *Pharmacol. Rev.*, 43: 109–142.

Nathan, C. (1992) Nitric oxide as a secretory product of mammalian cells. *FASEB J.*, 6: 3051–3064.

Steiner, J.P., Dawson, T.M., Fotuhi, M., Glatt, C.E., Snowman, A.M., Cohen, N. and Snyder, S.H. (1992) High brain densities of the immunophilin FKBP colocalized with calcineurin. *Nature (London)*, 358: 584–587.

Zhang, J., Dawson, V.L., Dawson, T.M. and Snyder, S.H. (1994) Nitric oxide activation of poly (ADP-ribose) synthetase in neurotoxicity. *Science*, 263: 687–689.

F.J. Seil (Ed.)
Progress in Brain Research, Vol 103

CHAPTER 31

Reactions of nitric oxide, superoxide and peroxynitrite with superoxide dismutase in neurodegeneration

Joseph S. Beckman, Jun Chen, John P. Crow and Yao Zu Ye

Department of Anesthesiology, University of Alabama at Birmingham, Birmingham, AL 25233, USA

Introduction

To be successful in any attempt to regenerate the nervous system, the processes responsible for the underlying neurodegeneration must be understood and controlled. In the past decade, phenomenal progress has been made in understanding the interrelations between excitatory neurotransmitter release and the resulting influx of calcium in toxicity. The mechanisms of calcium-mediated toxicity are complex because of the multiple processes that are activated. One of the newest hypotheses relates to the calcium-dependent production of nitric oxide by neurons as a cytotoxic mechanism (Beckman, 1991).

The history of nitric oxide in the neurosciences spans a brief five years. Glutamate-mediated neurotransmission was first linked with nitric oxide production by neurons by Garthwaite et al. (1988). The importance of nitric oxide as a retrograde messenger contributing to the formation of memory and development was shortly thereafter postulated by Williams et al. (1989) and modeled by Gally et al. (1990). In 1991, Shibuki and Okado demonstrated that nitric oxide was important for the development of long-term depression in brain. They also invented a simple electrode for measuring nitric oxide directly in cerebellar tissue slices and showed that brief electrical stimulation can produce 100 nM concentrations of nitric oxide. Many studies have since shown nitric oxide to participate in long-term potentiation (Böhme et al., 1991; O'Dell et al., 1991; Shulman and Madison, 1991).

Excitatory amino acids are also key initiators of neuronal death, and Garthwaite et al. (1988, 1991) proposed that nitric oxide production could also contribute to neuronal degeneration. Indeed, inhibition of nitric oxide synthesis can protect neurons in culture from glutamate toxicity and can reduce infarct volume in stroke models if administered in low concentrations (Nowicki et al., 1991; Nagafuji et al., 1992; Chen et al., 1994). Recently, Malinski and Taha (1992) have shown that cerebral ischemia in the middle cerebral territory of rats can lead to steady-state concentrations of nitric oxide in the 2–4 μM range (Malinski et al., 1993). However, not all laboratories have found inhibition of nitric oxide to be protective, and under some circumstances administration of nitric oxide donors is protective in stroke and myocardial ischemia models (Johnson et al., 1991; Yamamoto et al., 1992).

These inconsistencies can be largely resolved by a better understanding of the chemistry of nitric oxide in dilute aqueous solutions. In this paper, we wish to make three points:

1. Nitric oxide is far less reactive and toxic at physiologically relevant concentrations than commonly thought. Many investigators have been mis-

lead by using millimolar solutions of nitric oxide or various relatively uncharacterized 'nitric oxide' donors to study chemical reactivity and then equating the results with the reactivity of nitric oxide per se. In the present review, we will describe how low concentrations of nitric oxide do not react rapidly with oxygen to form nitrogen dioxide. Instead, nitric oxide is more likely to diffuse into red blood cells and be consumed by reaction with hemoglobin.

2. The reactivity and toxicity of nitric oxide is enormously increased by its near diffusion-limited reaction with superoxide to form peroxynitrite anion (Huie and Padmaja, 1993). From 1 to 5% of all oxygen consumed is partially reduced to produce the oxygen radical, superoxide ($O_2^{\cdot -}$). Normally, superoxide concentrations are kept at very low levels (10–100 pM) by large amounts of superoxide dismutase (SOD), an enzyme that rapidly scavenges superoxide. When produced at a high rate by cells under pathological conditions, nitric oxide is the one biological molecule capable of outcompeting SOD for superoxide. Peroxynitrite is a powerful oxidant, capable of damaging all major components of a cell.

3. Paradoxically, peroxynitrite reacts with SOD to form a powerful nitrating agent with the reactivity of nitronium ion (NO_2^+) and modifies tyrosine residues on proteins to form nitrotyrosine (Fig. 1) (Ischiropoulos et al., 1992a). Nitrotyrosine can not be phosphorylated by tyrosine kinases (Martin et al., 1990) and thus SOD-mediated injury may affect critical signal transduction pathways. We have proposed that this mechanism may account for the pathological action of SOD mutations in amyotrophic lateral sclerosis (ALS) (Beckman et al., 1993).

Limited reactivity of nitric oxide in vitro

The toxicity of nitric oxide per se at the low concentrations produced in vivo has been overestimated due to extrapolation from its reactivity at high concentrations. One must be extremely careful working with cylinders of pure nitric oxide because a leak will lead to the rapid formation of the orange gas, nitrogen dioxide, by the following reaction:

$$2\,NO + O_2 \rightarrow 2\,NO_2$$

Nitrogen dioxide is a powerful oxidant, and breathing concentrations above 300 ppm will lead to a slow death from pulmonary edema. However, the reaction depends upon the collision of two nitric oxides with oxygen, so the rate of forming toxic nitrogen dioxide falls rapidly with the square of nitric oxide concentration. While the orange brown color of nitrogen dioxide appears immediately when gaseous nitric oxide contacts air, its rate of formation is at least ten million times

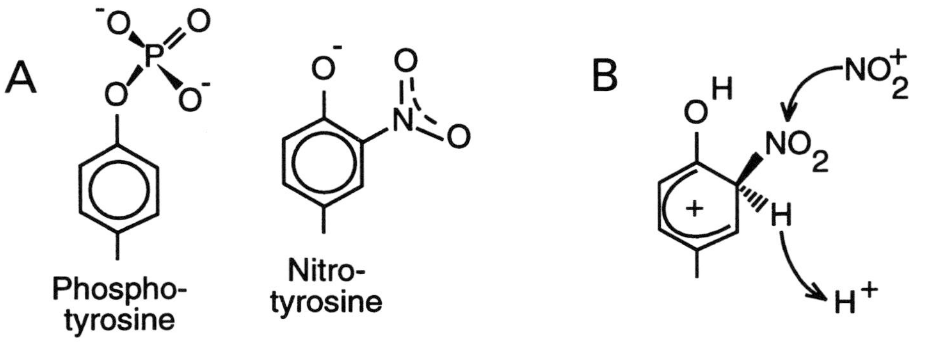

Fig. 1. (A) The structure of phosphotyrosine and nitrotyrosine. The nitro group involves a stable carbon-nitrogen bond, unlike phosphotyrosine, which is readily hydrolyzed. (B) Reaction of nitronium ion with tyrosine to form nitrotyrosine. The electrophilic nitronium attacks tyrosine through a cation intermediate, which releases a hydrogen ion to form nitrotyrosine.

slower at the maximum physiological nitric oxide concentrations (about 0.1 μM at peak levels) (Shibuki and Okada, 1991; Malinski and Taha, 1992). It takes over an hour for physiological concentrations of nitric oxide to decompose to nitrite and nitrate in solution. At low concentrations, similar to those which can be produced in vivo, nitric oxide can be safely administered for weeks in the gas phase to treat pulmonary hypertension. The interpretation of studies utilizing 100–1000 μM concentrations of nitric oxide as direct toxicity of nitric oxide is incorrect because of the rapid formation of nitrogen dioxide. The results will be quite different from a slow continuous exposure to physiologically relevant concentrations of nitric oxide (in the range of 0.01 to 10 μM) over many hours because of the slow formation of nitric oxide.

Nitrosothiols

Because of the inconvenience of working with nitric oxide, many studies have utilized nitrosothiols or other 'nitric oxide donors'. Each of these compounds must undergo a chemical reaction to release nitric oxide. For example, *S*-nitrosocysteine can release nitric oxide by a reaction occurring between two molecules:

$$2\ \text{Cys-S-NO} \rightarrow 2\ \text{NO} + \text{Cys-S-S-Cys}$$

However, this reaction depends upon the square of two cysteines reacting with each other. Nitrosothiols quickly react with other thiols to liberate nitric oxide, but the chemistry of these reactions still needs to be explored more fully. *S*-nitrosocysteine can also transfer the nitrosonium ion equivalent (NO^+) to other sulfhydryls and thus act as an effective sulfhydryl oxidant. Nitric oxide itself reacts slowly with thiols and nitrosothiols are not the product. Under anaerobic conditions, the nitric oxide is generally reduced to nitroxyl anion (NO^-) and eventually appears as nitrous oxide (N_2O). Nitrosothiols are clearly formed in vivo and have substantial biological effects (Stamler et al., 1992a,b,c; Kearney et al., 1993), but the mechanism is clearly more complex than nitric oxide reacting directly with a thiol.

SOD, cerebral ischemia and nitric oxide

Polyethylene glycol-conjugated superoxide dismutase (PEG-SOD) injected intravenously can reduce cerebral ischemic injury. We first observed protection by PEG-SOD in a prolonged global ischemia stroke model in gerbils (Beckman et al., 1986) and then in a more sophisticated middle cerebral artery stroke model in rats developed by Dr. Chung Hsu (Liu et al., 1989). PEG-SOD has recently been found to be protective in severe head trauma in humans (Muizelaar et al., 1993). In a recent randomized, blinded phase II study, treatment of severe head trauma patients (Glascow coma scale > 3) with 5,000 and 10,000 U/kg PEG-SOD resulted in a 50% decrease in morbidity and mortality compared to placebo-treated controls. The most striking effect was on the shorter duration of elevated intracranial pressure observed in patients receiving PEG-SOD.

Protection by moderate dosages of superoxide dismutase strongly implicates superoxide in toxicity, but superoxide is not a highly reactive molecule at neutral pH. The most commonly proposed mechanism to account for the toxicity of superoxide is the iron-catalyzed Haber-Weiss reaction. This is a complex cycle whereby superoxide reduces ferric iron and the resulting ferrous iron attacks hydrogen peroxide to form hydroxyl radical. This theory became widely accepted in part because there was no better explanation at the time for how SOD and catalase could protect tissue. However, there are several major problems with the Haber-Weiss reaction as an explanation for free radical toxicity. In particular, the reaction rate of hydrogen peroxide with ferrous iron is slow ($\approx 10^3\ M^{-1} \cdot s^{-1}$) and hydroxyl radical itself is so reactive that it tends to be rather nontoxic due to nonspecific side reactions (see Beckman and Siedow, 1985; Zhu et al., 1992, for further discussion).

When endothlium relaxing factor (EDRF) was identified as nitric oxide, we became interested in the reaction of nitric oxide with superoxide as a potential explanation for the apparent toxicity of superoxide. Both nitric oxide and superoxide are paramagnetic species that react by a diffusion-limited reaction ($6.7 \times 10^9\ M^{-1} \cdot s^{-1}$) to form peroxynitrite anion (Huie and Padmaja, 1993):

$$O_2^{\cdot -} + \cdot NO \rightarrow {}^{-}OONO$$

Nitric oxide is the only known biological molecule that can be produced in high enough concentrations and reacts fast enough to outcompete SOD for superoxide. In alkaline solutions, peroxynitrite anion is stable for months, but has a pK_a of 6.8 at 37°C. The protonated form, peroxynitrous acid (ONOOH), decays to form a species with the reactivity of hydroxyl radical (·OH) and nitrogen dioxide (NO_2) as intermediates by the following series of reactions:

$$(pK_a = 6.8) \quad (t_{1/2} < 1\ \text{sec})$$
$$^{-}OONO + H^{+} \leftrightarrow HOONO \rightarrow \text{'}HO^{\cdot} + NO_2\text{'}$$

However, direct oxidizing reactions of peroxynitrite appear to be far more toxic than the hydroxyl radical-like reactivity of peroxynitrite. We have extensively characterized the oxidative chemistry of peroxynitrite in terms of its thermodynamics (Koppenol et al., 1992), kinetics (Beckman et al., 1992) and types of reactions initiated (Beckman et al., 1990; Radi et al., 1991a,b, 1993; Bauer et al., 1992). We have shown that it is a major product of activated macrophages (Ischiropoulos et al., 1992b) and that it is highly toxic (Zhu et al., 1992). One surprising result that took several years to characterize was the reaction of peroxynitrite with SOD to form a nitrating species resembling nitronium ion (Ischiropoulos et al., 1990, 1992a; Beckman et al., 1992; Smith et al., 1992). This unusual reaction may explain the loss of protection at high dosages of SOD in ischemia and the actions of the SOD mutations in ALS.

Peroxynitrite reacts with superoxide dismutase

Peroxynitrite reacts with metal ions, including the metal centers in Mn, Fe and Cu,Zn forms of SOD, to produce the highly reactive and toxic nitronium ion (NO_2^+). Once in the active site, peroxynitrite forms a transient cuprous adduct:

$$\text{SOD-Cu}^{2+} \cdots {}^{-}OO\text{-}N = O \rightarrow \text{SOD-Cu}^{1+}O^{-} \cdots O = N^{+} = O$$

This intermediate complex can donate a nitronium ion (NO_2^+) to phenolics to form nitrophenols. After releasing hydroxyl ion, native SOD is regenerated and therefore acts catalytically:

$$\text{SOD-Cu}^{1+}O^{-} \cdots O = N^{+} = O + \text{tyrosine} \rightarrow \text{SOD-Cu}^{2+} + OH^{-} + NO_2\text{-tyrosine}$$

Cu,Zn SOD is not inactivated as a result of its reaction with peroxynitrite. SOD catalyzes the nitration of a wide range of phenolics, including tyrosines in lysozyme and histone. The implications from these data are: (a) exogenous SOD may also catalyze toxic reactions in tissues producing large amounts of nitric oxide and (b) SOD-catalyzed nitration reactions are specific and sensitive probes for measuring peroxynitrite in vivo.

High dosages of SOD lose efficacy in both cerebral and myocardial ischemia

Most animal studies utilizing SOD have been performed with a single dose because of the cost. In myocardial ischemia, 5-fold higher dosages of SOD reduce efficacy and may make injury worse. The effect is not due to toxicity of SOD itself, because much higher dosages of SOD are well tolerated in control animals. Dr. Chung Hsu (Washington University, St. Louis) has recently shown that the bell-shaped efficacy curve for PEG-SOD is even sharper in focal cerebral ischemia than reported for heart. Bell-shaped efficacy results were first reported in ischemic heart (Bernier et al., 1989; Omar et al., 1990 a,b).

Transgenic mice overexpressing native Cu,Zn SOD have been shown to exhibit abnormal proliferation of neuromuscular junctions (Avraham et al., 1988, 1990), similar to what is observed in ALS. These mice were originally developed as potential models of Down's syndrome, which exhibit a trisomy for chromosome 21 containing the SOD gene.

Higher amounts of SOD will not increase hydrogen peroxide production

One common misconception about the bell-shaped efficacy curve is that more SOD will increase the rate of hydrogen peroxide formation, resulting in damaging levels of hydrogen peroxide. The rate of forming hydrogen peroxide is limited by the rate of oxygen reduction to give superoxide (step 1), not by the dismutation of superoxide (step 2). The effect of adding more SOD is simply to lower the steady state concentration of superoxide to the level where the rate of dismutation is the same as the rate of oxygen reduction to superoxide:OC

$$O_2 \xrightarrow{1\,e^-} O_2^{\cdot -} \xrightarrow{SOD} 1/2\,O_2 + 1/2H_2O_2$$

In their original paper, McCord and Fridovich (1969) showed that the rate of forming hydrogen peroxide was independent of SOD concentration. Most other reactions of superoxide are rapidly outcompeted with only a small amount of SOD. The average intracellular concentration of SOD in a cell is 10–30 μM. Furthermore, hydrogen peroxide is toxic only at extremely high concentrations, which can never exist in the presence of catalase. It has always been troubling that concentrations of hydrogen peroxide used to show cytotoxicity are in the millimolar range, and even at these concentrations it can take exposures of up to an hour to get significant toxicity.

SOD minimizes reaction with peroxynitrite in *cis* conformation

The reaction rate of peroxynitrite with bovine Cu,Zn SOD was $10^5\ M^{-1} \cdot s^{-1}$ at low SOD concentrations, but the rate of nitration became independent of SOD concentration above 10 μM with a yield of only 9%. In contrast, peroxynitrite reacted directly with Fe^{3+} EDTA at a 20-fold slower rate ($5 \times 10^3\ M^{-1} \cdot s^{-1}$), but the reaction rate continued to accelerate as the concentration of iron (pseudo-first order with respect to Fe^{3+}) was increased. Because peroxynitrite anion is more stable in the *cis* conformation, its reaction with superoxide dismutase appears to be limited by the isomerization to the *trans* conformation, which is more likely to squeeze into the narrow active site of Cu,Zn SOD. At high SOD concentrations, phenolic nitration is limited by the rate of isomerization from *cis* to *trans* peroxynitrite, as well as by competing pathways for peroxynitrite decomposition.

Injury induces nitric oxide synthase in motor neurons

Peripheral nerve injury can induce the macrophage form of nitric oxide synthase to high levels (Solodkin et al., 1992). The macrophage remains the best characterized source of the inducible nitric oxide synthase. Its synthesis is induced by bacterial lipopolysaccharides, γ-interferon, and various interleukins with a lag time of a few hours. Transforming growth factor beta (TGF-β) downregulates expression of the inducible nitric oxide synthase. It seems that virtually all tissues can induce nitric oxide synthase. Tissue expressing the inducible isozyme can produce nitric oxide at rates a thousand-fold higher than typically produced by endothelium for signal transduction (Moncada et al., 1991), and this isoform appears to be constitutively active. The first evidence for nitric oxide synthase in spinal cord was based upon staining with nicotinamide-adenine dinucleotide phosphate (NADPH) diaphorase (Valtschanoff et al., 1992), which has a strong but not absolute correlation with nitric oxide synthase (Hope et al., 1991; Vincent and Hope, 1992). The distribution of nitric oxide has been confirmed with specific antibodies (Dun et al., 1992). However, motor neurons can be induced to express nitric oxide synthase (Wu, 1993). Microglia also produce nitric oxide via the high output nitric oxide (Boje and Arora, 1992). In addition, astrocytes and glia also can produce nitric oxide (Murphy et al., 1990; Galea et al., 1992). Surprisingly, the activity of neuronal nitric oxide synthase is high in human skeletal muscle (Nakane et al., 1993), which might contribute to injury of the neuromuscular junction.

Peroxynitrite is far more toxic than nitric oxide or hydroxyl radical generated by xanthine oxidase. Peroxynitrite (1 mM) kills in a few seconds, whereas exposure to 1 mM nitric oxide (aerobically or anaerobically), xanthine oxidase or hydrogen peroxide was essentially nontoxic (unpublished observations). Similar conclusions have been recently been published by Lipton et al. (1993) for cultured neurons, though the lethal dosage of peroxynitrite was only 20–50 μM compared to 250 μM for *E. coli*. Dawson et al. (1991, 1993a,b) also have found that SOD greatly reduces the toxicity of endogenous nitric oxide production after *N*-methyl-D-aspartic acid (NMDA) stimulation in their neuronal cell culture system, a finding consistent with peroxynitrite formation.

The peroxynitrite nitration hypothesis of ALS

Sherrington described the motor neuron as the final common pathway of the central nervous system, transforming neuronal action into activation of muscle. The neuromuscular junction distinguishes lower motor neurons from all other neurons and may contribute to the selective vulnerability of motor neurons in ALS. ALS is characterized principally by degeneration of large motor neurons in the ventral horn of the spinal cord and by degeneration of upper motor neurons in the cerebral cortex. Because muscle fibers are innervated by only a single motor neuron, other motor neurons normally rewire to the muscle fiber to take over the function of a damaged motor neuron. Muscle from ALS patients contains far more neuromuscular junctions than normal muscle. Remodeling of synapses and motor endplates may cause subsequent injury of adjacent motor neurons. This rewiring requires synaptic remodeling, a process that appears to involve nitric oxide (Gally et al., 1990). Nitric oxide may indirectly contribute to motor neuron destruction in ALS via Cu,Zn SOD. In addition to nitric oxide produced by neurons, nitric oxide as well as superoxide may be produced by reactive astrocytes and microglia that remove the cellular debris from degenerating motor neurons. Peripheral nerve injury and chronic inflammation have recently been shown to induce nitric oxide synthase in spinal cord (Solodkin et al., 1992; Verge et al., 1992). Furthermore, human skeletal muscle contains high concentrations of the neuronal form of nitric oxide synthase, which is probably localized in the neuromuscular junction (Nakane et al., 1993).

We propose that the Cu,Zn SOD mutants associated with familial ALS on chromosome 21 have a greater intrinsic ability to catalyze nitration by peroxynitrite of tyrosine residues on a key target in motor neurons. Because afflicted ALS patients have one normal SOD allele, superoxide scavenging should decrease by about 50%, which would at most double the steady state concentration of superoxide. Superoxide reacts with nitric oxide at a rate of $6.7 \times 10^9\ M^{-1} \cdot s^{-1}$, three times faster than with native SOD, to form the powerful oxidant, peroxynitrite ($ONOO^-$) (Huie and Padmaja, 1993). A doubling of the steady-state superoxide concentration will also double the rate of peroxynitrite formation. Peroxynitrite in turn reacts with SOD at $\approx 10^5\ M^{-1} \cdot s^{-1}$ to form a nitronium-like intermediate, which nitrates tyrosine residues (Fig. 1) (Beckman et al., 1992).

The mutations identified in ALS patients do not directly affect conserved amino acids forming the active site, but could slightly disrupt the active site pocket to allow greater access of peroxynitrite to the copper. Chemical modification of several amino acids in the active site allows SOD to react with peroxynitrite but greatly diminishes superoxide scavenging (Beckman et al., 1992). The details of the mutant effects of SOD upon structure are described in greater detail below. Thus, the SOD mutations may increase both the rate of peroxynitrite formation due to reduced scavenging of superoxide and nitration by peroxynitrite of critical cellular targets. Nitration of proteins will slowly injure motor neurons as well as other cells. However, motor neurons, among the largest in the central nervous system, cannot regenerate. The neuromuscular junction may also be another target that makes the motor neuron particularly susceptible.

Phosphorylation of tyrosine residues is a major signal transduction mechanism for most growth factors and is inhibited by nitration (Martin et al., 1990). One mechanism leading to ALS would involve disruption of signal transduction by growth factors. Skeletal muscle has been shown to produce two nerve growth factors, brain-derived neurotrophic factor (BDNF) and neurotrophin-3 (NT-3), that support the survival of motor neurons after injury. BDNF and NT-3 bind to the trkB receptor (Klein et al., 1991), which is a tyrosine kinase in the neuromuscular junction of motor neurons. Like most growth factor receptors, trkB phosphorylates itself, which is necessary for activation. The trkB receptor also is known to activate phospholipase Cγ-1 by phosphorylation (Widmer et al., 1993). The trkB receptor complex with BNDF is taken up by the motor neuron and appears to be transported to the cell body by retrograde transport (DiStefano et al., 1992). The trkB receptor is strongly upregulated after spinal cord injury (Frisen et al., 1992). There is a clear proliferation of motor end units in ALS, with some end units containing synaptic vesicles but not making contact with muscle. This suggests that the motor neuron in ALS might be suffering a deficiency of muscle-derived growth factors. It is also reminiscent of the proliferation of neuromuscular junctions observed in transgenic SOD mice (Avraham et al., 1988, 1990). Other potential tyrosine targets may affect kinases responsible for phosphorylation of neurofilaments, which have also been implicated in the pathogenesis of ALS. Thus, nitration of key tyrosine residues may lead to the gradual loss of motor neurons by several potential but as yet unknown mechanisms that need to be investigated.

As other motor neurons attempt to remodel, they become exposed to additional fluxes of nitric oxide and peroxynitrite, leading to their eventual demise. The continual recruitment and destruction of more neurons propagates the relentless progression of ALS. Upper motor neuron involvement might result from disruption of its synaptic connections to lower motor neurons. Further injury may result from the accumulation of microglia around degenerating Betz cells in the motor cortex (Hammer et al., 1979). Understanding whether such a nitration cycle occurs in ALS can lead to better therapeutic intervention by suggesting methods to break the cycle, such as selective inhibition of nitric oxide synthase found in or around motor neurons. Nitration of tyrosine residues may also be involved in other forms of neurodegeneration.

Acknowledgements

This work was supported by NIH grants HL46407, NS24338, and HL48676. J.S.B. is an Established Investigator of the American Heart Association.

References

Avraham, K., Schickler, M., Sapoznoikov, D., Yarom, R. and Groner, Y. (1988) Down's syndrome: abnormal neuromuscular junction in tongue of transgenic mice with elevated levels of human Cu/Zn-superoxide dismutase. *Cell*, 54: 823–829.

Avraham, K., Sugarman, H., Rotshenker, S. and Groner, Y. (1990) Down's syndrome: morphological remodelling and increased complexity in the neuromuscular junction of transgenic CuZn-superoxide dismutase mice. *J. Neurocytol.*, 20: 208–215.

Bauer, M., Beckman, J.S., Bridges, R. and Matalon, S. (1992) Peroxynitrite inhibits sodium transport in rat colonic membrane vesicles. *Biochim. Biophys. Acta*, 1104: 84–87.

Beckman, J.S. (1991) The double edged role of nitric oxide in brain function and superoxide-mediated pathology. *J. Dev. Physiol.*, 15: 53–59.

Beckman, J.S. and Siedow, J.N. (1985) Bactericidal agents generated by the peroxynitrite-catalyzed oxidation of *para*-hydroquinones. *J. Biol. Chem.*, 260: 14604–14609.

Beckman, J.S., Campbell, G.A., Hannan, J., Karfias, C.S. and

Freeman, B.A. (1986) Involvement of superoxide and xanthine oxidase with death due to cerebral ischemia-induced seizures in gerbils. In: G. Rotilio (Ed.), *Superoxide and Superoxide Dismutase in Chemistry, Biology and Medicine*, Elsevier, Amsterdam, pp. 602–607.

Beckman, J.S., Beckman, T.W., Chen, J., Marshall, P.M. and Freeman, B.A. (1990) Apparent hydroxyl radical production from peroxynitrite: implications for endothelial injury by nitric oxide and superoxide. *Proc. Natl. Acad. Sci. USA*, 87: 1620–1624.

Beckman, J.S., Ischiropoulos, H., Zhu, L., van der Woerd, M., Smith, C., Chen, J., Harrison, J., Martin, J.C. and Tsai, M. (1992) Kinetics of superoxide dismutase and iron catalyzed nitration of phenolics by peroxynitrite. *Arch. Biochem. Biophys.*, 298: 438–445.

Beckman, J.S., Carson, M., Smith, C.D. and Koppenol, W.H. (1993) ALS, SOD and peroxynitrite. *Nature (Lond.)*, 364: 584.

Bernier, M., Manning, A.S. and Hearse, D.J. (1989) Reperfusion arrhythmias: dose-related protection by anti-free radical interventions. *Am. J. Physiol.*, 256: H1344-H1352.

Böhme, G.A., Bon, C., Stutzmann, J.M., Doble, A. and Blanchard, J.C. (1991) Possible involvement of nitric oxide in long-term potentiation. *Eur. J. Pharmacol.*, 199: 379–381.

Boje, K.M. and Arora, P.K. (1992) Microglial-produced nitric oxide and reactive nitrogen oxides mediate neuronal cell death. *Brain Res.*, 587: 250–256.

Chen, J., Conger, K.A., Tan, M.J. and Beckman, J.S. (1994) Nitroarginine reduces infarction after middle cerebral artery occlusion in rats. In: A. Hartmann, F. Yatsu and W. Kuschinsky (Eds.), *Basic Mechanisms of Cerebral Ischemia*, Springer-Verlag, Berlin, in press.

Dawson, V.L., Dawson, T.M., London, E.D., Brent, D.S. and Snyder, S.H. (1991) Nitric oxide mediates glutamate neurotoxicity in primary cortical cultures. *Proc. Natl. Acad. Sci. USA*, 88: 6368–6371.

Dawson, V., Dawson, T., Bartley, D., Uhl, G. and Snyder, S. (1993a) Mechanisms of nitiric oxide mediated neurotoxicity in primary brain cultures. *J. Neurosci.*, 13: 2651–2661.

Dawson, V., Dawson, T., Uhl, G. and Snyder, S. (1993b) Human immunodeficiency virus type 1 coat protein neurotoxicity mediated by nitric oxide in primary cortical cultures. *Proc. Natl. Acad. Sci. USA*, 90: 3256–3259.

DiStefano, P.S., Friedman, B., Radziejewski, C., Alexander, C., Boland, P., Schick, C.M., Lindsay, R.M. and Wieland, S.J. (1992) The neurotrophins BDNF, NT-3 and NGF display distinct patterns of retrograde axonal transport in peripheral and central neurons. *Neuron*, 8: 983–993.

Dun, N.J., Dun, S.L., Forstermann, U. and Tseng, L.F. (1992) Nitric oxide synthase immunoreactivity in rat spinal cord. *Neurosci. Lett.*, 147: 217–220.

Frisen, J., Verge, V., Cullheim, S., Persson, H., Fried, K., Middlemas, D., Hunter, T., Hokfelt, T. and Risling, M. (1992) Increased levels of trkB mRNA and trkB protein-like immunoreactivity in the injured rat and cat spinal cord. *Proc. Natl. Acad. Sci. USA*, 89: 11282–11286.

Galea, E., Feinstein, D. and Reis, D. (1992) Induction of calcium-indepedent nitric oxide synthase activity in primary rat glial cultures. *Proc. Natl. Acad. Sci. USA*, 89: 10945–10949.

Gally, J.A., Montague, P.R., Reeke Jr., G.N. and Edelman, G.M. (1990) The NO hypothesis: possible effects of a short-lived, rapidly diffusible signal in the development and function of the nervous system. *Proc. Natl. Acad. Sci. USA*, 87: 3547–3551.

Garthwaite, J. (1991). Glutamate, nitric oxide and cell-cell signalling in the nervous system. *Trends Neurosci.*, 14: 75–82.

Garthwaite, J., Charles, S.L. and Chess-Williams, R. (1988) Endothelium-derived relaxing factor release on activation of NMDA receptors suggests role as intercellular messenger in the brain. *Nature (Lond.)*, 336: 385–388.

Hammer, R., Tomiyasu, U. and Scheibel, A. (1979) Degeneration of the human Betz cell due to amyotrophic lateral sclerosis. *Exp. Neurol.*, 63: 336–346.

Hope, B.T., Michael, G.J., Knigge, K.M. and Vincent, S.R. (1991) Neuronal NADPH diaphorase is a nitric oxide synthase. *Proc. Natl. Acad. Sci. USA*, 88: 2811–2814.

Huie, R.E. and Padmaja, S. (1993) The reaction rate of nitric oxide with superoxide. *Free Rad. Res. Commun.*, 18: 195–199.

Ischiropoulos, H., Chen, J., Tsai, J.H.M., Martin, J.C., Smith, C.D. and Beckman, J.S. (1990) Peroxynitrite ($ONOO^-$) reacts with superoxide dismutase to give the reactive nitronium ion. *Free Rad. Biol. Med.*, 9(Suppl. 1): 131.

Ischiropoulos, H., Zhu, L., Chen, J., Tsai, H.M., Martin, J.C., Smith, C.D. and Beckman, J.S. (1992a) Peroxynitrite-mediated tyrosine nitration catalyzed by superoxide dismutase. *Arch. Biochem. Biophys.*, 298: 431–437.

Ischiropoulos, H., Zhu, L. and Beckman, J.S. (1992b) Peroxynitrite formation from activated rat alveolar macrophages. *Arch. Biochem. Biophys.*, 298: 446–451.

Johnson G., III, Tsao, P. and Lefer, A. (1991) Cardioprotective effects of authentic nitric oxide in myocardial ischemia with reperfusion. *Crit. Care Med.*, 19: 244–252.

Kearney, J., Simon, D., Stamler, J., Jaraki, O., Schaftsein, J., Vita, J. and Loscalzo, J. (1993) NO forms an adduct with serum albumin that has endothelium-derived relaxing factor-like properties. *J. Clin. Inv.*, 91: 1582–1589.

Klein, R., Nanduri, V., Jing, S., Lamballe, F., Tapley, P., Bryant, S., Cordon-Cardo, C., Jones, K., Reichardt, L. and Barbacid, M. (1991) The trkB tyrosine protein kinase is a receptor for brain-derived neurotrophic factor and neurotrophin-3. *Cell*, 66: 395–403.

Koppenol, W.H., Moreno, J.J., Pryor, W.A., Ischiropoulos, H.

and Beckman, J.S. (1992) Peroxynitrite: a cloaked oxidant from superoxide and nitric oxide. *Chem. Res. Toxicol.*, 5: 834–842.

Lipton, S.A., Choi, Y.-B., Pan, Z.-H., Lei, S.Z., Chen, H.-S.V., Sucher, N.J., Loscalzo, J., Singel, D.J. and Stamler, J.S. (1993) A redox-based mechanism for the neuroprotective and neurodestructive effects of nitric oxide and related nitroso-compounds. *Nature (Lond.)*, 364: 626–631.

Liu, T.H., Beckman, J.S., Freeman, B.A., Hogan, E.L. and Hsu, C.Y. (1989) Polyethylene glycol-conjugated superoxide dismutase and catalase reduce ischemic brain injury. *Am. J. Physiol.*, 256: H589–H593.

Malinski, T. and Taha, Z. (1992) Nitric oxide release from a single cell measured in situ by a porphyrinic-based microsensor. *Nature (Lond.)*, 358: 676–678.

Malinski, T., Bailey, F., Zhang, Z.G. and Chopp, M. (1993) Nitric oxide measured by a porphyrinic microsensor in rat brain after transient middle cerebral artery occlusion. *J. Cereb. Blood Flow Metab.*, 13: 355–358.

Martin, B.L., Wu, D., Jakes, S. and Graves, D.J. (1990) Chemical influences on the specificity of tyrosine phosphorylation. *J. Biol. Chem.*, 265: 7108–7111.

McCord, J.M. and Fridovich, I. (1969) Superoxide dismutase: an enzymic function for erythrocuprein (hemocuprein). *J. Biol. Chem.*, 244: 6049–6055.

Moncada, S., Palmer, R.M.J. and Higgs, E.A. (1991) Nitric oxide: physiology, pathophysiology, and pharmacology. *Pharmacol. Rev.*, 43: 109–142.

Muizelaar, J., Marmarou, A., Young, H., Schoi, S., Wolf, A., Schneider, R. and Kontos, H. (1993) Improving the outcome of severe head injury with the oxygen radical scavenger polyethylene glycol-conjugated superoxide dismutase: a phase II trial. *J. Neurosurg.*, 78: 375–382.

Murphy, S., Minor, R.L., Jr., Wel, G. and Harrison, D.G. (1990) Evidence for an astrocyte-derived vasorelaxing factor with properties similar to nitric oxide. *J. Neurochem.*, 55: 349–351.

Nagafuji, T., Matsui, T., Koide, T. and Asano, T. (1992) Blockade of nitric oxide formation by *Nω*-nitro-L-arginine mitigates ischemic brain edema and subsequent cerebral infarction in rats. *Neurosci. Lett.*, 147: 159–162.

Nakane, M., Schmidt, H., Pollock, J., Forstermann, U. and Murad, F. (1993) Cloned human brain nitric oxide synthase is highly expressed in skeletal muscle. *FEBS Lett.*, 316: 175–180.

Nowicki, J.P., Duval, D., Poignet, H. and Scatton, B. (1991) Nitric oxide mediates neuronal death after focal cerebral ischemia in the mouse. *Eur. J. Pharmacol.*, 204: 339–340.

O'Dell, T.J., Hawkins, R.D., Kandel, E.R. and Arancio, O. (1991) Tests of the roles of two diffusible substances in long-term potentiation: evidence for nitric oxide as a possible early retrograde messenger. *Proc. Natl. Acad. Sci. USA*, 88: 11285–11289.

Omar, B.A. and McCord, J.M. (1990) The cardioprotective effect of Mn-superoxide dismutase is lost at high doses in the postischemic isolate rabbit heart. *Free Rad. Biol. Med.*, 9: 473–478.

Omar, B.A., Gad, N.M., Jordan, M.C., Striplin, S.P., Russell, W.J., Downey, J.M. and McCord, J.M. (1990) Cardioprotection by Cu,Zn-superoxide dismutase is lost at high doses in the reoxygenated heart. *Free Rad. Biol. Med.*, 9: 465–471.

Radi, R., Beckman, J.S., Bush, K.M. and Freeman, B.A. (1991a) Peroxynitrite-induced membrane lipid peroxidation. The cytotoxic potential of superoxide and nitric oxide. *Arch. Biochem. Biophys.*, 288: 481–487.

Radi, R., Beckman, J.S., Bush, K.M. and Freeman, B.A. (1991b) Peroxynitrite-mediated sulfhydryl oxidation: the cytotoxic potential of superoxide and nitric oxide. *J. Biol. Chem.*, 266: 4244–4250.

Radi, R., Cosgrove, T.P., Beckman, J.S. and Freeman, B.A. (1993) Peroxynitrite-induced luminol chemiluminescence. *Biochem. J.*, 290: 51–57.

Shibuki, K. and Okada, D. (1991) Endogenous nitric oxide release required for long-term synaptic depression in the cerebellum. *Nature (Lond.)*, 349: 326–329.

Shulman, E.M. and Madison, D.V. (1991) A requirement for the intercellular messenger nitric oxide in long-term potentiation. *Science*, 254: 1503–1506.

Smith, C.D., Carson, M., Van der Woerd, M., Chen, J., Ischiropoulos, H. and Beckman, J.S. (1992) Crystal structure of peroxynitrite-modified bovine Cu,Zn superoxide dismutase. *Arch. Biochem. Biophys.*, 299: 350–355.

Solodkin, A., Traub, R.J. and Gebhart, G.F. (1992) Unilateral hindpaw inflammation produces a bilateral increase in NADPH-diaphorase hisotchemical staining in the rat lumbar spinal cord. *Neuroscience*, 51: 495- 499.

Stamler, J.S., Jaraki, O., Osborne, J., Simon, D.I., Keaney, J., Vita, J., Singel, D., Valeri, C.R. and Loscalzo, J. (1992a) Nitric oxide circulates in mammalian plasma primarily as an *S*-nitroso adduct of serum albumin. *Proc. Natl. Acad. Sci. USA*, 89: 7674–7677.

Stamler, J.S., Simon, D.I., Osborne, J.A., Mullins, M.E., Jaraki, O., Michel, T., Singel, D.J. and Loscalzo, J. (1992b) *S*-Nitrosylation of proteins with nitric oxide: synthesis and characterization of biologically active compounds. *Proc. Natl. Acad. Sci. USA*, 89: 444–448.

Stamler, J.S., Singel, D.J. and Loscalzo, J. (1992c) Biochemistry of nitric oxide and its redox-activated forms. *Science*, 258: 1898–1902.

Valtschanoff, J.G., Weinberg, R.J. and Rustioni, A. (1992) NADPH diaphorase in the spinal cord of rats. *J. Comp. Neurol.*, 321: 209–222.

Verge, V., Xu, Z., Xu, X.-J. and Wiesenfeld-Hallin, Z. (1992) Marked increase in nitric oxide synthase mRNA in rat dorsal root ganglia after peripheral axotomy: in situ hybridization and functional studies. *Proc. Natl. Acad. Sci. USA*, 89: 11617–11621.

Vincent, S. and Hope, B. (1992) Neurons that say NO. *Trends Neurosci.*, 15: 108–113.

Widmer, H., Kaplan, D., Rabin, S., Beck, K., Hefti, F. and Knusel, B. (1993) Rapid phosphorylation of phospholipase $C\gamma 1$ by brain-derived neurotrophic factor and neurotrophin-3 in cultures of embryonic rat cortical neurons. *J. Neurochem.*, 60: 2111–2123.

Williams, J.H., Errington, M.L., Lynch, M.A. and Bliss, T.V.P. (1989) Arachidonic acid induces a long-term activity-dependent enhancement of synaptic transmission in the hippocampus. *Nature (Lond.)*, 341: 739–742.

Wu, W. (1993) Expression of nitric-oxide synthase (NOS) in injured CNS neurons as shown by NADPH diaphorase histochemistry. *Exp. Neurol.*, 120: 153–159.

Yamamoto, S., Golanov, E.V., Berger, S.B. and Reis, D.J. (1992) Inhibition of nitric oxide synthesis increases focal ischemic infarction in rat. *J. Cereb. Blood Flow Metab.*, 12: 717–726.

Zhu, L., Gunn, C. and Beckman, J.S. (1992) Bactericidal activity of peroxynitrite. *Arch. Biochem. Biophys.*, 298: 452–457.

F.J. Seil (Ed.)
Progress in Brain Research, Vol 103

CHAPTER 32

The role of free radicals in NMDA-dependent neurotoxicity

Laurent Fagni[1], Mireille Lafon-Cazal[1], Gérard Rondouin[2], Olivier Manzoni[1], Mireille Lerner-Natoli[2] and Joel Bockaert[1]

[1]CNRS UPR 9023, CCIPE, Rue de la Cardonille, 34094 Montpellier Cedex 5, and [2]Laboratoire de Médecine Expérimentale CNRS UPR 9008, INSERM U.249, Bd. Henri IV, 34000 Montpellier, France

Introduction

Glutamate is a major neurotransmitter in the brain and stimulates several types of receptors. These have been classified according to their molecular structure and pharmacology (Nakanishi, 1992). One can distinguish ionotropic receptor/channels and G protein coupled receptors. Three subtypes of the former family have been named according to their most selective agonists: kainate, α-amino-3-hydroxy-5-methyl-isoxazole-4-propionate (AMPA) and *N*-methyl-D-aspartate (NMDA) receptors. The NMDA receptor subtype is also distinguishable from the other subtypes by its Ca^{2+} permeability. Prolonged Ca^{2+} entry through this receptor/channel complex can induce neuronal death. A mechanism such as this may play a role in ischemia, brain trauma, amyotrophic lateral sclerosis and possibly Huntington and Alzheimer diseases (for reviews, see Choi, 1988; Meldrum and Garthwaite, 1990; Olney, 1991).

The cellular mechanisms involved in these neuronal disorders are still not fully understood. Stimulation of NMDA receptors in the brain results in free radical production, such as NO, synthesized by a Ca^{2+}/calmodulin-dependent NO synthase (NOS) (Bredt et al., 1991, 1992), and superoxide ion ($O_2^{\cdot -}$), which is produced through a different Ca^{2+}-dependent mechanism (Lafon-Cazal et al., 1993a). Based on in vitro studies, the highly toxic hydroxyl free radical ($^{\cdot}OH$) could then be generated either via a metal-catalysed decomposition of $O_2^{\cdot -}$ and H_2O_2 production (Halliwell and Gutteridge, 1985), or from the metal-independent cleavage of peroxinitrite ion ($ONOO^-$), the resulting product of the interaction of NO and $O_2^{\cdot -}$ (Beckman et al., 1990).

There is some uncertainty as to which of these free radicals plays the major role in NMDA-mediated neurotoxicity. In addressing this issue, we first examined whether such radicals could directly interact with the NMDA receptor itself. We found that NO inhibits NMDA responses and this should reduce neurotoxic effects mediated by excessive NMDA receptor stimulation (Manzoni et al., 1992a). In a second series of experiments, we examined the possible protective role of NO against NMDA-mediated neurotoxicity and epilepsy in freely moving animals (Rondouin et al., 1992, 1993). Finally, we demonstrated in cultured neurons that under NMDA receptor stimulation, $O_2^{\cdot -}$ is formed and that trapping $O_2^{\cdot -}$ with nitrone protects against NMDA-induced neurotoxicity (Lafon-Cazal et al., 1993a,b).

Materials and methods

Primary cultures

Cultures of cerebellar granule cells were prepared from one-week-old mice as previously described (Van-Vliet et al., 1989). Cultures were grown in 25 mM KCl in order to improve cell survival under normal conditions. Cytosine arabinoside (32 μM) was added 48 h after plating to prevent proliferation of nonneuronal cells. This provided cultures enriched in neurons (92% of cells were granule cells, less than 5% were glial cells and 3% were GABAergic interneurons). Granule cells were identified by their small size (5-10 μm) and long neurites. Experiments were performed on 10-day-old cultures either at 37°C for biochemical experiments or at room temperature for fura-2 ratio imaging and patch-clamp measurements.

Intracellular cyclic GMP determinations

For cyclic guanosine monophosphate (cGMP) measurements and all the following experiments, glycine (3 μM) was present and Mg^{2+} ions were omitted in the extracellular medium in order to fully activate NMDA receptors. Intracellular cGMP was determined in the presence of 3-isobutyl-1-methylxanthine (IBMX), a nonselective phosphodiesterase inhibitor, as previously described (Marin et al., 1992).

Fura-2 ratio imaging

Intracellular Ca^{2+} measurements were performed as described elsewhere (Manzoni et al., 1991). Briefly, neurons were loaded with the fluorescent Ca^{2+} chelator, fura-2-AM, and then washed. They were alternatively illuminated with 340 and 380 nm light and the emission was measured at 500 nm on an inverted microscope. Images were taken by a low-light-level camera and digitized. The whole-image treatments were performed using homemade software. Calcium levels were determined on the final image individually for each cell.

Patch-clamp recordings

For patch-clamp recordings, the culture medium was replaced by a solution containing 0.3 μM tetrodotoxin in order to block Na^+ currents. The recording pipette solution contained 140 mM CsCl in order to block K^+ currents. These conditions were ideal to record NMDA currents in both whole-cell and outside-out configurations. Drugs were applied using a rapid perfusion system that allowed us to change the environment of the recorded cell in less than 30 msec (for details see Fagni et al., 1991). NMDA current analyses were performed with the patch-clamp program of Axon Instruments.

Electron paramagnetic resonance experiments

Neurons were incubated in the presence of 5,5-dimethyl pyrroline-1-oxide (DMPO, 100 mM) and diethylenetriaminepentaacetic acid (DTPA, 0.5 mM), an iron-chelating agent. Following the exposure period, the incubation medium was immediately transferred into the cavity of an electron paramagnetic resonance (EPR) spectrometer. Spectra were acquired within 45 sec at 25°C. We verified that no EPR signal was obtained when the same compounds were added to the incubation medium in the absence of cells or with prekilled neurons.

Neurotoxicity experiments

Cells were incubated for 30 min at 37°C in physiological solution containing the substances to be tested. They were then washed and incubated again in the same original culture medium at 37°C for 24 h. The remaining living cells were surveyed by phase-contrast microscopy, then used for the fluorescein diacetate (FDA) method (Didier et al., 1990). The percentage of cell survival versus control was calculated.

In vivo experiments

In vivo experiments were performed in adult rats. Animals were chronically treated with the NOS inhibitor, L-N^{G}-nitroarginine (NOArg), injected intraperitoneally (25 mg/kg), while controls received vehicle. We verified that chronic treatment with NOArg completely inhibited NO synthesis. NMDA (100 μM) and nitroprusside (SNP, 10 μM), an NO donor, both stimulated cGMP formation in hippocampal slices of control rats. By contrast, in the NOArg-treated rats, only SNP stimulated cGMP formation, indicating that NO synthase but not guanylate cyclase activity was blocked following chronic treatment with NOArg (Rondouin et al., 1992).

To study the effect of NO depletion on the development of limbic epilepsy, a first group of rats chronically treated with NOS inhibitors were kindled. The kindling process consisted of electrical train stimulations delivered twice daily, over a period of 10 days, through a deep electrode positioned in the right amygdala with the minimal intensity required to trigger an electroencephalographically (EEG) recorded afterdischarge (AD threshold; Rondouin et al., 1992). At the end of the kindling session, when seizures were generalized, the NOArg treatment was stopped and replaced by a 4-day treatment with saline in order to examine a possible effect on the seizures of discontinuing treatment. The control rats received a 4-day treatment of NOS inhibitors in order to test the effect of NO depletion on these generalized seizures. Results were analyzed by comparing initial AD threshold, behavioral scores and AD duration in control and treated groups.

In a second series of experiments, at the end of the NOS inhibitor treatment, rats received 20 nmoles NMDA in the hippocampus (Lerner-Natoli et al., 1992). One week later the rats were killed and hippocampal slices were prepared for histological staining.

The last experiment was carried out to study the effects of chronic treatment with NOS inhibitor on both the electroclinical patterns and the histopathological consequences of limbic status epilepticus produced by an intraamygdala injection of 2.5 nmoles of kainic acid (Rondouin et al., 1993).

Results and discussion

Nitric oxide inhibits NMDA responses

The 3-morpholinosydnonimine (SIN-1) molecule spontaneously decomposes into NO and SIN-1C (Böhme et al., 1984). We found that SIN-1 can continuously produce a significant amount of NO to stimulate guanylate cyclase for at least 6 to 8 h (Fig. 1A). This NO donor was particularly interesting for the study of NMDA receptors because its breakdown product, SIN-1C, was absolutely inactive on this receptor. This was not the case for other NO donors such as nitroprusside (Manzoni et al., 1992b) or nitrosocysteine (unpublished data).

Both the increase in intracellular Ca^{2+} concentration measured with fura-2 by ratio imaging and the NMDA currents measured in the whole-cell configuration of the patch-clamp technique were blocked by SIN-1. The threshold concentration for these SIN-1 effects was around 1 μM, and 50% and 85% inhibition of NMDA responses was obtained at concentrations of 1 and 10 mM, respectively. NMDA responses were restored after washout of SIN-1. We showed that these inhibitory effects of SIN-1 were suppressed by hemoglobin (10 μM), a potent NO chelator, suggesting that the action of the drug was effectively mediated by NO (Manzoni et al., 1992a). AMPA responses in the same neurons were not affected by NO.

Since cultured cerebellar granule cells (Garthwaite, 1991) and striatal neurons (Marin et al., 1992) have been shown to produce NO upon stimulation of NMDA receptors, we tested whether endogenous production of NO could interfere with the NMDA receptor activity itself by incubating these cultured neurons in the presence of hemoglobin. This increased both NMDA-evoked elevation of intracellular Ca^{2+} and whole-cell NMDA currents (Manzoni et al., 1992a). Treatment of the neurons with NOArg, an inhibitor of NOS, potentiated NMDA responses. Conversely, treatment with L-arginine inhibited NMDA responses (Manzoni and Bockaert,

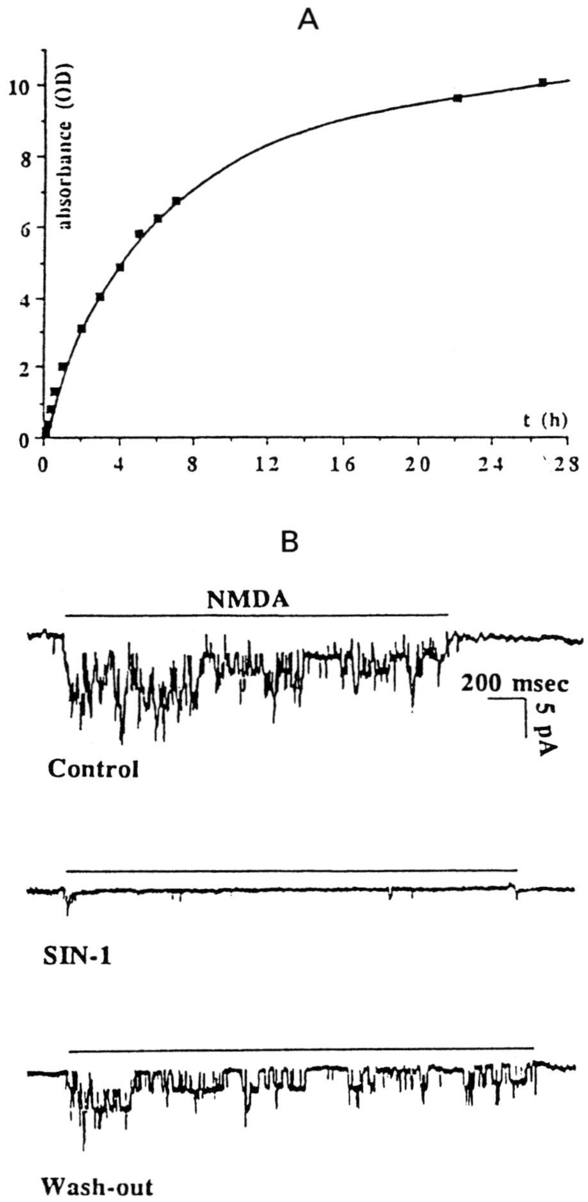

Fig. 1. SIN-1-generated NO (A) and blockade of NMDA receptors (B). (A) Kinetics of NO production by SIN-1. The kinetics of NO production (NO, NO_2 and NO_3 accumulation) by SIN-1 was studied using the method described by Ignarro et al. (1987). Measurements were performed with a physiological solution (pH 7.4) of 1 mM SIN-1. The exponential relation that we obtained shows that SIN-1 produced NO with a half-maximal saturation at 4 h and a plateau after 16 h. (B) Unitary NMDA currents recorded in an outside-out patch. NMDA was applied at a concentration of 100 μM and SIN-1 at a concentration of 1 mM. Holding potential was -60 mV. Note the reversible blockade of NMDA currents by the NO donor, SIN- 1.

1993). Altogether, these experiments show that endogenous NO tonically blocks NMDA receptors.

The mode of action of NO on the NMDA receptor is still controversial. Lipton and colleagues (Lei et al., 1992) have recently proposed that NO blocks the NMDA receptor by nitrosylation of putative sulfhydryl residues of the so-called redox modulatory site of this receptor complex (Aizenman et al., 1989). This hypothesis was mainly based on the observation that alkylation of the sulfhydryl groups suppressed the inhibition of the receptor by NO in cortical neurons (Lei et al., 1992). However, in other preparations (Hoyt et al., 1992), including our cultured cerebellar granule cells (unpublished data), alkylation of the redox modulatory receptor site did not affect NO-induced inhibition of NMDA responses. Therefore this model cannot be taken as a general rule for the action of NO in all preparations.

Because NO activates guanylate cyclase, we tested whether NO blocked NMDA receptors through cGMP production. Application of dibutyryl-cGMP, a cGMP analog that diffuses into cells, in the presence of 1 mM isobutyl methyl xanthine (IBMX), an inhibitor of phosphodiesterases, only partially inhibited the NMDA-induced intracellular Ca^{2+} rise. Addition of 1 mM cGMP in the presence of IBMX in the whole-cell recording pipette solution did not block NMDA currents. In the same cell, extracellular application of SIN-1 still inhibited NMDA currents and in the same proportion as the absence of intracellular cGMP. This clearly indicated that the inhibitory effects of SIN-1 did not require cGMP production (Manzoni et al., 1992a).

We also examined whether other second messengers were involved in the SIN-1-induced blockade of NMDA receptors. This was investigated in excised patches (outside-out configuration) where no more intracellular messenger is left in the patch. Application of SIN-1 on outside-out patches decreased the opening probability of NMDA channels, indicating a direct action of NO on the receptor complex (Fig. 1B). This effect did not result from alteration of the NMDA binding site since binding of ^{3}H-CGS 19755, an NMDA receptor ligand, was not significantly displaced by SIN-1 (Manzoni et al., 1992a). The most likely hypothesis was that NO blocked NMDA receptors by altering the gating process of the receptor/channel complex. Specific studies are in progress in our laboratory to elucidate the exact mechanisms involved in this receptor blockade by NO in cultured cerebellar granule cells.

SIN-1 is thought to produce $O_2^{\cdot -}$, in parallel to NO (Hogg et al., 1992). Therefore, the question was raised as to whether $O_2^{\cdot -}$ rather than NO could mediate the observed inhibitory effects of SIN-1 on NMDA responses. This hypothesis was unlikely since SOD, which transforms $O_2^{\cdot -}$ into H_2O_2, did not modify the inhibitory action of SIN-1. We also tested the effects of H_2O_2 itself. This drug rather facilitated NMDA responses. In view of these results, we will conclude that NO, rather than other free radicals, blocks NMDA receptors. This is particularly interesting if we consider the fact that the endogenous neuronal production of NO results mainly from activation of NMDA receptors themselves. Thus, neurons could regulate their own NMDA activity and consequently their own NO production via this feedback inhibitory process (Fig. 2). Of course, since NO is a diffusible molecule, this model would also apply for a paracrine action of NO on neighboring cells.

Protective effect of endogenous NO against NMDA-mediated neurological disorders

Since NO blocks NMDA receptors, we examined whether this molecule could protect against neurological disorders resulting from overstimulation of NMDA receptors, as in epilepsy. Kindling is an experimental model of limbic epilepsy that can be overcome by treating animals with NMDA receptor antagonists (McNamara et al., 1990). Briefly, kindled seizures

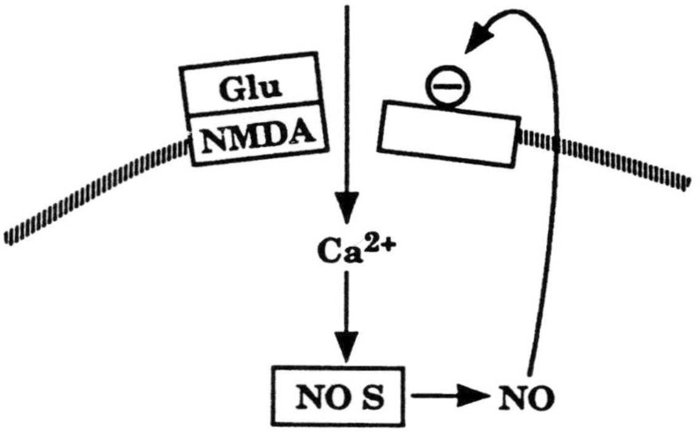

Fig. 2. Feedback inhibition of NMDA receptors by NO. NOS, NO synthase.

were induced in rats by applying repetitive stimulations as described in the methods section. The kindling phenomenon was quantified by measuring the AD threshold and duration in the amygdala and the severity of behavioral seizures in animals chronically treated with NOArg inhibitors, as described. We found that chronic NOArg treatment did not significantly modify the AD threshold, while ADs and progression of seizure severity developed more rapidly until the 10th day. After this period of time, kindling developed as in untreated rats. On the other hand, the NOArg treatment did not modify the severity of seizures in previously kindled rats. Since NO blocks NMDA receptors, we will tentatively conclude that the kindling rate increase might result from an enhanced neuronal excitability that can be attributed to the blockade of a tonic inhibition of NMDA receptors mediated by endogenous NO (Rondouin et al., 1992).

Finally, in the case of severe long-lasting seizures, i.e., status epilepticus, the electrical patterns recorded on EEG during induction of status epilepticus were not different in control and NOArg-treated animals. However, after 2–4 h of status epilepticus evolution, the electrical and behavioral signs were dramatically worsened in the treated animals, most of them dying during seizures. Histological observations showed that seizure-related damage was considerably increased in limbic structures, particularly in hippocampus (Fig. 3A) (Rondouin et al., 1993). Here again, we propose that the complete suppression of NO formation in the brain relieved a retrograde tonic inhibition of NMDA receptors and facilitated development of generalized seizures and amino acid mediated neurodegeneration.

In these in vivo experiments, specific measurements showed that NOArg treatment did not dramatically alter systolic arterial pressure (126.8 $\pm$ 3.2 mmHg before the treatment and 143.2 $\pm$ 7.7 mmHg 2 h before status epilepticus induction; $n = 8$). Nevertheless, the NOArg treatment may

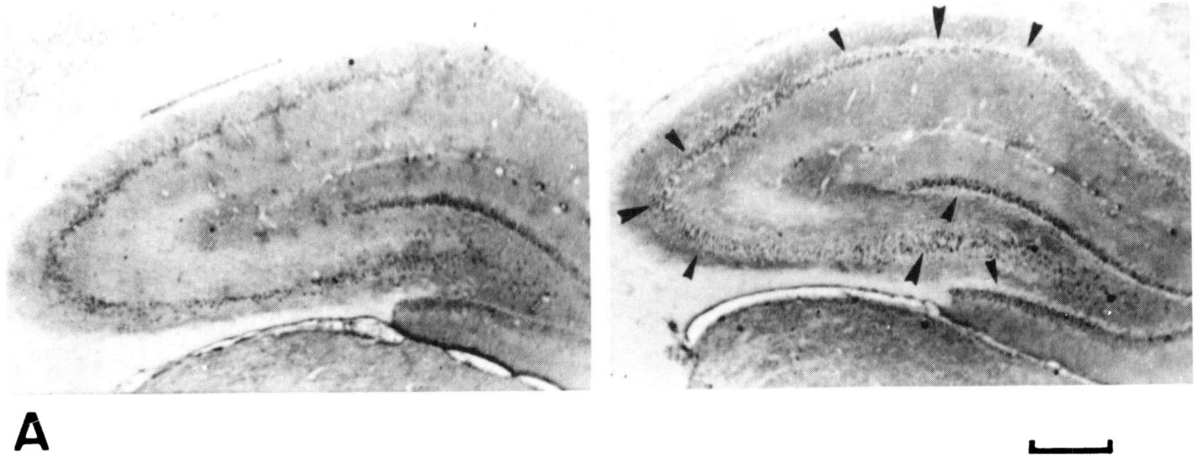

A

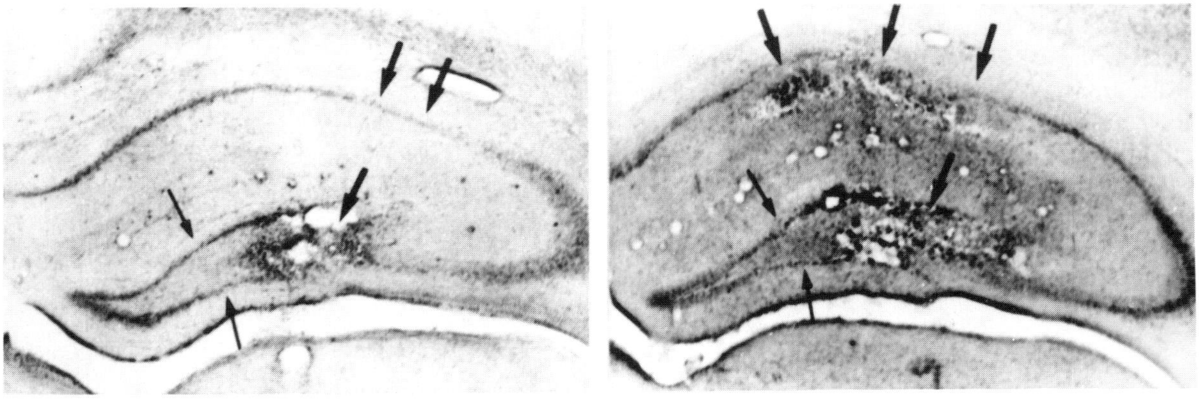

B

Fig. 3. In vivo excitotoxicity. (A) Hippocampal coronal sections (50 μm) stained with hemalum-eosine showing ongoing neurodegeneration after 4 h of status epilepticus in rats pretreated either with saline (left) or NOArg (right) (bar = 500 μm). Note the prominence of neuronal damage in the rat treated with NOArg (25 mg/kg twice daily for 4 days) compared to the control. Arrowheads indicate intense pycnosis and edema in CA1, CA3 and CA4 hippocampal areas and in the infragranular zone of the dentate gyrus. (B) Coronal sections (50 μm) of hippocampus, stained with cresyl violet, one week after local injection of 20 nM of NMDA in rats treated either with saline (left) or with NOArg (right) (bar = 500 μm). Both animals show neuronal loss and surrounding gliosis in CA1 and CA4 areas and dentate gyrus (arrows), indicating that the NOArg treatment did not protect hippocampal or granular neurons against NMDA toxicity.

have altered vascular tone in cerebral microvessels and such a change may have contributed to worsen neuronal injuries. Specific experiments are needed to verify this hypothesis.

The role of free radicals in NMDA-mediated neurotoxicity

There is a body of evidence suggesting that NOS activity plays a major role in glutamate-mediated neurotoxicity (Dawson et al., 1991; Nowicki et al., 1991; Moncada et al., 1992; but see Lipton et al., 1993). However, this hypothesis does not fit well with our observations of a blockade of NMDA-mediated responses (including neuronal injuries) by NO. In order to examine whether endogenous production of NO could be responsible for NMDA neurotoxicity, we performed in vivo experiments, originally designed to search for a protective effect of NOS inhibitors.

Rats were treated for 4 days with NOArg before intrahippocampal injection of NMDA (20 nmoles). Surprisingly, treated rats, like control rats, displayed severe tonic-clonic seizures. Histological observations indicated extensive lesions in all hippocampal regions (Fig. 3B) (Rondouin et al., 1993). These results do not confirm the current hypothesis of an involvement of NO in NMDA-mediated toxicity, at least in hippocampal neurons in vivo, and question the neuroprotective properties of NOS inhibitors. On the other hand, they are consistent with a blockade of NMDA receptors by endogenous NO and NMDA-mediated neurological disorders eventually induced by overproduction of NO.

In view of these results, we investigated which could be the key messenger in NMDA-induced neurotoxicity. An obvious hypothesis was that other free radicals, different from NO, generated by NMDA-induced neuronal activity, could mediate deleterious cellular effects and neuronal death. We addressed this issue on cultured cerebellar granule neurons using biochemical and EPR techniques. In these experiments, both NMDA and SIN-1 (both at 100 μM) stimulated NO-mediated cGMP accumulation in cerebellar neurons, SIN-1 being 10-times more potent than NMDA (Fig. 4A). Nevertheless only NMDA was neurotoxic (50% neurodegeneration, Fig. 4B). At 100 μM, NOArg completely blocked NMDA-induced cGMP production but only slightly reduced (10%) NMDA-mediated neuronal death. This series of experiments further suggested that NO was not the messenger for the neurotoxic effects of NMDA in neurons (Lafon-Cazal et al., 1993b).

The EPR technique allows direct detection of paramagnetic species such as free radicals. Because of the too short lifetime of such molecules, spin traps were used to stabilize and detect these species. This was achieved with the nitrone, DMPO, which yields the more stable paramagnetic nitroxide free radicals, DMPO-OOH and DMPO-OH, when it combines with $O_2^{\cdot -}$ and $^{\cdot}OH$, respectively (Finkelstein et al., 1980). A strong EPR signal was detected 15 to 30 min consecutive to NMDA receptor stimulation, consisting of DMPO-OOH as the major species. This suggested that $O_2^{\cdot -}$ was generated by the brief NMDA receptor stimulation. This was confirmed by suppression of the DMPO-OOH signal in the presence of superoxide dismutase (SOD; which converts $O_2^{\cdot -}$ into H_2O_2) (Lafon-Cazal et al., 1993a,b). One can conclude from these observations that NMDA receptor stimulation mainly leads to formation of $O_2^{\cdot -}$ (Lafon-Cazal et al., 1993b).

Exogenous production of $O_2^{\cdot -}$ through decomposition of xanthine-xanthine oxidase (XA-XO) produced an EPR signal similar to that seen with NMDA receptor stimulation. XA-XO induced neuronal death similar to that mediated by NMDA, suggesting that neuronal degeneration was mediated by $O_2^{\cdot -}$ or a related species. Interestingly, neurotoxicity induced by XA-XO, but not that induced by NMDA, was suppressed in the presence of SOD. Conversely, the more lipophilic compound, DMPO, greatly reduced both XA-XO- and NMDA-induced neurotoxicity (Lafon- Cazal et al., 1993b). These observations indicated that intracellularly generated $O_2^{\cdot -}$ was likely to initiate neurotoxic events.

Based on in vitro experiments, peroxynitrite ions ($ONOO^-$) have been proposed to be formed

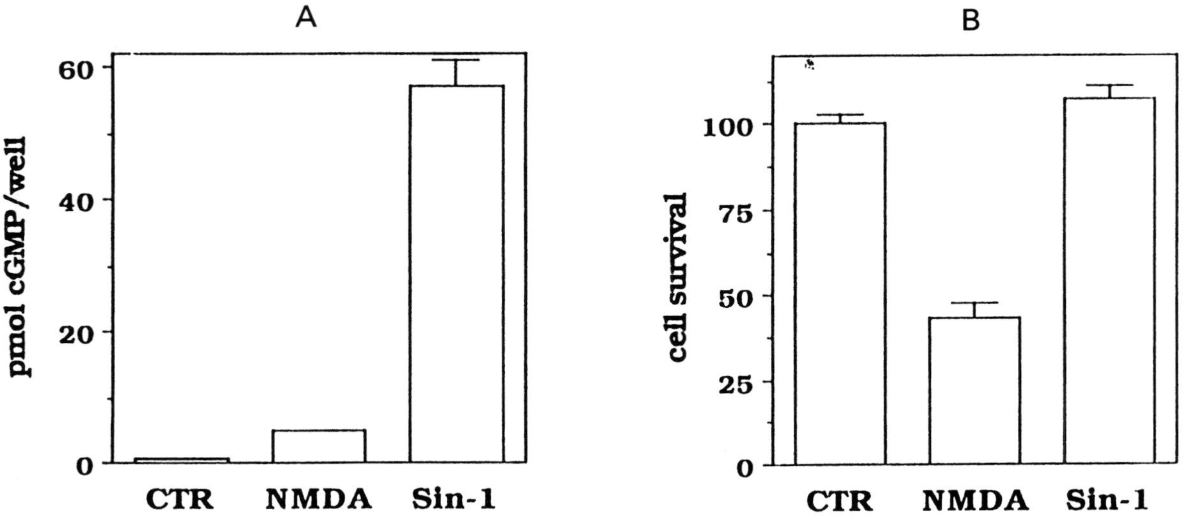

Fig. 4. Formation of NO/cGMP (A) and neurotoxicity (B) induced by the NOS activator, NMDA (0.1 mM) and the NO donor SIN-1 (0.1 mM) in cerebellar granule neurons maintained for 10 days in culture. (A) The production of cGMP was evaluated by radioimmunoassay after a 5 min incubation of the neurons in the presence of each drug and IBMX (1 mM). (B) Cell survival was measured 24 h after a 30 min incubation of the neurons in the presence of each drug. Data are expressed as mean ± SEM of tripiclate measurements performed in at least three different experiments.

when NO combines with $O_2^{\cdot-}$. Once formed, $ONOO^-$ decomposes into $^{\cdot}OH$ and $NO_2^{\cdot}$ (Beckman et al., 1990; Hogg et al., 1992; Lowenstein and Snyder, 1992). It has been claimed that $ONOO^-$ and $^{\cdot}OH$ could be more neurotoxic than NO itself by initiating lipid peroxidation and sulfhydryl oxidation (Radi et al., 1991a,b). According to this hypothesis, one would predict that combination of $O_2^{\cdot-}$ with NO-generating compounds would produce a substantial amount of $ONOO^-$, which then would induce neuronal death. This was not the case in our preparation; the neurotoxicity induced by XA-XO was not potentiated by 300 μM SIN-1 (Lafon-Cazal et al., 1993b). These observations imply that $ONOO^-$ was not a major neurotoxic compound in cerebellar granule cells.

As NMDA stimulates arachidonic acid in cultured neurons (Dumuis et al., 1988), arachidonic acid was tested and also found to generate DMPO-OOH (Lafon-Cazal et al., 1993a). Moreover the NMDA-induced signal was suppressed in the presence of mepacrine, a phospholipase A_2 (an arachidonic acid releasing enzyme) inhibitor. This result suggested that arachidonic acid could be one of the sources of $O_2^{\cdot-}$ generated by NMDA receptor stimulation (Fig. 5).

Conclusion

In cerebellar granule cells, endogenous production of NO tonically blocks NMDA receptors.

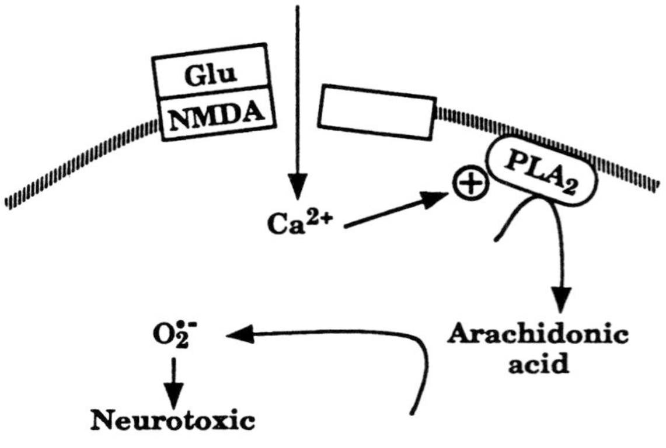

Fig. 5. NMDA-mediated neurotoxicity would depend upon activation of phospholipase A_2 (PLA_2) and $O_2^{\cdot-}$ production.

Superoxide ions seem to be more efficient than NO at inducing NMDA neurotoxicity. Under our experimental conditions, blocking NO formation did not prevent glutamate neurotoxicity in vitro or vivo. On the contrary, complete depletion of NO synthesis increased the deleterious action of NMDA on neurons, probably by suppressing the negative feedback exerted by NO on NMDA receptors.

In vitro studies showed that purified nitric oxide synthase can produce oxygenated free radicals such as $O_2^{\cdot -}$ when L-arginine concentrations are low (Heinzel et al., 1992; Pou et al., 1992). However, this was not the case under our experimental conditions, as indicated by the production of NO and cGMP upon NMDA receptor stimulation, because neurons are usually not depleted in L-arginine. Moreover, under such conditions NOArg did not suppress NMDA-induced $O_2^{\cdot -}$ production. Activation of phospholipase A_2 induced by NMDA receptor stimulation (Dumuis et al., 1988) may be an important although not exclusive step in the generation of oxygen radicals and neuronal death.

Acknowledgements

We would like thank Angie Turner-Madeuf and Jean-Marie Michel for their technical assistance. SIN-1 was generously provided by Hoechst Laboratories, Paris, France.

References

Aizenman, E., Lipton, S.A. and Loring, R.H. (1989) Selective modulation of NMDA responses by reduction and oxidation. *Neuron*, 2: 1257–1263.

Beckman, J.S., Beckman, T.W., Chen, J., Marshall, P.A. and Freeman, B.A. (1990) Apparent hydroxyl radical production by peroxinitrite: implications for endothelial injury from nitric oxide and superoxide. *Proc. Natl. Acad. Sci. USA*, 87: 1620–1624.

Böhme, E., Grossmann, G., Herz, J., Mülsch, A., Spies, C. and Günter, S. (1984) Regulation of cyclic GMP formation by soluble guanylate cyclase: stimulation by NO-containing compounds. In: P. Greengard (Ed.), *Advances in Cyclic Nucleotide and Protein Phosphorylation Research*, Vol. 17, Raven Press, New York, pp. 259–267.

Bredt, D.S., Ferris, C.D. and Snyder, S.H. (1992) Nitric oxide synthase regulatory sites. *J. Biol. Chem.*, 267: 10976–10981.

Bredt, D.S., Hwang, P.H., Glatt, C., Lowenstein, C., Reed, R.R. and Snyder, S.H. (1991) Cloned and expressed nitric oxide synthase structurally resembles cytochrome P-450 reductase. *Nature (Lond.)*, 352: 714–718.

Choi, D.W. (1988) Calcium-mediated neurotoxicity: relationship to specific channel types and role in ischemic damage. *Trends Neurosci.*, 11: 465–468.

Dawson, V.L., Dawson, T.M., London, E.D., Bredt, D.S. and Snyder, S.H. (1991) Nitric oxide mediates glutamate neurotoxicity in primary cortical culture. *Proc. Natl. Acad. Sci. USA*, 88: 6368–6371.

Didier, M., Heaulme, M., Soubrié, P., Bockaert, J. and Pin, J.-P. (1990) Rapid, sensitive and simple method for the quantification of both neurotoxic and neurotrophic effects of NMDA on cultured cerebellar granule cells. *J. Neurosci. Res.*, 27: 25–35.

Dumuis, A., Sebben, M., Haynes, L., Pin, J.P. and Bockaert, J. (1988) NMDA receptors activate the arachidonic acid cascade system in striatal neurons. *Nature (Lond.)*, 336: 68–70.

Fagni, L., Bossu, J.-L. and Bockaert, J. (1991) Activation of a large-conductance Ca^{2+}-dependent K^+-channel by stimulation of glutamate phosphoinositide-coupled receptors in cultured cerebellar granule cells. *Eur. J. Neurosci.*, 3: 778–789.

Finkelstein, E., Rosen, G.M. and Rauckman, E.J. (1980) Spin trapping of superoxide and hydroxyl radical: pratical aspects. *Arch. Biochem. Biophys.*, 200: 1–16.

Garthwaite, J. (1991) Glutamate, nitric oxide and cell-cell signalling in the nervous system. *Trends Neurosci.*, 14: 60–67.

Halliwell, B. and Gutteridge, J.M.C. (1985) Oxygen radicals and the nervous system. *Trends Neurosci.*, 8: 22–26.

Heinzel, B., John, M., Klatt, P., Böhme, E. and Mayer, B. (1992) Ca^{2+}/calmodulin-dependent formation of hydrogen peroxide by brain nitric oxide synthase. *Biochem. J.*, 281: 627–630.

Hogg, N., Darley-Usmar, V.M., Wilson, M.T. and Moncada, S. (1992) Production of hydroxyl radicals from the simultaneous generation of superoxide and nitric oxide. *Biochem. J.*, 281: 419–424.

Hoyt, K.R., Tang, L.-H., Aizenman, E. and Reynolds, I.J. (1992) Nitric oxide modulates NMDA-induced increases in intracellular Ca^{2+} in cultured rat forebrain neurons. *Brain Res.*, 592: 310–316.

Ignarro, L.J., Buga, G.M., Wood, K.S., Byrns, R.E. and Chaudhuri, G. (1987) EDRF produced and released from artery and vein is nitric oxide. *Proc. Natl. Acad. Sci. USA*, 84: 9265–9669.

Lafon-Cazal, M., Pietri, S., Culcasi, M. and Bockaert, J. (1993a) NMDA-dependent superoxide production and neurotoxicity. *Nature (Lond.)*, 364: 535–537.

Lafon-Cazal, M., Culcasi, M., Gaven, F., Pietri, S. and Bockaert, J. (1993b) Nitric oxide, superoxide and peroxinitrite: putative mediators of NMDA-induced cell death in cerebellar granule cells. *Neuropharmacology*, 32: 1259–1266.

Lei, S.Z., Pan, Z.-H., Aggarwal, S.K., Chen, H.-S.V., Hartman, J., Sucher, N.J. and Lipton, S.A. (1992) Effect of nitric oxide production on the redox modulatory site of the NMDA receptor-channel complex. *Neuron*, 8: 1087–1099.

Lerner-Natoli, M., Rondouin, G., deBock, F. and Bockaert, J. (1992) Chronic NO synthase inhibition fails to protect hippocampal neurones against NMDA toxicity. *NeuroReport*, 3: 1109–1112.

Lipton, S.A., Choi, Y.-B., Pan, Z.-H., Lei, S.Z., Chen, H.-S.V., Sucher, N.J., Loscalzo, J., Singel, D.J. and Stamler, J.S. (1993) A redox-based mechanism for the neuroprotective and neurodegenerative effects of nitric oxide and related nitroso-compounds. *Nature (Lond.)*, 364: 626–632.

Lowenstein, C.J. and Snyder, S.H. (1992) Nitric oxide, a novel biological messenger. *Cell*, 70: 705–707.

Manzoni, O. and Bockaert, J. (1993) Nitric oxide synthase activity endogenously modulates NMDA receptors. *J. Neurochem.*, 61: 368–370.

Manzoni, O.J.J., Poulat, F., Do, E., Sahuquet, A., Sassetti, I., Bockaert, J. and Sladeczek, F.A.J. (1991) Pharmacological characterization of the quisqualate receptor coupled to phospholipase C (Qp) in striatal neurons. *Eur. J. Pharmacol. (Mol. Pharmacol. Sec.)*, 207: 231–241.

Manzoni, O., Prézeau, L., Marin, P., Deshager, S., Bockaert, J. and Fagni, L. (1992a) Nitric oxide induced blockade of NMDA receptors. *Neuron*, 8: 653–662.

Manzoni, O., Prezeau, L., Desagher, S., Sahuquet, A., Sladeczek, F., Bockaert, J. and Fagni, L. (1992b) Sodium nitroprusside blocks NMDA receptors via formation of ferrocyanide ions. *NeuroReport*, 3: 77–80.

Marin, P., Lafon-Cazal, M. and Bockaert, J. (1992) A nitric oxide-synthase activity selectively stimulated by NMDA receptors via protein kinase C activation in mouse striatal neurons. *Eur. J. Neurosci.*, 4: 425–432.

McNamara, J.O., Bonhaus, D.W., Nadler, J.V. and Yeh, G.C. (1990) *N*-Methyl-D-aspartate receptors and the kindling model. In: J. Wada (Ed.), *Kindling*, Vol. 4, Plenum Press, New York, pp. 197–208.

Meldrum, B. and Garthwaite, J. (1990) Excitatory amino acid neurotoxicity and neurodegenerative disease. *Trends Pharmacol. Sci.*, 11: 379–387.

Moncada, C., Lekieffre, D., Arvin, B. and Meldrum, B. (1992) Effect of NO synthase inhibition on NMDA- and ischemia-induced hippocampal lesions. *NeuroReport*, 3: 530–532.

Nakanishi, S. (1992) Molecular diversity of glutamate receptors and implications for brain function. *Science*, 258: 597–603.

Nowicki, J.P., Duval, D., Poignet, A. and Scatton, B. (1991) Nitric oxide mediates neuronal death after focal cerebral ischemia in the mouse. *Eur. J. Pharmacol.*, 204: 339.

Olney, J.W. (1991) Excitotoxicity and neuropsychiatric disorders. In: P. Ascher, D.W. Choi and Y. Christen (Eds.), *Glutamate, Cell Death and Memory*, Springer-Verlag, New York, pp. 77–101.

Pou, S., Pou, W.S., Bredt, D.S., Snyder, S.H. and Rosen, G.M. (1992) Generation of superoxide by purified brain nitric oxide synthase. *J. Biol. Chem.*, 267: 24173–24176.

Radi, R., Beckman, J.S., Bush, K.M. and Freeman, B.A. (1991a) Peroxinitrite oxidation of sulfhydryls. The cytotoxic potential of superoxide and nitric oxide. *J. Biol. Chem.*, 266: 4244–4250.

Radi, R., Beckman, J.S., Bush, K.M. and Freeman, B.A. (1991b) Peroxinitrite-induced membrane lipid peroxidation. The cytotoxic potential of superoxide and nitric oxide. *Arch. Biochem. Biophys.*, 288: 481–487.

Rondouin, G., Lerner-Natoli, M., Manzoni, O., Lafon-Cazal, M. and Bockaert, J. (1992) A nitric oxide (NO) synthase inhibitor accelerates amygdala kindling. *NeuroReport*, 3: 805–808.

Rondouin, G., Bockaert, J. and Lerner-Natoli, M. (1993) L-Nitroarginine, an inhibitor of NO synthase, dramatically worsens limbic epilepsy in rats. *NeuroReport*, 4: 1187–1190.

Van-Vliet, B.J., Sebben, M., Dumuis, A., Gabrion, J., Bockaert, J. and Pin, J.-P. (1989) Endogenous amino acid release from cultured cerebellar neuronal cells: effect of tetanus toxin on glutamate release. *J. Neurochem.*, 52: 1229–1239.

F.J. Seil (Ed.)
Progress in Brain Research, Vol 103

CHAPTER 33

Regulation by neuroprotective factors of NMDA receptor mediated nitric oxide synthesis in the brain and retina

Akinori Akaike[1], Yutaka Tamura[2], Kaori Terada[2] and Noritaka Nakata[2]

[1]*Department of Pharmacology, Faculty of Pharmaceutical Sciences, Kyoto University, Kyoto 606-01, Japan*
[2]*Department of Neuropharmacology, Faculty of Pharmacy and Pharmaceutical Sciences, Fukuyama University, Fukuyama 729-02, Japan*

Introduction

Excitatory amino acids (EAAs) such as glutamate are acknowledged as the primary neurotransmitters that mediate synaptic excitation in the vertebrate central nervous system (CNS). Glutamate satisfies the main criteria for classification as a neurotransmitter: presynaptic localization; specific release by physiological stimuli; identical action to the endogenous transmitter, including response to antagonists; and the existence of mechanisms to terminate transmitter action rapidly (Gasic and Hollmann, 1992). In addition to its role in neurotransmission, glutamate can also act as a neurotoxin (Choi et al., 1987; Bresnick, 1989). Glutamate has been postulated to play an important role in the pathogenesis of the neuronal cell loss which is associated with several neurological disease states in the CNS. Thus, glutamate has a dual action on CNS neurons, acting as an excitatory neurotransmitter at physiological concentrations and as a neurotoxic substance when it is present in excess.

Glutamate receptors are divided into two major subgroups: ionotropic receptors and metabotropic receptors. On pharmacological and physiological grounds, ionotropic receptors have been grouped into two subtypes: NMDA and non-NMDA receptors. Non-NMDA receptors are further grouped into subgroups such as KA (kainate) and AMPA (α-amino-3-hydroxy-5-methyl-4-isoxazole propionate) receptors, formerly known as quisqualate receptors. The NMDA receptor has been postulated to be the predominant route of glutamate neurotoxicity in several regions in the CNS, including the cerebral cortex and the retina. NMDA receptor mediated glutamate cytotoxicity involves Ca^{2+} influx into cells via ligand gated ion channels in the NMDA receptors. Recent studies on cultured cortical neurons have suggested that the radical form of nitric oxide (NO) mediates the NMDA receptor mediated neurotoxicity of glutamate (Dawson et al., 1991; Tamura et al., 1992; Lipton et al., 1993). NO, apparently identical to the endothelium-derived relaxing factor in blood vessels, is also formed in brain tissues (Garthwaite et al., 1988; Garthwaite, 1991). Immunocytochemical studies demonstrated the presence of constitutive NO synthase in the brain, including the cerebral cortex (Bredt et al., 1990). NMDA receptor activation causes Ca^{2+} influx, after which cytosolic Ca^{2+}, working in conjunction with calmodulin, turns on the synthesis of NO. As NO gas easily permeates the cell membrane, it diffuses to adjacent cells, resulting in the appropriate physiological responses and/or glutamate-related cell death. This suggests that NO is a key substance in NMDA receptor mediated glutamate neurotoxicity in the CNS, although this evidence does not exclude the possible involvement of other mediators in glutamate-induced neurotoxicity.

The actions of glutamate as an excitatory neurotransmitter are regulated by many other endogenous substances, such as inhibitory neurotransmitters and neuromodulators. Suppression of the control by those substances on glutamate-induced excitation causes severe dysfunction of CNS activity. For example, convulsive drugs, which block the inhibitory actions of either GABA or glycine, are known to induce clonic and tonic convulsions, respectively. Therefore, excitatory actions of glutamate and other EAAs should receive tonic regulation by inhibitory neurotransmitters and neuromodulators to maintain normal neuronal activities in the CNS. Meanwhile, the cytotoxic effects of EAAs, including glutamate, have a crucial role in the pathogenesis of neuronal degeneration. This suggests that neurons in the CNS are exposed to both the excitatory and cytotoxic effects of glutamate. Then, it is possible that the neurotoxic action of glutamate is also regulated by other endogenous substances in physiological and/or pathological conditions. In other words, certain neurotransmitters, neuromodulators or other endogenous substances may possess a neuroprotective action against EAA cytotoxicity to promote cell survival in the CNS.

On the basis of the above mentioned hypothesis, we have used the term 'neuroprotective factor' for endogenous substances having protective actions against glutamate neurotoxicity. We have previously found, using primary cultures, that cholecystokinin (CCK) and dopamine prevented glutamate cytotoxicity in the cerebral cortex and the retina, respectively (Tamura et al., 1992; Kashii et al., 1994). The evidence suggests that the mechanisms of neuroprotective actions of CCK and dopamine are linked with NO formation triggered by NMDA receptors. We have postulated that these substances are a putative neuroprotective factor against glutamate cytotoxicity in the corresponding regions in the CNS. Therefore, this study focuses primarily on the neuroprotective actions of CCK and dopamine against cytotoxicity mediated by glutamate and NO.

CCK-induced protection of cortical neurons

Glutamate cytotoxicity in cultured cortical neurons

Brief exposure to glutamate produces delayed cell death in cultured cortical neurons over the next few hours (Choi, 1987; Choi et al., 1987). Because NMDA antagonists protect cells from glutamate cytotoxicity in cortical cultures, NMDA receptors are generally accepted to play crucial roles in glutamate-induced cytotoxicity in cortical neurons (Hartley and Choi, 1989). Therefore, we have examined the neurotoxic effects of glutamate on cultured cortical neurons.

Dissociated murine cortical cell cultures were prepared following the method described by Dichter (1978), with some modification. Single cells mechanically dissociated from whole cerebral cortex of fetal rats (16–18 days gestation) were maintained for 10–14 days (Akaike et al., 1991). Neurotoxicity induced by EAAs was quantified using trypan blue exclusion, as mentioned previously (Tamura et al., 1992, 1993). In our previous studies (Akaike et al., 1991; Tamura et al., 1992, 1993), the neurotoxic effects of glutamate on cultured rat cortical neurons were studied in detail. A 10 min exposure to 0.5–1 mM glutamate followed by a 1 h incubation with glutamate-free medium was established as the appropriate conditions under which to examine glutamate cytotoxicity and drug-induced protection. As shown in Fig. 1, a brief glutamate exposure followed by 1 h incubation induced cytotoxicity both in the presence and in the absence of Mg^{2+}, whereas a brief NMDA exposure induced cytotoxicity only in the absence of Mg^{2+}. The glutamate cytotoxicity and NMDA cytotoxicity were completely abolished by removing Ca^{2+} from the

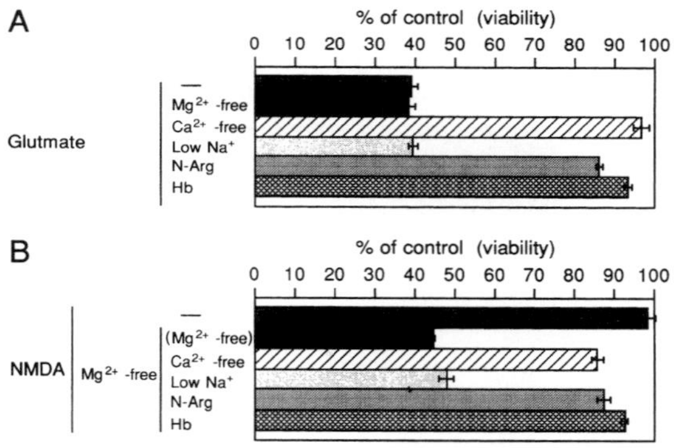

Fig. 1. Effects of cations and NO-related agents on cytotoxicity induced by glutamate (1 mM) and NMDA (1 mM) in cortical cultures. Experiments were performed following the methods described previously (Akaike et al., 1991; Tamura et al., 1992). Cultures were exposed to EAAs for 10 min followed by a 1 h incubation with EAA-free medium. In Mg^{2+}-free and Ca^{2+}-free conditions, the divalent cations were removed from both the EAA-containing and the EAA-free media. In the low Na^+ condition, cultures were incubated in the medium containing 27 mM Na^+. N-Arg (300 μM) and hemoglobin (Hb, 20 μM) were added to the EAA-containing medium.

incubation medium. By contrast, EAA cytotoxicity was not affected by the reduction of the Na^+ concentration in the incubation medium.

The neurotoxic effects of glutamate were ameliorated by NMDA antagonists such as dizocilpine (MK-801), 3-[(±)-2-carboxypiperazin-4-yl]propyl-1-phosphonic acid (CPP), ifenprodil and its derivative, SL 82.0715 (Tamura et al., 1993). These drugs at 0.01 to 10 μM protected cells from glutamate cytotoxicity in a dose-dependent manner, and a concentration of 1 μM was required for over 50% protection. All four antagonists showed protective effects against glutamate cytotoxicity with similar dose-response relationships.

These findings indicate that glutamate acts on both NMDA and non-NMDA receptors of cultured cortical neurons. Glutamate depolarizes the cells via non-NMDA receptors, then induces inward Ca^{2+} currents via an NMDA receptor-ion channel complex as Mg^{2+}-induced blockade of NMDA receptor gated ion channels decreases by depolarization (Collingridge and Lester, 1989).

Involvement of nitric oxide in glutamate cytotoxicity

The following two agents are acknowledged as a useful probe to estimate the role of NO. N^{ω}-Nitro-L-arginine (N-Arg, identical to L-N^{G}-nitro arginine) is a selective NO synthase inhibitor (Moore et al., 1990; Dwyer et al., 1991). Hemoglobin is also widely used since this compound traps NO in the incubation medium (Dawson et al., 1991; Tamura et al., 1992). Simultaneous application of N-Arg with EAA prevented the cytotoxicity induced by glutamate and NMDA (Fig. 1). Hemoglobin (20 μM) also prevented EAA-induced cytotoxicity. This indicates that NO mediates the cytotoxicity induced by a brief glutamate exposure in the cortical cultures.

Recently, Lipton et al. (1993) have shown evidence indicating the presence of alternative redox states of NO: the radical form ($NO^{\cdot}$) and the ionic form (NO^+). $NO^{\cdot}$ produces neurotoxicity when it yields peroxynitrite ($ONOO^-$) by reaction with superoxide anion ($O_2^{\cdot -}$). Contrarily, NO^+ induces neuroprotection by reaction with redox modulatory sites of NMDA receptors. Superoxide dismutase (SOD) prevents the reaction of $NO^{\cdot}$ and $O_2^{\cdot -}$ by eliminating $O_2^{\cdot -}$ from the incubation medium. On the other hand, ascorbate inhibits the formation of NO^+ by its reducing effect. Thus, SOD and ascorbate play crucial roles in NO-mediated glutamate cytotoxicity. As shown in Fig. 2, NMDA cytotoxicity was prevented by SOD but exacerbated by ascorbate. The ascorbate-induced potentiation of NMDA cytotoxicity was prominent when the cultures were treated with the low concentration (200 μM) of NMDA. The cytotoxicity of *S*-nitrosocysteine (SNOC), an NO-generating agent (Lei et al., 1992), was similarly affected by SOD and ascorbate. These findings suggest the existence of two kinds of actions of NO which is released following NMDA receptor stimulation: neurotoxic action in combination with superoxide and neuroprotective action by its oxidated form, NO^+. Since ascorbate reduces NO^+ to yield $NO^{\cdot}$, the inhibitory effect of NO^+ on the NMDA receptors decreases in the presence of ascorbate. Thus, it is likely that the radi-

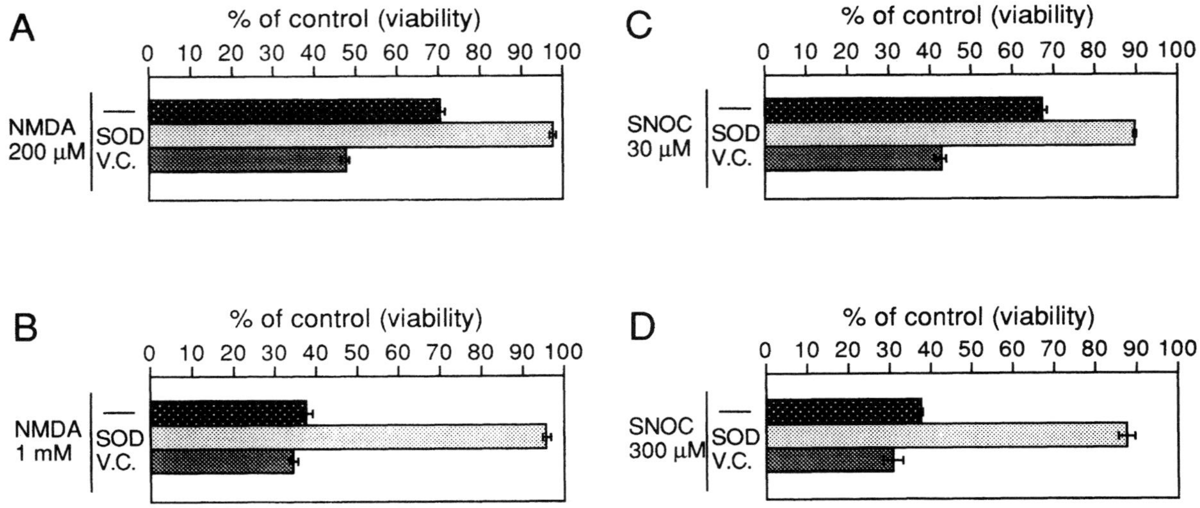

Fig. 2. Effects of SOD (100 U/ml) and ascorbate (400 μM, V.C.) on cytotoxicity induced by NMDA (200 μM in A, 1 mM in B) and SNOC (30 μM in C and 300 μM in D) in cortical cultures. Cultures were exposed to either NMDA or SNOC for 10 min followed by a 1 h incubation with standard medium. NMDA was added to the Mg^{2+}-free medium. SOD and V.C. were added to the NMDA- or SNOC-containing medium.

cal form but not the ionic form of NO mediates glutamate cytotoxicity in the cortical cultures.

Fig. 3 summarizes the mechanisms of NMDA receptor mediated glutamate cyotoxicity in cerebral cortical cultures. Activation of NMDA receptor gated ion channels by glutamate causes a Ca^{2+} influx. Since neuron-type NO synthase is a Ca^{2+} and calmodulin requiring enzyme (Bredt and Snyder, 1990), Ca^{2+} working in conjunction with the regulatory protein, calmodulin, activates NO synthase and facilitates the formation of NO, which in turn reacts with superoxide to yield peroxynitrite and mediates glutamate cyototoxicity.

Mechanism of neuroprotective action of CCK

High concentrations of CCK were found in the cerebral cortex of the rat and other species (Barden et al., 1981; Beinfeld et al., 1981). CCK-like immunoreactivity occurs predominantly in the nonpyramidal bipolar cells. The addition of a depolarizing concentration of K^+ or glutamate evoked the release of CCK-like immunoreactivity from the cerebral cortex, whereas the addition of GABA decreases the resting release of CCK-like immunoreactivity (Yaksh et al., 1987). Electrophysiological studies have demonstrated that CCK-related peptides produced excitation of neurons in a wide region of the CNS, including the cerebral cortex (Phillis and Kirkpatrick, 1980; Chiodo et al., 1987), hippocampus (Brooks and Kelly, 1985) and nucleus accumbens (White and Wang, 1984). These findings suggest that CCK acts as an excitatory neurotransmitter or modulator in the CNS, including the cerebral cortex. Among the CCK-related peptides, sulfated CCK octapeptide (CCK-8S) is the predominant form of the endogenous CCK-related peptides in the cerebral cortex (Rehfeld, 1978; Dockray, 1980). CCK receptors were divided into two subclasses: CCK_A and CCK_B receptors (Chang and Lotti, 1986). CCK_A and CCK_B receptors have been formerly considered to be peripheral and central types, respectively. However, recent studies have demonstrated that both types of CCK receptors are distributed in the CNS (Hill and Woodruff,

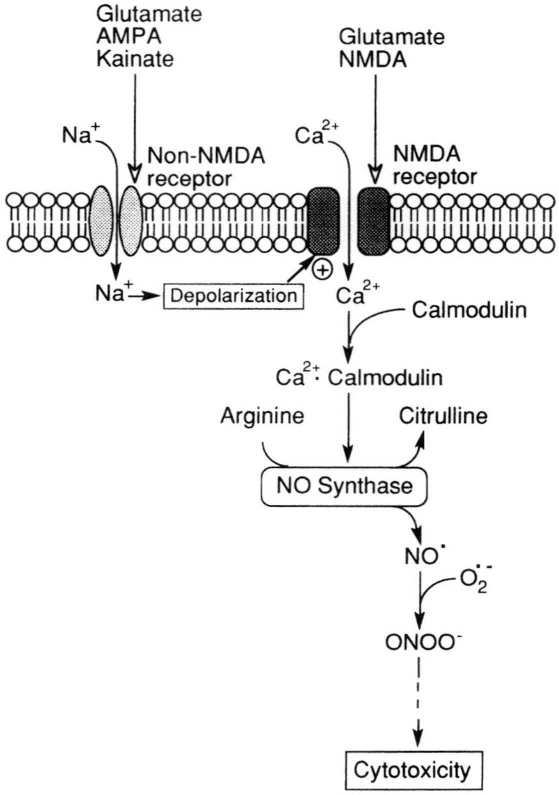

Fig. 3. Schematic representation of presumed mechanisms of NMDA receptor mediated glutamate cytotoxicity.

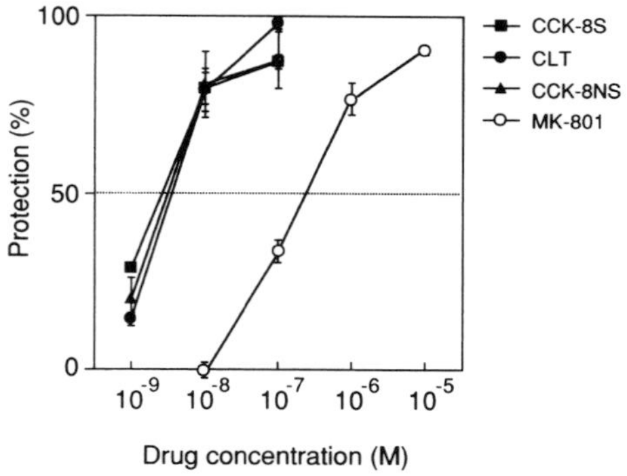

Fig. 4. Dose-response relationships of the neuroprotective effects of CCK-related peptides and NMDA antagonists in cortical cultures. CLT, ceruletide; IFN, ifenprodil. Protection in the ordinate was calculated using the following equation: Protection (%) $= ([D - G]/[C - G]) \times 100$, in which D is the viability of the cultures treated with drug and glutamate, G is the viability after glutamate and C is the viability of nontreated cultures. (From Akaike et al., 1991.)

1990). CCK-8S and ceruletide, the CCK-related decapeptide, have been reported to act as agonists of both the CCK_A and CCK_B receptors. CCK-octapeptide desulfated form (CCK-8NS) and CCK-tetrapeptide (CCK-4) are relatively selective agonists of CCK_B receptors. To date, selective CCK_A receptor agonists have not been found.

The effects of CCK-8S and related peptides on glutamate cytotoxicity were assessed using primary cultures obtained from rat cerebral cortex (Akaike et al., 1991; Tamura et al., 1992). Figure 4 summarizes the effects of the CCK-related peptides and NMDA antagonists. We tested three CCK receptor agonists: CCK-8S, CCK-NS and ceruletide. All of these peptides protected against glutamate-induced cytotoxicity at concentrations of 10–100 nM. At 100 nM, ceruletide was most effective, but CCK-8S and CCK-8NS also provided more than 70% protection. Thus, the effective concentration of CCK-related peptides was 10–100-times lower than that of the NMDA antagonists. The relatively selective CCK_B receptor agonist, CCK-8NS, showed protection which was similar in potency to that of CCK-8S itself. This finding suggested that the subtype of CCK receptors related to the neuroprotective effects of CCK-related peptides was the CCK_B receptor. Then, we examined the effects of nonpeptide antagonists for either CCK_A receptors, L-364718 (identical to MK-329; Chang et al., 1986), or CCK_B receptors, L-365260 (Lotti and Chang, 1989). L-364718 at 10 nM (10^{-8} M) did not affect the protective effect of 100 nM CCK-8S against glutamate neurotoxicity. By contrast, L-365260 at 10 nM (10^{-8} M) completely abolished the CCK-8S-induced neuroprotection.

Since NMDA receptors play a crucial role in glutamate cytotoxicity in cortical cultures, we compared the effects of CCK-related peptides (100 nM) and MK-801 (10 μM) on the cytotoxicity induced by a brief exposure to NMDA (Fig. 5A). All of these agents prevented NMDA-induced cytotoxicity with a similar magnitude.

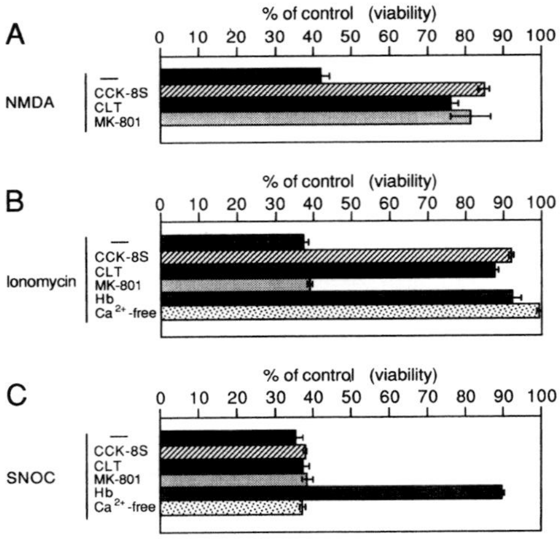

Fig. 5. Effects of CCK-related peptides on cytotoxicity induced by NMDA (1 mM, A), ionomycin (1 μM, B) and SNOC (300 μM, C) in cortical cultures. Cultures were exposed to these agents for 10 min followed by an incubation with standard medium for 1 h. CCK-related peptides (100 nM) and MK-801 (10 μM) were added to both the 10 min and the 1 h incubation media. Hemoglobin (Hb, 20 μM) was added only to the 10 min incubation medium. In Ca^{2+}-free conditions, Ca^{2+} was removed from both the 10 min and the 1 h incubation media.

Although there is no evidence that CCK-related peptides directly attenuate the ligand binding of NMDA receptors, CCK_B receptors may indirectly interact with NMDA receptors via intracellular messenger systems. Therefore, we examined the effects of CCK-related peptides on the cytotoxicity induced by a brief exposure to ionomycin. Ionomycin is a calcium ionophore that induces a persistent Ca^{2+} influx. Concentration-dependent cytotoxicity was induced by a brief exposure of cortical cultures to ionomycin at 10 nM to 1 μM followed by a 1 h incubation with ionomycin-free medium, though the viability of cultures was not affected immediately after a 10 min exposure to ionomycin. Ionomycin-induced cytotoxicity was mediated by Ca^{2+} since Ca^{2+} removal from the incubation medium completely abolished ionomycin cytotoxicity (Fig. 5B). NO presumably mediates ionomycin cytotoxicity as it does in glutamate cytotoxicity since ionomycin-induced cytotoxicity was prevented by hemoglobin (20 μM). Thus, ionomycin directly induces the Ca^{2+} influx to promote NO formation by skipping the step of NMDA receptor activation in the scheme shown in Fig. 3. CCK-related peptides (100 nM) but not MK-801 (10 μM) prevented ionomycin-induced cytotoxicity, indicating that CCK inhibits Ca^{2+}-induced intracellular responses without affecting NMDA receptor activity.

Agents which spontaneously release NO in aqueous solution have been widely used to determine the NO-induced effects on neuronal cells. We employed SNOC as an NO-generating agent to examine the effects of CCK-related peptides on NO-induced cytotoxicity. A 10 min exposure to SNOC followed by a 1 h incubation with SNOC-free medium markedly reduced the viability of the cultures. SNOC-induced cytotoxicity was prevented by hemoglobin (20 μM) but not by Ca^{2+} removal from the incubation medium. If CCK_B receptor stimulation facilitated the activities of the intracellular systems to protect cells from NO toxicity, CCK-related peptides should reduce SNOC-induced cytotoxicity. However, neither CCK-8S nor ceruletide affected SNOC cyototoxicity (Fig. 5C).

Then, the Ca^{2+} influx induced by NMDA receptor stimulation could be affected by CCK-related peptides. In order to examine this possibility, we assessed the cytosolic Ca^{2+} concentration using rhod-2, a fluorescent indicator for cytosolic Ca^{2+} (Minta et al., 1989). NMDA added in the absence of Mg^{2+} elevated the cytosolic Ca^{2+} concentration (Fig. 6A). MK-801 (10 μM) significantly reduced the NMDA-induced Ca^{2+} influx. However, neither CCK-8S (100 nM) nor ceruletide (100 nM) affected the NMDA-induced Ca^{2+} influx. This indicates that CCK receptor stimulation does not inhibit the ligand-induced activation of the NMDA receptor-ion channel complex.

These findings suggest that the neuroprotective effect of CCK-related peptides is caused by its inhibitory action on NO formation, but not by reduction of the Ca^{2+} influx or NO cytotoxicity. To confirm this speculation, NO released from the cerebral cortex was measured using the isolated thoracic aorta as a biological sensor of NO (Tamura et al., 1992). Both the brain tissues and aorta were acutely isolated from rats each weighing 200–300 g. Glutamate (10 mM) added in the presence of the brain tissues induced persistent relaxation of phenylephrine-induced contracture (Fig. 6B). Either CCK-8S (100 nM) or ceruletide (100 nM) was added following the glutamate-induced relaxation. CCK-related peptides completely abolished the glutamate-induced relaxation within 10 min. Sodium nitroprusside added after the addition of the CCK-related peptides elicited a prompt relaxation, the magnitude of which was approximately 100% of the CCK restored contraction.

Together with the findings mentioned above, we conclude that CCK_B receptor stimulation causes suppression of a step in NO formation by NO synthase (see Fig. 3). However, the precise mechanisms linked with the CCK_B receptors are yet to be determined. Molecular cloning of CCK receptors has revealed that both CCK_A and CCK_B receptors have seven putative transmembrane domains (Wank et al., 1992). Therefore, the CCK_B receptor is presumably a member of the guanine nucleotide-binding regulatory protein coupled receptor superfamily, although the second messenger systems related to CCK_B receptors are yet to be determined. Further study is required to determine the intracellular mechanisms of the neuroprotective action of CCK-related peptides.

Dopamine-induced protection of retinal neurons

Glutamate cytotoxicity in cultured retinal neurons

The neurotoxicity of glutamate was originally demonstrated in the retina by Lucas and Newhouse (1957) over 30 years ago. Recent evidence indicates that glutamate has both excitatory and excitotoxic actions in the retina as it does in the other brain regions such as the cerebral cortex, hippocampus and cerebellum (Olney 1982; Bresnick, 1989). A brief glutamate exposure has been demonstrated to produce delayed death in retinal neurons (Facci et al., 1990; Zeevalk and Nicklas, 1992). NMDA receptors have been regarded as the predominant route of retinal glutamate neurotoxicity (Abu El-Asrar et al., 1992).

Primary cultures of retinal neurons were obtained from retinas of fetal rats (16–19 day gestation) as described by Kashii et al. (1994). Several types of cells were observed during the first week in vitro. However, after 7–14 days in vitro, the majority of the isolated cells were multipolar cells with neuron-like shapes, such as bipolar or tripolar cells. Throughout the period, nonneuronal-like or glia-like cells were usually absent from the cultures. Immunocytochemical study demonstrated that more than 80% of the total isolated cells were stained with anti-neurofilament protein antibody. By contrast, fewer than 0.1% of the cells were stained by anti-glial fibrillary acidic protein antibody. To identify further the neuronal cell type, cell type-specific monoclonal antibodies against rat retinal neurons were used as a specific cellular probe. HPC-1 antigen is an integrated membrane protein which is present exclusively in amacrine cells in the retina (Akagawa et al., 1990). The HPC-1 monoclonal antibody reacted with 50–60% of the total population of isolated cells in retinal cultures. Cell surface glycoprotein Thy-1 is mainly present in the ganglion cells in the retina (Beale and Osborne, 1982). Isolated cells were not stained by the anti-Thy-1 antibody, although small populations of cells found in clusters were stained with anti-Thy-1 antibody. However, the cells located in clusters were excluded from the study. These observations indicate that the retinal cultures maintained in this study consisted mainly of neuronal cells, including amacrine cells.

The neurotoxic effects of EAAs and SNOC, an NO-generating agent, on retinal cultures were quantitatively assessed using the trypan blue exclusion method (Fig. 7). A brief exposure of the cells to either glutamate (1 mM), NMDA (1 mM) or SNOC (500 μM) followed by a 1 h incubation in a standard medium caused a marked reduction of the cell viability. Cytotoxicity induced by glutamate and NMDA was prevented by Ca^{2+} removal

A

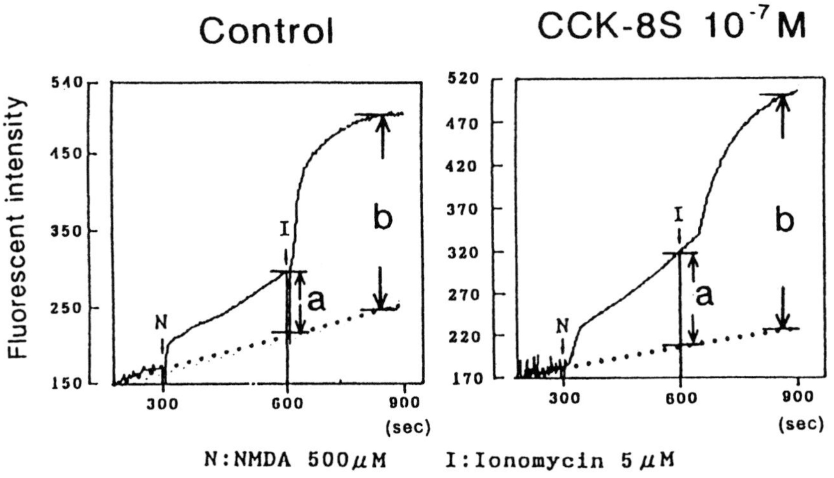

	Estimated NMDA-induced Ca^{2+} influx
	a / b (%)
Non-treated	46.6+ 8.8
CCK-8S 10^{-7}M	42.5+ 5.3
CLT 10^{-7}M	46.3+15.3
MK-801 10^{-5}M	12.9+ 4.7*

*p<0.05

B

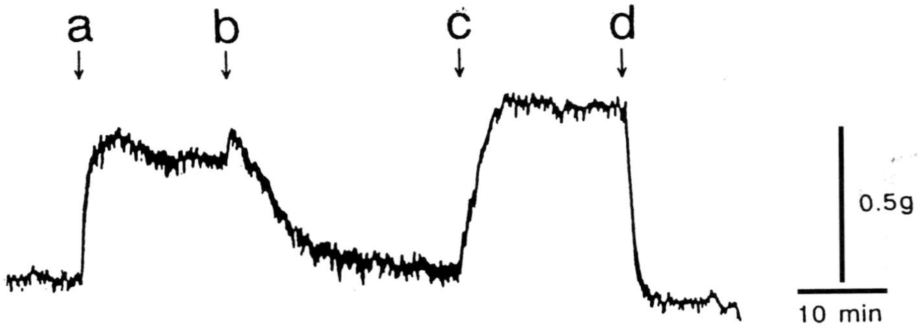

from both the EAA-containing and the EAA-free media. EAA cytotoxicity was prevented by N-Arg and hemoglobin. SNOC-induced cytotoxicity was also prevented by hemoglobin. These findings indicate that the cytotoxicity induced by a brief glutamate exposure involves mechanisms similar to that observed in cortical cultures (Fig. 3). Thus,

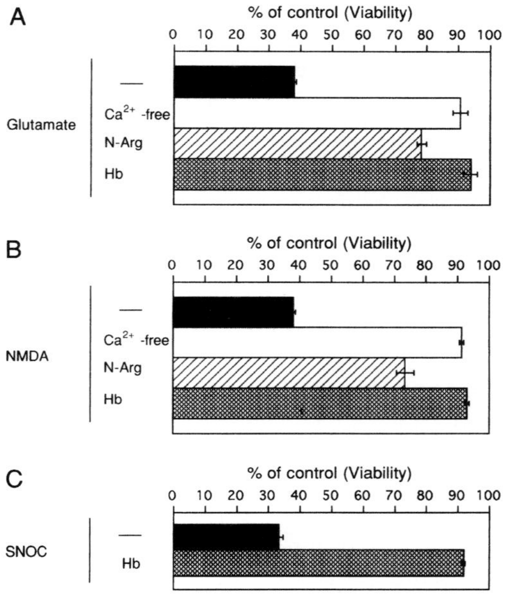

Fig. 7. Effects of cations and NO-related agents on cytotoxicity induced by glutamate (1 mM, A), NMDA (1 mM, B) and SNOC (500 μM, C) in retinal cultures. Cultures were exposed to EAAs or SNOC for 10 min followed by a 1 h incubation with standard medium. NMDA was added to Mg^{2+}-free medium. In Ca^{2+}-free conditions, Ca^{2+} was removed from both the EAA-containing and the EAA-free media. N-Arg (300 μM) and hemoglobin (Hb, 20 μM) were added to EAA- or SNOC-containing medium.

the NMDA receptor appeared to be a major cause of the delayed death induced by a brief exposure to glutamate, as observed in cortical cultures. NADPH diaphorase-positive cells, which are regarded as NO synthase-positive cells, were found in the inner nuclear layer of the retina (Sandell, 1985). L-Arginine-dependent NO formation was demonstrated in bovine retinal tissues (Venturini, 1991). The findings and the present observations indicate that NO plays an important role in NMDA receptor mediated cytotoxicity in the retina.

Dopamine-induced protection of retinal cultures

Dopamine is present in the highest concentration among the monoamine neurotransmitters in the mammalian retina (Hadjiconstantinou and Neff, 1984; Pycock, 1985). Dopamine is synthesized in amacrine and/or interplexiform cells and released upon membrane depolarization in a calcium-dependent manner (Djamgoz and Wagner, 1992). Thus, it appears to act as a neurotransmitter or modulator in the retina, but its role as a chemical messenger has not yet been fully elucidated.

The addition of dopamine (100 μM) to the glutamate-containing medium and the glutamate-free incubation medium prevented the cytotoxicity induced by a brief glutamate exposure. To prevent oxidation of dopamine during incubation at 37°C, addition of an antioxidant such as sodium metabisulfite to a dopamine-containing solution was required. Sodium metabisulfite (50 μM) did not affect the viability of non-treated and glutamate-treated cultures. The concomitant addition of dopamine (100 μM) and

Fig. 6. Effects of CCK on NMDA-induced Ca^{2+} influx (A) and formation of NO-like factor induced by glutamate (B). The procedures of experiments were as previously described (Tamura et al., 1992). (A) Cytosolic Ca^{2+} was assessed using rhod-2. Upper traces represent examples of intracellular Ca^{2+} changes induced by NMDA in the absence (Control) and presence of CCK-8S. CCK-8S, ceruletide (CLT) and MK-801 were added to the medium 2 min before NMDA application. Arrows N and I in the recording traces respectively indicate the addition of NMDA (0.5 mM) and ionomycin (5 μM). In the traces, 'a' and 'b' are regarded as NMDA-induced Ca^{2+} influx and total Ca^{2+} influx, respectively. (B) The isolated thoracic aorta was incubated with minced cerebral tissues. a, phenylephrine (100 μM); b, glutamate (10 mM); c, CCK-8S (100 nM); d, sodium nitroprusside (500 μM). (From Tamura et al., 1992.)

sodium metabisulfite (50 μM) did not affect the viability of the cultures. Dopamine at concentrations of 1 to 100 μM prevented glutamate-induced neurotoxicity in dose-dependent fashion (Fig. 8A). Maximal protection was observed at a concentration of 100 μM of dopamine. Dopamine at this concentration showed neuroprotection similar in potency to that of MK-801 (10 μM). These observations indicate that dopamine protects retinal cultures against glutamate cytotoxicity.

Receptor binding studies have shown that D_1 receptors are less sensitive to dopamine than are D_2 receptors (Creese et al., 1983). Biochemical studies of the dopamine-induced effects on the intracellular cAMP level have demonstrated that the maximal responses mediated by D_1 receptors are not induced by dopamine until concentrations of more than 40 μM are reached (Stoof and Kebabian, 1981). In an electrophysiological study of the caudate nucleus, 1 μM dopamine induced D_2 receptor mediated excitation, whereas 100 μM dopamine is required to induce D_1 receptor mediated inhibition of neuronal activities (Akaike et al., 1987). Physiological studies of the retina are also generally consistent with the reported pharmacological affinity of dopamine receptor subtypes (Witokovsky and Dearry, 1991). To further determine the receptor subtype mediating the dopamine-induced effects, selective agonists and antagonists of either D_1 or D_2 receptors were used. As shown in Fig. 8B, SCH 23390, a selective D_1 receptor antagonist (Hyttel, 1983; Iorio et al. 1983), inhibited the protective effect of dopamine. However, domperidone, a selective D_2 receptor antagonist (Baudry et al., 1979; Laduron and Leysen, 1979), did not affect the dopamine-induced protection. SKF38393, a selective D_1 receptor agonist (O'Boyle and Waddington, 1984), induced protective effects against glutamate cytotoxicity. By contrast, quinpirole, a D_2 receptor agonist (Titus et al., 1983), did not affect glutamate cytotoxicity. Therefore, it is indicated that D_1 receptors mediate dopamine-induced protection of retinal neurons against glutamate neurotoxicity.

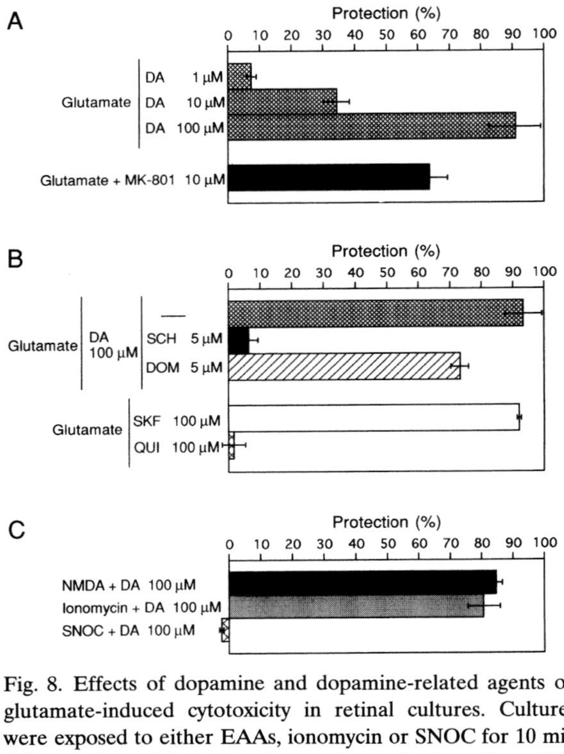

Fig. 8. Effects of dopamine and dopamine-related agents on glutamate-induced cytotoxicity in retinal cultures. Cultures were exposed to either EAAs, ionomycin or SNOC for 10 min followed by a 1 h incubation with standard medium. Dopamine and dopamine-related agents were added to both 10 min and 1 h incubation media. DA, dopamine; DOM, domperidone; SCH, SCH23390; SKF, SKF38393; and QUI, quinpirole. Protection in the abscissa was calculated using the equation in the legend to Fig. 4. (From Kashii et al.,1994.)

As shown in Fig. 8C, dopamine (100 μM) prevented the cytotoxicity induced by NMDA and ionomycin. However, the same concentration of dopamine did not affect the cytotoxicity induced by an NO-generating agent, SNOC. This finding is quite similar with that obtained on CCK-related peptides in cortical cultures (Fig. 5). In the rat retina, the D_1 receptors are related to the stimulation of adenylate cyclase similar to that in the striatum, whereas the D_2 receptors are coupled negatively to adenylate cyclase (Qu et al., 1989; Nowak et al., 1990). This suggests that dopamine D_1 receptor stimulation causes suppression of a step in NO formation by NO synthase through cAMP as a second messenger.

Conclusion

Recent studies in cultured CNS neurons have provided evidence suggesting the existence of endogenous factors which regulate glutamate neurotoxicity. Nerve growth factor (NGF) promotes cell survival in various types of neurons (Cheng and Mattson, 1991). NGF also ameliorates glutamate cyototoxicity in cortical cultures, though the protective action is not as prominent as that of NMDA receptor antagonists (Shimohama et al., 1994). Other neurotransmitters, such as acetylcholine and GABA, exacerbate glutamate cytotoxicity (Mattson, 1989; Erdo et al., 1991). CCK and dopamine appeared to induce strong neuroprotection against glutamate cytotoxicity in cultured cortical and retinal neurons, respectively. Neither substance has a direct interaction with NMDA receptors. These findings suggest that the neuroprotective actions of CCK and dopamine are linked to the step of NO formation, which is triggered by NMDA receptor stimulation. Therefore, we have proposed that CCK and dopamine are putative neuroprotective factors in the cerebral cortex and retina, respectively. These substances may have a role in promoting cell survival in life-regulatory functions in the CNS.

Acknowledgements

The study on the retinal cultures is collaborative research with Dr. S. Kashii, Dr. M. Takahashi, Dr. M. Mandai, Dr. H. Shimizu, Dr. M. Kikuchi, Dr. Y. Honda (Department of Ophthalmology, Faculty of Medicine, Kyoto University, Japan), Dr. M. Sasa (Department of Pharmacology, School of Medicine, Hiroshima University, Japan) and Dr. H. Ujihara (Department of Pharmacology, School of Medicine, Yamaguchi University, Japan). This work was supported in part by a Grant-in-Aid for Scientific Research from the Ministry of Education, Science and Culture, Japan.

References

Abu El-Asrar, A.M., Morse, P.H., Maimone, D., Torczynski, E. and Reder, A.T. (1992) MK-801 protects retinal neurons from hypoxia and the toxicity of glutamate and aspartate. *Invest. Ophthalmol. Vis. Sci.*, 33: 3463–3468.

Akagawa, K., Takada, M., Hayashi, H. and Uemura, K. (1990) Calcium- and voltage-dependent potassium channel in the rat retinal amacrine cells identified in vitro using a cell type-specific monoclonal antibody. *Brain Res.*, 518: 1–5.

Akaike, A., Ohno, Y., Sasa, M. and Takaori S. (1987) Excitatory and inhibitory effects of dopamine on neuronal activity of the caudate nucleus neurons in vitro. *Brain Res.*, 418: 262–272.

Akaike, A., Tamura, Y., Sato, Y., Ozaki, K., Matsuoka, R., Miura, S. and Yoshinaga, T. (1991) Cholecystokinin-induced protection of cultured cortical neurons against glutamate neurotoxicity. *Brain Res.*, 557: 303–307.

Barden, N., Merand, Y., Rouleau, D., Moore, S., Dockray, G.J. and Dupont, A. (1981) Regional distribution of somatostatin and cholecystokinin-like immunoreactivities in rat and bovine brain. *Peptides*, 2: 299–302.

Baudry, M., Martres, M.P. and Schwartz, J.C. (1979) ^{3}H-domperidone: a selective ligand for dopamine receptors. *Naunyn-Schmiederberg's Arch. Pharmacol.*, 308: 231–237.

Beal, R. and Osborne, N. (1982) Localization of the Thy-1 antigen to the surfaces of rat retinal ganglion cells. *Neurochem. Int.*, 4: 581–595.

Beinfeld, M.C., Meyer, D.K., Eskay, R.L., Jensen, R.T. and Brownstein, M.J. (1981) The distribution of cholecystokinin in the central nervous system of the rat as determined by radioimmunoassay. *Brain Res.*, 212; 51–57.

Bredt, D.S. and Snyder, S.H. (1990) Isolation of nitric oxide synthase, a calmodulin-requiring enzyme. *Proc. Natl. Acad. Sci. USA*, 87: 682–685.

Bredt, D.S., Hwang, P.M. and Snyder, S.H. (1990) Localization of nitric oxide synthase indicating a neural role for nitric oxide. *Nature (Lond.)*, 347: 768–770.

Bresnick, G.H. (1989) Excitotoxins: a possible new mechanism for the pathogenesis of ischemic retinal damage. *Arch. Ophthalmol.*, 107: 339–341.

Brooks, P.A. and Kelly, J.S., (1985) Cholecystokinin as a potent excitant of neurons of the dentate gyrus of rats. *Ann. N.Y. Acad. Sci.*, 448: 361–374.

Chang, R.S.L. and Lotti, V.J. (1986) Biochemical and pharmacological characterization of an extremely potent and selective non-peptide cholecystokinin antagonist. *Proc. Natl. Acad. Sci. USA*, 83: 4923–4926.

Chang, R.S.L., Lotti, V.J., Chen, T.B. and Kunkel, K.A. (1986)

Characterization of binding [^{3}H]-(±)L-364,718: a new potent, non-peptide cholecystokinin antagonist radioligand selective for peripheral receptors. *Mol. Pharmacol.*, 30: 212–217.

Cheng, B. and Mattson, M.P. (1991) NGF and bFGF protect rat hippocampal and human cortical neurons against hypoglycemic damage by stabilizing calcium homeostasis. *Neuron*, 7: 1031–1041.

Chiodo, L.A., Freeman, A.S. and Bunney, B.S., (1987) Electrophysiological studies on the specificity of the cholecystokinin antagonist proglumide. *Brain Res.*, 410: 205–211.

Choi, D.W. (1987) Ionic dependence of glutamate neurotoxicity. *J. Neurosci.*, 7: 369–379.

Choi, D.W., Maulucci-Gedde, M. and Kriegstein, A. (1987) Glutamate neurotoxicity in cortical cell culture. *J. Neurosci.*, 7: 357–368.

Collingridge, G.L. and Lester, R.A.J. (1989) Excitatory amino acid receptors in the vertebrate central nervous system. *Pharmacol. Rev.*, 40: 143–210.

Creese, I., Sibely, D.R., Hamblin, M.W. and Leff, S.E. (1983) The classification of dopamine receptors: relationship to radioligand binding. *Annu. Rev. Neurosci.*, 6: 43–71.

Dawson, V.L., Dawson, T.M., London, E.D., Bredt, D.S. and Snyder, S.H. (1991) Nitric oxide mediates glutamate neurotoxicity in primary cortical cultures. *Proc. Natl. Acad. Sci. USA*, 88: 6368–6371.

Dichter, M.A. (1978) Rat cortical neurons in cell culture: culture methods, cell morphology, electrophysiology, and synapse formation. *Brain Res.*, 149: 279–293.

Djamgoz, M.B.A. and Wagner, H.-J. (1992) Localization and function of dopamine in the adult vertebrate retina. *Neurochem. Int.*, 20: 139–191.

Dockray, G.J. (1980) Cholecystokinin in rat cerebral cortex: identification, purification and characterization by immuno-chemical methods. *Brain Res.*, 188: 155–165.

Dwyer, M.A., Bredt, D.S. and Snyder, S.H. (1991) Nitric oxide synthase: irreversible inhibition by L-N^G-nitroarginine in brain in vitro and in vivo. *Biochem. Biophys. Res. Commun.*, 176: 1136–1141.

Erdo, S.L., Michler, A. and Wolff, J.R. (1991) GABA accelerates excitotoxic cell death in cortical cultures: protection by blockers of GABA-gated chloride channels. *Brain Res.*, 542: 254–258.

Facci, L., Leon, A. and Skaper, S.D. (1990) Excitatory amino acid neurotoxicity in cultured retinal neurons: involvement of *N*-methyl-D-aspartate (NMDA) and non-NMDA receptors and effect of ganglioside GM1. *J. Neurosci. Res.*, 27: 202–210.

Garthwaite, J., (1991) Glutamate, nitric oxide and cell-cell signalling in the nervous system. *Trends Neurosci.*, 14: 60–67.

Garthwaite, J., Charles, S.L. and Chess-Williams, R., (1988) Endothelium-derived relaxing factor release on activation of NMDA receptors suggests role as a messenger in the brain. *Nature (Lond.)*, 336:385–388.

Gasic, G.P. and Hollmann, M. (1992) Molecular neurobiology of glutamate receptors. *Annu. Rev. Physiol.*, 54: 507–536.

Hadjiconstantinou, M. and Neff, N.H. (1984) Catecholamine systems of retina: a model for studying synaptic systems. *Life Sci.*, 35: 1135–1147.

Hartley, D.M. and Choi, D.W. (1989) Delayed rescue of *N*-methyl-D-aspartate receptor-mediated neuronal injury in cortical culture. *J. Pharmacol. Exp. Ther.*, 250: 752–758.

Hill, D.R. and Woodruff, G.N. (1990) Differentiation of central cholecystokinin receptor binding sites using the non-peptide antagonists MK-329 and L-365,260. *Brain Res.*, 526: 276–283.

Hyttel, J. (1983) SCH23390 – the first selective dopamine D-1 antagonist. *Eur. J. Pharmacol.*, 91: 153–154.

Iorio, L.C., Barnett, A., Leitz, F.H., Houser, V.P. and Korduba, C.A. (1983) SCH23390, a potential benzazepine antipsychotic with unique interactions on dopaminergic systems. *J. Pharmacol. Exp. Ther.*, 226: 462–468.

Kashii, S., Takahashi, M., Mandai, M., Shimizu, H., Honda, Y., Sasa, M., Ujihara, H., Tamura, Y., Yokota, T. and Akaike, A. (1994) Protective action of dopamine against glutamate neurotoxicity in the retina. *Invest. Ophthalmol. Vis. Sci.*, 35: 685–695.

Laduron, P.M. and Leysen, J.E. (1979) Domperidone, a specific in vitro dopamine antagonist, devoid of in vivo central dopaminergic activity. *Biochem. Pharmacol.*, 28: 2161–2165.

Lei, S.Z., Pan, Z.-H., Aggarwal, S.K., Chen, H.-S.V., Hartman, J., Sucher, N.J. and Lipton, S.A. (1992) Effects of nitric oxide protection on the redox modulatory site of the NMDA receptor-channel complex. *Neuron*, 8: 1087–1099.

Lipton, S.A., Choi, Y.-B., Pan, Z.-H., Lei, S.Z., Chen, H.-S. V., Sucher, N.J., Loscalzo, J., Singel, D.J. and Stamler, J.S. (1993) A redox-based mechanism for the neuroprotective and neurodestructive effects of nitric oxide and related nitroso-compounds. *Nature (Lond.)*, 364: 626–632.

Lotti, V.J. and Chang, R.S.L. (1989) A new potent and selective non-peptide gastrin antagonist and brain cholecystokinin receptor (CCK-B) ligand: L-365,260. *Eur. J. Pharmacol.*, 162: 273–280.

Lucas, D.R. and Newhouse, J.P. (1957) The toxic effect of sodium L-glutamate on the inner layer of the retina. *Arch. Ophthalmol.*, 58: 193–201.

Mattson, M.P. (1989) Acetylcholine potentiates glutamate-induced neurodegeneration in cultured cortical neurons. *Brain Res.*, 497: 402–406.

Minta, A., Kao, J.P.Y. and Tsien, R.Y., (1989) Fluorescent indicators for cytosolic calcium based on rhodamine and fluorescein chromophores. *J. Biol. Chem.*, 264: 8171–8178.

Moore, P.K., Al-Swayeh, O.A., Chong, N.W.S., Evans, R.A. and Gibson, A. (1990) L-N^G-nitro arginine (L-NOARG), a novel L-arginine reversible inhibitor of endothelium-dependent vasodilation in vitro. *Br. J. Pharmacol.*, 99: 408–414.

Nowak, J.S., Sek, B. and Schorderet, M. (1990) Bidirectional regulation of cAMP generating system by dopamine-D_1

and D_2-receptors in the rat retina. *J. Neural. Transm. Gen. Sect.*, 81: 235–240.

O'Boyle, K.M. and Waddington, J.L. (1984) Selective and stereospecific interactions of R-SK & F 38393 with (^{3}H)pifultixol but not (^{3}H)spiperone binding to D_1 and D_2 receptors: comparison with SCH23390. *Eur. J. Pharmacol.*, 98: 433–436.

Olney, J.W. (1982) The toxic effects of glutamate and related compounds in the retina and the brain. *Retina*, 2: 341–359.

Phillis, J.W. and Kirkpatrick, J.R. (1980) The actions of motilin, luteinizing hormone releasing hormone, cholecystokinin, somatostatin, vasoactive intestinal peptide, and other peptides on rat cerebral cortical neurons. *Can. J. Physiol. Pharmacol.*, 58: 612–623.

Qu Z.-X., Fertel, R., Neff, N.H. and Hadjiconstantinou, M. (1989) Pharmacological characterization of rat retinal dopamine receptors. *J. Pharmacol. Exp. Ther.*, 248: 621–625.

Pycock, C.J. (1985) Retinal neurotransmission. *Surv. Ophthalmol.*, 29: 355–365.

Rehfeld, J.F. (1978) Immunological studies on cholecystokinin II. Distribution and molecular heterogeneity in the central nervous system and small intestine of man and hog. *J. Biol. Chem.*, 253: 4022–4030.

Sandell, J.H. (1985) NADPH diaphorase cells in the mammalian inner retina. *J. Comp. Neurol.*, 238: 466–472.

Shimohama, S., Ogawa, N., Tamura, Y., Akaike, A., Tsukahara, T., Iwata, H. and Kimura, J. (1994) Protective effect of nerve growth factor against glutamate-induced neurotoxicity in cultured cortical neurons. *Neurosci. Lett.*, in press.

Stoof, J.C. and Kebabian, J.W. (1981) Opposing roles for D-1 and D-2 dopamine receptors in efflux of cyclic AMP from rat neostriatum. *Nature (Lond.)*, 294: 366–368.

Tamura, Y., Sato, Y., Akaike, A. and Shiomi, H. (1992) Mechanisms of cholecystokinin-induced protection of cultured cortical neurons against *N*-methyl-D-aspartate receptor-mediated glutamate cytotoxicity. *Brain Res.*, 592: 317–325.

Tamura, Y., Sato, Y., Yokota, T., Akaike, A., Sasa, M. and Takaori, S. (1993) Ifenprodil prevents glutamate cytotoxicity via polyamine modulatory sites on *N*-methyl-D-aspartate receptors in cultured cortical neurons. *J. Pharmacol. Exp. Ther.*, 265: 1017–1025.

Titus, D.R., Kornfeld, E.C., Jones, N.D., Clemens, J.A., Smalstig, E.B., Fuller, R.W., Hahn, R.A., Hynes, M.D., Mason, N.R., Wong, D.T. and Foreman, M.M. (1983) Resolution and absolute configuration of an ergline-related dopamine agonist, trans-4,4a,5,6,7,8,8a,9-octahydro-5-propyl-1H(or 2H)-pyraolo(3,4-g)quinoline. *J. Med. Chem.*, 26: 1112–1116.

Venturini, C.M., Knowles, R.G, Palmer, R.M.J. and Moncada, S. (1991) Synthesis of nitric oxide in the bovine retina. *Biochem. Biophys. Res. Commun.*, 180: 920–925.

Wank, S.A., Pisegna, J.R. and De Weerth, A. (1992) Brain and gastrointestinal cholecystokinin receptor family: structure and functional expression. *Proc. Natl. Acad. Sci. USA*, 89: 8691–8695.

White, F.J. and Wang, R.Y. (1984) Interactions of cholecystokinin octapeptide and dopamine on nucleus accumbens neurons. *Brain Res.*, 300: 161–166.

Witokovsky, P. and Dearry, A. (1991) Functional roles of dopamine in the vertebrate retina. *Prog. Retinal Res.*, 11: 247–292.

Yaksh, T.L., Furui, T., Kanawati, I.S. and Go, V.L.W. (1987) Release of cholecystokinin from rat cerebral cortex in vivo: role of GABA and glutamate receptor systems. *Brain Res.*, 406: 207–214.

Zeevalk, G.D. and Nicklas, W.J. (1992) Developmental differences in antagonism of NMDA toxicity by the polyamine site antagonist ifenprodil. *Dev. Brain Res.*, 65: 147–155.

Subject Index